# The Art of Limb Alignment

Twelfth Edition

Shawn C. Standard, MD
John E. Herzenberg, MD
Philip K. McClure, MD
*Editors*

# The Art of Limb Alignment

**Case Example on the Cover:**
Planning and execution of retrograde lengthening for a male with a bone age of 14.5 and a history of physeal fracture of the distal femur with subsequent growth arrest. Left panel: Initial imaging demonstrates leg length discrepancy and distal femoral growth arrest with severe valgus deformity. Center panel: Planning for deformity correction and lengthening using the modified reverse planning method based on the predicted length of the contralateral side after completion of natural growth. Right panel: Final position after retrograde lengthening with a magnetic intramedullary lengthening nail. Note the overlengthening of the right to accommodate future growth of the unaffected left side.

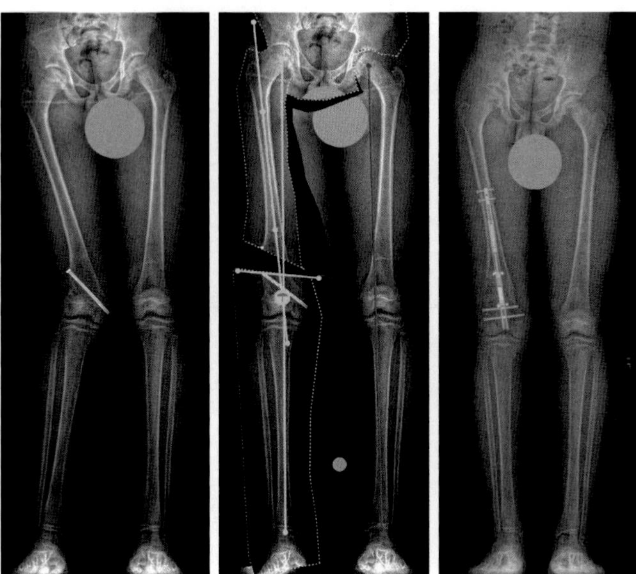

International Center for Limb Lengthening (ICLL)
Rubin Institute for Advanced Orthopedics (RIAO)
Sinai Hospital of Baltimore
2401 West Belvedere Avenue
Baltimore, Maryland 21215 USA
1-410-601-BONE (2663)
1-844-LBH-RIAO toll-free
www.LimbLength.org

Baltimore Limb Deformity Course:
www.DeformityCourse.com

Facebook page for apps created by the ICLL:
www.facebook.com/LimbLengthApps

Follow the ICLL and RIAO on social media:
Facebook: www.facebook.com/LimbLengthMD
Twitter: www.twitter.com/LimbLengthMD
www.twitter.com/RIAOResearch
Instagram: www.instagram.com/LimbLengthMD

**Recommended citation format for this book:**
Standard SC, Herzenberg JE, McClure PK, eds. *The Art of Limb Alignment.* 12th ed. Baltimore, MD: Rubin Institute for Advanced Orthopedics, Sinai Hospital of Baltimore; 2023.

**Example citation format for a chapter in this book:**
Standard SC. Normal limb alignment. In: Standard SC, Herzenberg JE, McClure PK, eds. *The Art of Limb Alignment.* 12th ed. Baltimore, MD: Rubin Institute for Advanced Orthopedics, Sinai Hospital of Baltimore; 2023:1-18.

ISBN: 9798852531957

**© 2023 Rubin Institute for Advanced Orthopedics, Sinai Hospital of Baltimore**
This work is subject to copyright law. All rights are reserved. Duplication or reprinting of this work is allowed only with permission. For permission, contact mbacon@lifebridgehealth.org. **Disclaimer:** In view of the possibility of human error or changes in medical science, the authors do not warrant that the information contained in this book is accurate or complete, and they are not responsible for any errors or omissions or the results obtained from the use of such information.

# Preface for the Twelfth Edition

For more than 31 years, we have taught limb correction surgery at the annual Baltimore Limb Deformity Course (www.DeformityCourse.com). We have used these hands-on experiences with our students to guide us when creating this book. *The Art of Limb Alignment* is a concise guide for beginners starting on their journey to master the art of limb alignment. Understanding limb alignment and malalignment is a critical task for surgeons who treat lower extremity deformities. The first step is to characterize the deformity: Is the bone angulated? In what direction is the bone angulated? What is the level of the deformity? Where is the apex of the deformity? What is the magnitude of the deformity? Is the bone short? Is it rotated on its axis? All these questions must be answered before correcting the problem.

In a new Chapter 16 for this twelfth edition, planning and considerations for internal lengthening are discussed. The anatomy of the mechanical intramedullary lengthening nail and its different variations are reviewed. A walkthrough is provided for determining the placement of the osteotomy and proper nail length. Planning cases are provided for retrograde femoral lengthening and tibial lengthening in adults. A substantial section on pediatric considerations for internal lengthening is also included; it contains the intraoperative technique and postoperative protocol for the more recent development of extramedullary internal lengthening.

This edition also includes noteworthy updates to multiple chapters. Chapter 3 features 12 all-new illustrations. Chapter 11 has been revised to include four examples of calculating total limb length discrepancy with the Three Line Method, with four new illustrations to accompany them. Finally, Chapter 12 has been overhauled to include modifications to the classic reverse planning technique that was introduced in 2009. Extensive illustrations are provided for both the classic and modified methods, and the steps of planning a case are depicted in detail with 17 images from digital planning software.

Several different deformity planning software programs exist. We are unable to provide specific instructions for all of them and have focused the contents of this book on using Bone Ninja, created at our institution and available as an iPad app educational tool through the App Store. However, Bone Ninja is not distinctly necessary for the planning and concepts outlined within this book.

*The Art of Limb Alignment* is intentionally short, concise, and we hope, easy to grasp. The theme is that of student and teacher (sensei) embarking on a voyage to master the art of limb alignment.

Enjoy the journey!

## Contributors

**Michael J. Assayag** International Center for Limb Lengthening, Rubin Institute for Advanced Orthopedics, Sinai Hospital of Baltimore, Baltimore, MD, USA

**Janet D. Conway** International Center for Limb Lengthening, Rubin Institute for Advanced Orthopedics, Sinai Hospital of Baltimore, Baltimore, MD, USA

**John E. Herzenberg** International Center for Limb Lengthening, Rubin Institute for Advanced Orthopedics, Sinai Hospital of Baltimore, Baltimore, MD, USA

**Bradley M. Lamm** Foot and Ankle Deformity Center and Fellowship, Paley Orthopedic and Spine Institute, West Palm Beach, FL, USA

**Philip K. McClure** International Center for Limb Lengthening, Rubin Institute for Advanced Orthopedics, Sinai Hospital of Baltimore, Baltimore, MD, USA

**Kelsey J. Millonig** East Village Foot and Ankle Surgeons, Des Moines, IA, USA

**Noman A. Siddiqui** International Center for Limb Lengthening, Rubin Institute for Advanced Orthopedics, Sinai Hospital of Baltimore, Baltimore, MD, USA

**Shawn C. Standard** International Center for Limb Lengthening, Rubin Institute for Advanced Orthopedics, Sinai Hospital of Baltimore, Baltimore, MD, USA

## Acknowledgments

John E. Herzenberg provided editorial assistance for the classic textbook, *Principles of Deformity Correction*, by Dror Paley (Springer Verlag, 2002). This 800+ page work is an excellent resource for deformity correction surgery, but it can be rather intimidating in its size and scope. *The Art of Limb Alignment* is intended to be an easy introduction to the essential concepts and will hopefully stimulate the motivated student to then delve deeper into the intricacies of deformity analysis and planning.

We would like to thank Bradley M. Lamm, DPM, and Kelsey J. Millonig, DPM, for their contributions to this book. We would also like to give a heartfelt thank you to the staff of the Academic and Research Support Services Department for their invaluable help in putting together the Baltimore Limb Deformity Course and this book. The team includes Robert Farley (Medical Editor), Joy Marlowe (Medical Illustrator), Gary Trout (Graphic Designer), Alvien Lee (Medical Photographer), and Madeline Bacon (Manager of Academic and Research Programs).

# Table of Contents

## Definitions of Acronyms and Abbreviations

ABC — **A**pex of the deformity; **B**one cut; **C**orrection
ADTA — anterior distal tibial angle
aLDFA — anatomic lateral distal femoral angle
aLPFA — anatomic lateral proximal femoral angle
aMPFA — anatomic medial proximal femoral angle
AP — anteroposterior
CIA — calcaneal inclination angle
DPHA — dorsal proximal hallux angle
DPMA — dorsal proximal metatarsal angle
DPPA — dorsal proximal phalangeal angle
HAA — hallux abductus angle
HIA — hallux interphalangeal angle
IMA — intermetatarsal angle
JLCA — joint line convergence angle
LAT — lateral
LDHA — lateral distal hallux angle
LDMA — lateral distal metatarsal angle
LDTA — lateral distal tibial angle
LLD — limb length discrepancy
MAA — metatarsus adductus angle
MAD — mechanical axis deviation
MAP — For frontal plane deformity analysis:
- **M**easure MAD
- **A**nalyze joint angles
- **P**ick the bone

MAP — For sagittal plane deformity analysis:
- **M**easure MAD and anterior cortical lines
- **A**nalyze joint angles
- **P**ick the bone

MAP — For determination of LLD:
- **M**easure LLD
- **A**nalyze length of bone segments
- **P**ick the shortened bone segment

mIMA — mechanical intermetatarsal angle
mLDFA — mechanical lateral distal femoral angle
mLPFA — mechanical lateral proximal femoral angle
MPFA — medial proximal femoral angle
MPHA — medial proximal hallux angle
MPMA — medial proximal metatarsal angle
MPPA — medial proximal phalangeal angle
MPTA — medial proximal tibial angle
NSA — neck shaft angle
PDFA — posterior distal femoral angle
PDHA — plantar distal hallux angle
PDMA — plantar distal metatarsal angle
PMA — plafond malleolar angle
PPTA — posterior proximal tibial angle
SJLA — sagittal joint line angle
SMAA — sagittal mechanical axes angle
TCA — talocalcaneal angle

# Chapter 1

# Normal Limb Alignment

Shawn C. Standard, MD

## Alignment in the Frontal Plane

The development of limb alignment in the frontal plane during childhood has been described by Salenius and Vankka (Fig. 1).[1] These authors defined normal alignment as a final femoral-tibial angle of 5° or 6° valgus established by 7 years of age. However, the femoral-tibial angle is an indirect measurement of true limb alignment. It does not allow for analysis or quantification of the location of the mechanical forces traveling through the knee while standing.

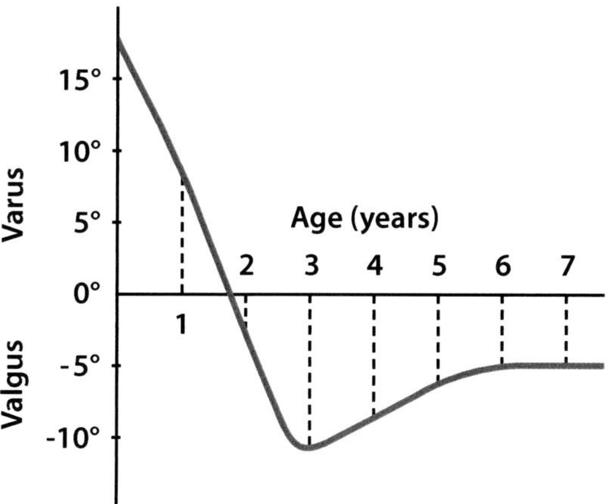


**Fig. 1:** Graph shows the typical change that is observed in the femoral-tibial angle during childhood. Note that by age 7 years, the femoral-tibial angle has stabilized with an average value of 5° or 6° valgus.

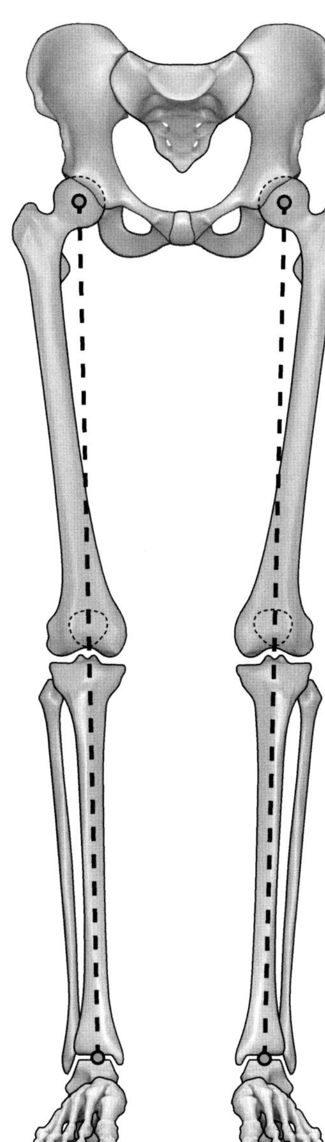

**Fig. 2:** The mechanical axis of the lower limb on a full length standing AP view x-ray is defined as a line connecting the center of the femoral head with the center of the ankle joint. In a normal limb, the mechanical axis should pass through the zone that lies between 3 mm medial to the center of the knee joint and 3 mm lateral to the center of the knee joint. In general, perfect alignment is defined as when the mechanical axis passes through the center of the knee. In other words, collinearity of the hip, knee, and ankle represents perfect alignment.

© 2023 Sinai Hospital of Baltimore

Normal parameters for alignment in the frontal plane have been established that take into account the mechanical forces on the lower limbs. To determine frontal plane alignment, examine a full length standing anteroposterior (AP) view x-ray of the lower limb with the knee joint maximally extended. True normal limb alignment is defined as the collinearity of the center of the hip, knee, and ankle joints. The mechanical axis of the lower limb in the frontal plane is defined as a straight line connecting the center of the femoral head to the center of the ankle (Fig. 2). The mechanical axis allows for a direct analysis of limb alignment. In most individuals with normal limbs, the mechanical axis passes slightly medial to the center of the knee. The goal of corrective surgery is a mechanical axis that passes directly through the center of the knee. Some people with normal limbs have a mechanical axis that falls up to 17 mm medial to the center of

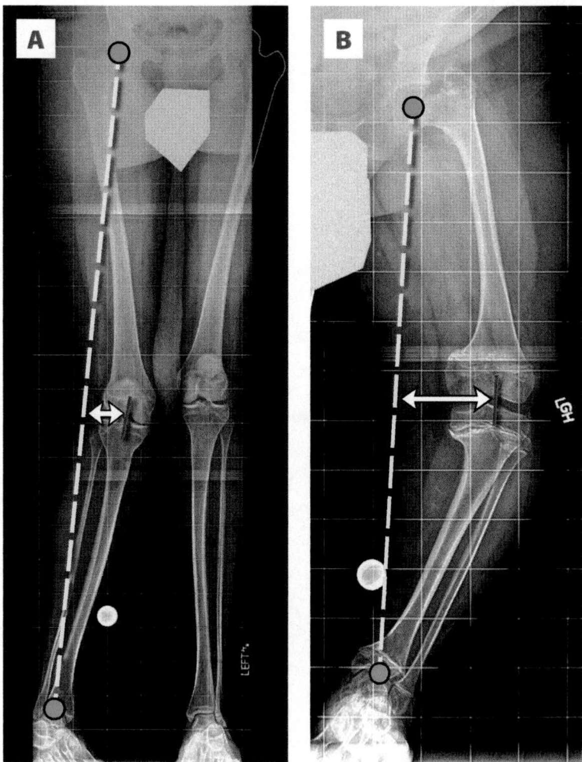


**Fig. 3: A**, The mechanical axis is termed "deviated" if it passes outside of the normal zone. If the mechanical axis (*yellow line*) is lateral to the center of the knee (*red line*), then a valgus deformity is present. **B**, If the mechanical axis (*yellow line*) is medial to the center of the knee (*red line*), then a varus deformity is present.

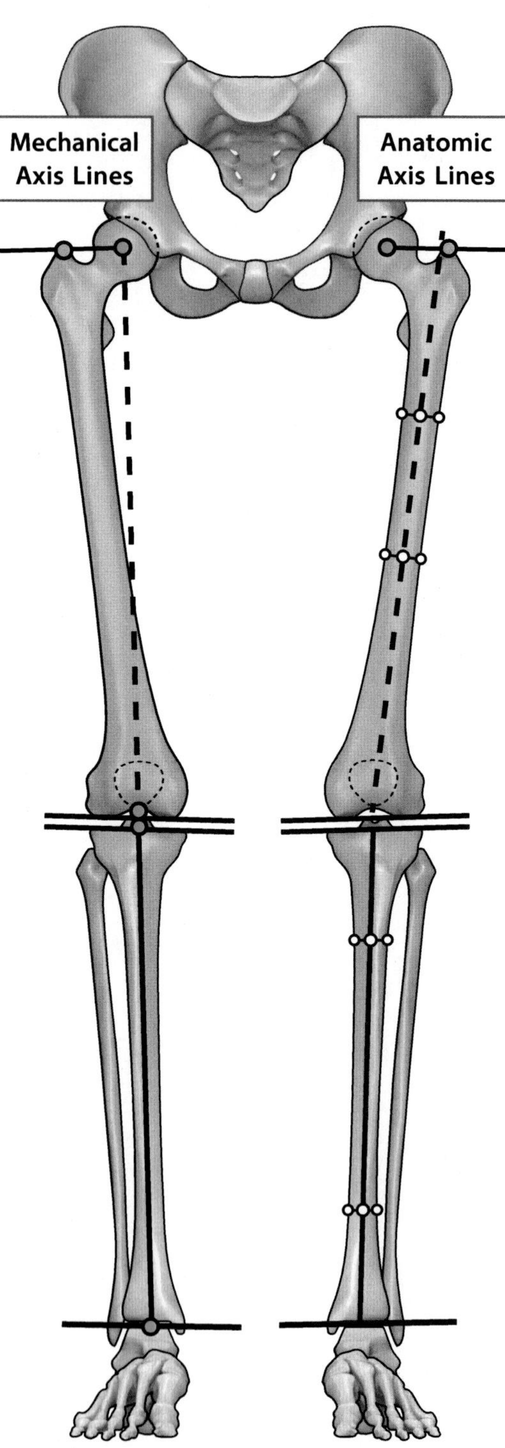


**Fig. 4:** The mechanical axis of the individual bones on the AP view is a straight line connecting the center of the proximal joint to the center of the distal joint. The anatomic axis of a bone segment is defined as the mid-diaphyseal line of the bone and can be a straight line or a curved line.

the knee, but these individuals may be more prone to medial compartment arthritis as they age.

When the mechanical axis does not pass through the center of the knee, the limb is said to have mechanical axis deviation (MAD). To determine the MAD, measure the perpendicular distance between the center of the knee joint and the mechanical axis. When the mechanical axis is lateral to the center of the knee joint, it is called valgus (Fig. 3A). When the mechanical axis is medial to the center of the knee joint, it is called varus (Fig. 3B). Normal MAD falls within 3 mm medial and 3 mm lateral of the center of the knee.

Which factors contribute to the mechanical alignment? The mechanical alignment of the lower limb is formed by the additive effects of the shape of the femur and tibia and by the joint alignment

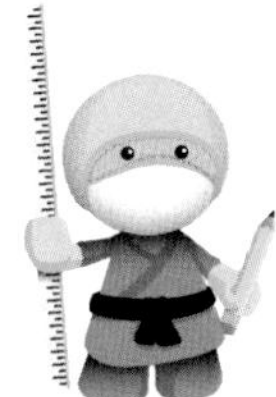

***Sensei says,***
*"Balance is achieved when the mechanical axis of the limb in the frontal plane passes through the center of the knee (MAD = 0)."*

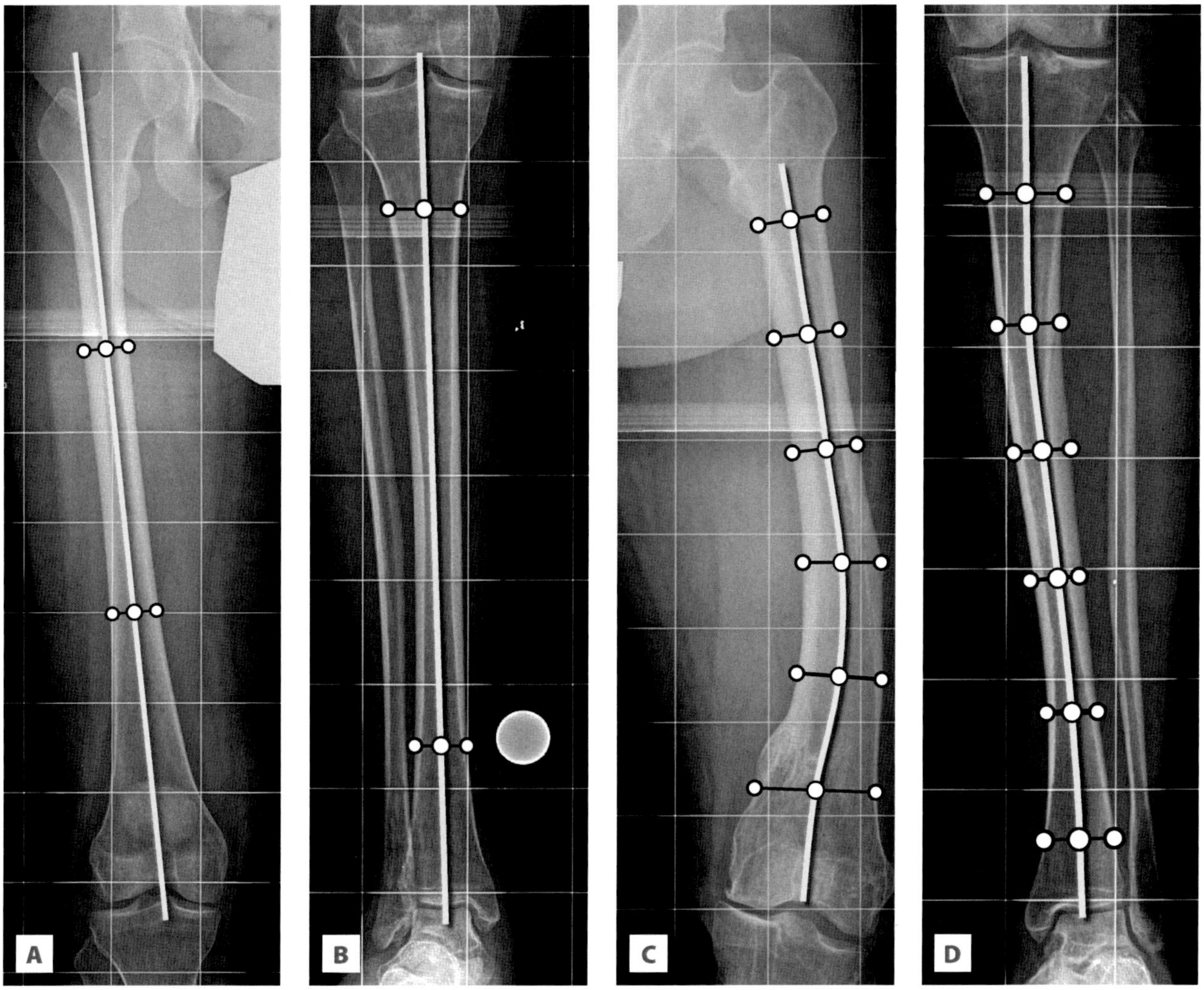

**Fig. 5:** The anatomic axis on an AP view x-ray can either be straight (**A** and **B**) or curved (**C** and **D**) depending on the shape of the bone. Panels **A** and **B** show normal bones. Panel **C** shows a pathologic abnormal bone and panel **D** shows a variation of normal.

*© 2023 Sinai Hospital of Baltimore*

of the hip, knee, and ankle. The femur and tibia each have a mechanical axis and an anatomic axis. The hip, knee, and ankle each have a joint line that represents the plane of that joint in space. The intersection of the joint line and the femoral or tibial axis (mechanical or anatomic) forms a joint angle. These joint angles are the major factors that determine the overall alignment of the lower limb. After you determine these angles, you can conduct a detailed analysis of limb alignment.

The mechanical axis of a bone segment is defined as a straight line connecting the center of the proximal joint to the center of the distal joint (Fig. 4). The mechanical axis of the bone is always a straight line. The anatomic axis of a bone segment is defined as the mid-diaphyseal line of the bone. The anatomic axis can be a straight line or a curved line (Fig. 5). The normal anatomic axis of the femur in the frontal plane should be straight. The normal anatomic axis of the femur in the sagittal plane is curved. Figure 5 shows normal and abnormal anatomic axes in the frontal plane. A non-linear anatomic axis can exist in a bone with a normal mechanical axis and concurrent normal mechanical joint angles. A non-linear anatomic axis may represent a true deformity, but a joint angle analysis must still be performed.

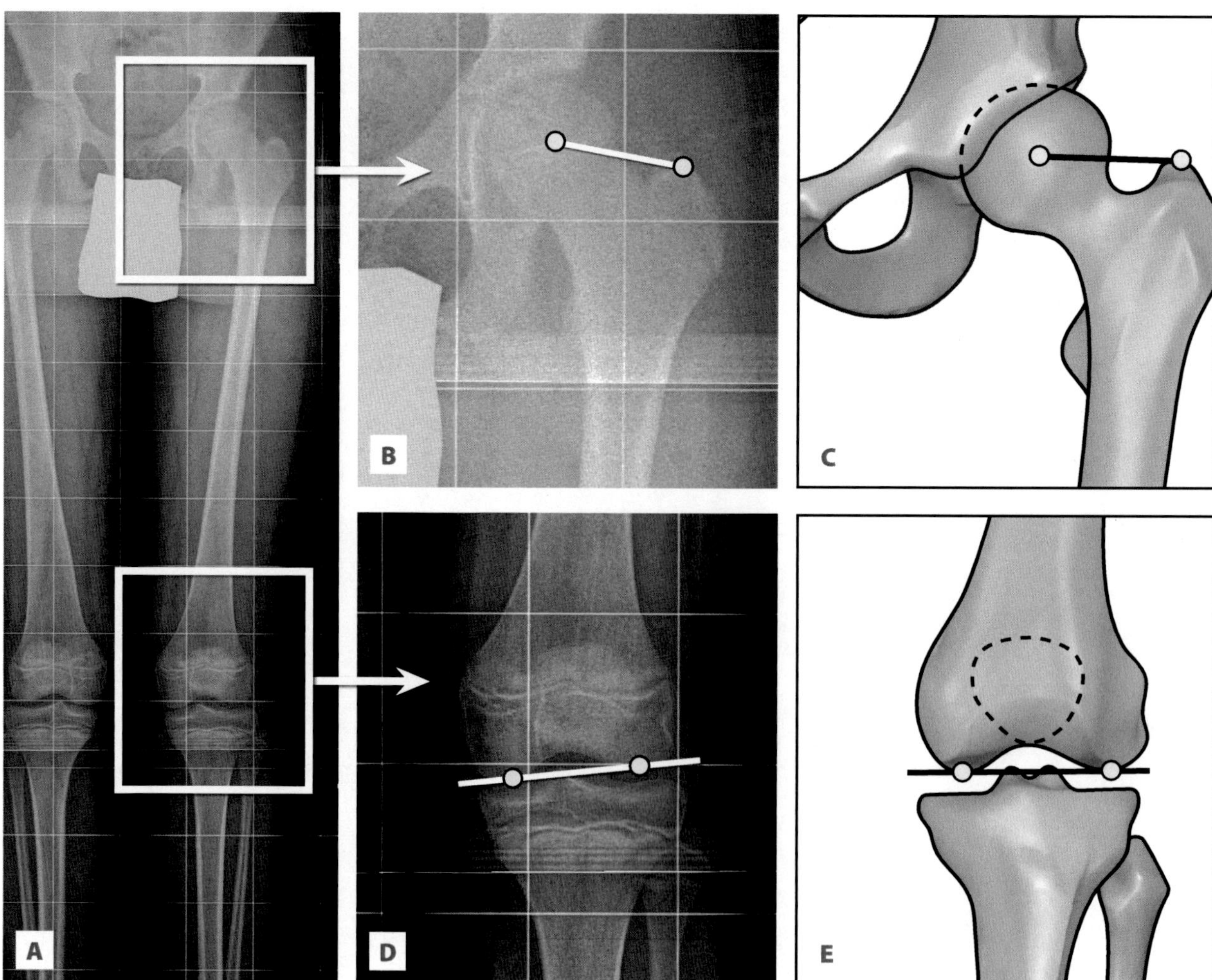


**Fig. 6: A**, The joint lines of the proximal and distal femur on an AP view x-ray are formed by placing two points in specific locations for each joint. A joint line is formed by connecting the two points. **B** and **C**, The points for the proximal femur are placed at the center of the femoral head and the tip of the greater trochanter. **D** and **E**, The distal femoral points are placed at the convexity of the medial and lateral femoral condyles.

Each joint has a defined line that represents that joint's position in space (Fig. 6). In the frontal plane, the hip joint line (i.e., proximal femoral line) is formed by connecting a point from the tip of the greater trochanter to a point at the center of the femoral head (Fig. 6B and 6C). The tip of the greater trochanter is difficult to identify in the skeletally immature patient. This will decrease the accuracy of the proximal femoral joint line and must be taken into account. The distal femoral joint line is formed by connecting points placed at the apex of the medial and lateral femoral condyles (Fig. 6D and 6E). The proximal tibial joint line (Fig. 7) is formed by connecting points on the concavity of the medial and lateral tibial plateaus directly under the apex of the femoral condyles (Fig. 7B and 7C). The ankle (i.e., distal tibial) joint line is formed by connecting points on the medial and lateral aspect of the distal tibial plafond (Fig. 7D and 7E).

The intersection of the mechanical and anatomic axes with the joint lines creates joint angles. To form joint angles, draw the mechanical or anatomic axes of the femur or tibia so that they intersect the joint lines. Each angle has an average and range of values that is considered to be normal based on average population values (Fig. 8, Tables 1 and 2).

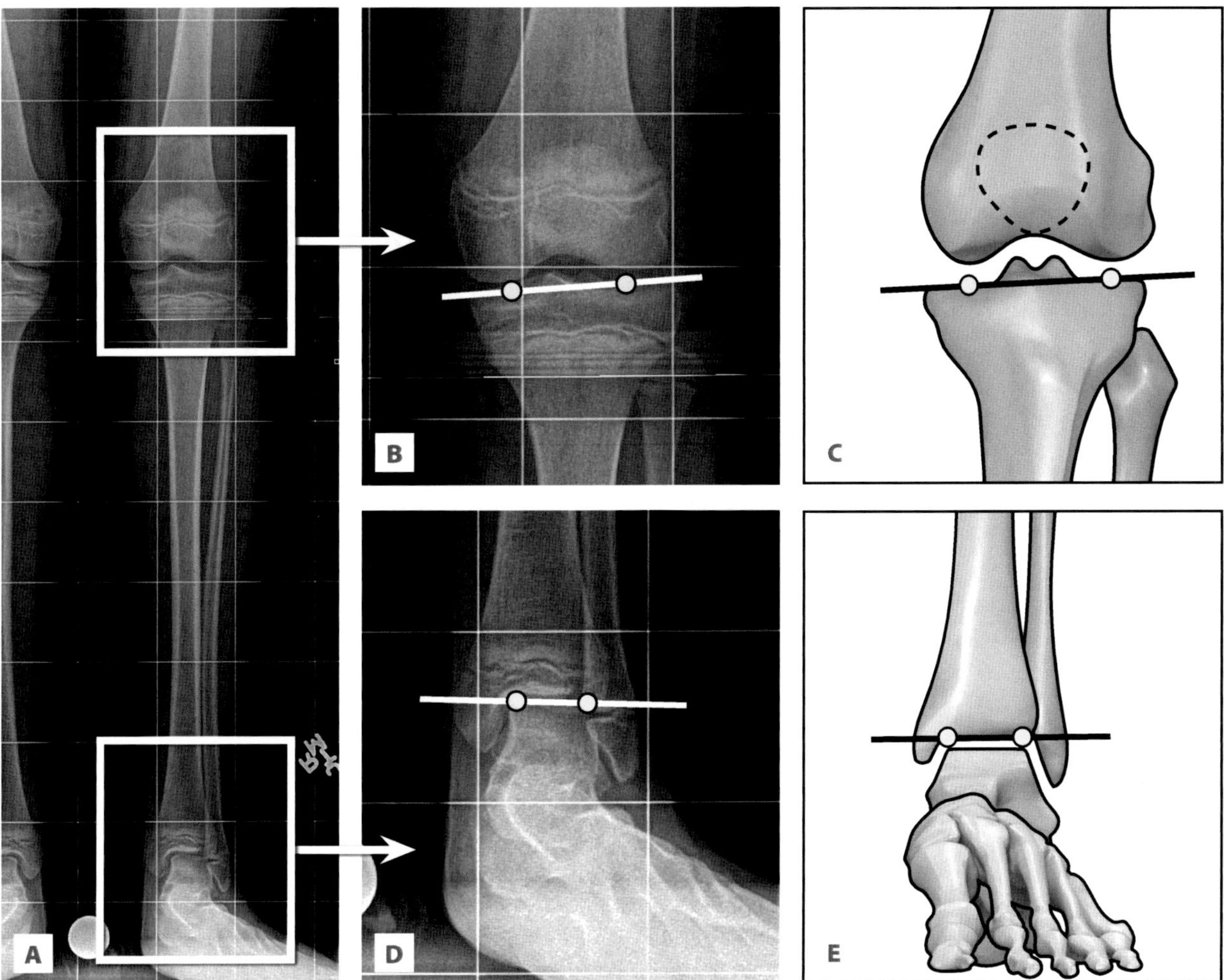


**Fig. 7: A**, Proximal and distal tibial joint lines on an AP view x-ray are formed by placing two points in specific locations for each joint. A joint line is formed by connecting the two points. **B** and **C**, Proximal tibial points are placed on the concavity of the medial and lateral tibial plateau. **D** and **E**, Distal tibial points are placed on the medial and lateral aspect of the distal tibial plafond or the proximal talar dome.

© 2023 Sinai Hospital of Baltimore

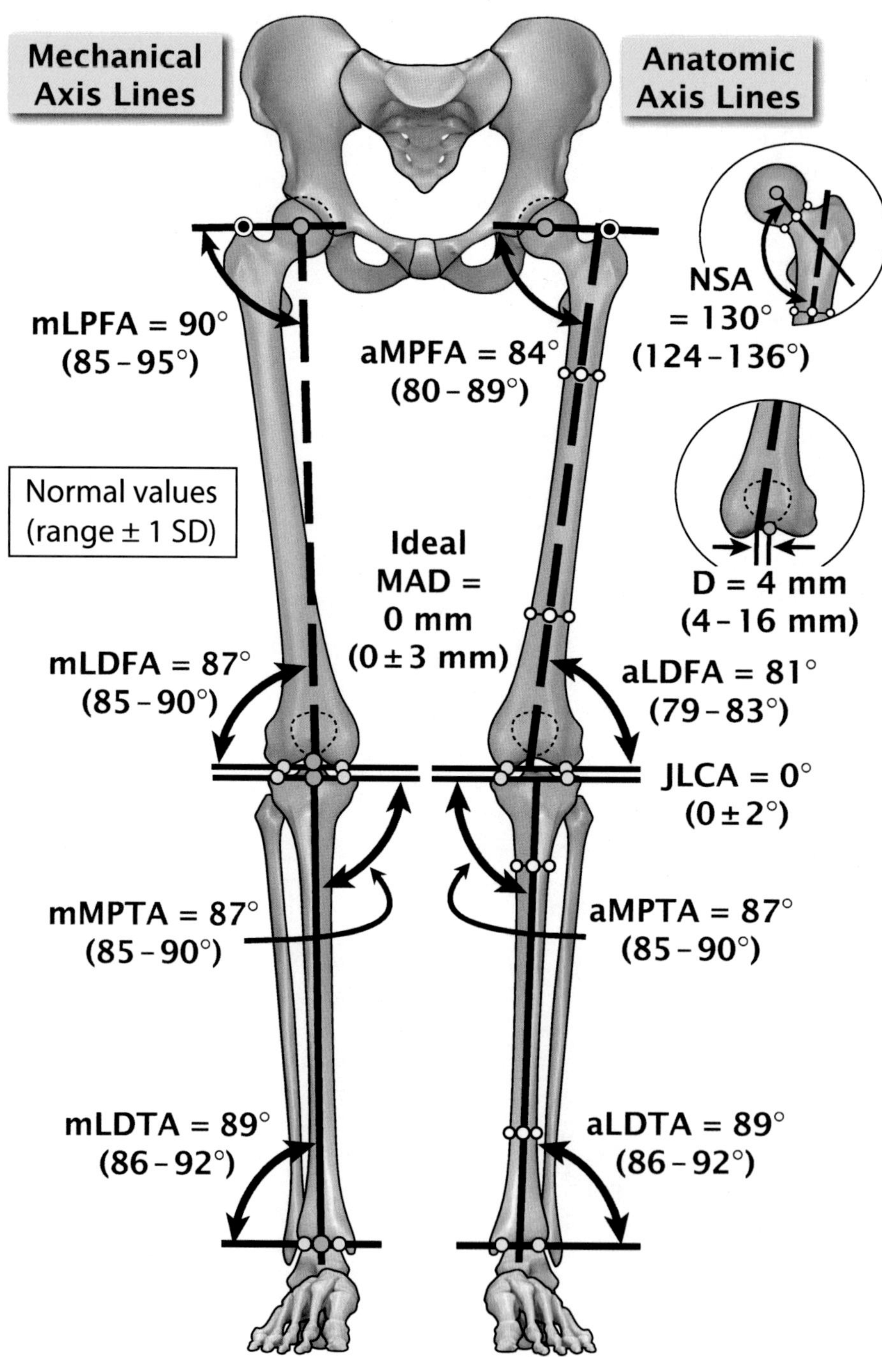


**Fig. 8:** Mechanical and anatomic joint angles, including the average normal values and ranges, are shown. aLDFA, anatomic lateral distal femoral angle; aLDTA, anatomic lateral distal tibial angle; aMPFA, anatomic medial proximal femoral angle; aMPTA, anatomic medial proximal tibial angle; D, distance; JLCA, joint line convergence angle; MAD, mechanical axis deviation; mLDFA, mechanical lateral distal femoral angle; mLDTA, mechanical lateral distal tibial angle; mLPFA, mechanical lateral proximal femoral angle; mMPTA, mechanical medial proximal tibial angle; NSA, neck shaft angle.

The system for naming the joint angles in the frontal plane consists of five components:

- **a** or **m:** designates whether the anatomic (a) or mechanical (m) axis is being used
- **M** or **L:** designates whether the angle is medial (M) or lateral (L) to the axis
- **P** or **D:** designates whether the angle is located at the proximal (P) or distal (D) end of the axis
- **F** or **T:** designates whether the femur (F) or tibia (T) is being measured
- **A:** Stands for angle (A)

**Table 1. Frontal Plane Joint Angles Created by the Mechanical Axis Lines**

| Acronym of Joint Angle | Complete Name of Joint Angle | Average Normal Value and Range |
|---|---|---|
| mLPFA | mechanical lateral proximal femoral angle | 90° (85–95°) |
| mLDFA | mechanical lateral distal femoral angle | 87° (85–90°) |
| mMPTA | mechanical medial proximal tibial angle | 87° (85–90°) |
| mLDTA | mechanical lateral distal tibial angle | 89° (86–92°) |

**Table 2. Frontal Plane Joint Angles Created by the Anatomic Axis Lines**

| Acronym of Joint Angle | Complete Name of Joint Angle | Average Normal Value and Range |
|---|---|---|
| aMPFA | anatomic medial proximal femoral angle | 84° (80–89°) |
| aLDFA | anatomic lateral distal femoral angle | 81° (79–83°) |
| aMPTA | anatomic medial proximal tibial angle | 87° (85–90°) |
| aLDTA | anatomic lateral distal tibial angle | 89° (86–92°) |

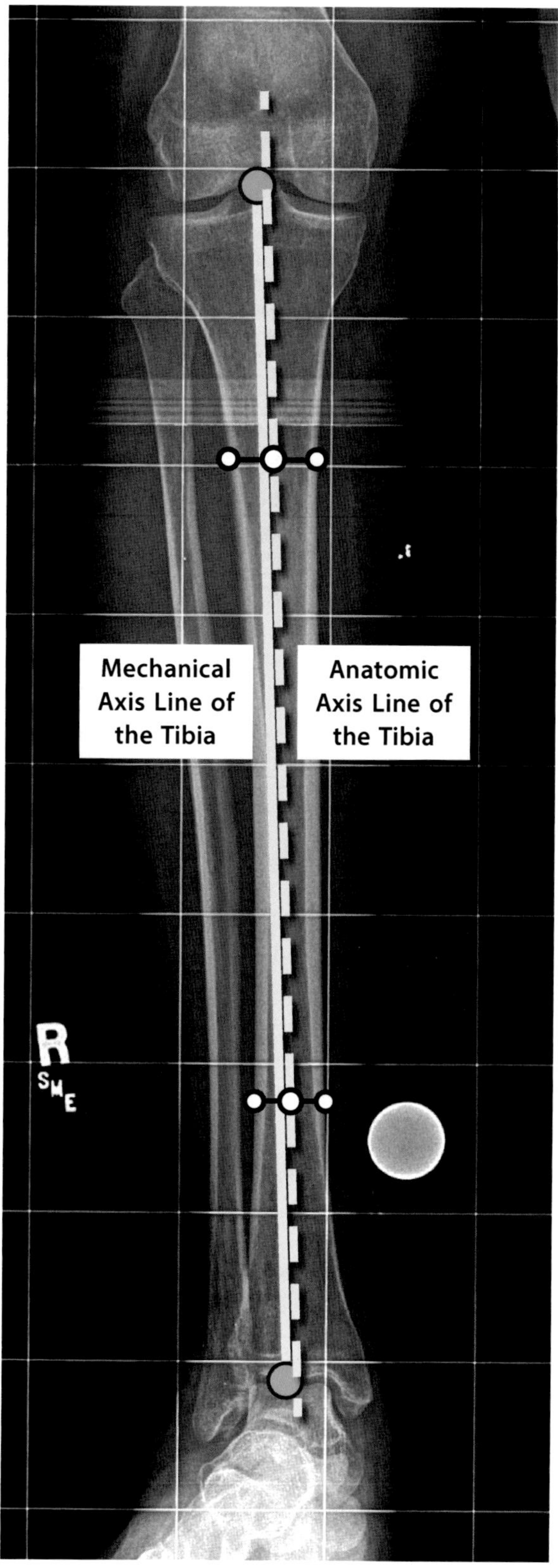


**Fig. 9:** In a normal tibia, the mechanical axis and the anatomic axis are essentially the same axis.

© 2023 Sinai Hospital of Baltimore

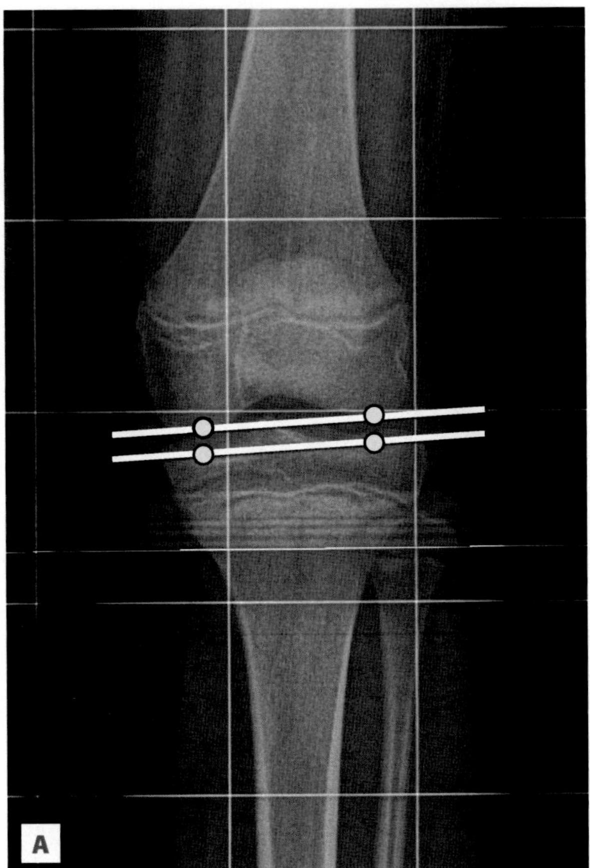


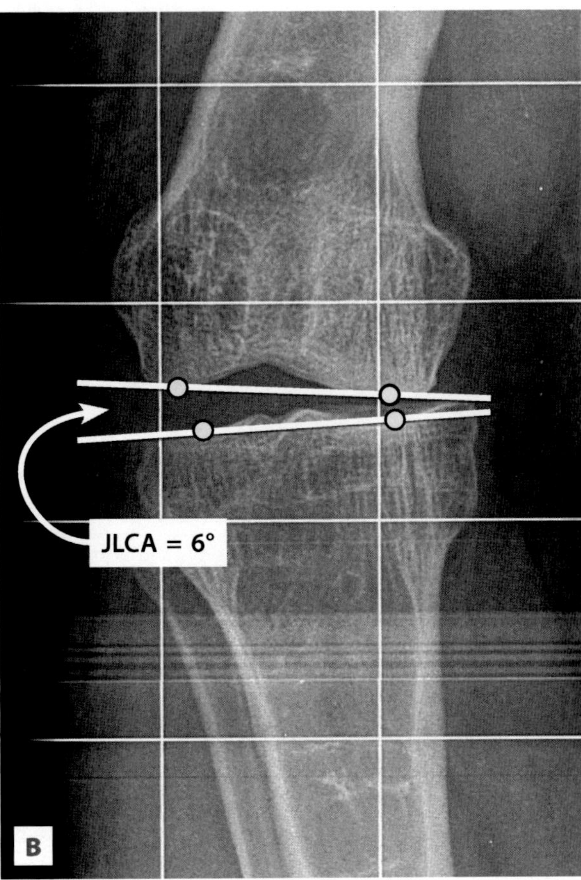


**Fig. 10: A,** The joint line convergence angle (JLCA) is formed by the distal femoral and proximal tibial joint lines. In a normal limb, these two lines are parallel with a range of normal of ±2°. **B,** The JLCA is 6°, which denotes laxity in the lateral collateral ligament secondary to the abnormal medial mechanical axis. The joint laxity exacerbates the varus deformity.

**Table 3. Additional Frontal Plane Joint Angles**

| Acronym of Joint Angle | Complete Name of Joint Angle | Average Normal Value and Range |
|---|---|---|
| JLCA | joint line convergence angle | 0±2° |
| AMA of the femur | anatomic-mechanical angle of the femur | 7° (5–9°) |
| NSA | neck shaft angle | 130° (124–136°) |

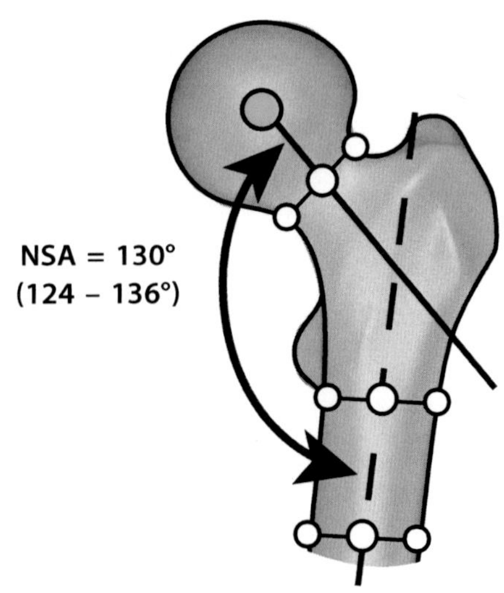


**Fig. 11:** The neck shaft angle should be approximately 130°.

In a normal tibia, the mechanical and anatomic axes are essentially the same axis (Fig. 9). This means that the mechanical and anatomic medial proximal tibial angle (i.e., mMPTA, aMPTA) and the mechanical and anatomic lateral distal tibial angle (i.e., mLDTA, aLDTA) each have the same average normal values and ranges (Fig. 8). Therefore, the anatomic and mechanical joint angles of the tibia do not need to be differentiated and are referred to simply as medial proximal tibial angle (MPTA) and lateral distal tibial angle (LDTA). Note that the abbreviations "a" for anatomic and "m" for mechanical are generally not included in these tibial joint angles.

In a normal femur, the anatomic and mechanical axes are different, so we must differentiate between the anatomic and mechanical joint angles. In practice, the mechanical femoral angles are used more often than the anatomic femoral angles. Therefore, the mLDFA is often referred to as simply the LDFA (i.e., the "m" for "mechanical" is not included in the acronym). The anatomic LDFA is always designated as aLDFA (i.e., including the abbreviation "a" for "anatomic").

Three additional angles must be defined in the frontal plane: the joint line convergence angle (JLCA), the femoral anatomic-mechanical angle (AMA), and the neck shaft angle (NSA). These angles play a role in assessing the presence of a deformity and aid in deformity correction planning.

The joint line convergence angle is the angle created by the distal femoral joint line and the proximal tibial joint line (Fig. 10A, Table 3). Normally, these lines should be parallel with a range of normal being 0 ± 2°. However, if there is a significant angulation between these two joint lines (>2°), then ligamentous laxity or loss of cartilage space about the knee joint may be contributing to the deformity (Fig. 10B).

Another useful angle in the frontal plane is the neck shaft angle (Fig. 11, Table 3). First, a line is created by connecting the center of the femoral head and the center of the femoral neck. The NSA is the angle created by this previously drawn line and the anatomic axis of the femur. The angle should be 130° with a range of normal from 124 to 136°.

The femoral anatomic-mechanical angle is the angle created by the anatomic axis and the

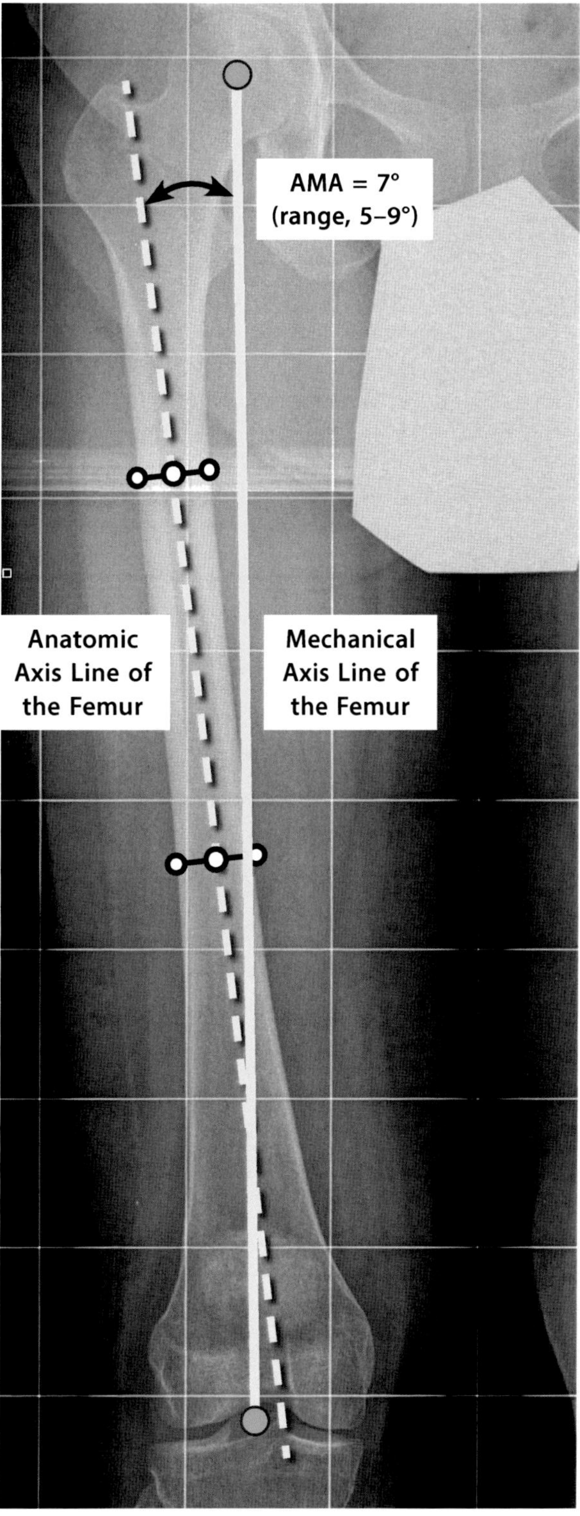


**Fig. 12:** The intersection of the femoral mechanical axis and femoral anatomic axis forms the anatomic-mechanical angle. Normally, this angle should be 7° (range, 5–9°).

© 2023 Sinai Hospital of Baltimore

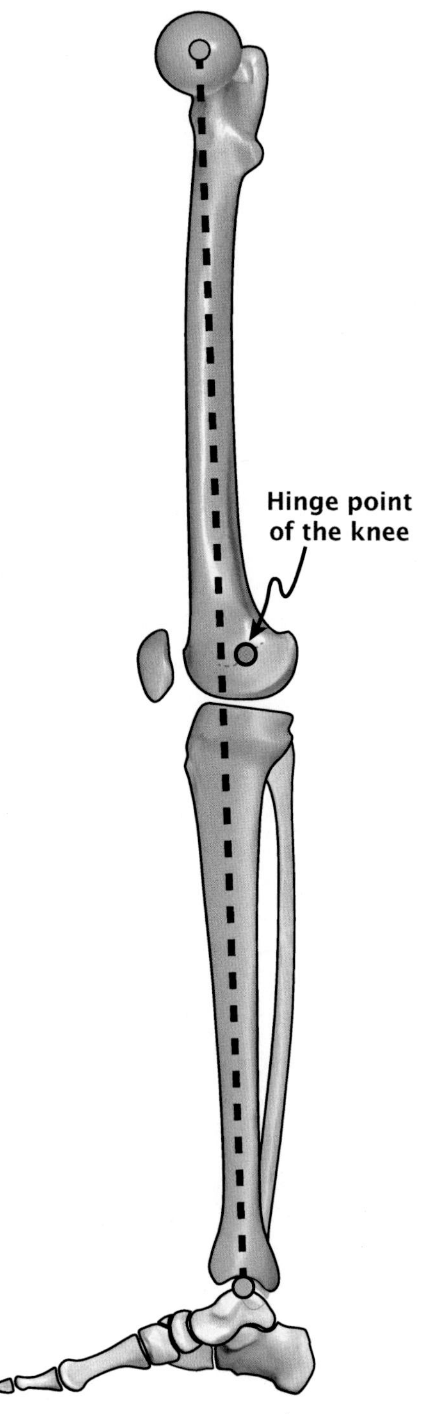


**Fig. 13:** On a lateral view x-ray, the sagittal plane mechanical axis is defined as a line from the center of the femoral head to the center of the ankle joint. The normal sagittal plane mechanical axis passes slightly anterior to the hinge point of the knee (*purple point*) and is within the anterior confines of the distal femur. This allows the knee to "lock" in full extension so that the quadriceps muscle can relax.

mechanical axis of the femur (Fig. 12, Table 3). Normally, this angle should be approximately 7° with a range of normal from 5° to 9°. Note that the femoral anatomic axis intersects the distal joint line 4 to 16 mm medial to the center of the joint. This angle is useful when analyzing the femur and will be described in more detail in subsequent chapters. This AMA is also becoming more important with the advent of intramedullary lengthening and the creation of secondary post-lengthening deformities.

## Alignment in the Sagittal Plane

The sagittal plane is examined using a full length standing lateral view x-ray of the lower limb with the knee joint maximally extended. Just like the frontal plane, the sagittal plane has a mechanical axis of the limb that extends from the center of the femoral head to the center of the ankle (Fig. 13). This mechanical axis should pass slightly anterior to the hinge point of the knee (purple dot). In children, the hinge point of the knee may be approximated by the intersection of the posterior femoral cortex and the physis/physeal scar (Fig. 14A–C). In skeletally mature patients, the hinge point of the knee may be approximated by the intersection of the Blumensaat line and the posterior femoral cortex (Fig. 14D and 14E).

Although the ideal sagittal plane mechanical axis passes slightly anterior to the hinge point of the knee, it is considered within the range of normal if it stays within the zone that lies between the hinge point of the knee and the anterior confines of the distal femur. An abnormal sagittal plane mechanical axis will fall posterior to the hinge point of the knee or anterior to the confines of the distal femur (Fig. 15).

When the mechanical axis of the limb passes slightly anterior to the hinge point of the knee, the knee can "lock" when the lower limb is fully extended, which allows the quadriceps muscle to rest during prolonged standing (Fig. 13). If the lower extremity has a "fixed flexion" deformity at the knee and the mechanical axis is posterior to the hinge point of the knee, then the individual will have to activate the quadriceps muscle constantly (Fig. 15A). This constant activation of the quadriceps muscle can result in fatigue, patella-femoral pain, and gait disturbance. If the mechanical axis of the limb passes anterior to the confines of the distal femur, a hyperextension deformity is present (Fig. 15B).

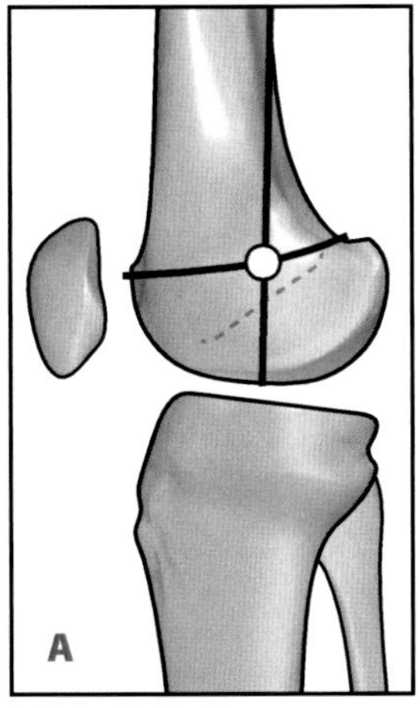


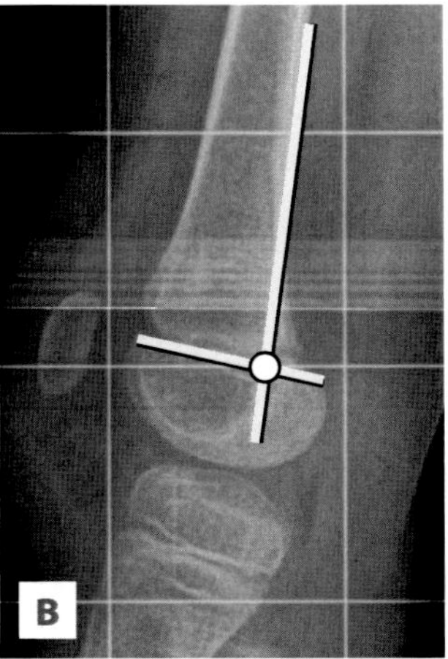


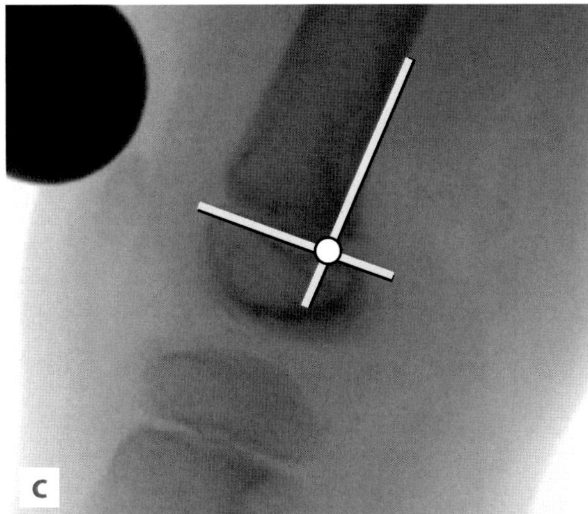


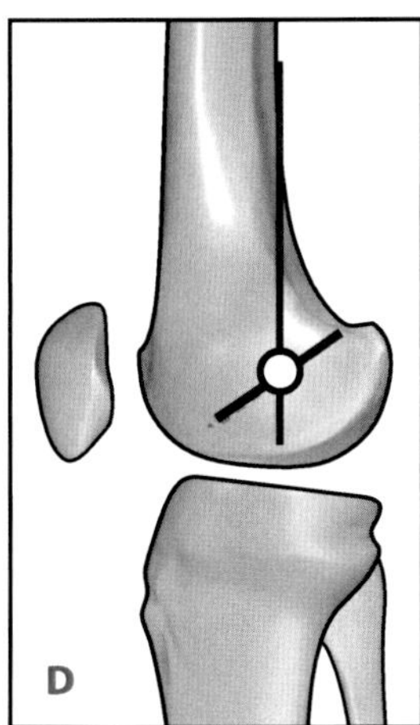


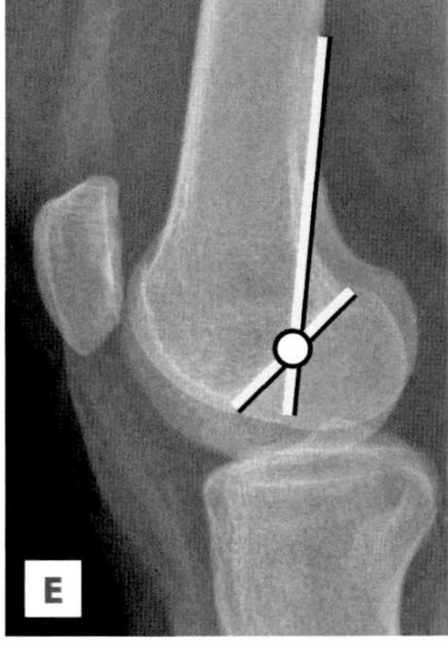


**Fig. 14: A–C**, In children, the hinge point of the knee is defined as the intersection of the posterior femoral cortex and the distal femoral physis/physeal scar. **D** and **E**, In adults, the hinge point of the knee is at the intersection of the posterior femoral cortex and the Blumensaat line.

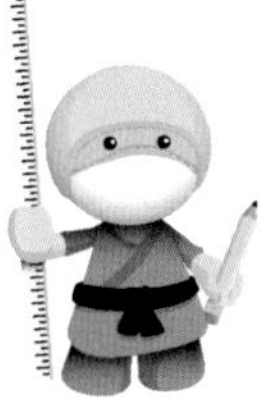

***Sensei says,***
*"He who cannot lock knee in full extension will quickly tire during the journey."*

In the sagittal plane, we use a "true" mechanical axis of the limb (described above as the center of the femoral head to the center of the ankle) to analyze sagittal plane MAD (Fig. 16A). However, we use a "modified" mechanical axis of each limb segment to draw the joint angles (Fig. 16B). When we draw the modified mechanical axis of the femur or tibia, we do not use the center of the distal femur or center of the proximal tibia. By convention, we use other points of reference on the joint lines to draw these modified mechanical axes, which can also be called segmental mechanical axes.

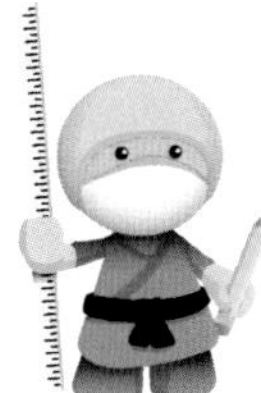

***Sensei says,***
*"He who measures the sagittal joint angles must use the modified mechanical axes of the femur and of the tibia."*

The sagittal plane joint lines and the modified mechanical axes of the femur and of the tibia create joint angles. The designation as mechanical (m) or anatomic (a) for the sagittal plane joint angles is not needed. The system for naming three of the joint angles in the sagittal plane consists of four components:

- **P** or **A:** designates whether the angle is posterior (P) or anterior (A) to the axis
- **P** or **D:** designates whether the angle is located at the proximal (P) or distal (D) end of the axis
- **F** or **T:** designates whether the femur (F) or tibia (T) is being measured
- **A:** Stands for angle (A)

To draw the modified mechanical axis of the femur, first draw the distal femoral joint line.

© 2023 Sinai Hospital of Baltimore

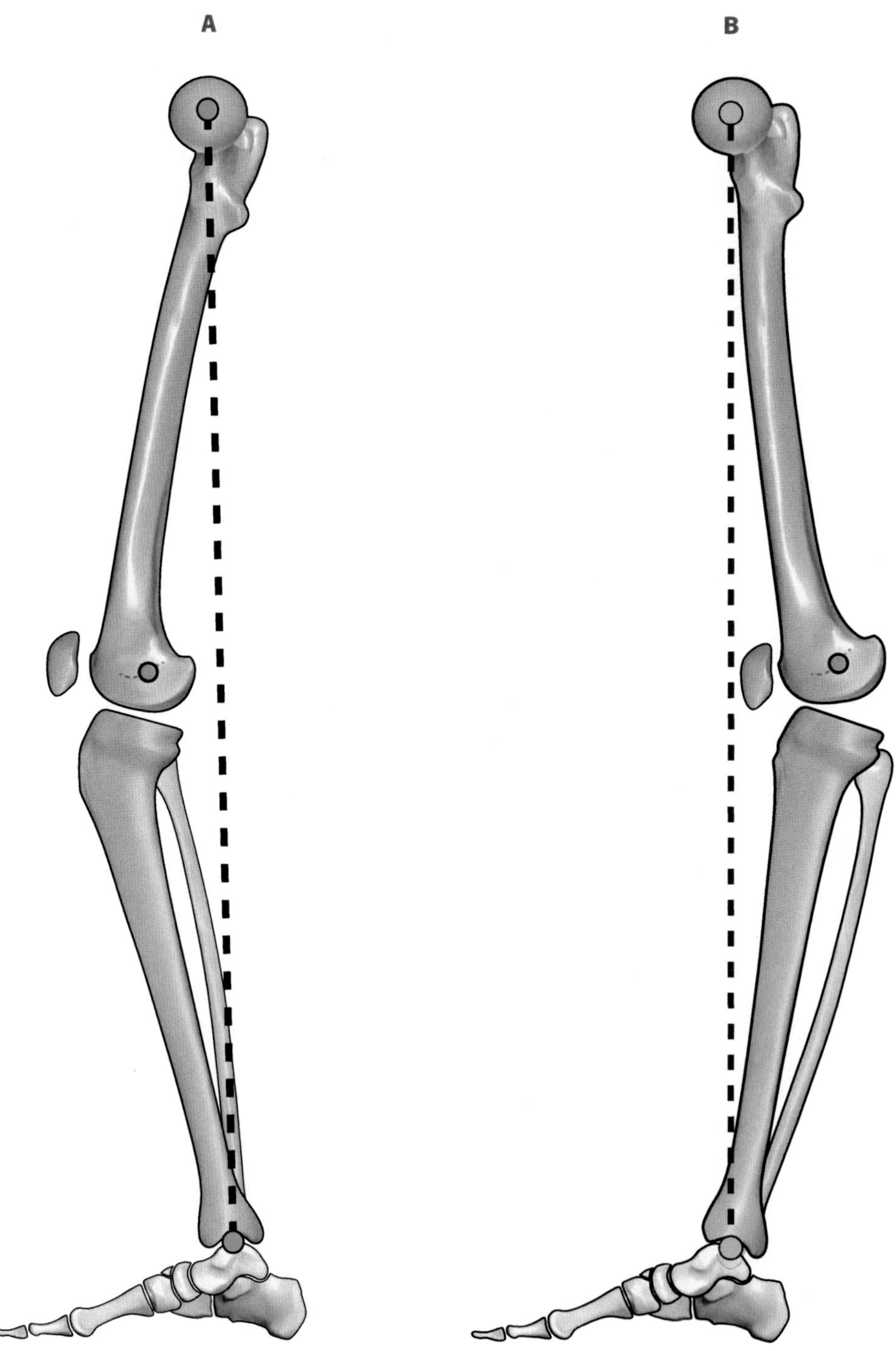


**Fig. 15: A**, If the mechanical axis is posterior to the hinge point of the knee (*purple point*), then the individual will have to activate the quadriceps muscle constantly. **B**, If the mechanical axis is anterior to the distal femoral cortex, then the limb has a hyperextension deformity.

To draw the distal femoral joint line in a skeletally mature patient, connect two points that are placed at the anterior and posterior aspects of the physeal scar (Fig. 17A and 17B). To draw the distal femoral joint line in a child, connect two points that are placed at the anterior and posterior aspect of the open distal femoral physis. Then place a point on the distal femoral joint line that is 1/3 of the total length of the joint line from the anterior cortex (Fig. 17C). To draw the sagittal plane modified mechanical axis of the femur, connect a point at the center of the femoral head to the 1/3 point on the distal femoral joint line (Fig. 17D). The intersection of this modified mechanical axis and the joint line creates the posterior distal femoral angle (PDFA) (Fig. 18). In the same way that the normal joint angles have been established in the frontal plane, the sagittal plane joint angles each have an average normal value and a range (Fig. 18, Table 4).

To draw the modified mechanical axis of the tibia, first draw the proximal tibial joint line. The proximal tibial joint line is formed by connecting points on the anterior and posterior aspect of the tibial plateau (Fig. 19A and 19B). This joint line can be difficult to delineate due to the presence of the tibial spines. Then place a point on the proximal tibial joint line that is 1/5 of the total length of the proximal tibial joint line from the anterior cortex (Fig. 19C). Next, draw the distal tibial joint line by connecting points placed on the anterior and posterior "beaks" of the distal tibia (Fig. 19D and 19E). Place a point at the center of the distal tibial joint line (Fig. 19F). To draw the sagittal plane modified mechanical axis of the tibia, connect the point on the proximal joint line to the point on the distal joint line (Fig. 19G). This axis line creates the posterior proximal tibial angle (PPTA) and anterior distal tibial angle (ADTA) (Fig. 18, Table 4).

Note that the points on the joint lines that are used to draw the modified mechanical axis of each limb segment are not selected arbitrarily. In a normal tibia, the mid-diaphyseal line intersects the proximal joint

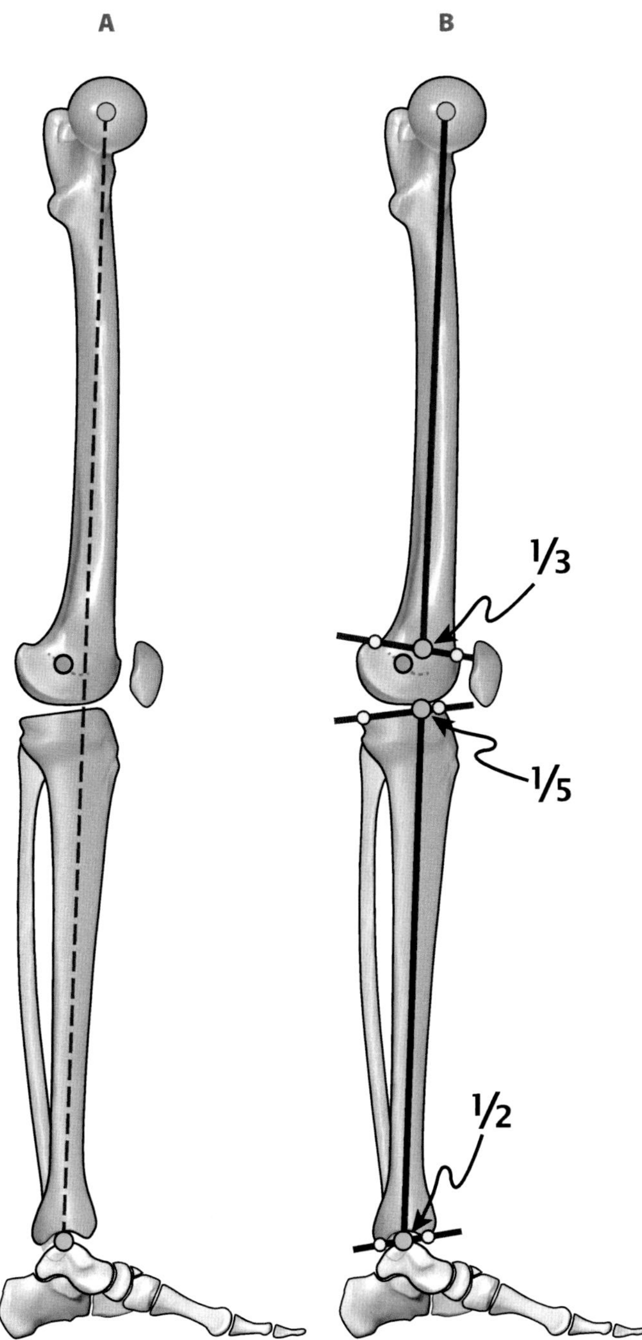


**Fig. 16: A**, The "true" mechanical axis of the limb is used to determine sagittal plane MAD. **B**, The "modified" mechanical axis lines of the femur and of the tibia are used to analyze the joint angles.

© 2023 Sinai Hospital of Baltimore

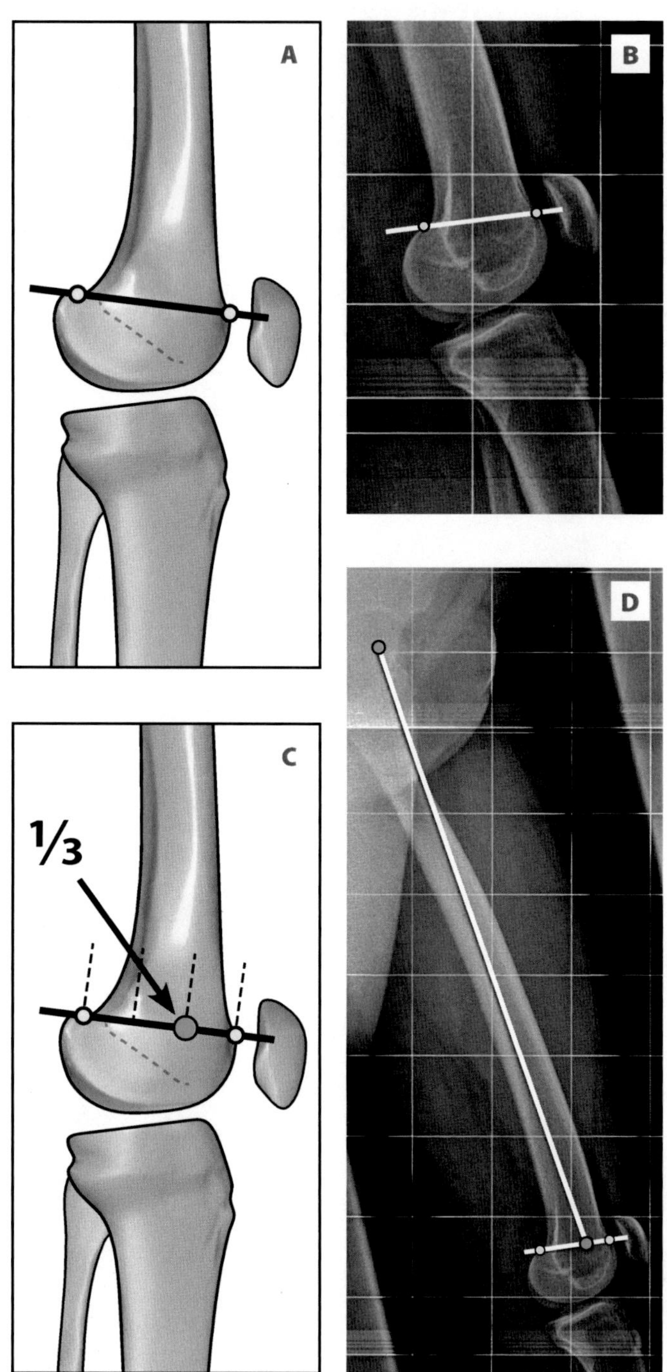


Fig. 17: A and B, In adults, the distal femoral joint line is created by connecting points at the anterior and posterior margins of the physeal scar. C, Place a point on the distal femoral joint line that is 1/3 of the total length of the joint line back from the anterior cortex. D, Draw the sagittal plane modified mechanical axis of the femur by connecting a point at the center of the femoral head to the point on the distal femoral joint line that is 1/3 of the total length of the joint line from the anterior cortex.

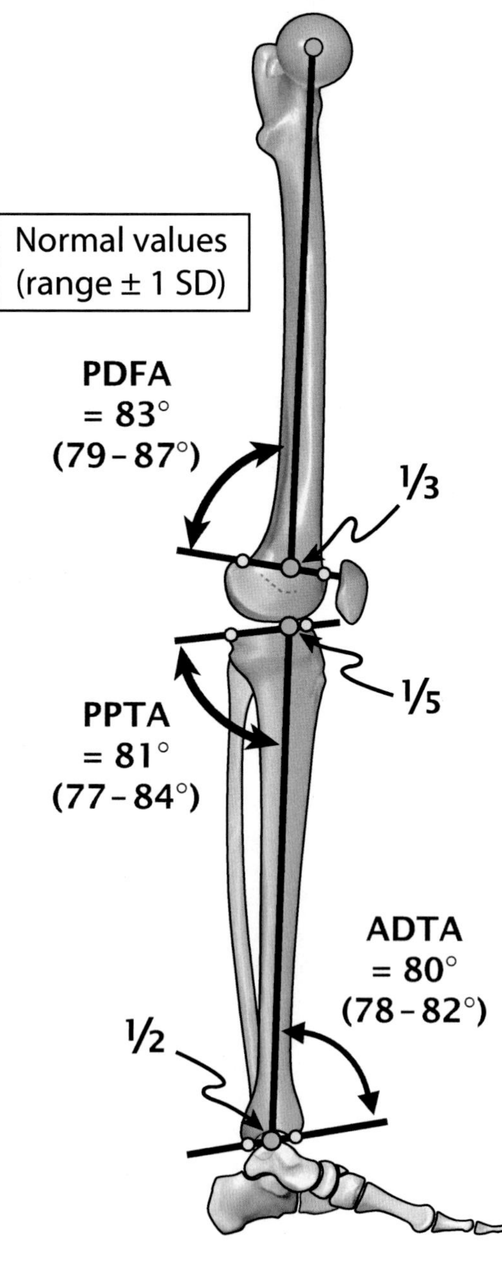


Fig. 18: Normal values and ranges for the sagittal plane joint angles are shown. The modified femoral and tibial mechanical axes are used to draw these angles. PDFA, posterior distal femoral angle, PPTA, posterior proximal tibial angle, ADTA, anterior distal tibial angle.

line at 1/5 of the total length of the proximal tibial joint line from the anterior cortex and at 1/2 of the total length of the distal tibial joint line (Fig. 20). In a normal femur, the mid-diaphyseal line of the distal third of the femur intersects the joint line at 1/3 of the total length of the distal femoral joint line from the anterior cortex (Fig. 20). This convention was developed to allow the use of the distal femoral mid-diaphyseal line and the tibial mid-diaphyesal line during joint angle analysis and planning. It is also helpful if you have a lateral view x-ray of the femur that does not visualize the entire femur. When your x-ray only visualizes the distal femur, you can draw the femoral modified mechanical axis by using the anatomic axis of the distal one-third of the femur.

**Table 4. Sagittal Plane Joint Angles**

| Acronym of Joint Angle | Complete Name of Joint Angle | Average Normal Value and Range |
|---|---|---|
| PDFA | posterior distal femoral angle | 83° (79–87°) |
| PPTA | posterior proximal tibial angle | 81° (77–84°) |
| ADTA | anterior distal tibial angle | 80° (78–82°) |
| SJLA | sagittal joint line angle | 16° ± 3° |
| SMAA | sagittal mechanical axes angle | 0° ± 2° |

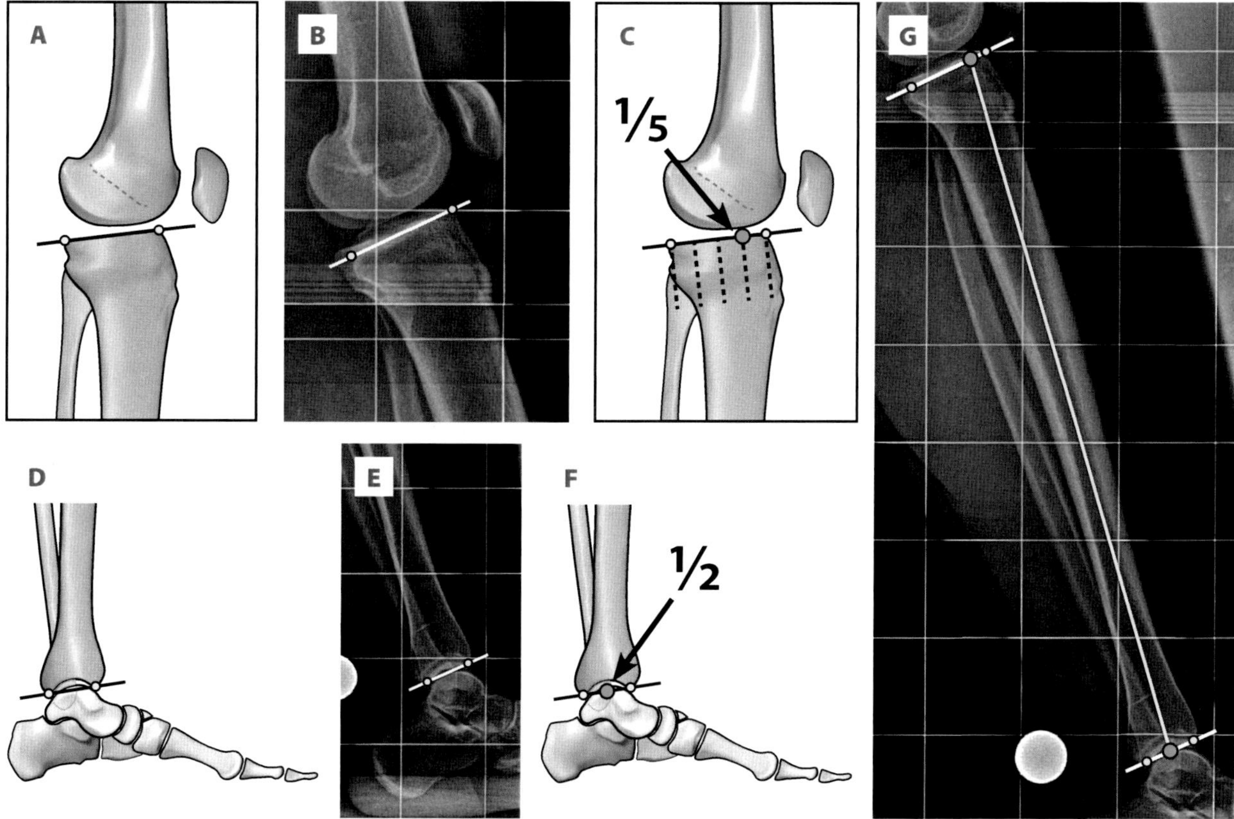


**Fig. 19:** **A** and **B**, Draw the proximal tibial joint line by connecting points placed on the anterior and posterior aspect of the tibial plateau. **C**, Place a point on the proximal tibial joint line that is 1/5 of the total length of the joint line from the anterior cortex. **D** and **E**, Draw the distal tibial joint line by connecting points placed on the anterior and posterior "beaks" of the distal tibia. **F**, Place a point at the center of the distal tibial joint line. **G**, Draw the sagittal plane modified mechanical axis of the tibia by connecting the point on the proximal tibial joint line to the point on the distal tibial joint line.

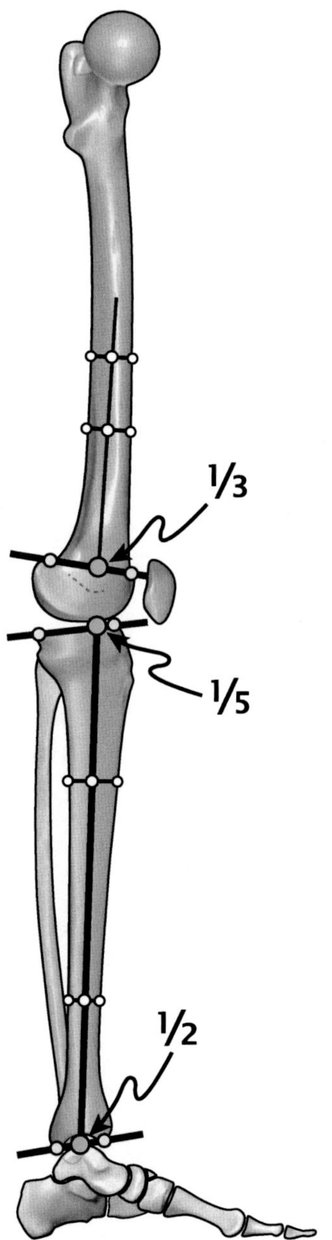


**Fig. 20:** In a normal femur, the mid-diaphyseal line of the distal third of the femur intersects the joint line at 1/3 of the total length of the distal femoral joint line from the anterior cortex. This is how the 1/3 point on the joint line was selected to be used when drawing the modified mechanical axis of the femur (Fig. 18). In a normal tibia, the mid-diaphyseal line intersects the proximal joint line at 1/5 of the total length of the proximal tibial joint line from the anterior cortex and at 1/2 of the total length of the distal tibial joint line. This is how the 1/5 and 1/2 points on the joint lines were selected to be used when drawing the modified mechanical axis of the tibia (Fig. 18).

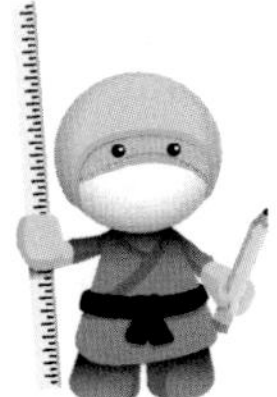

***Sensei says,***
*"In the sagittal plane, the modified mechanical axis of the femur and of the tibia intersect their respective joint lines at 1/3 of the distal femoral joint line, 1/5 of the proximal tibial joint line, and 1/2 of the distal tibial joint line from the anterior cortex."*

In addition to the PDFA, PPTA, and ADTA, two other angles are measured in the sagittal plane: the sagittal mechanical axes angle (SMAA) and the sagittal joint line angle (SJLA). Both the SMAA and the SJLA help analyze the confounding factor of knee motion in the sagittal plane.

The SMAA is the angle formed by the femoral and tibial modified mechanical axes (Fig. 21A). In a normal limb, the SMAA will be 0° (± 2°). The SMAA represents the overall position of the knee joint and will determine if the knee joint is in a neutral position (Fig. 21A), a flexion position (Fig. 21B), or a hyperextended position (Fig. 21C).

The SJLA is the angle that is formed by the distal femoral joint line and the proximal tibial joint line (Fig. 22). The average normal value of the SJLA is 16° ± 3° (Fig. 22). The normal value for the SJLA was determined by conducting a review of 130 normal full length standing lateral view x-rays (normal PDFA and PPTA, collinear tibial and femoral mechanical axes). An SJLA greater than 16° indicates extension while an SJLA less than 16° indicates flexion (Fig. 22).

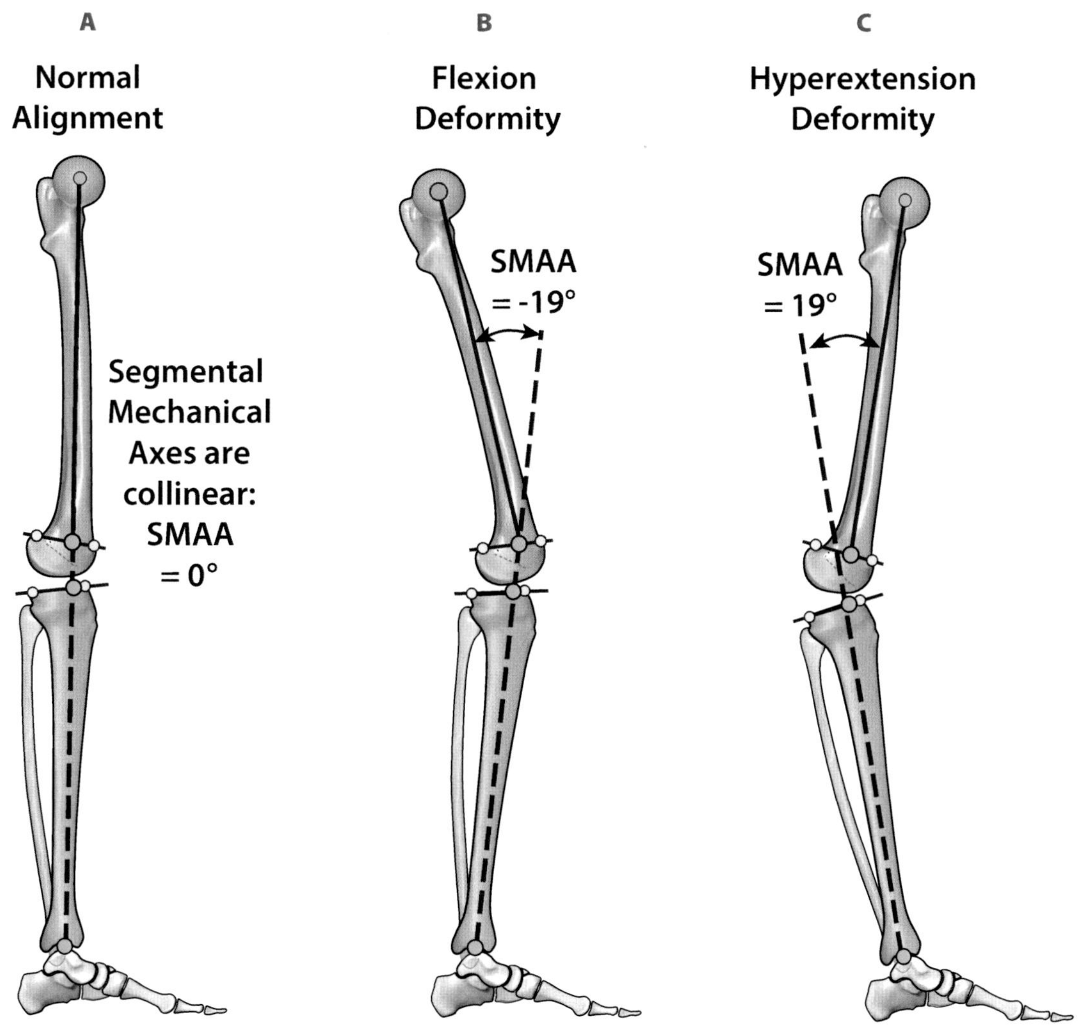


**Fig. 21:** Maximum extension views. **A**, Collinear modified mechanical axes of the femur and the tibia show that the sagittal mechanical axes angle (SMAA) is 0° and the limb has normal sagittal plane alignment. **B**, SMAA shows that a flexion deformity is present (SMAA = -19° flexion). **C**, SMAA shows that a hyperextension deformity is present (SMAA = 19° hyperextension).

© 2023 Sinai Hospital of Baltimore

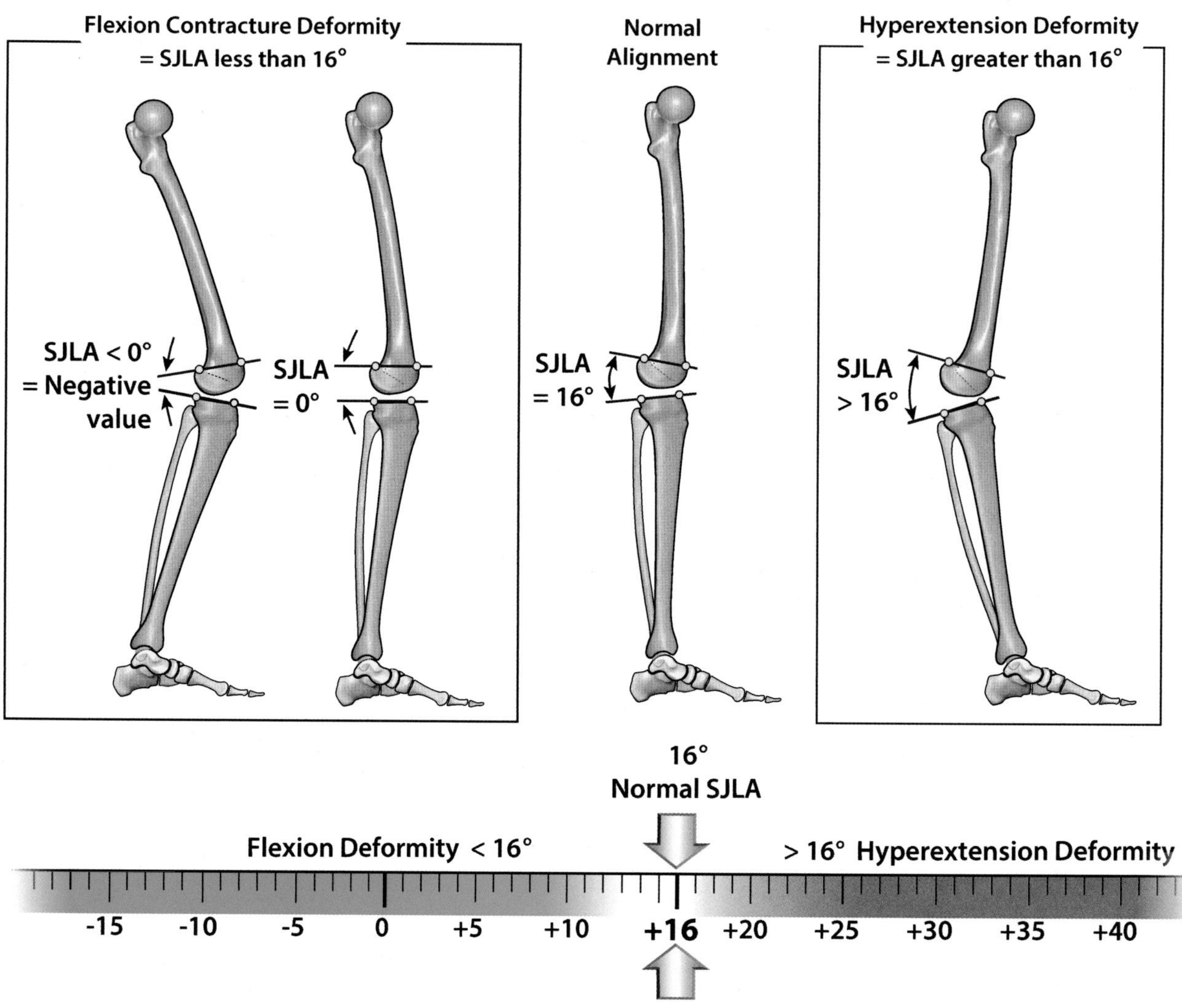


**Fig. 22:** A sagittal joint line angle (SJLA) less than 16° indicates flexion deformity while an SJLA greater than 16° indicates hyperextension deformity.

In the sagittal plane, both the bony alignment and soft-tissue characteristics must be evaluated because they influence the overall position of the limb in this plane. Bony and soft-tissue characteristics of the knee or ankle can add to or compensate for the deformity. A deformity in the sagittal plane can result from a bony deformity of the femur, the tibia, or both the femur and tibia. A sagittal plane deformity can also occur when soft-tissue abnormalities are present. Since the knee joint moves in the sagittal plane, soft-tissue contractures or laxity will contribute to or compensate for the bony deformities. A knee joint soft-tissue contracture will result in a "fixed flexion" deformity of the knee. Posterior capsular laxity may result in hyperextension of the knee. In the chapter entitled "Deformity Analysis in the Sagittal Plane," the five sagittal joint angles will be used to analyze bony deformities in the femur and tibia as well as the soft-tissue contributions to the deformity.

## Reference

1. Salenius P, Vankka E. The development of the tibiofemoral angle in children. J Bone Joint Surg Am. 1975;57(2):259-61.

# Chapter 2

# Natural History of Malalignment

Philip K. McClure, MD

Malalignment has long been assumed to be a primary cause of degenerative joint disease. In fact, it often seems to be a core component of orthopedic education and thought. However, close inspection of the literature leaves many opportunities to prove this assumption; our literature is currently very sparse on the long-term consequences of malalignment, particularly from a pediatric perspective. Data have been gathered from biomechanical analysis, animal models, cross-sectional cohort studies, and longitudinal studies. Data have also been extrapolated from studies evaluating the effects of realignment on symptoms and radiographic progression. Though the knee and ankle are linked in the mechanical environment, studies tend to focus on one or the other in general and hence are fairly easily separated into sections rather than discussed together.

## Knee

When considering mechanical axis deviation (MAD) of the knee, most orthopedic surgeons will quickly envision total knee replacement in someone with varus malalignment (i.e., severe medial degeneration with relatively spared lateral compartments). This picture is so ubiquitous that it is easy to assume that this is clearly the primary cause of degenerative arthritis. However, the literature is somewhat less clear. So much less clear, in fact, that systematic reviews have left a split decision between limited and strong data to support malalignment as a cause of arthritis.[1–5] Cohort studies have shown that malalignment is a risk factor for short-term progression of established arthritis, but extrapolating this to malalignment as the original cause is difficult.[6–8] To add to this difficulty, a recent study[9] found progressive distal femoral varus in an adult population, adding further doubt to the origin of malalignment that could lead to degeneration. Another interesting development of our understanding of malalignment and degeneration relates to gait lab data, with the indication that an increasing varus thrust can accentuate arthritic progression in severe disease.[10] In an attempt to understand whether lifelong malalignment leads to arthritis at the knee, we will take a pediatric perspective in which longitudinal data are king (and rare).

### Biomechanical Data

Biomechanical data allow us to understand forces across the knee in various settings. Several studies are available to support the concept that MAD is detrimental to the knee joint. McKellop et al.[11] simulated deformity in 5° increments in cadaveric specimens and measured contact pressures on either side of the joint. Proximal deformities generate much larger changes at the knee than distal, with up to 106% increase in medial force with 20° proximal varus, whereas a distal deformity of the same magnitude generated only a 26% increase in medial contact pressure. The role of the deformity level on the pathologic forces created is illustrated in Figure 1.

© 2023 Sinai Hospital of Baltimore

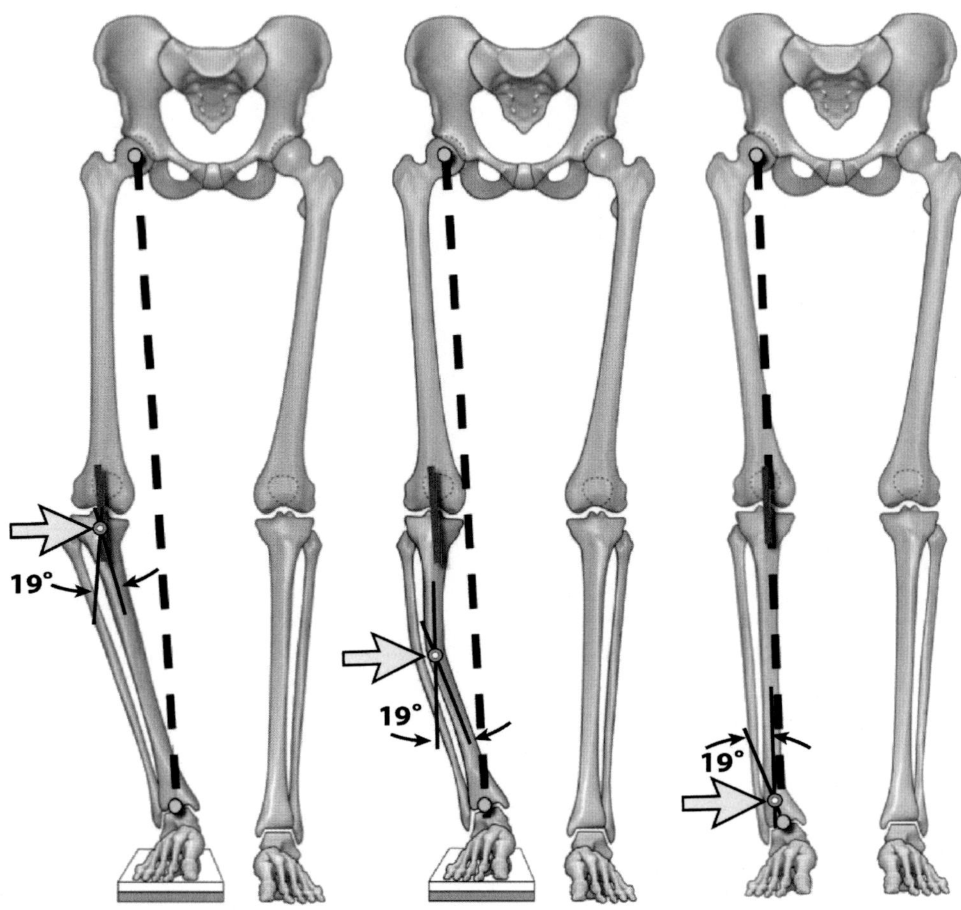


**Fig. 1:** Closer proximity to the knee joint yields higher mechanical axis deviation, despite unchanged angular deformity at the apex.

McKellop et al.[11] concluded that varus and valgus were equally detrimental to joint health. While multiple sources have concluded that normal alignment consists of slight medial MAD,[12-14] their biomechanical study[11] began with the mechanical axis simulated directly through the center of the knee, resulting in a slight valgus bias. This could explain why McKellop et al.[11] found equally deleterious effects of varus and valgus, while adult cross-sectional data implicate varus more consistently.

The sagittal plane has been nearly completely neglected. One study[15] did demonstrate increased posterior joint contact pressures with simulated increased posterior slope after high tibial osteotomy. The results showed decreased posterior contact pressures with increasing flexion. Additional data are needed in order to more fully evaluate the biomechanics of the sagittal plane.

## In Vivo Experimental Studies

Animal studies create a perfect opportunity to study long-term joint health, though they are not without problems when trying to extrapolate to the human experience. Wu et al.[16] analyzed the effect of deformity on the knee joints of New Zealand white rabbits. Twelve weeks after varus, valgus, or neutral osteotomies, there were histological changes in the synovium without any cartilage or meniscal damage. However, by 34 weeks, all deformed specimens demonstrated arthritic change in the overloaded compartment, with more severe degeneration in the varus model.[16]

In hopes of simulating increased contact pressure directly rather than through osteotomy, Ogata et al.[17] placed a compression spring into rabbit knees. They were able to modulate both magnitude and duration of stress in their experimental model. Higher magnitude of force and duration were both important, but they concluded that duration of force was more predictive than magnitude. This lends hope to realignment surgery as a preventative or palliative treatment; however, multiple mental leaps are required.

## Clinical Cross-Sectional Data

Long-term follow-up of pediatric disease is the ideal setting to evaluate the effects of MAD on arthritic risk. Such evaluation was carried out for Blount disease by Zayer.[18] In this series, no patients developed arthritis prior to age 30, regardless of alignment. Eleven of 27 knees developed arthritis after age 30, with a statistically insignificant increase in higher deformity magnitudes.[18]

Two authors pursued long-term outcomes of femoral malunion. Fifty-two children who sustained femoral fractures were reviewed by Palmu et al.[19] at a mean of 21 years after injury. Knee arthritis was detected in the injured limb of 6 patients and non-injured in one at a mean age of 34 years. Patients who were affected by arthritis had a higher degree of sagittal and coronal plane deformity than those without, with the sagittal plane being more strongly associated. In their cohort, a higher degree of sagittal deformity was present, which could have been the driving factor for stronger association. After age 11 years, the authors recommended angulation be kept under 10° in the sagittal plane and 5° in the coronal. The level of deformity relative to the knee was not correlated with arthritic change in their study.[19]

A similar conclusion was drawn by Kettelkamp et al.[20] Fourteen patients with 15 limbs were evaluated at an average 31-year follow-up (range, 10–60 years). Nine femoral fractures had residual varus from 3° to 25°, and all patients developed arthritis at an average age of 28 years. Varus deformity produced earlier arthritis than valgus, and all patients had arthritis in the overloaded compartment.[20] Again, the authors did not stratify outcomes according to the level of deformity or the overall MAD.

Twenty-nine-year follow-up was documented by Dietz and Merchant[21] for malunited tibial fractures in 37 children. A non-significant increase in arthritis was found in the injured limb. The authors concluded that deformity of less than 10° in the sagittal plane and 5° in the coronal plane were acceptable for tibial fractures, though they were unable to define a clear upper limit of acceptable deformity statistically.[21]

Adult tibial malunions have been reviewed by several authors. Two studies[22,23] demonstrated correlation with malunion and arthritis at an average of 8 to 24 years. Varus was more correlated with arthritis than valgus. Both studies concluded that anatomic alignment was ideal, with statistically increased risk of arthritis after malunion greater than 5°.[22,23] Not all studies have been so conclusive, with one demonstrating no increased risk at 28-year follow-up.[24] However, the group was highly selected and only 5 of 88 patients had proximal one-third fractures, which would have higher risk of degeneration based on extrapolation from biomechanical data. Only two patients had more than 15° of angular deformity.[24]

## Clinical Follow-up Data: Correction of Malalignment

No long-term comparative data have been reported of children whose limbs have been realigned versus children whose limbs have not. A large amount of data is available for realignment in symptomatic adults. Mean survival time for high tibial osteotomy in the setting of arthritis has been reported at 9.7 years, with 90% survival at 5- to 8-year follow-up.[25] Earlier realignment of the limbs of symptomatic patients has improved outcomes compared with later realignment of more severe disease.[26] Extrapolation of this data to the pediatric population and preventative surgical intervention are difficult, though it stands to reason that prevention would have a longer lasting effect than delayed treatment.

Regarding the natural history of a joint that has been surgically realigned, relatively few long-term studies are available to give guidance. "Regenerated" cartilage has been found on second look arthrotomy in the bed of previous defects after realignment.[27] While this may indicate an improved environment for cartilage, it is unclear what the long-term viability of this tissue will be. In animal models, it has been shown that the duration of pathologic

© 2023 Sinai Hospital of Baltimore

loading is critical to the development of arthritis.[28] While it remains unproven, it is reasonable to anticipate that earlier relief of the abnormal loading would correlate with better cartilage health in the long-term.

## Gait Lab Data

Orthopedics is inherently a specialty of dynamic movement; unfortunately, we are nearly entirely dependent on static data points when trying to help our patients. Full length standing images are an example of our attempts to solve dynamic problems with static images. The correlation between lower extremity angular deformity and joint overload during gait is not necessarily 1:1.[29] Compensatory gait patterns have been observed as a mechanism to cope with lower extremity deformity and joint overload.[30] Further study may eventually help elucidate why some patients progress to osteoarthritis and some do not, despite similar static images.

Proximal tibial osteotomy for medial arthritis has been studied by Wang et al.[31] through the lens of the gait lab. After high tibial osteotomy, patients with a high adduction moment had 64% good or excellent outcomes in their study while patients with low adduction moments experienced 100% good or excellent outcomes. An increased rate of deformity recurrence was also noted in the high moment group.[31]

Growth modulation for coronal deformity has also been studied in the gait lab. Eight patients were treated with growth modulation for idiopathic genu varum or valgum.[32] Preoperative to postoperative changes between static and dynamic studies correlated well. However, in both the preoperative and postoperative settings, there was little correlation between abnormal static alignment and dynamic loading abnormalities. Abnormal gait parameters after growth modulation were noted in two patients with previously normal gait labs.[32] Surgical indications should be carefully reviewed in patients with normal preoperative dynamics in the setting of static deformity.

Another study evaluating growth modulation with the gait lab showed different results with a larger number of patients.[33] In their study, static and dynamic studies correlated well and improved alongside each other during correction. Generation of pathologic gait parameters was not noted in their study. Patients were not reported to have normal gait analysis prior to implantation, however, indicating that further study of this concern is needed.[33]

## Patellofemoral Joint Considerations

The patellofemoral (PF) joint is known to be afflicted with arthritis at a high rate.[34,35] Multiple studies have evaluated the role of malalignment on patellofemoral degeneration. Weinberg et al.[36] reviewed anatomic and demographic factors associated with PF arthritis in a sample of 71 human skeletons. Valgus alignment, a shallow trochlea, and a lateralized tibial tubercle were associated with PF arthritis.[36]

Patellofemoral cartilage volume was evaluated in relation to mechanical alignment using serial magnetic resonance imaging evaluations and radiographs by Teichtahl et al.[37] Decreasing lateral patellar cartilage volume was noted in relation to increasing valgus alignment. The authors posited that this is due to increasing lateral loads in the PF joint.[37] An association between valgus alignment and PF arthritis was also noted in two large clinical studies.[8,38] Three-dimensional analysis of patellar spin during resisted knee extension exercises demonstrated internal spin with varus knees and external spin with valgus knees, indicating a complex relationship between patellar mechanics and coronal alignment.[39] Further study is needed to elucidate the contribution of mechanical alignment to PF disease.

## Correlating Knee Deformity Angles with MAD

Mechanical axis deviation is a familiar concept to many orthopedic surgeons as a continuous variable, though it has also been further categorized into zones of the knee.[40] Correlation between MAD and tibiofemoral angles, which are used in a significant percentage of the literature, is not necessarily direct. Depending on femoral neck orientation and segmental and femoral neck lengths, different angles may manifest variably when measuring MAD. The use of MAD for deformity measurement is more

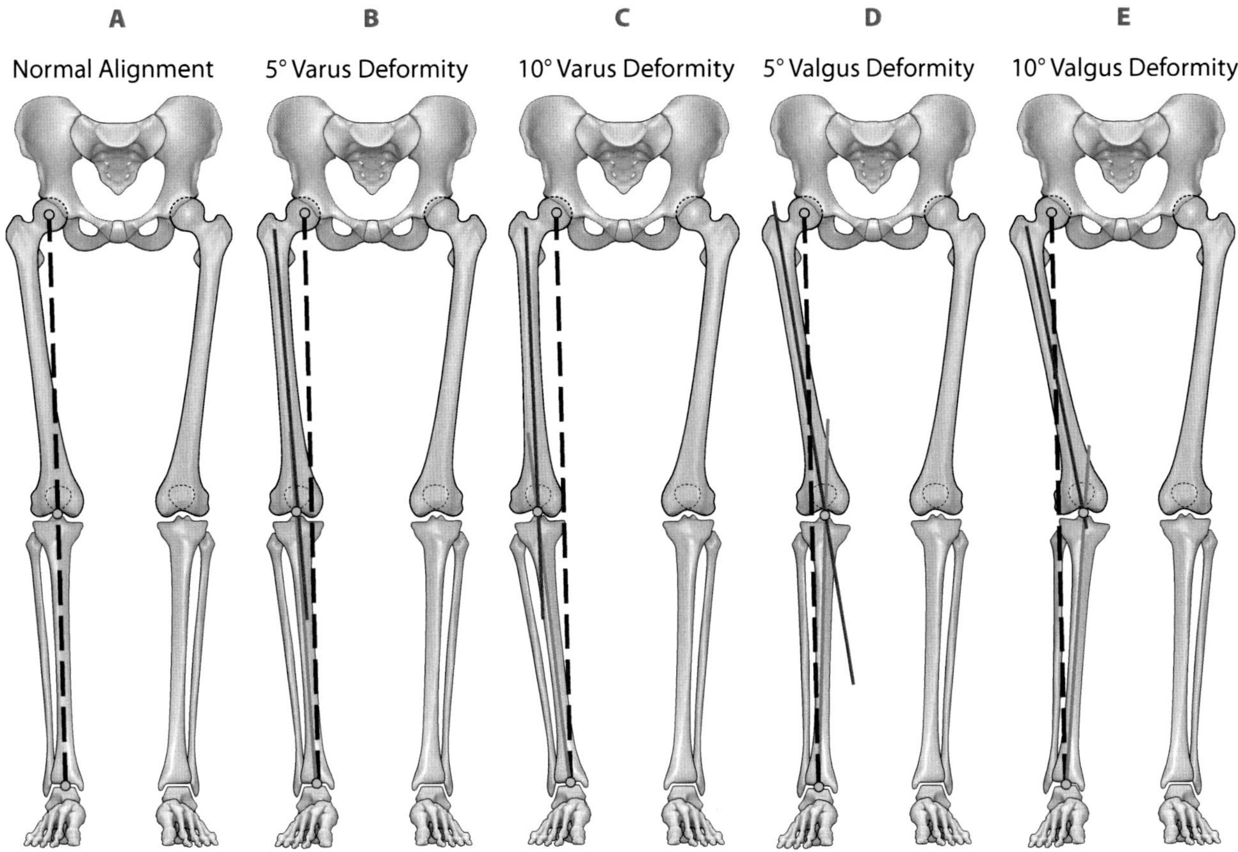


**Fig. 2: A**, Normal alignment with mechanical axis of the limb. **B** and **C**, Distal femoral varus deformity of 5° and 10°. **D** and **E**, Distal femoral valgus deformity of 5° and 10°. Panels **B** through **E** shown with associated femoral/tibial anatomic axes and overall mechanical axis.

sound from a strict mechanical standpoint, as the force experienced at the fulcrum is strongly related to the length of the lever arm. Therefore, direct correlation of MAD with the angles measured in many older papers is difficult. Based on the author's experience, 5° correlates well with the zone 1–2 border and 10° correlates well with zone 3 (Fig. 2).

## Ankle

The ankle joint is inherently different than the knee, both from the obvious anatomic variation and from a mechanical standpoint regarding pathologic forces on the joint due to MAD. The knee, as it is in the center of the limb, is subject to exaggerated local pressure due to long lever arms and is protected from shear forces by a complex network of intra-articular and extra-articular stabilizers. The ankle, as it is closer to the end of the limb, is largely spared from large lever arms of pathologic forces, but it is subject to shear forces as angulation is generated. The complex relationship of the multiple articulations in the hindfoot and midfoot is difficult to study using methods that account for all the variables. Biomechanical studies have examined the effect of malalignment on pathologic forces at the ankle.

Tarr et al.[41] demonstrated little effect on the ankle with deformities in the proximal and middle tibia. The authors felt that no significant changes occurred with 5° angulation in any direction. Larger effects were observed with deformities of 10° in the distal tibial region, with worse changes in the sagittal plane than the coronal plane.[41] McKellop et al.[42] examined the effects of simulated deformity at multiple levels and orientations in the tibia, with and without an immobilized subtalar joint. Their

© 2023 Sinai Hospital of Baltimore

findings[42] corroborated those of Tarr et al.,[41] with increasing effects of distal fractures, more severe changes in the sagittal plane than the coronal, and the addition of marked worsening after immobilization of the subtalar joint.

## Fracture Malunion

Initial outcome studies of tibial shaft fractures focused on hindfoot stiffness, which was primarily felt to be due to prolonged immobilization. Unfortunately, these studies did not evaluate malunion or degenerate changes specifically but noted that more severe injuries predisposed to worse ankle function.[43–45] This was primarily attributed to soft-tissue injury and scarring; radiographic outcomes were not discussed. Despite the fact that malunion was not considered, these studies are often referenced in malunion literature, likely due to the hindfoot stiffness identified with prolonged immobilization. No studies prior to 1969 considered malunion to be a significant problem.[46]

Teitz et al.[47] found no patients with symptomatic malunion of less than 5° varus, while 22% of patients with 5° or more were symptomatic at 2- to 4-year follow-up. Two of six patients older than 20 years with greater than 5° of varus malunion were noted to have symptomatic ankles with radiographic evidence of arthritis at 2 years.[47] Merchant and Dietz[48] found decreased ankle outcomes compared with knee outcomes after tibial malunion, but they failed to correlate this decrease with malalignment.

Intending to improve upon the analysis of Merchant and Dietz,[48] Puno et al.[22] evaluated 27 patients with 28 isolated extra-articular angular malunions of the tibia with a mean age of 44 years (range, 24–75 years). Worsening ankle outcomes were encountered above 4° of malorientation. Ankles were found to fare worse than knees regarding malalignment, though the study had lower degrees of deformity at the knee than the ankle. The authors concluded that the goal of treatment should be anatomic alignment, as there was no clear critical threshold below which arthrosis did not occur.[22] Kristensen et al.,[24] however, concluded that up to 15° could be tolerated without arthritis after reviewing 92 patients, 22 of whom had deformity greater than 10° at 28-year follow-up. None had radiographic arthritis in their report.[24]

Van der Schoot et al.[49] evaluated 88 patients with isolated tibial shaft fractures with average follow-up of 15 years. While they were able to demonstrate increased risk of radiographic degenerative changes with malunion greater than 4°, they found no relationship between malalignment and symptomatic arthritis.[49]

## Realignment of Distal Tibial Malunion

Stamatis et al.[50] reviewed 12 patients treated for ankle pain (with and without degenerative change) with supramalleolar osteotomy. At an average of 33 months follow-up, arthritic progression had halted and outcome scores improved.[50] Similar results have been reported in other studies, with improvement at 3 years and 5 years in most patients.[51,52]

A majority of patients with adult ankle arthritis demonstrate malalignment, but a significant minority present without malalignment. Ligamentous injuries and instability also play a significant role in degenerative disease of the ankle.[53] Graehl et al.[54] reported on adult patients with symptomatic malunion. Five of 8 improved after realignment osteotomy, one despite some degenerative changes. The authors concluded that this improvement demonstrated that at least a portion of symptoms came from malalignment.[54]

## Talar and Subtalar Hindfoot Malalignment

Cavovarus foot deformity is known to lead to degenerative ankle arthritis and introduces an additional component of complexity to ankle malalignment. Hindfoot malalignment has been assessed in biomechanical studies, with calcaneal position, soft-tissue integrity, and subtalar/midfoot motion contributing to forces across the ankle joint.[55–57] Further discussion of this multifactorial topic is beyond the intended scope of this chapter, though it is a meaningful component of ankle degeneration.

# Conclusion

To summarize available biomechanical, experimental, and clinical data, it is clear that deformity generates abnormal joint forces, which in animal models of the knee creates early degeneration and arthritic change. Clinical data support the concept that this is a relevant concern in the human knee, and several studies in the ankle generate similar concern. The long-term effects of malalignment correction remain unclear, particularly if pursued in a prophylactic manner. Based on extrapolation of data from joint salvage procedures and experimental studies, early realignment of the limbs of symptomatic individuals is expected to be beneficial.

## References

1. Chapple CM, Nicholson H, Baxter GD, Abbott JH. Patient characteristics that predict progression of knee osteoarthritis: a systematic review of prognostic studies. Arthritis Care Res (Hoboken). 2011;63(8):1115–25.

2. Bastick AN, Runhaar J, Belo JN, Bierma-Zeinstra SM. Prognostic factors for progression of clinical osteoarthritis of the knee: a systematic review of observational studies. Arthritis Res Ther. 2015;17:152.

3. Belo JN, Berger MY, Reijman M, Koes BW, Bierma-Zeinstra SM. Prognostic factors of progression of osteoarthritis of the knee: a systematic review of observational studies. Arthritis Rheum. 2007;57(1):13–26.

4. van Dijk GM, Dekker J, Veenhof C, van den Ende CH; Carpa Study Group. Course of functional status and pain in osteoarthritis of the hip or knee: a systematic review of the literature. Arthritis Rheum. 2006;55(5):779–85.

5. Tanamas S, Hanna FS, Cicuttini FM, Wluka AE, Berry P, Urquhart DM. Does knee malalignment increase the risk of development and progression of knee osteoarthritis? A systematic review. Arthritis Rheum. 2009;61(4):459–67.

6. Sharma L, Song J, Felson DT, Cahue S, Shamiyeh E, Dunlop DD. The role of knee alignment in disease progression and functional decline in knee osteoarthritis. JAMA. 2001;286(2):188–95.

7. Sharma L, Song J, Dunlop D, Felson D, Lewis CE, Segal N, Torner J, Cooke TD, Hietpas J, Lynch J, Nevitt M. Varus and valgus alignment and incident and progressive knee osteoarthritis. Ann Rheum Dis. 2010;69(11):1940–5.

8. Elahi S, Cahue S, Felson DT, Engelman L, Sharma L. The association between varus-valgus alignment and patellofemoral osteoarthritis. Arthritis Rheum. 2000;43(8):1874–80.

9. Matsumoto T, Hashimura M, Takayama K, Ishida K, Kawakami Y, Matsuzaki T, Nakano N, Matsushita T, Kuroda R, Kurosaka M. A radiographic analysis of alignment of the lower extremities--initiation and progression of varus-type knee osteoarthritis. Osteoarthritis Cartilage. 2015;23(2):217–23.

10. Sharma L, Chang AH, Jackson RD, Nevitt M, Moisio KC, Hochberg M, Eaton C, Kwoh CK, Almagor O, Cauley J, Chmiel JS. Varus thrust and incident and progressive knee osteoarthritis. Arthritis Rheumatol. 2017;69(11):2136–43.

11. McKellop HA, Sigholm G, Redfern FC, Doyle B, Sarmiento A, Luck JV Sr. The effect of simulated fracture-angulations of the tibia on cartilage pressures in the knee joint. J Bone Joint Surg Am. 1991;73(9):1382–91.

12. Moreland JR, Bassett LW, Hanker GJ. Radiographic analysis of the axial alignment of the lower extremity. J Bone Joint Surg Am. 1987;69(5):745–9.

13. Cooke D, Scudamore A, Li J, Wyss U, Bryant T, Costigan P. Axial lower-limb alignment: comparison of knee geometry in normal volunteers and osteoarthritis patients. Osteoarthritis Cartilage. 1997;5(1):39–47.

14. Hsu RW, Himeno S, Coventry MB, Chao EY. Normal axial alignment of the lower extremity and load-bearing distribution at the knee. Clin Orthop Relat Res. 1990;255:215–27.

© 2023 Sinai Hospital of Baltimore

15. Agneskirchner JD, Hurschler C, Stukenborg-Colsman C, Imhoff AB, Lobenhoffer P. Effect of high tibial flexion osteotomy on cartilage pressure and joint kinematics: a biomechanical study in human cadaveric knees. Winner of the AGA-DonJoy Award 2004. Arch Orthop Trauma Surg. 2004;124(9):575–84.

16. Wu DD, Burr DB, Boyd RD, Radin EL. Bone and cartilage changes following experimental varus or valgus tibial angulation. J Orthop Res. 1990;8(4):572–85.

17. Ogata K, Whiteside LA, Lesker PA, Simmons DJ. The effect of varus stress on the moving rabbit knee joint. Clin Orthop Relat Res. 1977;(129):313–8.

18. Zayer M. Osteoarthritis following Blount's disease. Int Orthop. 1980;4(1):63–6.

19. Palmu SA, Lohman M, Paukku RT, Peltonen JI, Nietosvaara Y. Childhood femoral fracture can lead to premature knee-joint arthritis. 21-year follow-up results: a retrospective study. Acta Orthop. 2013;84(1):71–5.

20. Kettelkamp DB, Hillberry BM, Murrish DE, Heck DA. Degenerative arthritis of the knee secondary to fracture malunion. Clin Orthop Relat Res. 1988;234:159–69.

21. Dietz FR, Merchant TC. Indications for osteotomy of the tibia in children. J Pediatr Orthop. 1990;10(4):486–90.

22. Puno RM, Vaughan JJ, Stetten ML, Johnson JR. Long-term effects of tibial angular malunion on the knee and ankle joints. J Orthop Trauma. 1991;5(3):247–54.

23. van der Schoot DK, Den Outer AJ, Bode PJ, Obermann WR, van Vugt AB. Degenerative changes at the knee and ankle related to malunion of tibial fractures. 15-year follow-up of 88 patients. J Bone Joint Surg Br. 1996;78(5):722–5.

24. Kristensen KD, Kiaer T, Blicher J. No arthrosis of the ankle 20 years after malaligned tibial-shaft fracture. Acta Orthop Scand. 1989 Apr;60(2):208–9.

25. Spahn G, Hofmann GO, von Engelhardt LV, Li M, Neubauer H, Klinger HM. The impact of a high tibial valgus osteotomy and unicondylar medial arthroplasty on the treatment for knee osteoarthritis: a meta-analysis. Knee Surg Sports Traumatol Arthrosc. 2013;21(1):96–112.

26. Floerkemeier S, Staubli AE, Schroeter S, Goldhahn S, Lobenhoffer P. Outcome after high tibial open-wedge osteotomy: a retrospective evaluation of 533 patients. Knee Surg Sports Traumatol Arthrosc. 2013;21(1):170–80.

27. Koshino T, Murase T, Saito T. Medial opening-wedge high tibial osteotomy with use of porous hydroxyapatite to treat medial compartment osteoarthritis of the knee. J Bone Joint Surg Am. 2003;85-A(1):78–85.

28. Reimann I. Experimental osteoarthritis of the knee in rabbits induced by alteration of the load-bearing. Acta Orthop Scand. 1973;44(4):496–504.

29. Farr S, Kranzl A, Pablik E, Kaipel M, Ganger R. Functional and radiographic consideration of lower limb malalignment in children and adolescents with idiopathic genu valgum. J Orthop Res. 2014;32(10):1362–70.

30. Stief F, Böhm H, Schwirtz A, Dussa CU, Döderlein L. Dynamic loading of the knee and hip joint and compensatory strategies in children and adolescents with varus malalignment. Gait Posture. 2011;33(3):490–5.

31. Wang JW, Kuo KN, Andriacchi TP, Galante JO. The influence of walking mechanics and time on the results of proximal tibial osteotomy. J Bone Joint Surg Am. 1990;72(6):905–9.

32. Böhm H, Stief F, Sander K, Hösl M, Döderlein L. Correction of static axial alignment in children with knee varus or valgus deformities through guided growth: Does it also correct dynamic frontal plane moments during walking? Gait Posture. 2015;42(3):394–7.

33. Stevens PM, MacWilliams B, Mohr RA. Gait analysis of stapling for genu valgum. J Pediatr Orthop. 2004;24(1):70–4.

34. Hinman RS, Crossley KM. Patellofemoral joint osteoarthritis: an important subgroup of knee osteoarthritis. Rheumatology (Oxford). 2007;46(7):1057–62.

35. Kim YM, Joo YB. Patellofemoral osteoarthritis. Knee Surg Relat Res. 2012;24(4):193–200.

36. Weinberg DS, Tucker BJ, Drain JP, Wang DM, Gilmore A, Liu RW. A cadaveric investigation into the demographic and bony alignment properties associated with osteoarthritis of the patellofemoral joint. Knee. 2016;23(3):350–6.

37. Teichtahl AJ, Wluka AE, Cicuttini FM. Frontal plane knee alignment is associated with a longitudinal reduction in patella cartilage volume in people with knee osteoarthritis. Osteoarthritis Cartilage. 2008;16(7):851–4.

38. Cahue S, Dunlop D, Hayes K, Song J, Torres L, Sharma L. Varus-valgus alignment in the progression of patellofemoral osteoarthritis. Arthritis Rheum. 2004;50(7):2184–90.

39. McWalter EJ, Cibere J, MacIntyre NJ, Nicolaou S, Schulzer M, Wilson DR. Relationship between varus-valgus alignment and patellar kinematics in individuals with knee osteoarthritis. J Bone Joint Surg Am. 2007;89(12):2723–31.

40. Stevens PM, Maguire M, Dales MD, Robins AJ. Physeal stapling for idiopathic genu valgum. J Pediatr Orthop. 1999;19(5):645–9.

41. Tarr RR, Resnick CT, Wagner KS, Sarmiento A. Changes in tibiotalar joint contact areas following experimentally induced tibial angular deformities. Clin Orthop Relat Res. 1985;(199):72–80.

42. McKellop HA, Llinás A, Sarmiento A. Effects of tibial malalignment on the knee and ankle. Orthop Clin North Am. 1994;25(3):415–23.

43. Ellis H. Disabilities after tibial shaft fractures; with special reference to Volkmann's ischaemic contracture. J Bone Joint Surg Br. 1958;40-B(2):190–7.

44. Merriam WF, Porter KM. Hindfoot disability after a tibial shaft fracture treated by internal fixation. J Bone Joint Surg Br. 1983;65(3):326–8.

45. McMaster M. Disability of the hindfoot after fracture of the tibial shaft. J Bone Joint Surg Br. 1976;58(1):90–3.

46. Brown PW, Urban JG. Early weight-bearing treatment of open fractures of the tibia. An end-result study of sixty-three cases. J Bone Joint Surg Am. 1969;51(1):59–75.

47. Teitz CC, Carter DR, Frankel VH. Problems associated with tibial fractures with intact fibulae. J Bone Joint Surg Am. 1980;62(5):770–6.

48. Merchant TC, Dietz FR. Long-term follow-up after fractures of the tibial and fibular shafts. J Bone Joint Surg Am. 1989;71(4):599–606.

49. van der Schoot DK, Den Outer AJ, Bode PJ, Obermann WR, van Vugt AB. Degenerative changes at the knee and ankle related to malunion of tibial fractures. 15-year follow-up of 88 patients. J Bone Joint Surg Br. 1996;78(5):722–5.

50. Stamatis ED, Cooper PS, Myerson MS. Supramalleolar osteotomy for the treatment of distal tibial angular deformities and arthritis of the ankle joint. Foot Ankle Int. 2003;24(10):754–64.


© 2023 Sinai Hospital of Baltimore

51. Pagenstert G, Knupp M, Valderrabano V, Hintermann B. Realignment surgery for valgus ankle osteoarthritis. Oper Orthop Traumatol. 2009;21(1):77–87.

52. Hongmou Z, Xiaojun L, Yi L, Hongliang L, Junhu W, Cheng L. Supramalleolar osteotomy with or without fibular osteotomy for varus ankle arthritis. Foot Ankle Int. 2016;37(9):1001–7.

53. Valderrabano V, Hintermann B, Horisberger M, Fung TS. Ligamentous posttraumatic ankle osteoarthritis. Am J Sports Med. 2006;34(4):612–20.

54. Graehl PM, Hersh MR, Heckman JD. Supramalleolar osteotomy for the treatment of symptomatic tibial malunion. J Orthop Trauma. 1987;1(4):281–92.

55. Resnick RB, Jahss MH, Choueka J, Kummer F, Hersch JC, Okereke E. Deltoid ligament forces after tibialis posterior tendon rupture: effects of triple arthrodesis and calcaneal displacement osteotomies. Foot Ankle Int. 1995;16(1):14–20.

56. Steffensmeier SJ, Saltzman CL, Berbaum KS, Brown TD. Effects of medial and lateral displacement calcaneal osteotomies on tibiotalar joint contact stresses. J Orthop Res. 1996;14(6):980–5.

57. Fortin PT, Guettler J, Manoli A 2nd. Idiopathic cavovarus and lateral ankle instability: recognition and treatment implications relating to ankle arthritis. Foot Ankle Int. 2002;23(11):1031–7.

# Chapter 3

# Patient History and Physical Examination of Lower Limb Deformity

Janet D. Conway, MD

Shawn C. Standard, MD

Care for a patient presenting with a deformity begins with a thorough history and physical examination. Radiographs are the final phase of the assessment and will be discussed in the chapter entitled "Obtaining X-rays of the Lower Limbs." Obtaining key facts from the history will allow you to make informed decisions about tackling deformity correction in the manner that is best for the patient. There are often multiple ways to correct the deformity, yet patients may be reluctant or unwilling to consider certain treatment options, such as revisiting external fixation methods if they have previously worn a hexapod for a prolonged period. Performing an in-depth assessment will result in more information to consider when planning and executing a treatment strategy. Keeping this chapter's methods in mind can be of benefit to both surgeon and patient.

## On Patient History: Thorough, but Focused

Carefully record the patient's chief complaint and concerns. Identify the causative factors of the lower limb deformity: congenital, developmental, iatrogenic, post-traumatic, and/or post-infective. Each broad classification brings certain characteristics and patterns that need to be identified and addressed. For example, a child presenting with a moderate lower limb deformity and limb length difference with a history of meningococcemia will require close evaluation of all extremities for possible multiple growth arrests and concurrent subtle deformities that might cause future problems. Patients with congenital or chromosomal abnormalities might require genetic counseling for further delineation of the exact diagnosis and potential inheritable patterns. Previous treatments and the current impact of the deformity are also important historical details.

When initially engaging a patient with a deformity, whether congenital or acquired, there are many details that the patient may feel are important and will want to tell you. The narrative presented by a patient can distract from obtaining the critical data that directly impacts your ability to effectively care for them. To ensure that you will not miss any essential information, an adult history checklist is provided in Table 1. A case sheet that may aid in the history collection and physical exam is provided in Figure 1.

© 2023 Sinai Hospital of Baltimore

A

Dr. ______________________

Patient Name

Date ______________________

## History

Smoking: No Yes ____________

DM: No Yes ____________

BC: No Yes ____________

BT: No Yes ____________

Steroids: No Yes ____________

Pain Meds: No Yes ____________

Living Situation: ____________

C/C/W: ____________

Stairs: No Yes ____________

Pets: No Yes ____________

Flaps: No Yes ____________

Vasc: No Yes ____________

Metal Allergy: No Yes ____________

Work: No Yes ____________

Other Medical Issues: ____________

## Homework

## Problems

## Solutions

B

## Physical Exam

| | | |
|---|---|---|
| *Height* | | |
| *Weight* | | |

| | R | L |
|---|---|---|
| *Sensation* | | |
| *Pulse* | | |
| *Hip:* | | |
| FFD | | |
| IR | | |
| ER | | |
| ABD | | |
| ADD | | |
| *Knee:* | | |
| KE | | |
| KF Supine | | |
| KF Prone | | |
| POP Angle | | |
| *Ankle:* | | |
| DF KE | | |
| DF KF | | |
| PF | | |
| *IT Band* | | |
| *Subtalar* | | |
| *TFA* | | |

## Radiology

*LLD*

| | R | L |
|---|---|---|
| *Coronal Angles:* | | |
| MAD | | |
| LDFA | | |
| JLCA | | |
| MPTA | | |
| LDTA | | |
| *Sagittal Angles:* | | |
| PDFA | | |
| PPTA | | |
| ADTA | | |
| SMAA | | |
| SJLA | | |
| *Leg Lengths:* | | |
| Tibia | | |
| Femur | | |
| Overall | | |
| Ratio | | |
| *Canal Diameters:* | | |
| Femur | | |
| Tibia | | |
| *From Lateral:* | | |
| Femoral Bow | | |

## Hardware Options

© 2023 Sinai Hospital of Baltimore

**Fig. 1:** Example of a new patient case sheet to bring into evaluation. Referring to a standardized document such as this, and using it to record information, is beneficial. **A**, front. **B**, back.

Histories of steroid use, smoking, diabetes, infection, and immunocompromise are important because these issues, when not addressed, lead to the unnecessarily increased potential of postoperative complications. Patients need to modify these risk factors when possible, especially for elective deformity surgery. Patients with diabetes preferably have their hemoglobin A1c (HbA1c) level below 7%. Smoking, especially nicotine use, should be stopped. Depending on the urgency of the surgery, the motivation of the patient, and the risk of complications considering all other issues present, the patient can be monitored with urine screenings to confirm nicotine cessation. Steroids can be tapered, and biologics need to be discontinued.

Alcohol and drug abuse are self-explanatory as far as sabotaging effects for your successful postoperative outcome. Daily alcohol use, even in small amounts, inhibits osteoblast formation and leads to poor bone healing. Furthermore, daily drinking can predispose your patient to postoperative delirium tremens (DTs).

Users of intravenous (IV) drugs are difficult patients and pose varied problems when managing their orthopedic infections. These patients typically present with preoperative methadone use and histories of addiction that complicate postoperative pain management. The quickest solution, requiring the least amount of patient cooperation, is usually the best choice.

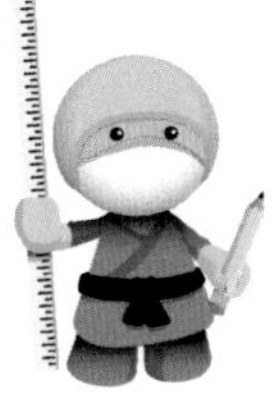

*Sensei says,*
*"The optimal path may be the one of least resistance."*

**Table 1. Past Medical History**

| Do you use/have you ever used: |
|---|
| Steroids |
| Blood thinners |
| Biologics |
| Cigarettes, chewing tobacco, marijuana, vaping |
| DMARDs or other similar immune modulators |
| Alcohol |
| Intravenous drugs |
| Ambulatory-assistive devices |
| Pain medication |
| Inferior vena cava (IFC) filter |
| **Any history of:** |
| Diabetes |
| Blood clots |
| Infection (random or postsurgical) |
| Allergy to metal |
| Immunocompromise |
| Plastic surgery or free flap surgery |
| Vascular surgery, angioplasty, or bypass grafts |
| Trauma |
| **Other:** |
| Ambulatory status |
| Live alone or with family |
| Work/school status |
| Stairs at home |
| Pets at home |
| Distance from hospital |
| Transportation arranged or accommodations needed |

An easy-to-use format is available in the new patient case sheet (Fig. 1). DMARD, disease-modifying anti-rheumatic drug.

If patients are already taking pain medication, it is advisable to engage in dialogue with their pain management physician for postoperative assistance. These patients will require higher doses of pain medication in the hospital; you may want the anesthesiologist to perform a regional nerve block to help with postoperative pain.

Blood clot history indicates an elevated risk of recurrence with any additional surgery. If the patient has an existing inferior vena cava (IVC) filter, do not assume you are safe from the occurrence of pulmonary embolism (PE); any prolonged indwelling IVC filter can induce collateral venous flow that could predispose the patient to another PE. A computed tomography venogram (CTV) should be obtained to preoperatively evaluate for this condition, and a vascular surgery consult is helpful.

Flap history (e.g., medial or lateral gastrocnemius flap, reverse sural, soleus, or free flap) is essential information that needs to be respected in any surgical approach. Lacking this medical history could result in a catastrophic mistake, such as an incision damaging the blood flow to the flap and causing a full-thickness loss of tissue over the bone. When the patient is unsure, previous operative reports should be obtained.

Vascular history, too, is critical. Previous angioplasty, bypass grafts, and arterial injuries must be documented. Preferably, these are preoperatively evaluated by a vascular surgeon. In these cases, the use of a tourniquet often is not an option.

The patient's ambulatory status and living situation (including the presence of stairs) are important factors that can impact the success of an outcome. Postoperatively, many patients who rely on the assistance of a walker, live alone, and/or have stairs in their home will need to transfer to a nursing facility and stay there for an extended period. When patients are already using a walker, performing additional surgery may not provide them with freedom from their assistive device. Expectations need to be managed.

Knowledge of any pets in the home is also an important part of the history; certain organisms may be obtained from animals, such as a dog carrying *Streptococcus canis*. There have been reports in the joint literature regarding these bacteria as a cause of arthroplasty infection. Similarly, patients with fish tanks may become infected with *Mycobacterium marinum*. Negative cultures do not guarantee that there is no infection. Some of these organisms do not grow on routine cultures in the laboratory and must be handled separately. Occasionally, bacteria need to be sent elsewhere for DNA testing when they cannot be grown. Being aware of the potential for an organism that is difficult to culture will allow you to send the proper intraoperative specimens, and thereby increase the chance of identifying an organism.

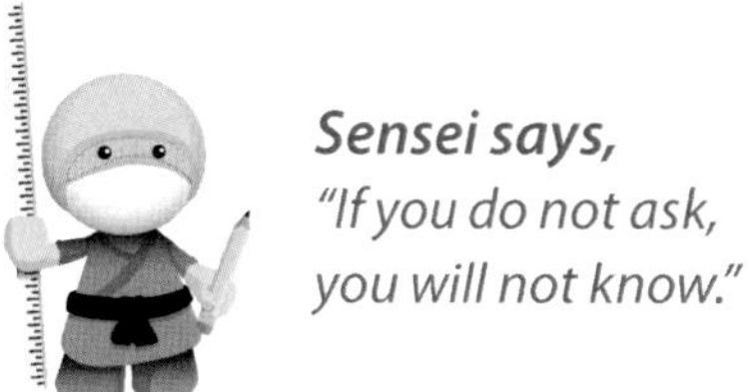

***Sensei says,***
*"If you do not ask, you will not know."*

## Pediatric Patient History Considerations

Similar to the preceding considerations for adults, pediatric patients have unique concerns for the physician to regard as they collect history and conduct examinations. First, the primary concern of the parents should be noted. The deformities and abnormal physical findings that are present may not correlate with the parents' focus. For example, a parent may be concerned about an apparent limb length discrepancy (LLD) when the child has a Trendelenburg gait due to underlying hip pathology. A pediatric history checklist that ensures that you will not miss any essential information is offered in Table 2.

It is recommended either to review the checklist in Table 2 with the parents, or otherwise have the parents fill out a questionnaire that includes the table's information. This will prevent the long clinic visit in which vital information is only shared at the very end—such as a parent stating the patient was born at 32 weeks or has a previously-diagnosed syndrome—thereby completely changing the clinical situation.

© 2023 Sinai Hospital of Baltimore

**Table 2.** Pediatric History Checklist

| Pregnancy and birth history |
|---|
| Prematurity |
| Abnormal prenatal ultrasounds |
| Neonatal sepsis |
| Presence of congenital deformities |
| Motor Milestones |
| Head control |
| Independent sitting |
| Age the patient began cruising and walking |
| Family History |
| Hip dysplasia |
| Early joint replacement |
| Limb deformity |
| Skeletal dysplasia |
| Syndromes |
| Pain |
| *Unlike adults, children rarely complain of pain, including pain that prevents play activities |
| Functional limitations |
| Past medical history |
| *Unlike adults, most children will not have significant medical history, but this must be checked |
| Cardiac or renal congenital abnormalities |
| Neurologic conditions: cerebral palsy, spina bifida, myopathy, developmental delay/autism, hypotonia |
| Bone dysplasia: achondroplasia, hypochondroplasia, MED, SED, pseudoachondroplasia, etc. |
| Rheumatologic conditions: JIA, lupus, ankylosing spondylitis |
| Hematologic conditions: sickle cell anemia, hemophilia, TAR |
| Oncologic conditions: ALL, osteosarcoma, chemotherapy |
| Previous infections or sepsis |
| Previous hospitalizations |
| Previous genetic evaluation |
| Specific diagnosed syndrome |
| Previous trauma |

ALL, acute lymphoblastic leukemia; JIA, juvenile idiopathic arthritis; MED, multiple epiphyseal dysplasia; SED, spondyloepiphyseal dysplasia; TAR, thrombocytopenia-absent radius.

## Adult and Pediatric Physical Examination Considerations

Every new patient must receive a detailed physical examination, with height and weight recorded. It is crucial to have a goniometer on hand for the exam. Normal ranges of motion (ROM) for individual joints are available in Table 3.

### Standing Posture and Gait Considerations

The physical exam should start with the patient standing. The patient's posture and standing position should be noted. Details such as obvious spine deformity, pelvic obliquity, knee flexion, foot position, and the need for an assistive device should be recorded. The examiner should observe the patient from the front, side, and behind. When examining the patient from the rear, the iliac crest should be palpated to check for pelvic obliquity. If an oblique pelvis is noted, 1-cm blocks should be placed under the short side until a level pelvis is achieved. The number of blocks will denote the clinical LLD present. This discrepancy could be an actual leg length difference or an apparent discrepancy due to joint contractures or spinal deformity. The delineation of a true vs. apparent LLD will become obvious when the detailed physical exam is completed and compared to long-standing radiographs. With the pelvis level, the patient should bend forward so the spine may be examined for obvious deformity. If spinal decompensation occurs by leveling the pelvis, a fixed pelvic obliquity is present. The fixed pelvic obliquity results from either underlying spinal deformity or hip deformity.

**Table 3.** Joint Range of Motion

| Joint | Measurement | Average Normal Value |
|---|---|---|
| Hip | Internal rotation | 35° |
| Hip | External rotation | 45° |
| Hip | Flexion | 120° |
| Hip | Extension | 30° |
| Hip | Abduction | 45° |
| Hip | Adduction | 20–30° |
| Knee | Extension | 0° |
| Knee | Flexion | 135° |
| Knee | Internal/external rotary motion | 10° |
| Ankle | Dorsiflexion | 20° |
| Ankle | Plantar flexion | 20° |
| Subtalar | Inversion | 5° |
| Subtalar | Eversion | 5° |

Adapted with permission from Hoppenfeld S. *Physical Examination of the Spine and Extremities.* East Norwalk, CT: Appleton-Century-Crofts; 1976.

© 2023 Sinai Hospital of Baltimore

After standing examination is completed, the patient's gait should be observed. During the gait assessment, details such as the presence of a limp, patella progression angle, foot progression angle, position of the knee at foot strike, foot position at foot strike, and the need for an assisted device should be recorded. Common abnormal findings include:

- Antalgic gait: Shortened stance phase denoting pain on weight bearing.
- An internal or external foot progression angle, denoting a rotational abnormality in the limb segment. This should be compared to the patella progression angle. Rotational abnormalities of the hip/femur, tibia/ankle, or the foot can produce an abnormal foot progression angle.
- An internal or external patella progression angle, denoting a rotational abnormality of the hip/femoral segment.
- Toe-down gait (also called toe-to-toe gait with no heel strike): This gait denotes either an equinus contracture of the foot and ankle or a compensatory gait for an LLD.
- Trendelenburg gait: A side lean during gait with obvious bending of the spine and lowering of the shoulder to the side of hip abductor weakness (Fig. 2).
- Vaulting gait: Denoting a leg length difference when the patient walks heel-to-toe on both the long and short leg, this gait causes a vertical height change of the head and shoulders as single-leg stance switches from the long leg to the short leg.

It is unquestionably imperative to perform a thorough inspection of the patient's walking. Additionally, it is suggested to ask the patient to walk quickly; speed can reveal otherwise subtle deformities, such as the Trendelenburg gait or posturing of the upper extremities. In very complex situations, a three-dimensional gait analysis should be performed to objectively assess the gait cycle.

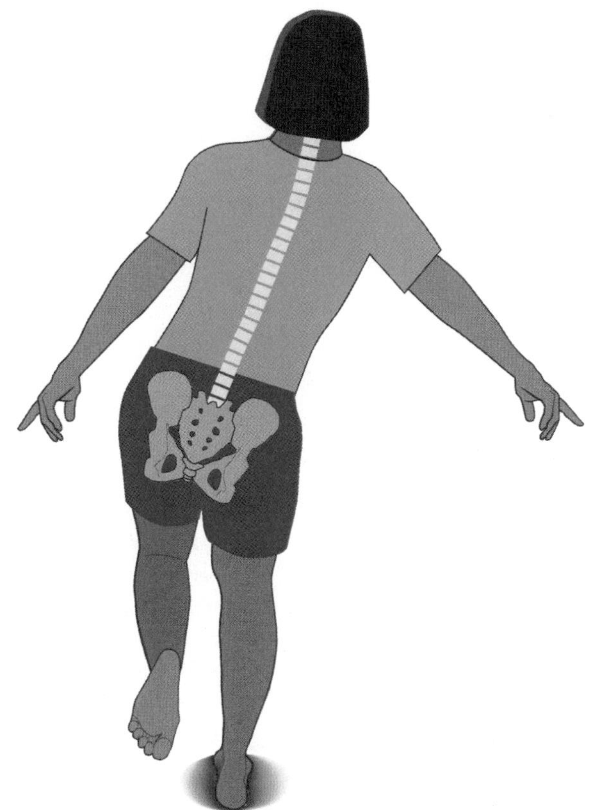

**Fig. 2:** Compensated Trendelenberg on the right hip.

## Hip Exam and Considerations

A careful hip examination is important when evaluating for fixed flexion deformities, abduction contractures, adduction contractures, rotational deformities, and abductor weakness.

### Flexion Contractures of the Hip

Flexion contractures of the hip can be subtle and result in apparent limb length discrepancies and gait disturbance. The hip is classically tested with the Thomas test (Fig. 3A). The patient is supine, with the uninvolved leg bent at the knee and flexed maximally at the hip, while the lumbar spine is flat on the exam table (knee-to-chest position for the "good" leg). The involved leg will be forced off the table if a contracture is present. The angle formed by the leg and the surface of the table is the magnitude of flexion deformity. Care must be taken not to let the patient's good leg come away from the chest, or for the lumbar spine to arch. Both motions attempt to compensate for the hip flexion contracture and will decrease the magnitude of the angle between the involved leg and the exam table, thereby hiding the true magnitude of the contracture.

The exact amount of extension of the hip can be tested in the same way, but with the patient positioned with their pelvis at the edge of the exam table and the involved leg hanging free (Fig. 3B). With the good leg in the same knee-to-chest position, the tested leg hangs, and the angle between the tested leg and surface of the exam table is the magnitude of hip extension. This also can be tested with the patient in the prone position, by raising the tested leg while maintaining pressure on the lower back/pelvis (Fig. 3C).

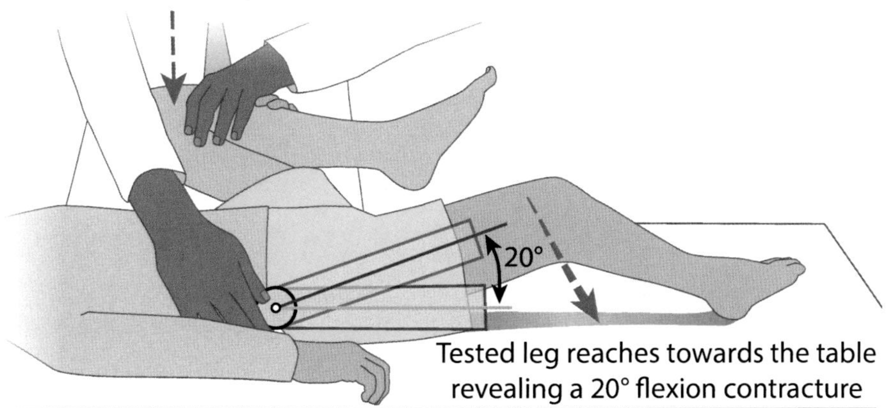


**Fig. 3A:** The classic Thomas test is performed with the patient supine and the uninvolved leg flexed to the patient's chest. The tested/involved leg should remain flat on the table. If the leg raises off the table, then a hip flexion deformity exists. The angle created by the surface of the table and the involved leg is the magnitude of the deformity. This example demonstrates a right hip flexion deformity of 20°.

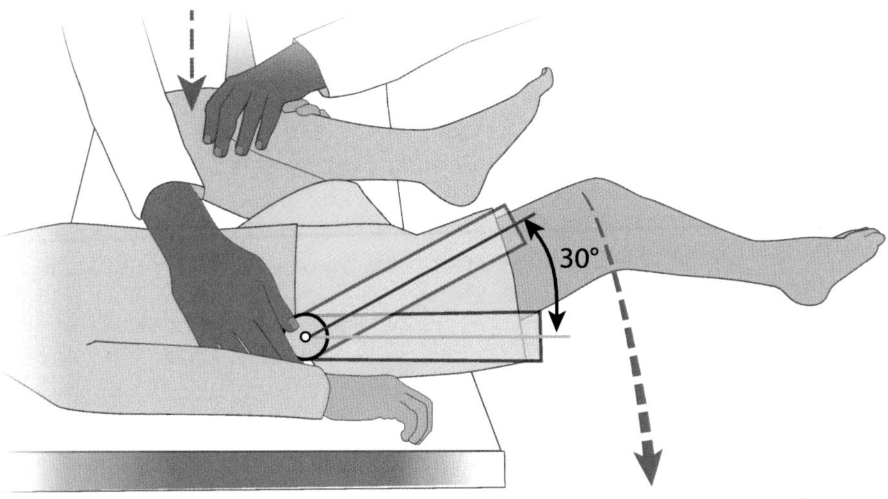


**Fig. 3B:** Hip extension can be measured with the patient in the same position as the Thomas test, but at the end of the exam table. This allows the measurement of true hip extension. In the classic position, a knee flexion contracture will block hip extension and give an erroneous appearance of a hip flexion contracture.

© 2023 Sinai Hospital of Baltimore

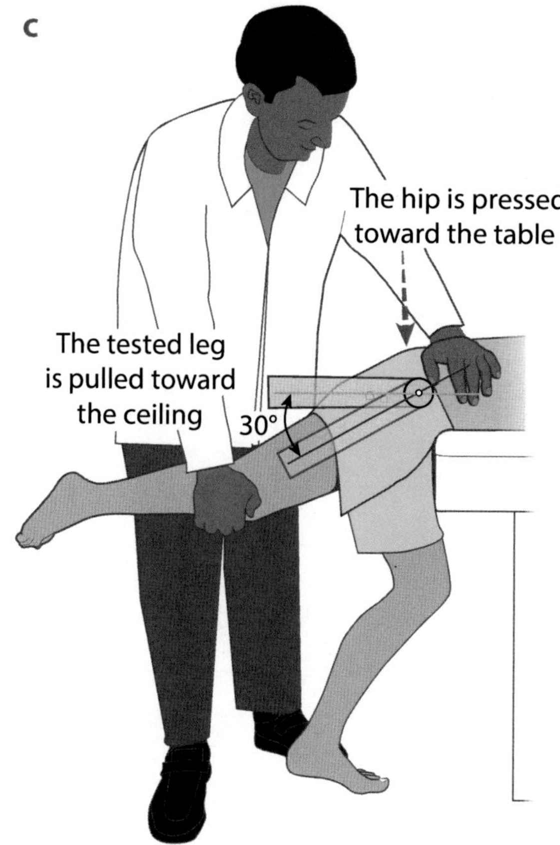


**Fig. 3C:** Placing the patient prone or at the end of the exam table is beneficial, as it will eliminate the effect of a concurrent knee flexion contracture.

## Abduction and Adduction Contractures of the Hip

Abduction and adduction contractures can result in apparent LLD. The best way to check for hip abduction and hip adduction motion is with the patient in a supine position.

### Hip Abduction:

The patient is placed supine, the uninvolved leg is stabilized in abduction, and the level of the anterior superior iliac spine (ASIS) prominences are noted. The tested leg is then gently abducted until the pelvis begins to shift. Once the pelvis shifts, there is no further hip motion but only spine/pelvic compensation. The angle between the center line of the body and the abducted leg before pelvic shift is the magnitude of hip abduction. The easiest way to stabilize the pelvis during this type of exam is to maximally abduct the uninvolved side before abducting the tested leg (Fig. 4).

### Hip Adduction:

With the patient supine, the uninvolved leg is lifted enough for the tested leg to be crossed underneath (Fig. 5). The tested leg is adducted until the pelvis begins to shift. The angle between the center line of the body and the tested leg is the magnitude of adduction of the hip.

True hip abduction and adduction may be difficult to ascertain in large patients or patients with excessive mobility of the pelvis and spine. To confirm the clinical test of hip abduction and hip adduction, a simple anteroposterior pelvis radiograph, with the patient in the tested position as described above, will allow objective measurement of these ranges of motion and reveal spine and pelvis compensation (Fig. 6).

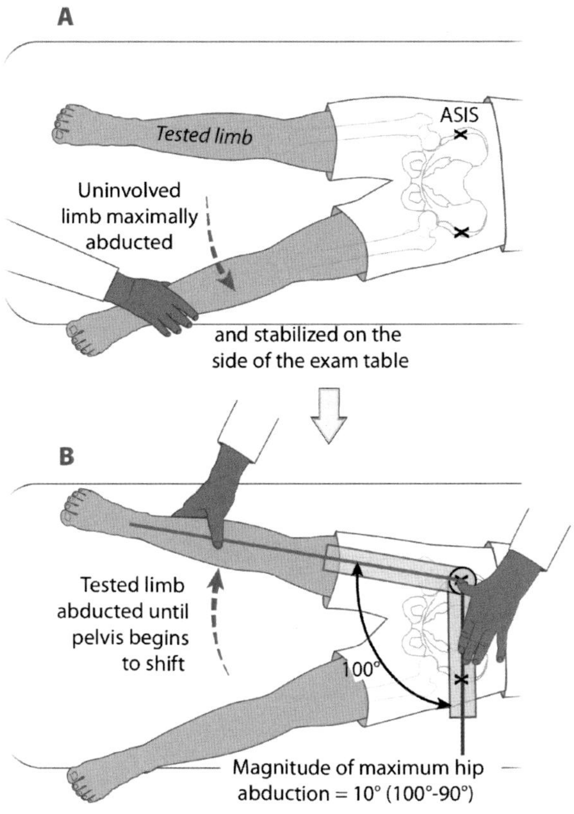


**Fig. 4:** **A**, Hip abduction is tested with the patient supine and the uninvolved hip maximally abducted and stabilized on the side of the exam table. **B**, The involved side is abducted until the pelvis begins to shift. A goniometer aligned with the anterior superior iliac spine and down the tested leg measures the magnitude of hip abduction.

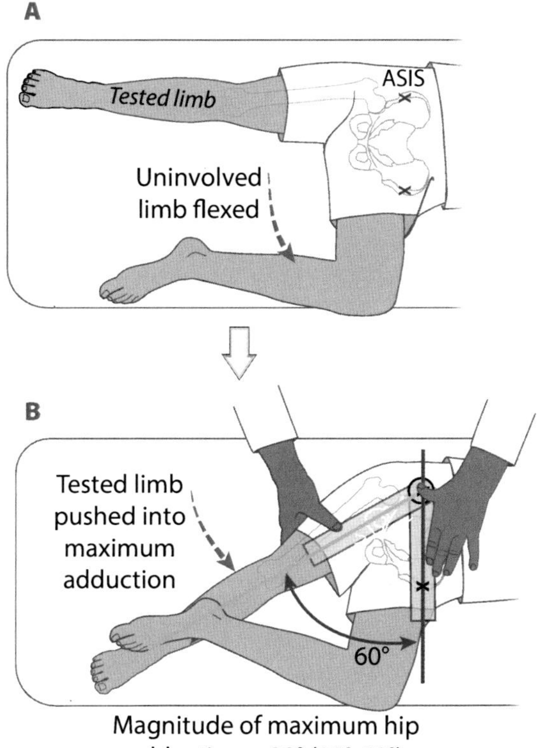


**Fig. 5:** **A**, Hip adduction is tested with the pelvis stabilized, the uninvolved leg flexed/lifted. **B**, The tested leg is pushed into adduction. A goniometer aligned with the anterior superior iliac spine and down the tested leg measures the magnitude of hip adduction.

© 2023 Sinai Hospital of Baltimore 

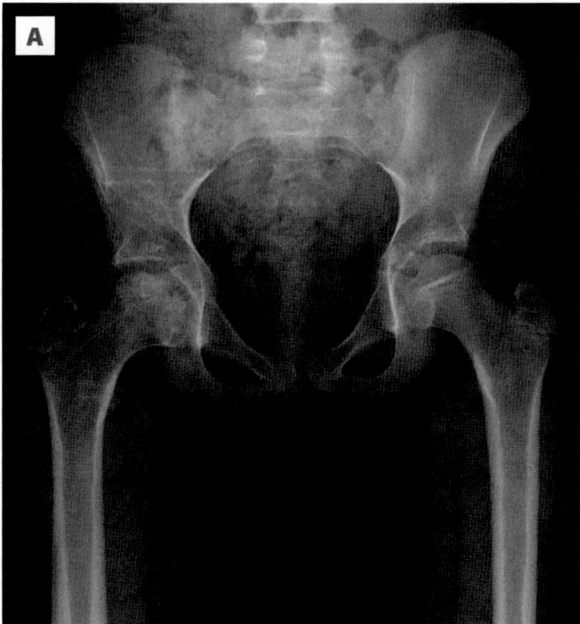


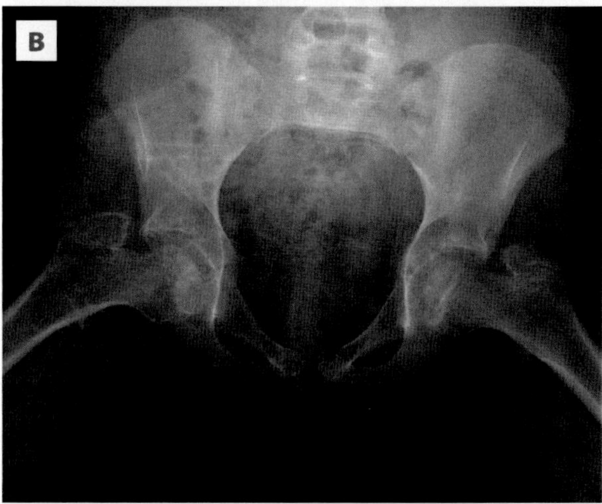


**Fig. 6: A**, Anteroposterior (AP) radiograph of pelvis. **B**, AP pelvis with maximum abduction. These x-rays allow for definitive and objective measurement of hip abduction. Example shown is a patient with Perthes disease.

## Rotational Profile of the Hip

### Hip Rotation:

Internal and external rotation of the hips is evaluated in the prone position (Figs. 7-10). This position places the hip in extension similar to normal gait. The knees should be flexed. Large tibial coronal deformities or posterior condylar deficiencies of the femur will alter measurements and should be noted during interpretation. Ensure the pelvis is level by firmly holding it flat on the table while rotating the femur. The leg on the tested side is allowed to rotate outward. The angle between an imaginary vertical line and the line of the rotated extremity represents the internal rotation of the hip/femur. The tested leg is then rotated inward, and the angle between the imaginary vertical line and the rotated extremity represents the external rotation of the hip/femur. Mismatched rotation and malrotation are shown in Figures 11 and 12.

The range of rotational motion in children can vary significantly. Typically, the rotation can range between 30-70° with the total arc of motion equal to 90-100°. If a child's total arc of motion is greater than 100°, this represents hypermobility.

## Hip Abductor Weakness

Hip abductor weakness and its clinical manifestations are poorly understood by many healthcare providers. In a single-leg stance, the hip abductor muscles on the side of the weight-bearing leg must contract to hold the pelvis level. With a horizontal pelvis, the spine remains straight and the shoulders level. If a patient stands on one leg while facing away from the examiner, the pelvis should remain horizontal and the spine straight. If abductor weakness is present, the pelvis will drop away from the weight-bearing leg because the abductor muscle cannot maintain a horizontal pelvic position. As the pelvis drops, the patient will shift their weight and lean over the weight-bearing leg to maintain balance and prevent a fall—this leaning over the weak hip is the Trendelenburg sign (Fig. 2). During gait, it is repeated every step during the stance phase on the side of the weak abductors and is called a Trendelenburg gait or Trendelenburg lurch. This type of gait is often misinterpreted by therapists and physicians as representing an LLD. If you apply an appropriate shoe lift to a patient with a concurrent hip abductor weakness and an LLD, the patient will continue to lean or lurch. The source of this type of gait must be explained carefully to patients and parents, as it will not be resolved with lengthening surgery.

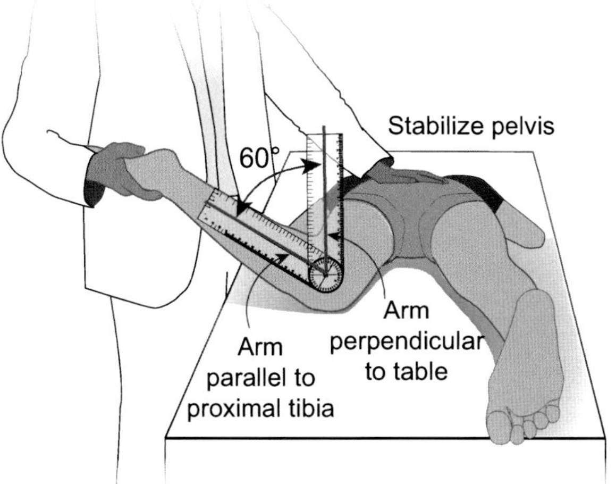


**Fig. 7:** Internal rotation of the left hip.

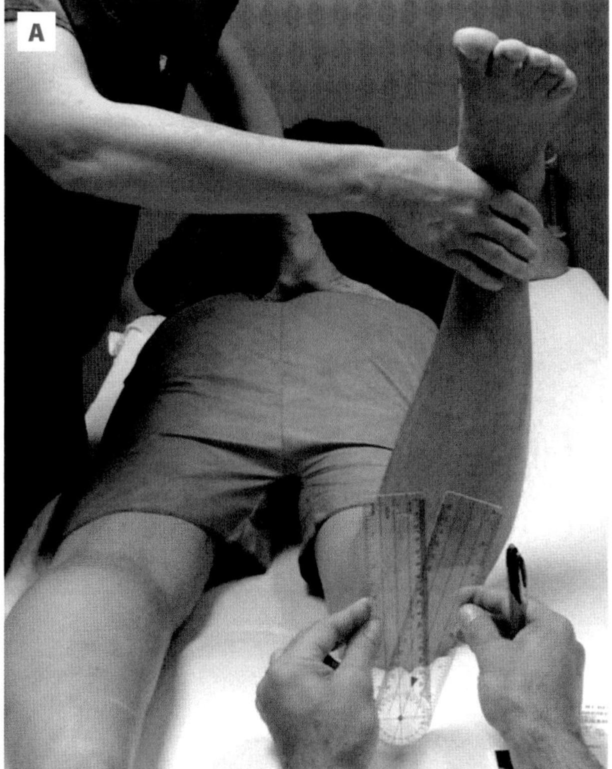


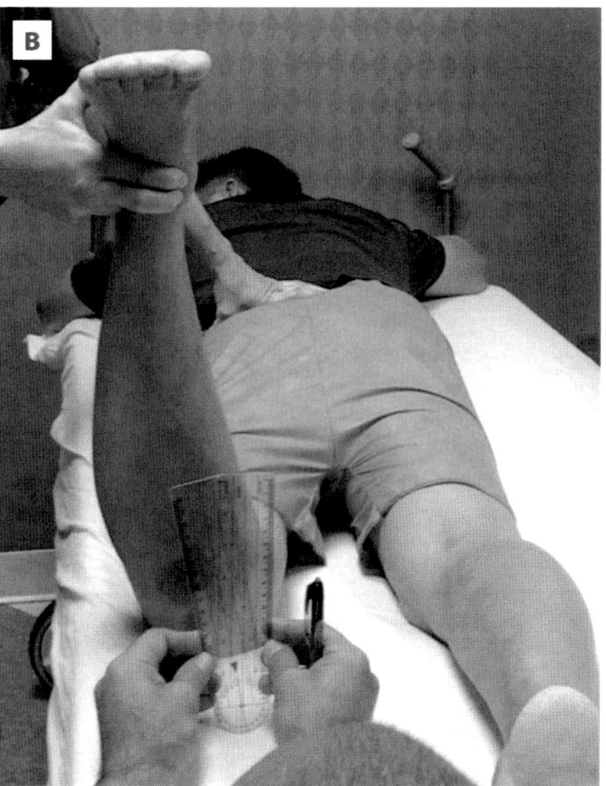


**Fig. 8:** Internal rotation of hip exam. Be careful not to under measure secondary to tibia vara. Center the goniometer at the patella with one arm perpendicular to the table, with the other arm of the goniometer parallel to the proximal tibia. **A**, Right leg. **B**, Left leg.

© 2023 Sinai Hospital of Baltimore

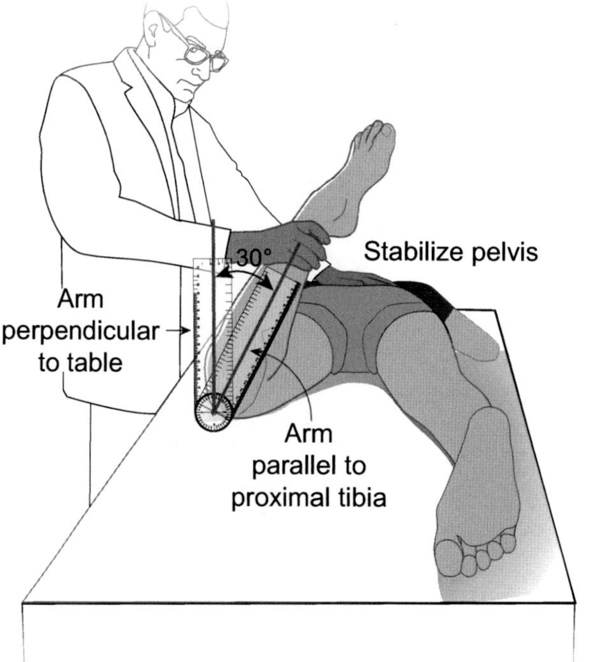


**Fig. 9:** External rotation of left hip.

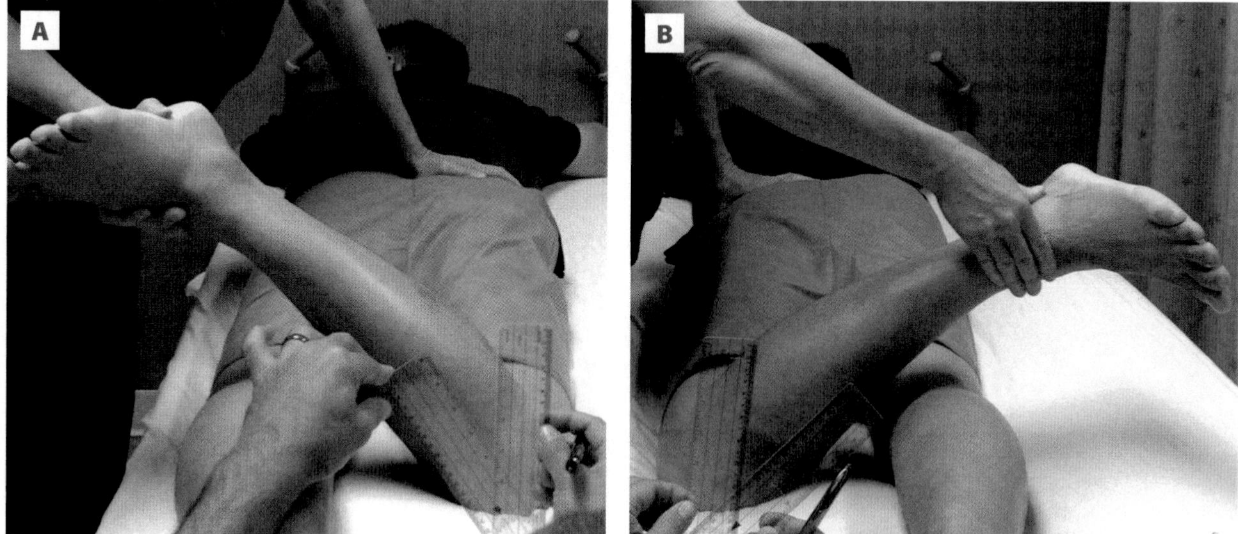


**Fig. 10:** External rotation of hip exam. Be careful not to overmeasure secondary to tibia vara. Center the goniometer at the patella with one arm perpendicular to the table, with the other arm of the goniometer parallel to the proximal tibia. **A**, Right leg. **B**, Left leg.

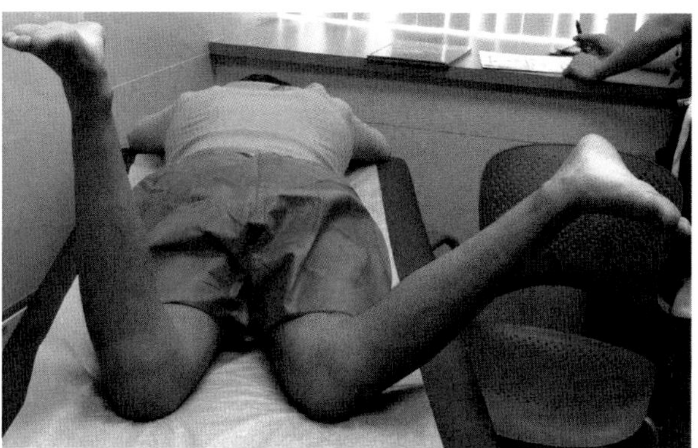

**Fig. 11:** Hip exam, continued. An example of mismatched internal rotation.

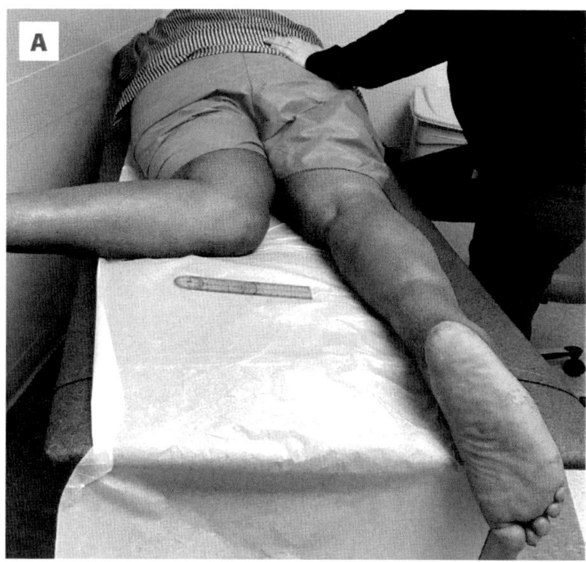



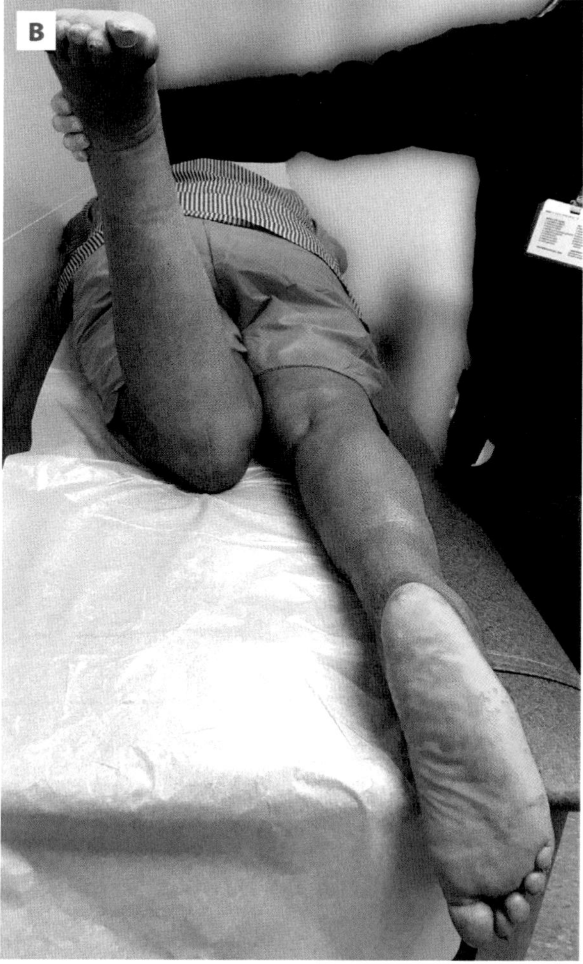



**Fig. 12:** Hip exam, continued. Left leg malrotation after hip fracture nailing. **A**, Internal rotation. **B**, Maximum external rotation.

## Pediatric Hip Strength Exam

For pediatric patients with underlying neurologic disease, the hip strength assessment is a crucial portion of the physical exam. The presence or absence of functional muscle groups will determine if the patient has the capacity for ambulation. The strength profile of the pediatric hip will help guide the physician's treatment options and allow parent expectations to be managed appropriately.

In the supine position, the patient demonstrates hip flexion, abduction, and adduction against resistance. In the sitting position, the patient should demonstrate hip flexion against gravity and resistance. The patient's hip extension should be tested in the prone position. When prone, the patient demonstrates active hip extension by lifting the leg off the exam table. In the standing position, the abductor strength is evaluated using a timed single-leg stance test. Patients should be able to hold the pelvis stable for at least 15 to 30 seconds while in single-leg stance.

## Hip Treatment Tips and Tricks

Fixed flexion contractures can be addressed with a hip flexor release, with or without iliopsoas recession. Another way to address a fixed flexion deformity is with an extension osteotomy using a plate or external fixator. In pediatric patients, botulinum toxin (Botox) injection of the iliopsoas muscle under ultrasound guidance is an effective minimally invasive technique to address hip flexion contractures.

© 2023 Sinai Hospital of Baltimore

Adduction contractures are easily treated with a percutaneous adductor tenotomy. In certain circumstances, Botox injection into the adductor muscles can resolve the contracture along with dedicated therapy, bracing, and stretching at home. Long-standing or severe adduction contractures usually require a more open and extensive release of the adductor longus muscle, adductor brevis muscle, and gracilis muscle. Abduction contractures, however, are more difficult to treat and need to be reconciled with physical therapy. Surgical treatment for abduction contractures is based upon the etiology and can be treated with abductor muscle sequential releases (either open or arthroscopically) of the iliotibial (IT) band, gluteus maximus, gluteus medius, and gluteus minimus.

Fixator-assisted derotational osteotomies can correct both excessive internal or external rotation by using a nail and an osteotomy in the proximal third of the femur. A proximal osteotomy—as opposed to a distal osteotomy—minimizes the effect that the derotation has on the quadriceps muscle alignment and patellar tracking.

Treatment for hip abductor weakness can be difficult and complex. First, a viable muscle must be present and confirmed with muscle testing, neurostimulation, or electromyography. Second, the hip structure must be evaluated to assess for abnormal femoral neck length (coxa breva) with concurrent greater trochanteric "overgrowth," acetabular dysplasia with hip joint subluxation and femoral head proximal migration, severe coxa vara, and malunions/nonunions of the proximal femur. Third, muscle balance must be maintained between the hip's abductors and adductors. A weakened hip abductor complex will be compromised and ineffective when there is a significant hip adductor contracture. Treatments for hip abductor weakness consist of aggressive therapy for strengthening, pelvic and proximal femoral osteotomies to correct structural abnormalities, and muscle balancing by addressing underlying hip adduction contractures (Figs. 13 and 14).

## Knee Exam and Considerations

The knee exam begins with the patient in the sitting position on the exam table. Passive extension of the knee is noted, and the amount of extension is recorded in degrees. Full extension of the knee is noted as 0°. If the knee hyperextends 10°, then this is noted as +10° of extension, whereas the knee that lacks 10° from full extension is noted as -10° of extension. If the patient automatically leans back during passive knee extension, hamstring tightness and contracture are present. The patient then actively extends the knee to allow assessment for a quadriceps lag. If the passive and active extensions are different, then a muscle weakness is present and is noted as quadriceps lag.

The supine examination of the knee is next. In this position, the patient's knee ROM is passively and actively demonstrated. The patient's passive knee extension is noted at three different positions of the hip. The passive knee extension should be assessed at neutral hip extension, 45°of hip flexion, and 90° of hip flexion. The knee extension with the hip in a neutral position simulates the knee's ability to extend during the stance phase of gait. Knee extension at 45° of hip flexion simulates the knee's ability to extend at the end of the swing phase of gait. The knee extension with the hip flexed at 90° is typically referred to as the popliteal angle and should be <30° (>30° short of full extension indicates hamstring tightness).

Abnormalities of knee ROM are categorized as hyperextension deformities and flexion deformities. These deformities can be caused by soft tissue problems, bony deformities, or a combination of both. Because the knee joint moves in the sagittal plane, this motion can either contribute to, or compensate for, underlying soft tissue and bony abnormalities. The complete assessment of the sagittal plane in limb deformity is addressed in the chapter entitled "Deformity Analysis in the Sagittal Plane."

While the patient is still supine, the stability of the knee is tested. The anterior and posterior translation of the knee is tested in 30° of flexion (Lachman test) and 90° of flexion (anterior and posterior drawer test). The varus and valgus stability of the knee are tested in full knee extension. In patients with hyperextension deformities, stability should be assessed in the "neutral" position as well as the hyperextended position. Any instability of the knee should be noted, and the dynamic effect should be assessed during the patient's gait

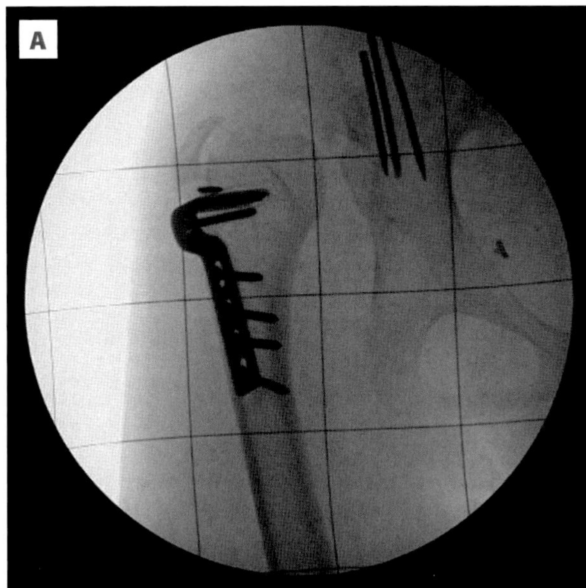


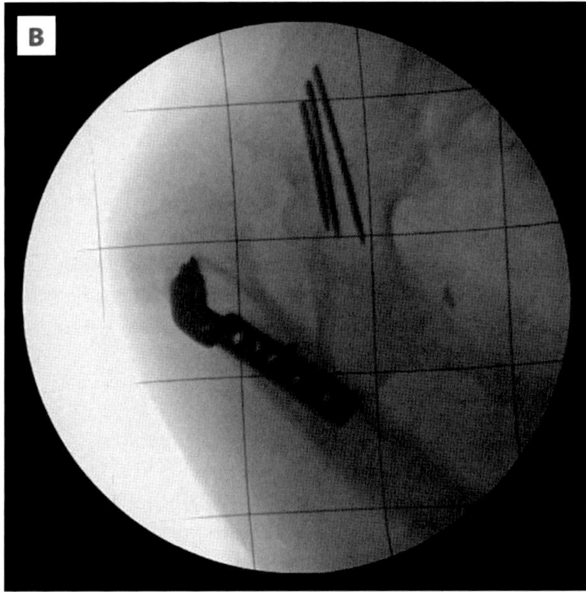


**Fig. 13:** Intraoperative fluoroscopic film comparison in preparation for a pelvic support osteotomy. **A**, The right hip in neutral position. **B**, The right hip in maximum adduction.

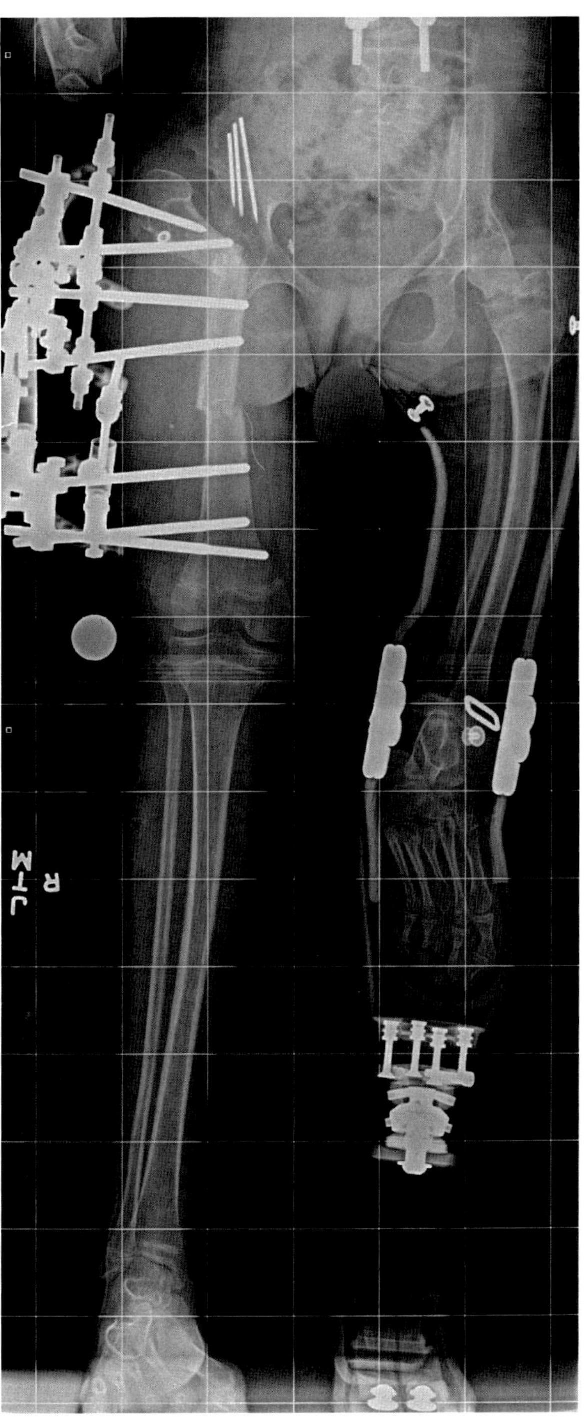

**Fig. 14:** Postoperative hip position after pelvic support osteotomy eliminating any further right hip adduction to prevent a Trendelenburg gait.

© 2023 Sinai Hospital of Baltimore

exam. The patella position at rest and the tracking during passive range of motion are recorded. Patella stability should be examined in full extension. Any apprehension with patella glide can denote medial or lateral instability. The notch sign, if present, denotes a subluxed or dislocated patella in flexion. When the knee is maximally flexed, the examiner's thumb is pressed into the center of the distal femur. If the notch can be palpated, the patella is translated either laterally or medially. In conditions such as congenital dislocation of the patella, posttraumatic dislocations of the patella, or congenital limb deficiency, it is typical for the patella to be displaced laterally. Medial displacement is rare but can occur after overzealous patella realignment surgery or severe soft tissue connective diseases (e.g., Ehlers-Danlos syndrome).

The knee examination continues in the prone position. Good prone knee flexion should allow the heel to touch (or almost touch) the buttocks. When there is a tight rectus femoris muscle, the prone knee flexion will result in the buttocks and pelvis tilting off the bed (positive Ely test). Tightness of the rectus femoris muscle may be overlooked if ROM is only performed in the supine position.

While in the prone position, the thigh-foot axis is assessed (Figs. 15-18). To perform this test, the patient's knee is bent to 90° and the foot and ankle are passively dorsiflexed to neutral. The examiner must not impart excessive inversion or eversion of the subtalar joint. The thigh-foot angle is the angle between the long axis of the thigh and the long axis of the foot. This angle denotes the rotation of the lower leg. An internal angle is denoted as a negative (-) degree and an external angle is denoted as a positive (+) degree. Typically, the normal rotational profile for a lower leg ranges from -15° to +25°. This test can be compromised by foot and ankle deformities.

## Knee Treatment Tips and Tricks

The possible treatments for abnormal findings in a knee examination are complex and extensive. The following are selected clinical tips and tricks for various treatments.

Extension lag (when active extension does not match passive extension): Quadriceps weakness can be a major contributor to producing flexion contractures. Mechanical reasons for quadriceps muscle weakness should be thoroughly evaluated. Underlying conditions (e.g., extensor mechanism scarring, quadriceps or patellar tendon tears, nerve injury, bony deformity, and soft tissue redundancy) can lead to quadriceps extension lag. Treatments such as dynamic extension bracing, aggressive therapy, soft tissue/scar release, osteotomies, and neuromuscular electrical stimulation can play a role in resolving lag.

Flexion contractures: A lack of full passive extension will become worse with any lengthening. Considerations in this situation depend upon the degree of the bony deformity, such as distal femoral procurvatum or proximal tibial procurvatum. If a distal femoral extension osteotomy is not needed to correct this, then a posterior capsular release with hamstring tenotomies can correct soft tissue flexion deformities ≤30°. Peroneal nerve decompression is always performed when correcting flexion deformities to prevent palsy.

Rectus femoris contracture: Physical therapy is important for stretching the rectus, especially before and during any amount of femoral lengthening. Botox can be used cautiously in these situations to improve and maintain knee ROM.

Tibial rotational abnormalities: Derotational tibial osteotomies may be performed either gradually or acutely. Proximal derotation is considered separately from distal. Proximally, acute correction can be performed ≤20° with prophylactic peroneal nerve decompression and anterior fasciotomy. Anything more severe than this should be performed gradually with nerve decompression, fasciotomy, and the addition of proximal and distal syndesmotic screw fixation. If a distal supramalleolar osteotomy is chosen, a tarsal tunnel release may be helpful to protect the posterior tibial nerve regardless of the derotation direction. This is particularly salient for revision procedures. With distal derotation, the peroneal nerve is at less risk and generally does not require decompression.

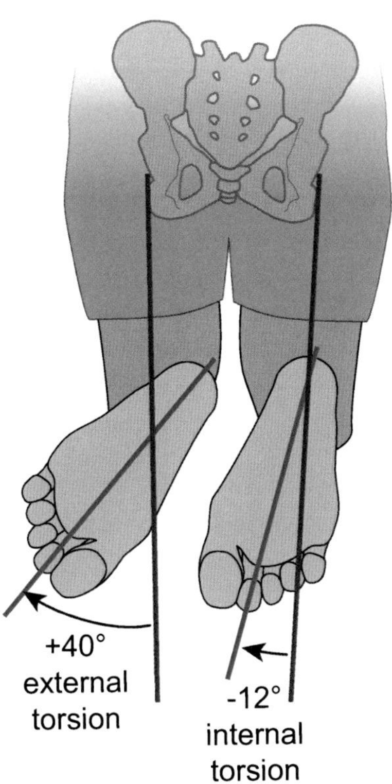


Fig. 15: Thigh-foot axis: tibial rotation. Center of goniometer on the heel, with one arm on the thigh to the ischial tuberosity, and the other arm of the goniometer on the center of the foot axis in line with the second metatarsal.

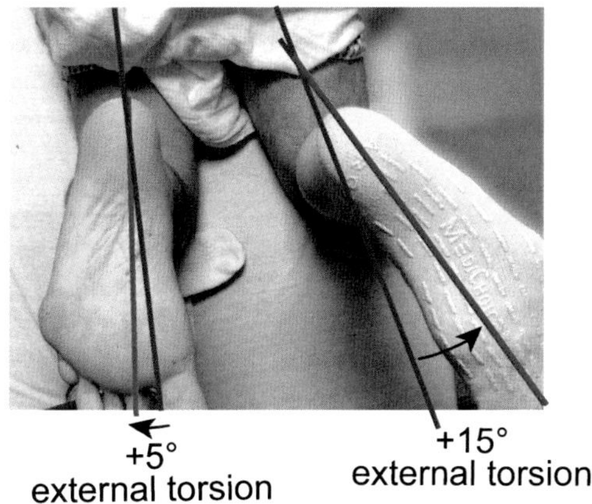


Fig. 16: External tibial torsion, right side.

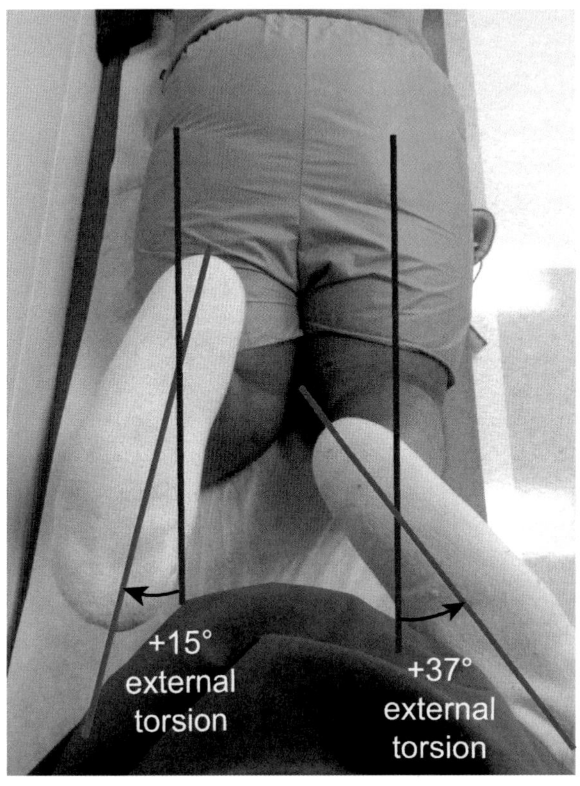


Fig. 17: Malrotation after total knee arthroplasty on the right.

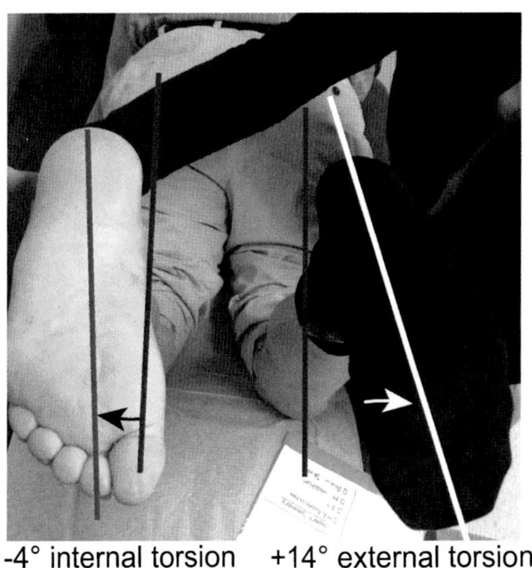


Fig. 18: Windswept feet with left internal tibial torsion.

## Ankle and Subtalar Exam and Considerations

### Ankle and Subtalar ROM

The patient should be either in a sitting or supine position. The ankle dorsiflexion and plantar flexion are tested both passively and actively. The normal range of motion for a typical ankle is 15-20° of dorsiflexion and 50-75° of plantar flexion.

It is essential for the examiner to "lock" the subtalar joint in varus before assessing the dorsiflexion. Subtalar joint motion can simulate dorsiflexion, especially with an equinus contracture. The passive ankle dorsiflexion is assessed with the knee bent as well as extended; this allows the soleus muscle's flexibility to be isolated. In the instance of an equinus contracture, the passive dorsiflexion of the ankle should be noted with the knee bent as well as extended, and the two should be compared. If the passive dorsiflexion is normal with the knee bent, then the contracture is isolated to the gastrocnemius muscle. If the passive range of the ankle is similar with the knee bent and extended, then the gastrocsoleus complex is contracted.

The patient should then be assessed in a standing position. The shape of the arch should be noted, as well as if the patient can achieve a foot-flat position. Next, the patient should be viewed from behind while they alternate between standing flat-footed and standing on their toes. This process should be repeated several times. The amount of dorsiflexion, subtalar motion, and arch shape should be recorded in both the foot-flat and toe-standing positions. If limited subtalar motion is noted, this joint needs to be examined carefully.

The subtalar joint is best assessed with the patient in the prone position and the knee flexed to 90° (Fig. 19). The subtalar joint is examined by manipulating the joint and determining the amount of varus and valgus motion present. With long-standing deformities, the subtalar joint is often contracted. The hindfoot's flexibility can also be inspected with the Coleman block test, by placing full weight on the heel and border of the foot while multiple toes hang in plantarflexion (Fig. 20).

### Ankle and Subtalar Stability

Ankle stability should be assessed with the patient seated in a relaxed position. The stabilizing ligaments of the ankle joint are examined with the anterior and posterior drawer test. Any overt shift or translation should be noted. The varus/valgus stability of the ankle is difficult to ascertain in the setting of a normal subtalar joint. Stress radiographs are necessary to objectively determine and assess varus and valgus instability of the ankle joint. Similarly, examination of the subtalar joint under stress radiographs or live fluoroscopy can determine overt hypermobility or instability.

### Ankle and Subtalar Treatment Tips and Tricks

If the gastrocnemius is tight, a gastrocnemius recession can be performed. When the ankle equinus is fixed regardless of the knee position, correction can be achieved with a tenoachilles lengthening (open or percutaneous) or a gastrocsoleus recession. Depending on the degree of equinus, a tarsal tunnel release will have to be performed to protect the posterior tibial nerve. If an acute equinus correction is >25-30°, a tarsal tunnel decompression should be performed. When the equinus is severe, a Z-lengthening of the tendon is done through the same incision as the tarsal tunnel release so that the stretch on the nerve with equinus correction can be assessed under direct vision. A posterior capsular release can also be done through this open incision. Any bone impingement to dorsiflexion is addressed through a separate anterior incision. When the equinus is too severe for acute correction, a posterior tibial nerve release is performed in combination with a percutaneous tenoachilles lengthening and frame application for a gradual correction.

In a patient with long-standing distal tibial varus deformity, the subtalar joint is compensatorily contracted in valgus to allow the foot to touch the floor when standing. Similarly, if the deformity is a long-standing distal tibial valgus, then the subtalar joint will be contracted in a compensatory varus position. Assessing the flexibility of the subtalar contracture is crucial when creating the deformity correction plan. During the preoperative

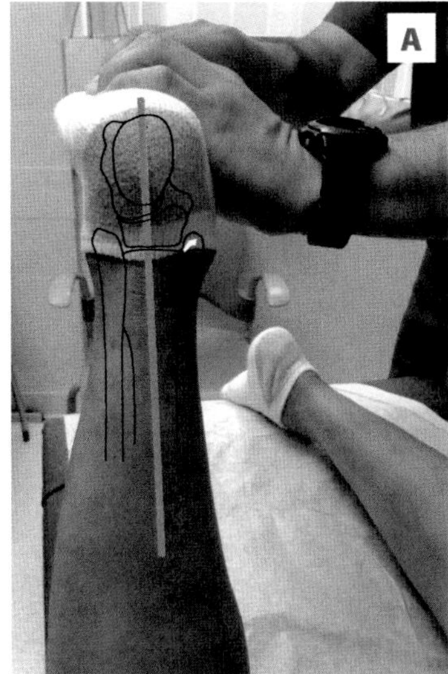


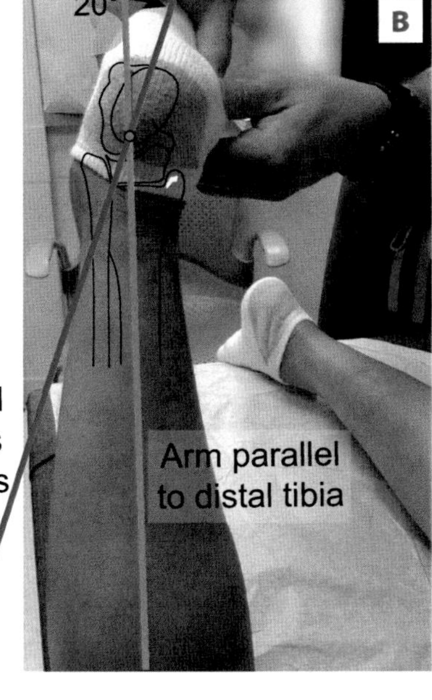


**Fig. 19:** Subtalar joint evaluation. **A**, Eversion. **B**, Inversion.

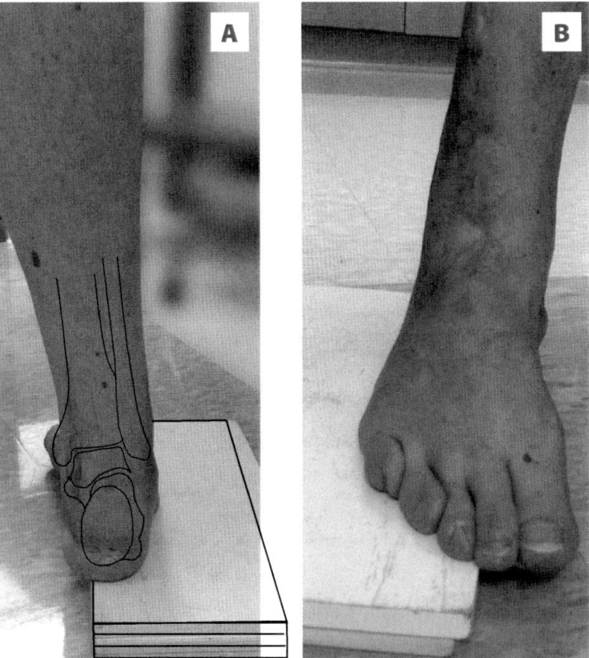


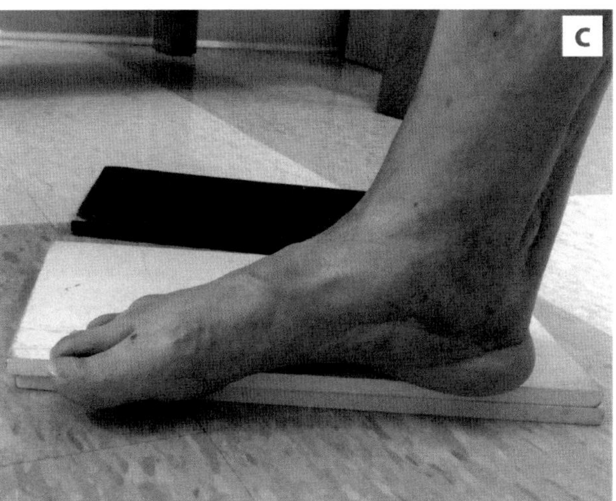


**Fig. 20:** Coleman block test to check for hindfoot flexibility and pronation of forefoot. **A**, Posterior view. **B**, Anterior view. **C**, Lateral view.

assessment, the subtalar joint should be able to be manipulated to match the deformity in the distal tibia. If the subtalar joint is flexible enough to match the deformity, then the foot will shift into a normal position after distal tibial correction. However, if the subtalar joint is contracted and not assessed, the surgeon will find a severe subtalar deformity after the tibial bony correction. This will result in a poorly positioned foot—and an unhappy patient.

A distal tibial deformity and concurrent subtalar joint contracture must be corrected simultaneously. Depending on the severity of the deformity, either a subtalar distraction or a hindfoot osteotomy with or without a midfoot osteotomy can be performed to restore the foot to a plantigrade position. Understanding the relationship of ankle and subtalar deformities will improve planning to correct all deformities present within the same

© 2023 Sinai Hospital of Baltimore

operative setting, and thereby effectively restore proper foot and ankle biomechanics.

## Skin and Soft Tissue Assessments

Preoperative planning for correction of complex limb deformity necessitates the detailed examination and assessment of the skin and soft tissues. Underlying dermatologic conditions and skin integrity must be reviewed. When dermatologic conditions are present, preoperative assessment and treatment should be performed by a dermatologist to maximize skin health before surgery. For patients with a history of multiple surgeries and poor soft tissues, all previous incisions need to be documented. A small skin bridge between new and old incisions could lead to necrosis. Creative strategies will need to be used when poor skin does not permit an incision, such as the provided examples of soft tissue stuck to bone (Fig. 21), necrotizing fasciitis (Fig. 22), and radiation necrosis (Fig. 23). These locations will have poor healing; any need to perform surgery through these areas will result in problems. Self-retaining retractors should be avoided in situations with poor soft tissue envelope. With at-risk wounds, a postoperative incisional wound vacuum is helpful to improve healing. When a poor soft tissue envelope cannot be avoided, backup plans such as fascial and muscle flaps should be planned for additional coverage. If the orthopedist is not comfortable performing rotational flaps, then a preoperative plastic surgery consult should be obtained. A gastrocnemius flap is pictured in Figure 24.

With the history of infection, sinus tracts are also important to note on the skin. These should be biopsied because sinus tracts can convert to a cutaneous squamous cell carcinoma called a Marjolin ulcer. If the biopsy proves to be positive, the orthopedic oncologist needs to be involved. Depending upon the sinus tract location, amputation may become necessary.

Other examination considerations that are important include evaluation for peripheral vascular status and chronic edema. The vascular evaluation can be as simple as noting the appearance of the distal extremity to include capillary refill, venous congestion, and color/texture of the skin. Palpate the dorsalis pedis and posterior tibial artery pulses. If there is concern about vascularity, then refer the patient to a vascular lab before considering lower extremity reconstruction. Incisions in a limb with poor blood flow or edema will not heal.

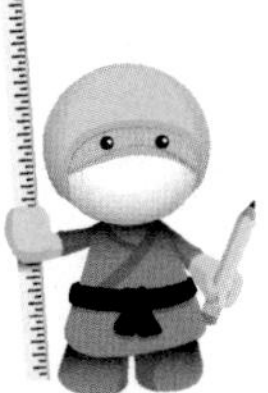

***Sensei says,***
*"If the skin is poor, the long journey will be arduous and bear little fruit."*

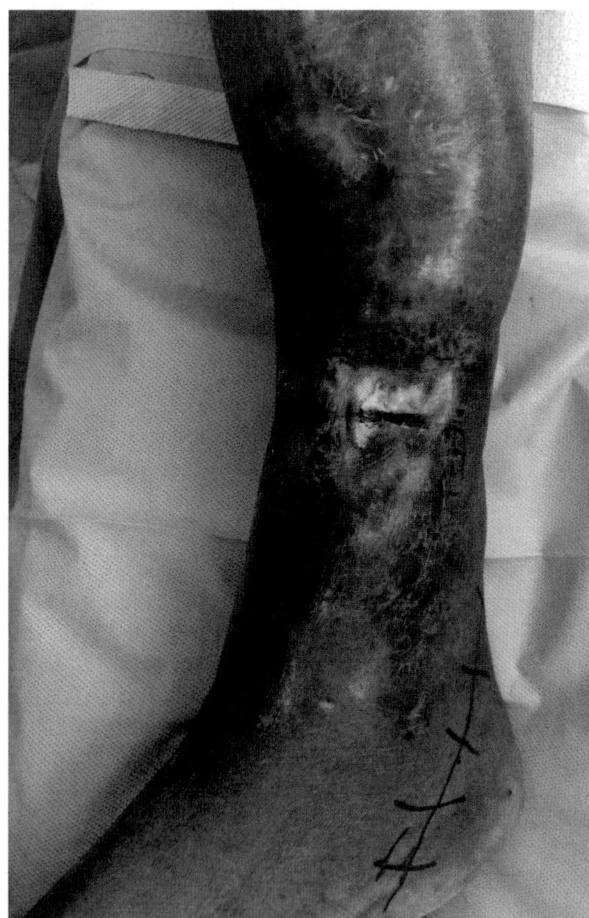

**Fig. 21:** Soft tissue examination. Soft tissue stuck to the bone. Avoid this area.

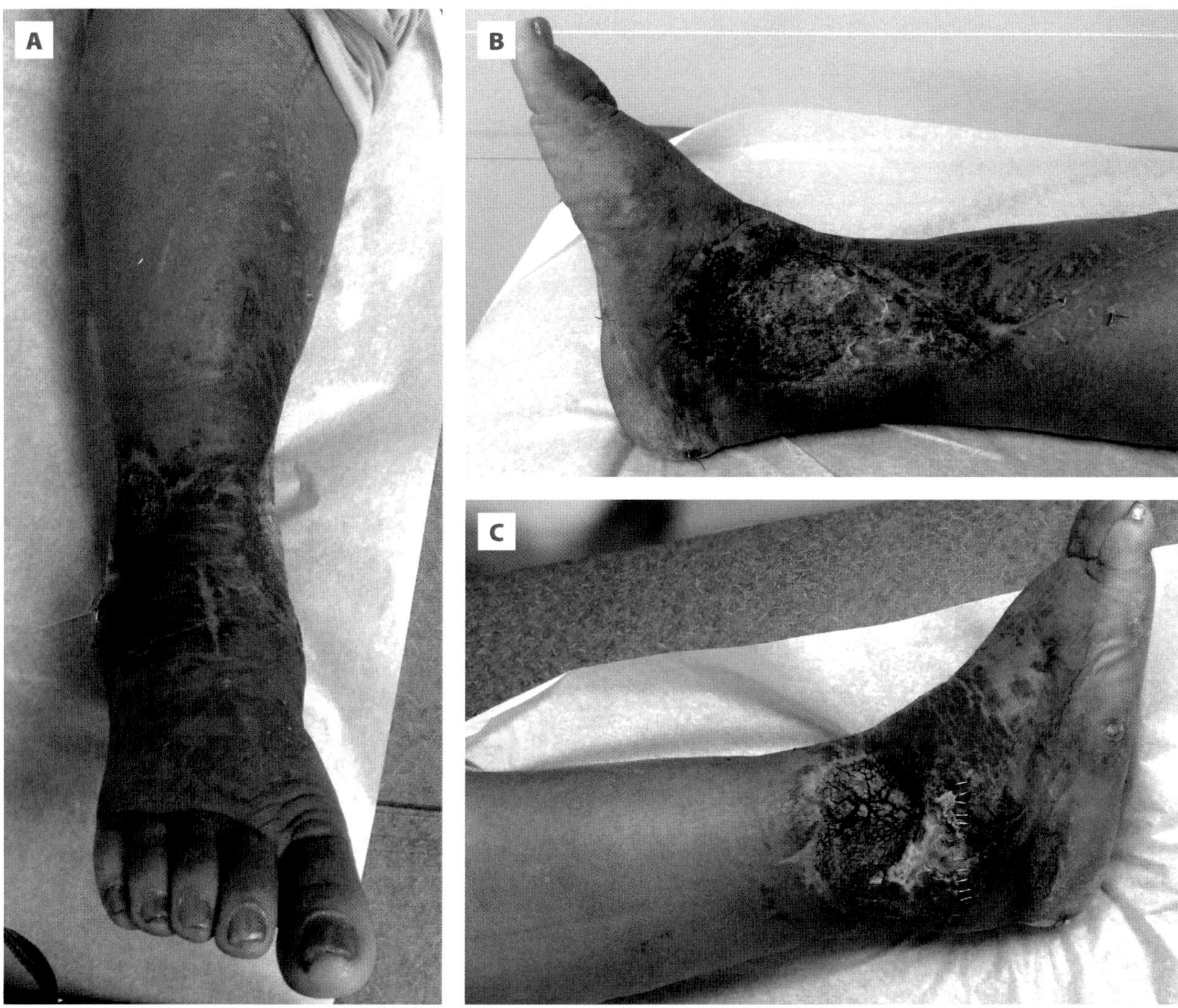


**Fig. 22:** Soft tissue examination, continued. A revision ankle fusion can be performed through a pristine transachilles approach instead of the skin that was damaged from necrotizing fasciitis. **A**, Anterior view. **B**, Medial view. **C**, Lateral view.

© 2023 Sinai Hospital of Baltimore

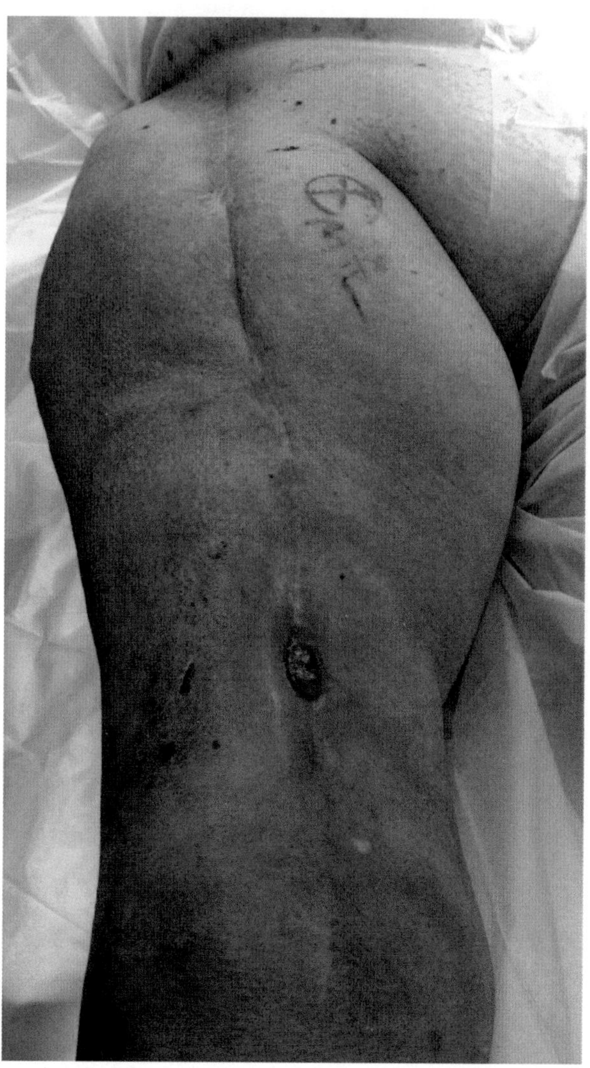

**Fig. 23:** Soft tissue examination, continued. A fibrotic and hard anterior thigh envelope secondary to radiation necrosis.

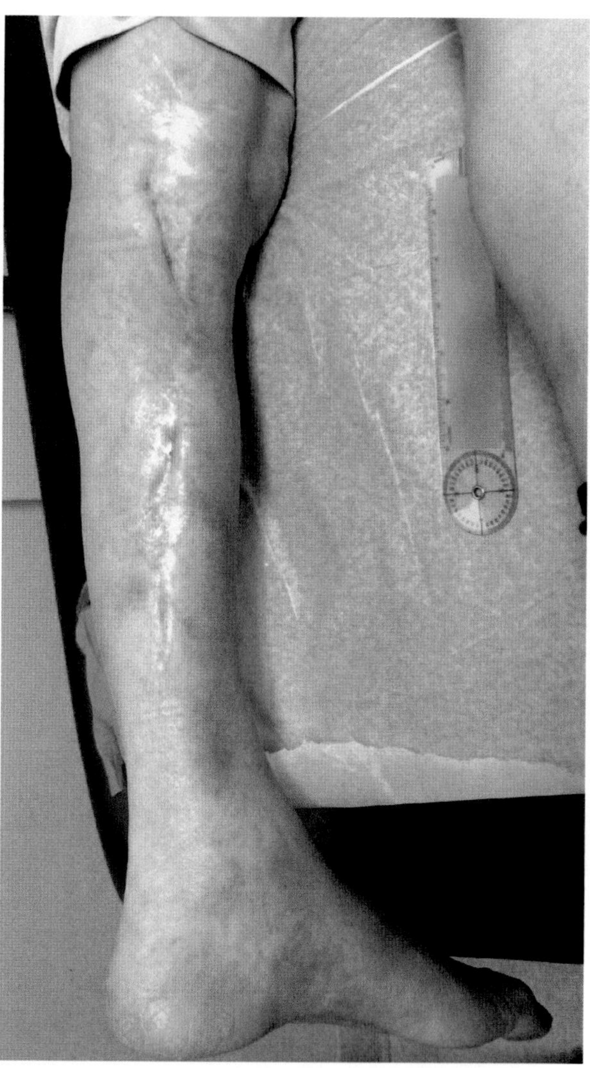

**Fig. 24:** Soft tissue examination, continued. Posterior view of previous gastrocnemius flap.

## Planning Ahead for Surgery

A checklist for patients who are preparing for surgery is available in Table 4. Some to-do items are standard and should be obvious before any procedure, such as cardiac and medical clearances, vitamin D level and supplementation, and crossmatching for significant blood loss cases. Additional preparations (weight loss, smoking cessation, and diabetic management) will contribute to a more successful outcome for the patient. If the patient lives alone, then planning for postoperative home help is vital. Otherwise, the patient will need to decide upon a rehabilitation destination where they can relocate for recovery. Checking their insurance plans is also imperative, as certain carriers will not pay for home antibiotics and those patients with infections may need to transfer to a facility postoperatively and stay there for several weeks.

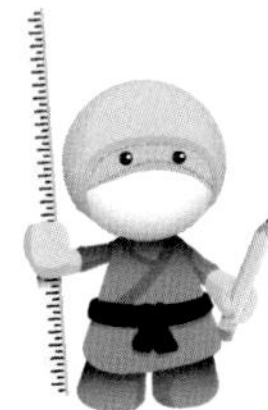

*Sensei says,*
*"It is better to prevent a problem from occurring than it is to act after it arises."*

No surgery candidate is ever ideal. It is up to the surgeon to decide what factors from the checklist, if any, are dealbreakers. It also will be necessary to determine which problems may be too difficult to manage (e.g., weight loss) before a limb deformity or infection surgery.

**Table 4.** Checklist to Optimize the Patient for Surgery

| Checklist to Optimize the Patient for Surgery |
|---|
| Weight loss |
| Hemoglobin A1c (HbA1c) level <7% |
| Stop smoking |
| Decrease narcotics usage |
| Decrease alcohol usage |
| Vascular evaluation |
| Cardiac clearance |
| Medical clearance |
| Immunology profile |
| +/- Hematology/rheumatology/ immunology referral |
| Computed tomography (CT) scan |
| Vitamin D level and supplementation |
| Postoperative recovery plans |
| Rehab versus homecare |

© 2023 Sinai Hospital of Baltimore

# Chapter 4

# Obtaining X-rays of the Lower Limbs

Shawn C. Standard, MD

An essential aspect of deformity evaluation and correction is reliable and reproducible x-rays. In this chapter, we will discuss how to obtain appropriate x-rays of the lower extremity to conduct a detailed deformity analysis. Poorly positioned x-rays should be rejected because they provide inaccurate information when conducting the analysis.

A magnification marker should be used in every x-ray. The magnification marker that we use is a 2.54-cm (1-inch) steel sphere. The magnification marker should be placed in the same plane as the bone of interest. If the magnification marker is taped in front of or behind the bone of interest, then magnification error will occur. Magnification error affects measurements of length but does not affect angular measurements.

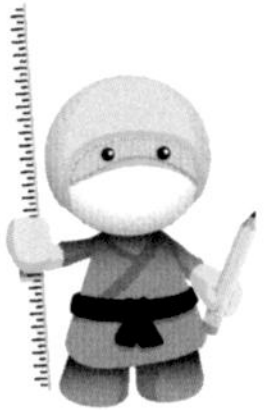

*Sensei says,*
*"He who uses an erroneous map will be lost before the journey begins."*

## Full Length Standing X-rays

The standard views of the lower extremity include full length standing anteroposterior (AP) and lateral view x-rays. Full length standing x-rays can be obtained on 36-inch (91.4 cm), 48-inch (121.9 cm), or 51-inch (129.5 cm) plain film cassettes. Alternatively, 14 inch × 17 inch (35.6 cm × 43.2 cm) computerized radiography (CR) cassettes can be used: two overlapping CR cassettes for pediatric patients and three overlapping CR cassettes for adult or adolescent patients. Special stitching software is required when using CR cassettes for digital x-rays.

It can be challenging to obtain a full length standing x-ray of a large or obese patient. Digital x-rays allow for significant manipulation of brightness and contrast, but a large soft-tissue overlap will decrease the detail and quality of the x-ray. To overcome the problem of decreased visualization of the proximal femur and pelvis, the x-ray technologist must ask the patient to lift up the excessive anterior soft tissue (i.e., panniculus) and compress the soft tissue with moderate force while exhaling. This will allow for better visualization of the hips and pelvis.

© 2023 Sinai Hospital of Baltimore

## Full Length Standing AP View X-ray

The full length standing AP view includes both lower extremities in the x-ray and includes each limb from the top of the iliac crest to the ankle (Fig. 1A). The patient stands with both feet flat on the floor, both knees maximally extended, and the patellae in the forward position (Fig. 1B). The central ray is perpendicular to the cassette and is aimed between the knees. The distance from the x-ray tube to the film cassette, called the source to image-receptor distance (SID), is 110 inches (279.4 cm) (Fig. 1C–D). If there is a limb length discrepancy, 1-cm blocks are placed under the short leg until both iliac crests appear to be level. The x-ray technologist should note on the x-ray the number of blocks (if any) that were used.

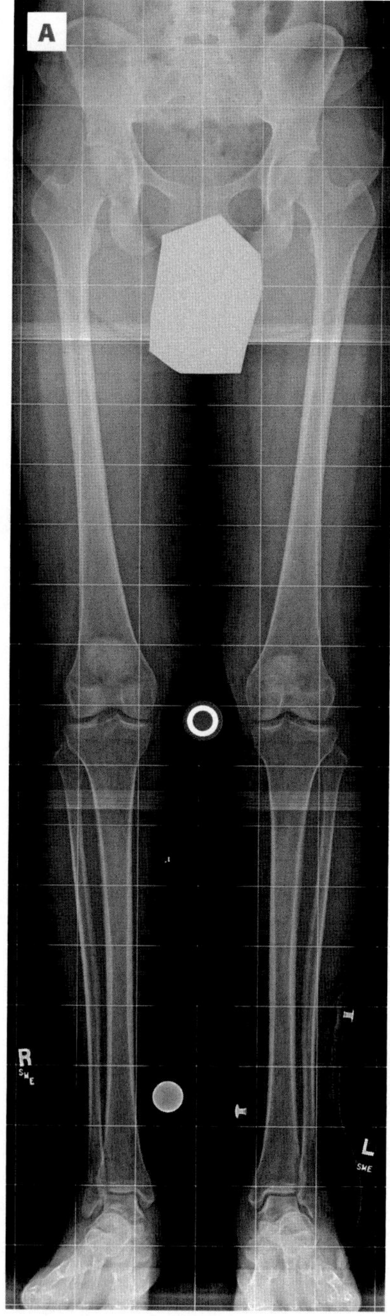


**Fig. 1: A**, Example of a well-positioned, full length standing AP view x-ray that includes both extremities on one film. The pelvis to the ankle is visible for each limb. Both lower extremities are oriented with patellae facing forward. A magnification marker is positioned next to the tibia. The central ray is aimed between the knees (*red circle*).

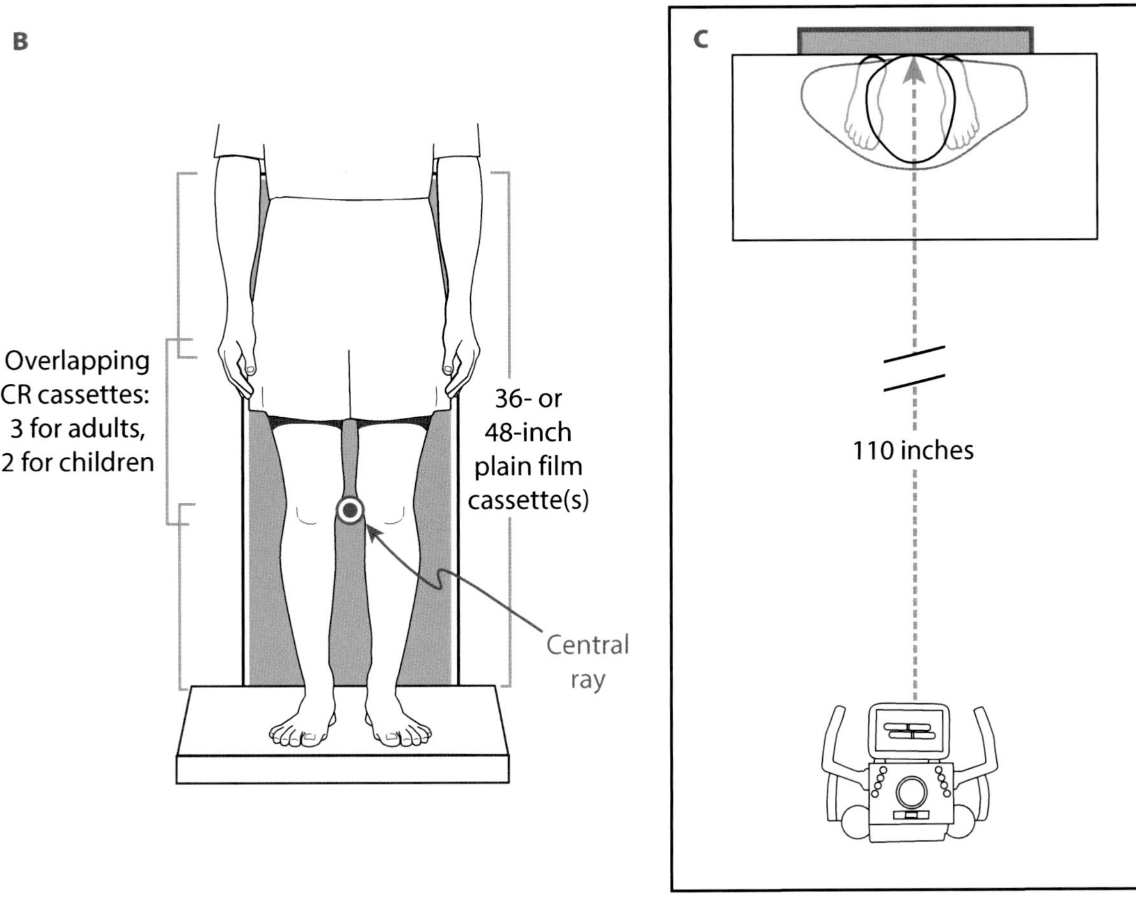


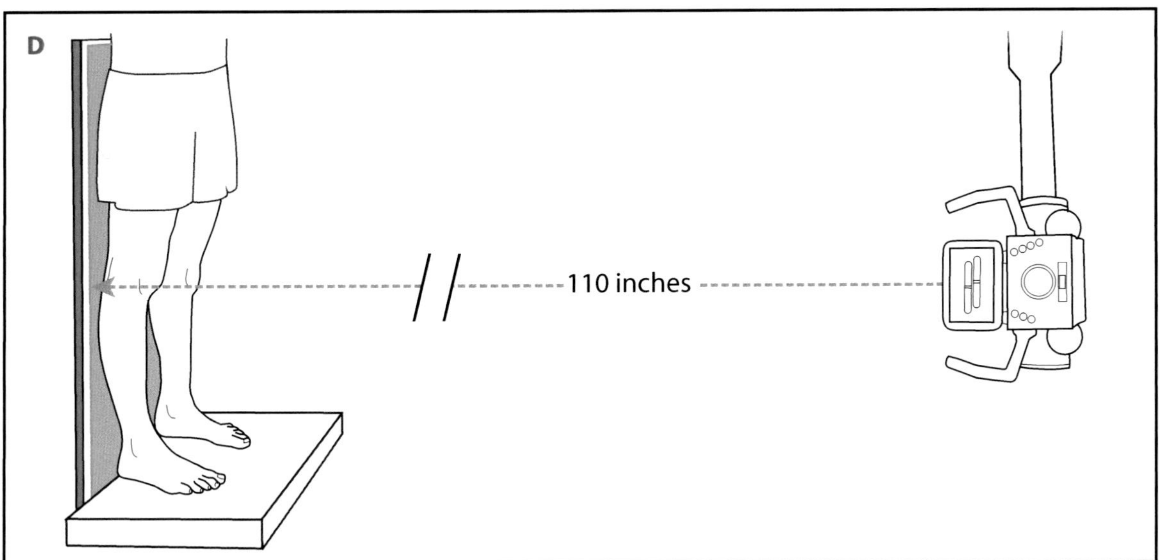


**Fig. 1 (continued): B**, For a full length standing AP view x-ray, the central ray is aimed between the knees (*red circle*). A plain film cassette or overlapping CR cassettes can be used. Both legs should appear in the x-ray. The patient is standing with each patella rotated forward and with the knees maximally extended. If necessary, blocks should be used to level the pelvis. **C**, The central ray is perpendicular to the cassette. **D**, The central ray is aimed at the level of the knee joint.

## Full Length Standing Lateral View X-ray

The full length standing lateral view x-ray includes one limb from the hip joint to the ankle joint (Fig. 2A). This x-ray is often obtained incorrectly, which limits the visualization of the proximal femur and hip. To obtain this lateral view, the foot is planted so that it is flat on the ground and the lateral aspect of the foot is against the cassette (Fig. 2B). Then the heel and knee of this limb are externally rotated 10° with the knee maximally extended. The patient then pivots the opposite leg and the rest of the body 45° away from the planted leg (Fig. 2C). This position moves the patient's body away from the limb of interest enabling visualization from the femoral head to the ankle joint. The central ray is perpendicular to the cassette and aimed at the knee. The SID is 110 inches (279.4 cm). Poorly positioned full length standing lateral view x-rays should be rejected because they can simulate a knee flexion contracture or hide hyperextension.

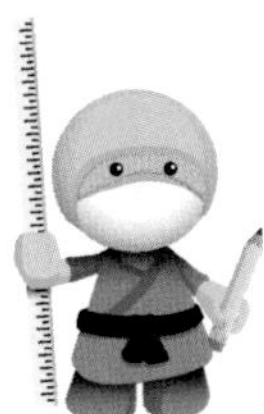

*Sensei says,*
*"To ensure a perfect lateral view of the knee, slightly externally rotate the planted leg approximately 10° to obtain distal femoral condylar overlap."*

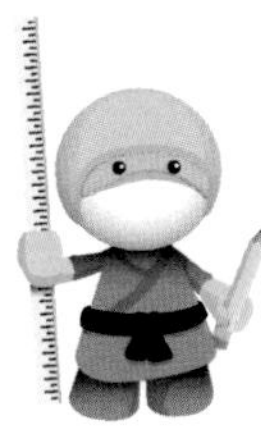

*Sensei says,*
*"If full length standing AP and lateral view x-rays reveal significant deformity at the hip, knee, or ankle joint, then additional x-ray views should be obtained in which the central ray is aimed at the joint of interest."*

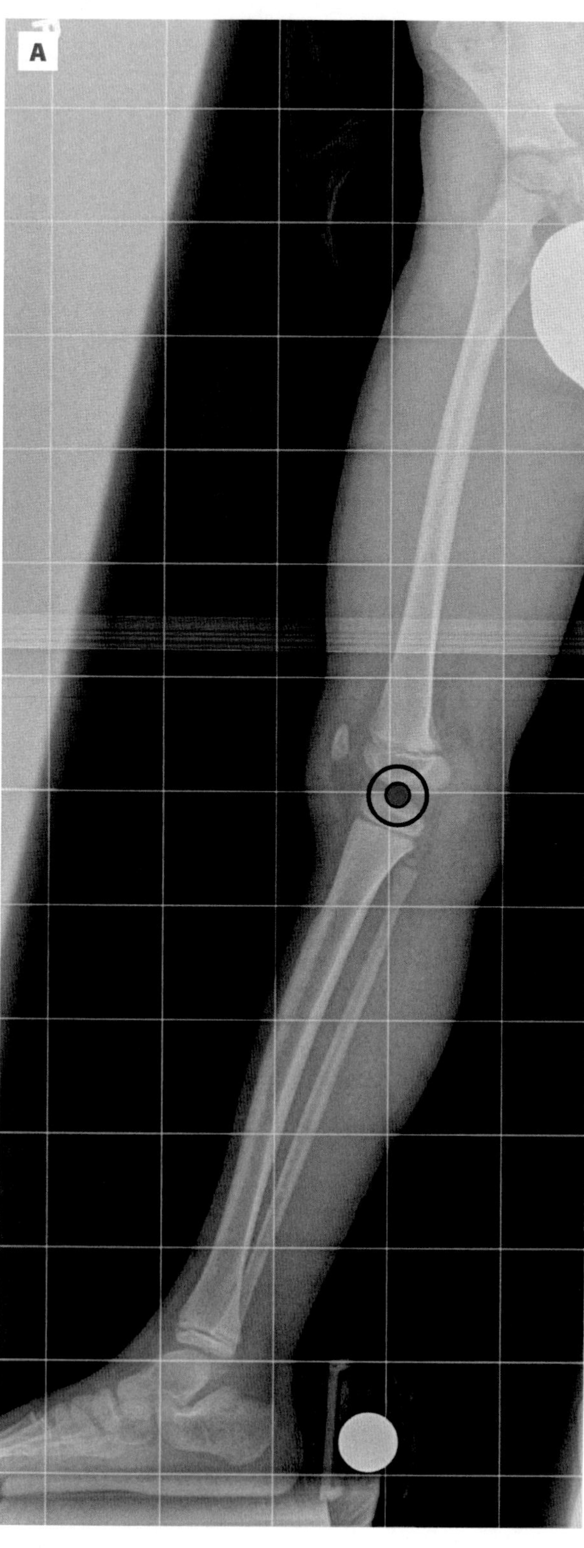


**Fig. 2: A**, Example of a well-positioned, full length standing lateral view x-ray with a fully extended knee. The femoral head to the ankle of this limb is visible. The central ray is aimed at the knee joint (*red circle*).

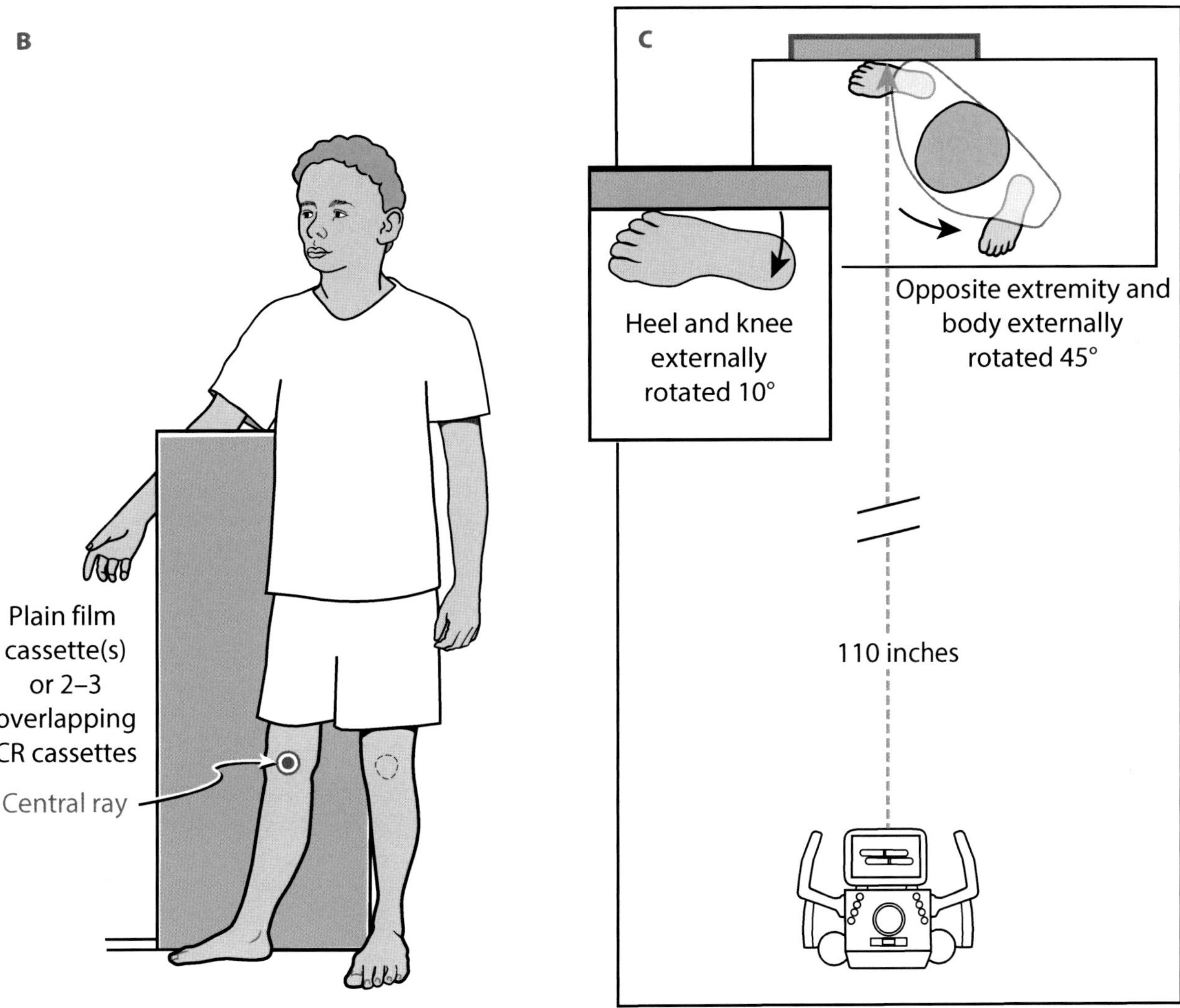


**Fig. 2 (continued): B,** For a full length standing lateral view x-ray, the central ray is aimed at the knee joint (*red circle*). **C,** The patient plants the limb of interest so that the lateral aspect of the foot is against the cassette and the knee is fully extended. The patient externally rotates the heel and knee 10°. Then the patient pivots the contralateral limb and the rest of the body 45° away from the planted leg. This allows for complete visualization of the lower extremity from the femoral head to the ankle joint. The central ray should be perpendicular to the cassette and aimed at the knee joint.

© 2023 Sinai Hospital of Baltimore

## Summary

- Always take two orthogonal views
- Use cassettes that are large enough to visualize the limb(s) from the pelvis to the ankle joint(s).
- SID = 110 inches (279.4 cm)
- Knees should be maximally extended.
- Feet flat on the floor
- Obese patients must lift up and compress excessive anterior soft tissue.
- AP View Limb Position: Patellae forward
- AP View: 1-cm blocks for limb length discrepancy placed incrementally until iliac crests are level. Number of blocks used should be noted on the x-ray.
- Lateral View Limb Position: Patella 10° externally rotated so that the femoral condyles overlap

***Remember:***

- *Do not accept inadequate films. If necessary, the physician should provide assistance with positioning.*
- *Physicians should assist in the training of x-ray technologists in order to have proper and useful views.*
- *On every x-ray, use a magnification marker that is placed in the plane of the bone of interest.*
- *The central ray should be aimed at the joint of interest.*

# Chapter 5

# Obtaining X-rays of the Ankle and Foot for Deformity Analysis

Bradley M. Lamm, DPM

Noman A. Siddiqui, DPM

Multiplanar x-rays of the ankle and foot should be obtained separately from full length standing x-rays to accurately assess deformities about the foot and ankle. All x-rays except for the medial oblique view of the foot should be taken while the foot is in a full weightbearing, plantigrade position when possible (unless contraindicated due to recent surgery or patient safety). If full weightbearing is not feasible, the x-rays can be obtained in a simulated plantigrade, weightbearing position. We use 14 inch × 17 inch (35.6 cm × 43.2 cm) computerized radiography (CR) cassettes when obtaining x-rays of the foot and ankle. For two of the x-ray views, it is important for the entire tibia to be visualized on the x-ray (i.e., AP view ankle, mortise lateral view ankle). The SID is 40 inches (101.6 cm) for all foot and ankle x-rays (Bontrager KL, Lampignano JP. *Textbook of Radiographic Positioning and Related Anatomy.* 6th edition. St. Louis: Elsevier Mosby, 2005: p 223).

## X-rays of the Ankle

X-rays of the ankle consist of the following views (Table 1):

- AP
- Mortise
- Mortise Lateral

### AP View of the Ankle

The AP view of the ankle should include the tibia and is obtained while the patient stands with the knee fully extended (Fig. 1). If patients are unable to bear weight, they may sit. The heel touches the cassette posteriorly. The central ray of the x-ray is centered at the ankle joint (midway between the malleoli) and perpendicular to the radiographic cassette. The SID is 40 inches (101.6 cm).

© 2023 Sinai Hospital of Baltimore

**Table 1.** Obtaining Ankle X-rays

| Type of Ankle X-ray | Cassette with Dimensions of 14 inches x 17 inches (35.6 cm x 43.2 cm) | SID 40 inches (101.6 cm) | mAs/kVp 4.0/56 | Central Ray Considerations | Patient Positioning | Tibia Included |
|---|---|---|---|---|---|---|
| AP | √ | √ | √ | Central ray aimed perpendicular to the cassette and between malleoli at the level of the ankle joint | Posterior heel placed against cassette with knee fully extended | √ |
| Mortise | √ | √ | √ | Central ray aimed perpendicular to the cassette and between malleoli at the level of the ankle joint | Posterior heel placed against cassette with knee fully extended; foot internally rotated 15° | |
| Mortise Lateral | √ | √ | √ | Central ray aimed perpendicular to the cassette and between malleoli at the level of the ankle joint | Lateral aspect of foot placed against cassette; forefoot internally rotated 15° | √ |

AP, anteroposterior; SID, source to image-receptor distance; mAs, milli amps per second; kVp, kilovoltage potential.

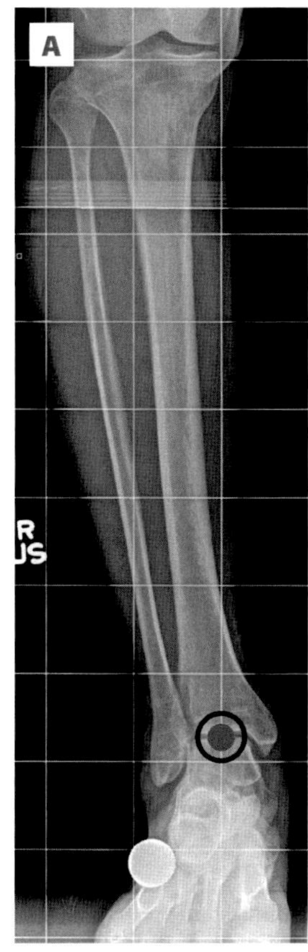


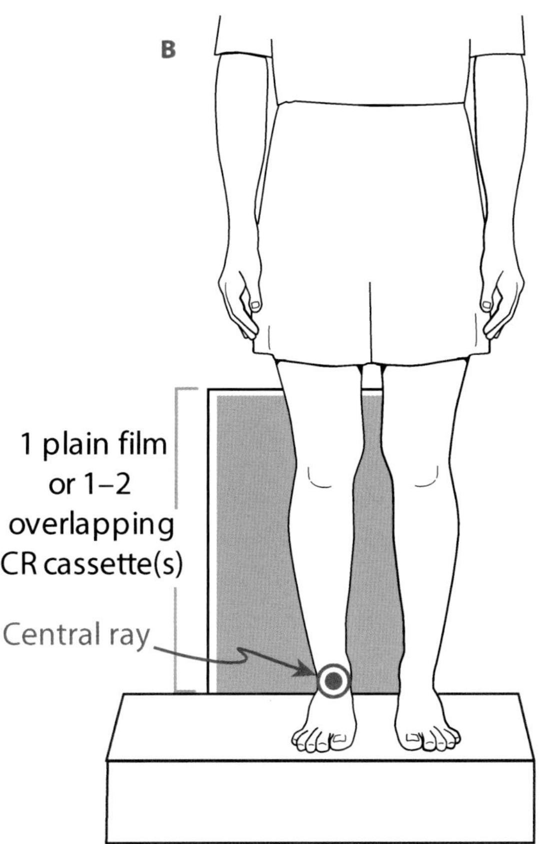


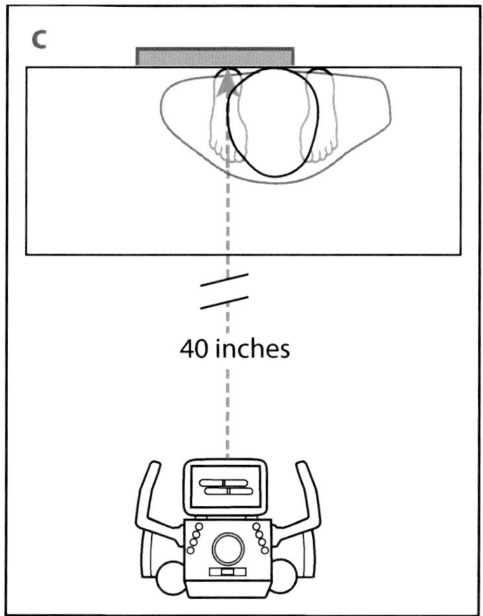


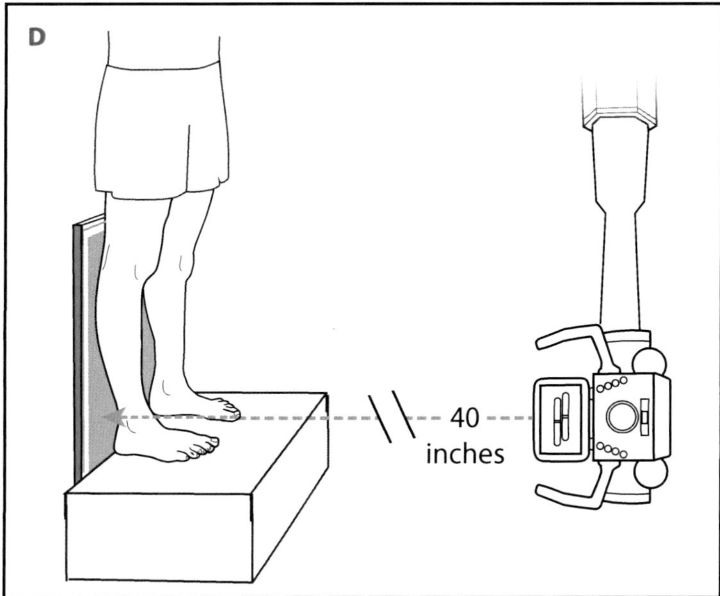


**Fig. 1:** **A**, Example of a well-positioned AP view ankle x-ray to include the tibia. The central ray is aimed midway between the malleoli (*red circle*). **B**, For an AP view ankle x-ray to include the tibia, 1 or 2 overlapping CR cassettes are used. The central ray is aimed midway between the malleoli (*red circle*). **C**, The central ray is aimed perpendicular to the cassette. **D**, The patient stands full weightbearing with the knee extended. The central ray is aimed at the level of the ankle joint.

© 2023 Sinai Hospital of Baltimore

## Mortise View of the Ankle

For the mortise view of the ankle, the patient positioning and beam orientation are similar to the AP view of the ankle except that the foot is internally rotated 15° (Fig. 2). The central ray is aimed at the ankle joint between the malleoli, and it is perpendicular to the radiographic cassette. The SID is 40 inches (101.6 cm).

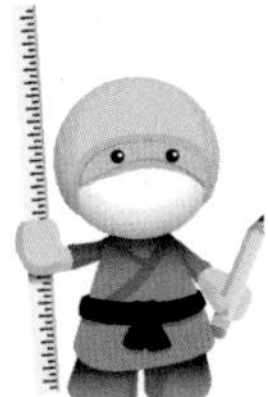

*Sensei says,*

*"The mortise view is obtained to visualize the entire ankle joint congruity and not typically used to measure angles or distances."*

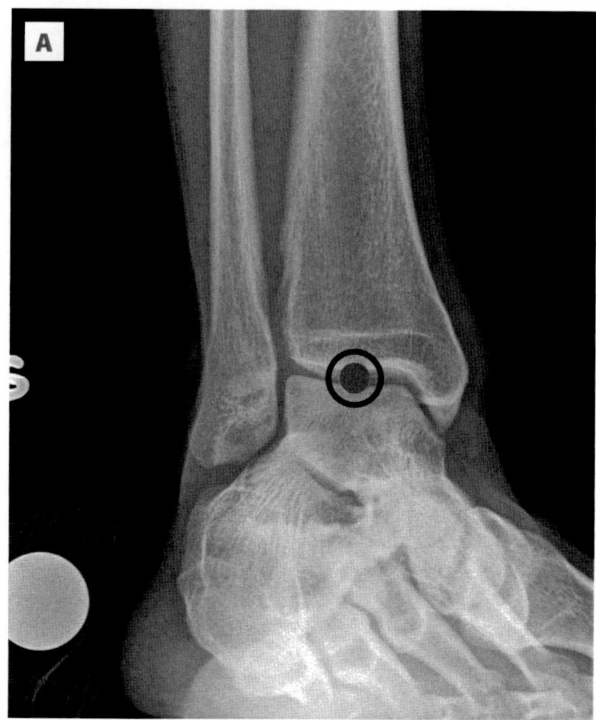


**Fig. 2: A**, Example of a well-positioned, mortise view ankle x-ray. The central ray is aimed midway between the malleoli (*red circle*).

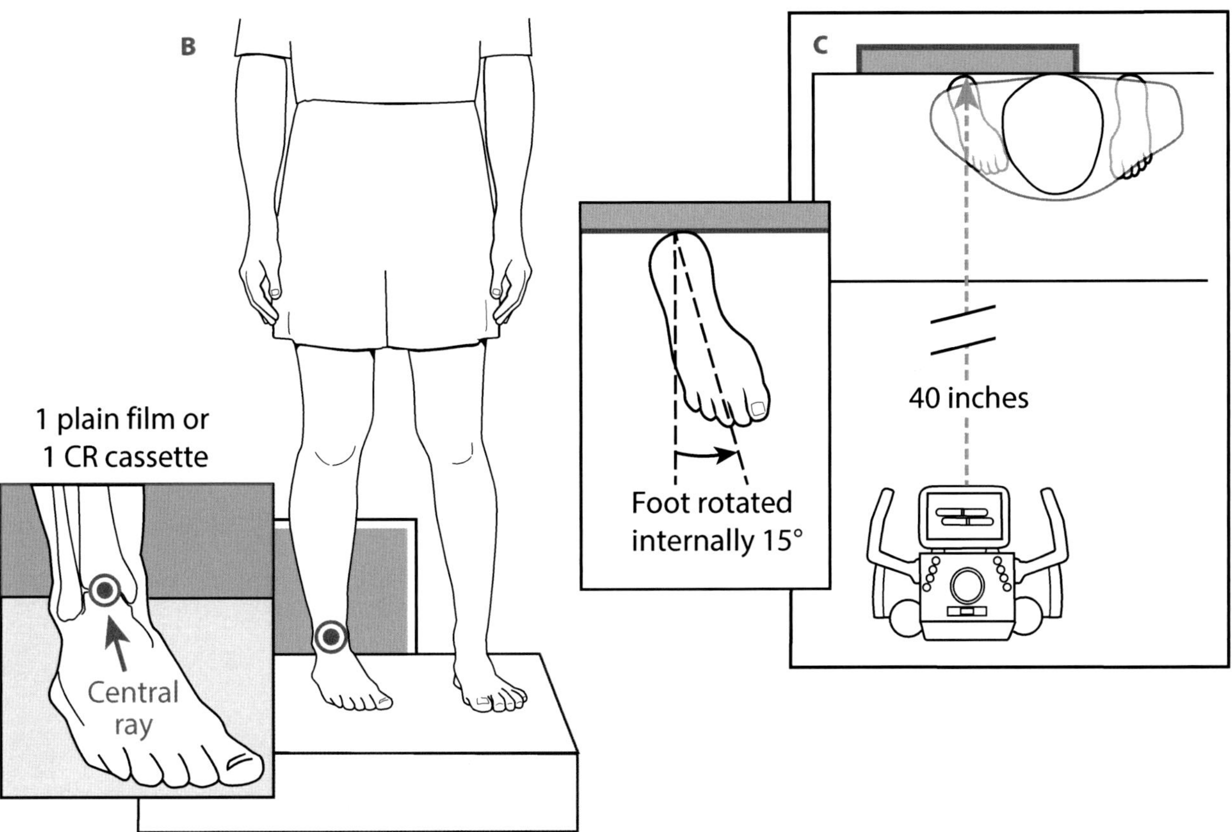


**Fig. 2 (continued): B**, The patient stands full weightbearing and the central ray is aimed midway between the malleoli (*red circle*). **C**, The patient stands full weightbearing with the foot internally rotated 15°. The central ray is aimed perpendicular to the cassette at the level of the ankle joint.

*© 2023 Sinai Hospital of Baltimore*

## Mortise Lateral View of the Ankle

A mortise lateral view of the ankle should include the tibia. The x-ray is obtained by first placing the lateral aspect of the foot against the radiographic cassette (Fig. 3). Then the forefoot is internally rotated 15° while weightbearing. The patient should take a small step backwards with the contralateral foot to move the body away from the field of view. The central ray is perpendicular to the radiographic cassette and is aimed at the ankle malleoli, which allows the malleoli to overlap on the x-ray. The SID is 40 inches (101.6 cm).

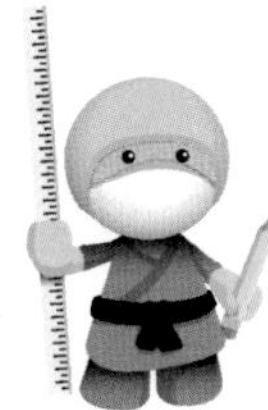

*Sensei says,*

*"The technologist or surgeon should request a cassette that is large enough (14 inches × 17 inches [35.6 cm × 43.2 cm]) to capture the entire tibia on the AP and mortise lateral views with the central ray aimed at the ankle joint. When these ankle views include the tibia, the mechanical and anatomic axis lines of the tibia can be precisely drawn, which results in accurate ankle joint lines, angular measurements, and planning."*

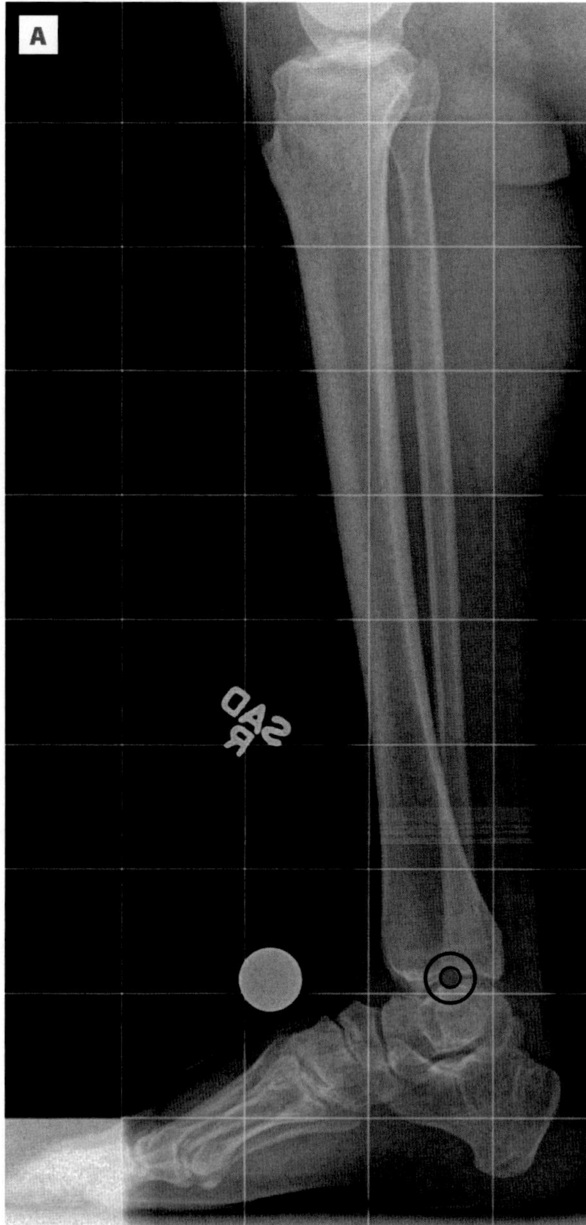


**Fig. 3: A**, Example of a well-positioned mortise lateral view ankle x-ray. The central ray is aimed at the malleoli (*red circle*).

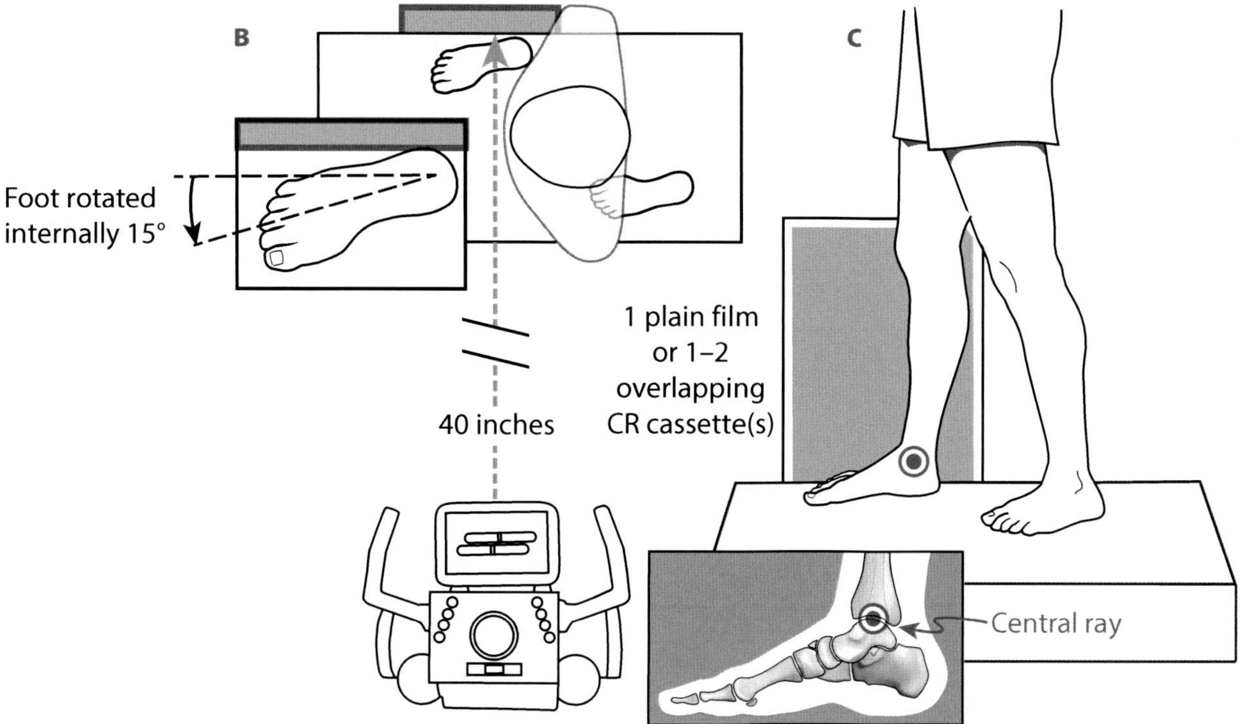


**Fig. 3 (continued): B**, For a mortise lateral view ankle x-ray that includes the tibia, the patient stands full weightbearing with the lateral aspect of the foot against the radiographic cassette. Then the forefoot is internally rotated 15°. The central ray is perpendicular to the cassette. **C**, The central ray is aimed at the malleoli (*red circle*). This positioning allows the malleoli to overlap in the image.

© 2023 Sinai Hospital of Baltimore

## X-rays of the Foot

X-rays of the foot consist of the following views (Table 2):

- AP
- Medial Oblique (MO)
- Lateral

### AP View of the Foot

The AP view of the foot is obtained while the patient stands with the knee fully extended (Fig. 4). If unable to bear weight, the patient may sit. The cassette is placed on the floor, and the patient stands with the foot on the center of the cassette. The patient should take a small step to the side to allow the ipsilateral ankle to be out of the field of view. The central ray should be aimed at the third cuneiform and angled 15° proximal or cephalad. The SID is 40 inches (101.6 cm).

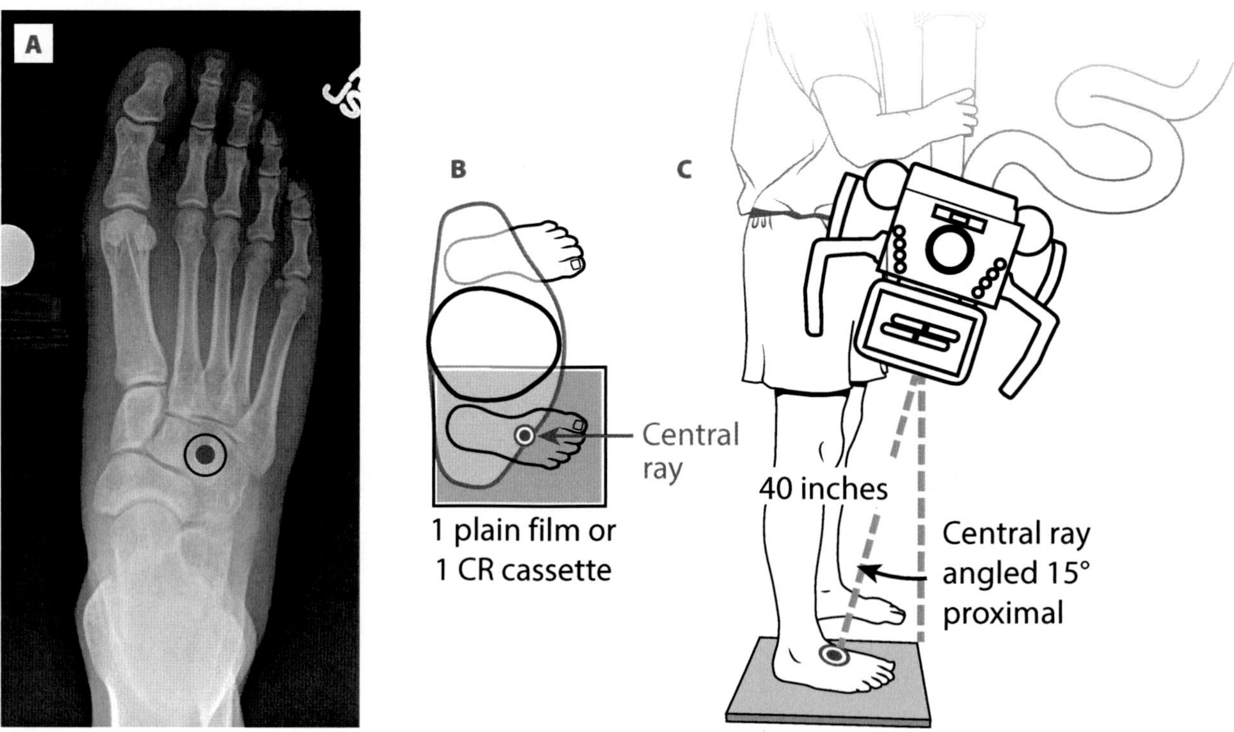


**Fig. 4: A**, Example of a well-positioned AP view foot x-ray. The central ray should be aimed at the third cuneiform (*red circle*). **B**, For an AP view of the foot, the cassette is placed on the floor. The patient stands with the foot placed on the center of the cassette. **C**, The patient stands with the knee fully extended. The central ray is aimed at the third cuneiform (*red circle*) and angled 15° proximal.

**Table 2.** Obtaining Foot X-rays

| Type of Foot X-ray | Cassette with Dimensions of 14 inches x 17 inches (35.6 cm x 43.2 cm) | SID 40 inches (101.6 cm) | mAs/kVp 5.0/60 | mAs/kVp 4.0/56 | Central Ray Considerations | Patient Positioning | Tibia Included |
|---|---|---|---|---|---|---|---|
| AP | √ | √ | | √ | Central ray directed at third cuneiform and aimed 15° proximal | Foot placed on center of the cassette, which is on the floor; knee fully extended | |
| Medial Oblique | √ | √ | | √ | Central ray perpendicular to cassette and aimed at third cuneiform | Foot placed on center of cassette, which is on the floor; leg tilted 30° from central ray; foot internally rotated 15° to the cassette; Goal = 45° angle between plantar surface of foot and central ray | |
| Lateral | √ | √ | | √ | Central ray aimed perpendicular to the cassette and directed at third cuneiform | Lateral aspect of foot placed against cassette with ankle in neutral position | |
| Long Leg Calcaneal Axial | √ | √ | √ | | Central ray 45° to the cassette and aimed at subtalar joint | Foot placed on center of cassette, which is on the floor | Only distal half of tibia |
| Hindfoot Alignment | √ | √ | √ | | Cassette is placed in 20° angulated slot in plexiglass box; central ray directed perpendicular to cassette and aimed at the ankle joint | Patient stands on elevated x-ray plexiglass box | Only distal half of tibia |

AP, anteroposterior; SID, source to image-receptor distance; mAs, milli amps per second; kVp, kilovoltage potential.

© 2023 Sinai Hospital of Baltimore

## Medial Oblique View of the Foot

To obtain an MO view of the foot, the cassette is placed on the floor. The patient stands with the foot of interest on the center of the cassette and the other foot on the floor (Fig. 5). The central ray is perpendicular to the cassette and aimed at the third cuneiform. Then the knee is fully extended, the entire leg to include the foot is tilted 30° from the central ray, and the foot is internally rotated or pronated an additional 15° from the cassette. The goal of this positioning is to achieve a 45° angle between the plantar surface of the foot and the central ray. The SID is 40 inches (101.6 cm).

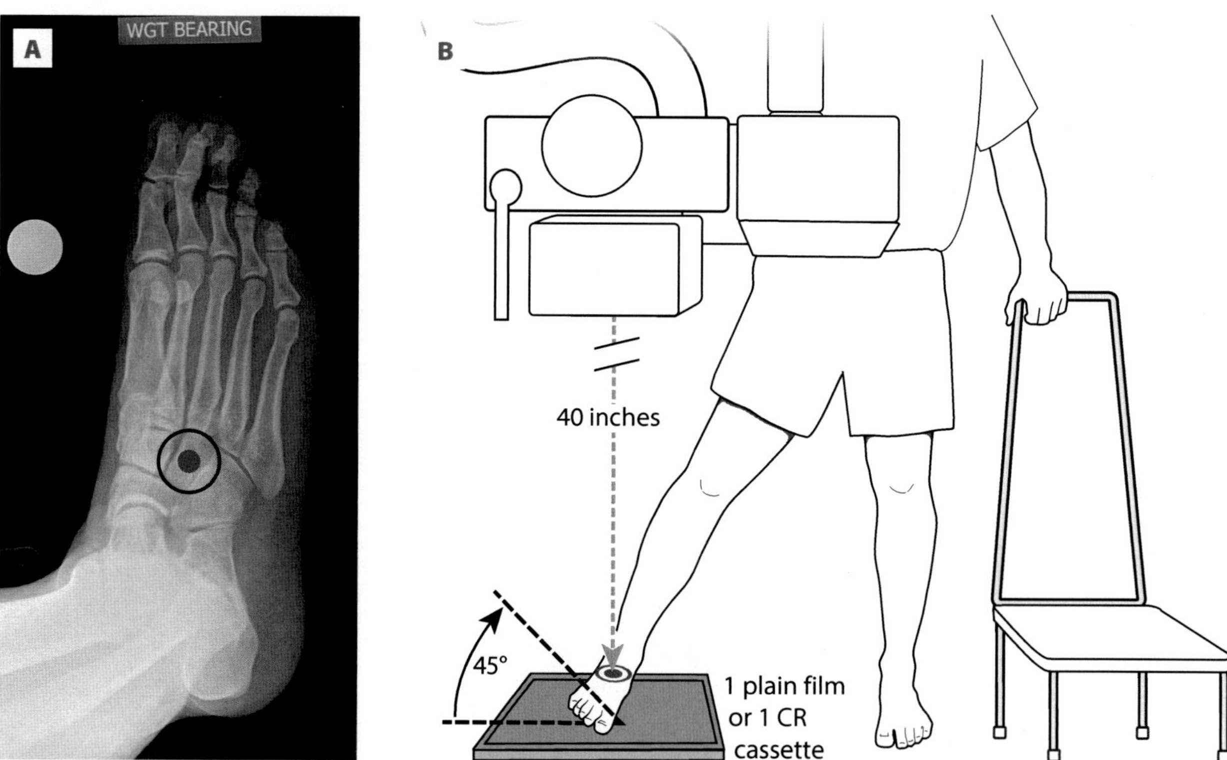


**Fig. 5: A,** Example of a well-positioned medial oblique view x-ray of the foot. The central ray should be aimed at the third cuneiform (*red circle*). **B,** To obtain a medial oblique view x-ray of the foot, the cassette is placed on the floor. The patient stands with the foot of interest placed on the center of the cassette. The central ray is perpendicular to the cassette and aimed at the third cuneiform (*red circle*). Then the knee is fully extended, the leg is tilted 30° from the central ray, and the foot is internally rotated or pronated an additional 15° from the cassette.

## Lateral View of the Foot

The lateral view of the foot is obtained by placing the lateral aspect of the patient's foot against the cassette while weightbearing (Fig. 6). The ankle is in a neutral position. The patient should take a small step backwards with the contralateral foot to move the patient's body away from the field of view. The central ray is perpendicular to the cassette and is aimed at the third cuneiform. The SID is 40 inches (101.6 cm).

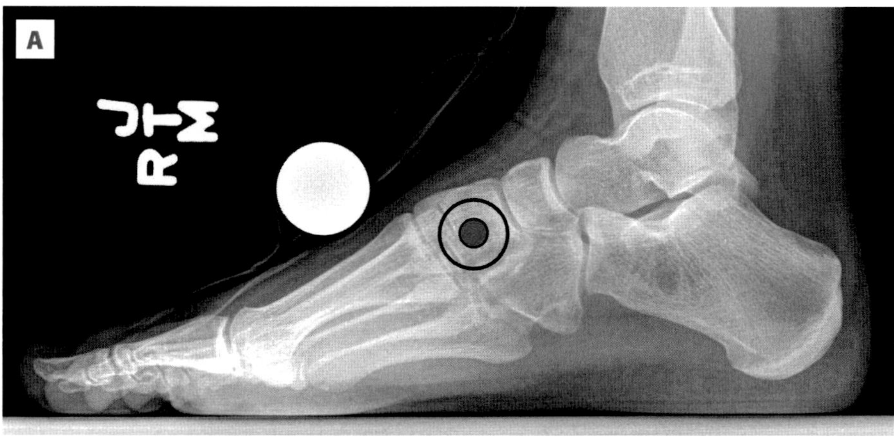


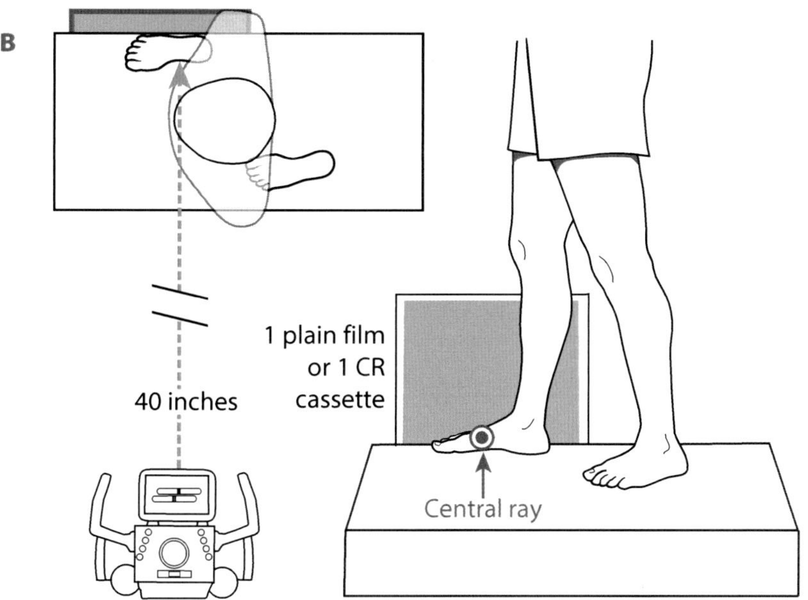


**Fig. 6: A**, Example of a well-positioned lateral view x-ray of the foot. The central ray should be aimed at the third cuneiform (*red circle*). **B**, To obtain a lateral view x-ray of the foot, the lateral aspect of the patient's foot is placed against the cassette while weightbearing. The ankle is in a neutral position. The patient should take a small step backwards with the contralateral foot. The central ray is perpendicular to the cassette and is aimed at the third cuneiform (*red circle*).

© 2023 Sinai Hospital of Baltimore

## Additional X-rays of the Foot

### Long Leg Calcaneal Axial View X-ray

The long leg calcaneal axial view is also referred to as a Harris heel view to include the distal tibia (Fig. 7). To obtain this x-ray, the cassette is placed on the floor. The patient stands with the foot of interest on the center of the cassette and the other foot placed anteriorly on the floor (i.e., other foot is one step ahead of the foot of interest). The central ray is 45° to the cassette and is aimed at the subtalar joint in a posterior-anterior orientation. The radiographic cassette should be large enough to capture the distal half of the tibia. The goal is to visualize the subtalar joint, the calcaneal tuber, and the relationship of the tibia to the calcaneus. The SID is 40 inches (101.6 cm).

A

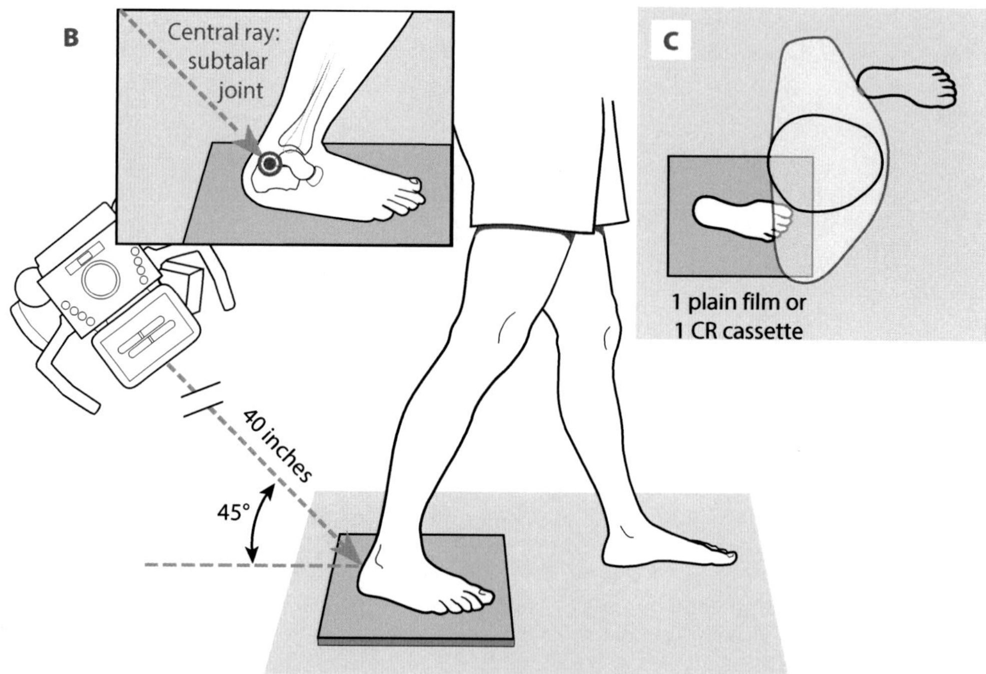


**Fig. 7: A**, Example of a well-positioned long leg calcaneal axial view x-ray that includes the distal tibia. The central ray is aimed at the subtalar joint (*red circle*). **B**, To obtain a long leg calcaneal axial view x-ray, the cassette is placed on the floor and the patient stands with the foot of interest on the center of the cassette. The other foot is placed anteriorly on the floor. The central ray is 45° to the cassette and is aimed at the subtalar joint (*red circle*) in a posterior-anterior orientation. **C**, Bird's eye view of positioning for a long leg calcaneal axial view x-ray.

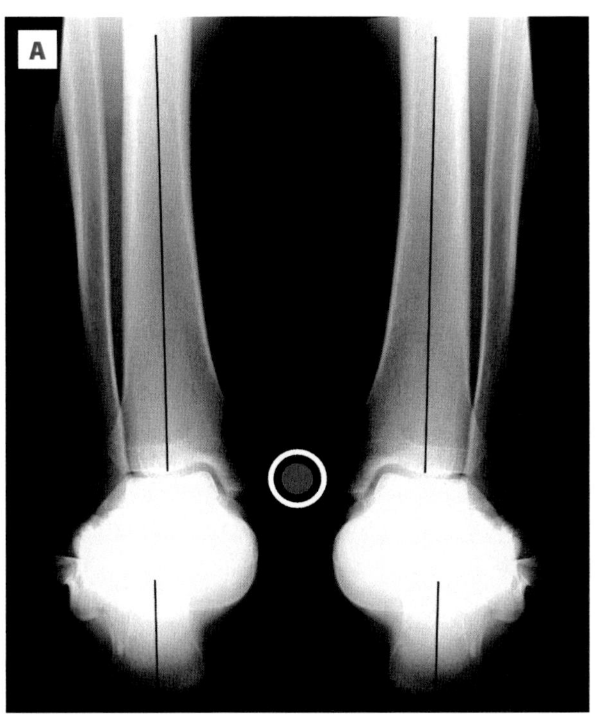


## Hindfoot Alignment View X-ray

The hindfoot alignment view or Saltzman view x-ray is obtained by utilizing a special elevated x-ray plexiglass box (Fig. 8). The view should include both tibiae and feet. The patient stands full weightbearing on the plexiglass box in a comfortable angle and base of gait. The x-ray cassette is placed in a slot that is in front of the patient and is angulated 20°. The central ray is aimed between the ankle joints in a posterior-anterior orientation. The beam is directed 20° from the surface of the plexiglass box so that it is perpendicular to the radiographic cassette. The goal is to visualize the ankle joint and the angular and translational relationship of the tibia to the calcaneus. The SID is 40 inches (101.6 cm).

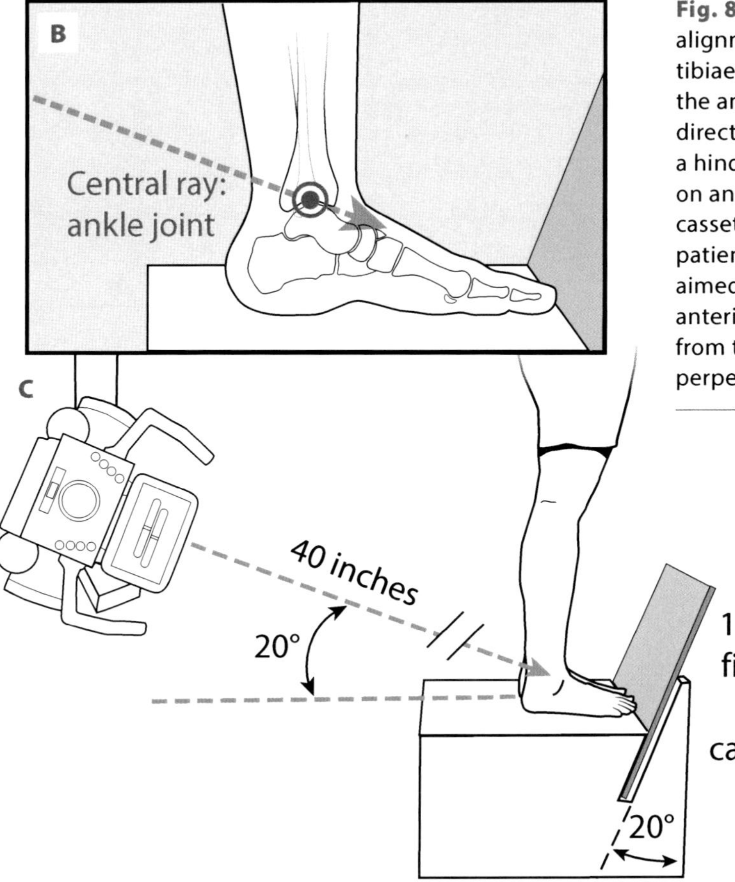


**Fig. 8:** **A**, Example of a well-positioned hindfoot alignment view x-ray that includes both distal tibiae and feet. The central ray is aimed between the ankle joints (*red circle*). **B**, The central ray is directed at the level of the ankle joints. **C**, To obtain a hindfoot alignment view x-ray, the patient stands on an elevated plexiglass x-ray box. The x-ray cassette is placed in a slot that is in front of the patient and is angulated 20°. The central ray is aimed between the ankle joints in a posterior-anterior orientation. The beam is directed 20° from the surface of the plexiglass box so that it is perpendicular to the radiographic cassette.

© 2023 Sinai Hospital of Baltimore

## Summary

- To accurately assess foot and ankle deformities, obtain separate weightbearing foot and ankle x-rays (do not use only full length standing x-rays of the lower extremity)
- When possible, the foot should be in a full weightbearing, plantigrade position except for the medial oblique view of the foot.
- The entire tibia should be included in the AP view of the ankle and the mortise lateral view of the ankle.
- Stress views are critical to use when joint instability is present.

***Remember:***

- *Do not accept inadequate films. If necessary, the physician should provide assistance with positioning.*
- *Physicians should assist in the training of x-ray technologists in order to have proper and useful views.*
- *On every x-ray, use a magnification marker that is placed in the plane of the bone of interest.*
- *The central ray should be aimed at the joint of interest.*

# Chapter 6

# Deformity Analysis and Osteotomy Strategies: Frontal Plane

Shawn C. Standard, MD

To analyze deformities using the full-length standing AP and lateral view x-rays, we recommend using the mnemonic MAP the ABCs. This approach simplifies the steps needed to analyze a deformity. This mnemonic will help you to approach lower limb analysis in a consistent manner. The mnemonic "MAP" helps you perform a systematic initial screening in the clinic. The mnemonic "ABC" is used to formulate a preoperative plan. Together, "MAP the ABCs" will help direct each surgeon to the ultimate destination of correct and accurate deformity assessment (Table 1).

After the first example, osteotomy rules and considerations will be reviewed. These osteotomy concepts will pertain to both the frontal and sagittal planes. This chapter is an overview of the frontal plane deformity analysis. Sagittal plane analysis, as well as the exact methods of axis planning wherein the surgeon defines the apex of deformity for both the frontal and sagittal planes, will be explained in great detail within subsequent chapters.

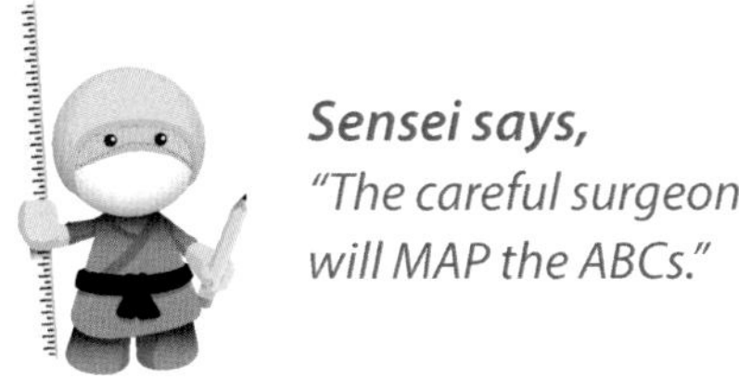


## MAP the ABCs

The goal of this analytical approach is to answer the questions: Is there a deformity? Which bone segment is abnormal? Where is the apex of the deformity? What is the magnitude and direction of the deformity? One must take into account limb length discrepancy (LLD), which will be discussed later in this book. With the answers to these questions, you can accurately plan the osteotomy and correction strategy.

© 2023 Sinai Hospital of Baltimore

**Table 1. Summary of MAP the ABCs**

**MAP**

**M** = Measure the Mechanical Axis Deviation (MAD)

**A** = Analyze the joint angles

**P** = Pick the deformed bone

**ABC**

**A** = Apex of deformity

**B** = Bone cut (choose the level of the osteotomy)

**C** = Correction

Acute Correction:

Use angulation, rotation, and translation to align the proximal and distal axes.

Gradual Correction:

Using a Hinged Device: Locate the obtuse angle that is created by the intersection of the proximal and distal axes. Draw a line that bisects this obtuse angle and passes through the apex. This line is called the correction bisector line (C-level). The point of hinge rotation (thumbtack) must always be placed on the C-level. Angulate the bone segment about the thumbtack until the proximal and distal axes are aligned.

Using a Hexapod Device: Perform a three-dimensional gradual correction to align two axes or two points in space.

**Table 2. Frontal Plane Joint Angles of Left Limb**

| Angle | Measurements | Average Normal Value and Range |
|---|---|---|
| LPFA | 87° | 90° (85–95°) |
| LDFA | **96°** | 87° (85–90°) |
| MPTA | **74°** | 87° (85–90°) |
| LDTA | 89° | 89° (86–92°) |
| JLCA | 0° | 0° (0±2°) |

## MAP: An Overview

### M = Measure the MAD

First, ask yourself, "Is there a deformity?" Although a deformity can be evident just by clinical observation or superficial review of the x-ray, the presence of a deformity needs to be quantified by starting with "M," which stands for "measure the MAD (mechanical axis deviation)."

To determine the MAD, review an AP view full-length standing x-ray. Draw a mechanical axis line from the center of the femoral head to the center of the ankle. The ideal mechanical axis passes through the middle of the knee, thus the MAD is the distance measured between the mechanical axis and the center of the knee joint (Fig. 1). In obvious deformities, measuring the MAD allows you to objectively measure and document the preoperative deformity.

### A = Analyze the joint angles

The next step in the analysis is the "A" of the acronym: analyze the joint angles. This analysis will allow you to determine which limb segment is contributing to the deformity. First, draw the joint lines for the proximal and distal femur and the proximal and distal tibia. Next, draw the mechanical axis of the femur and the tibia. Finally, measure the appropriate joint orientation angles and compare them with the population normal (Table 2) or the normal opposite limb.

### P = Pick the deformed bones

The evaluation continues with the "P" in the acronym "MAP," which stands for picking the bone segment that is contributing to the deformity. Select the bone based on the above joint angle analysis and any clinically relevant factors.

Note: If there is a MAD present with obvious clinical deformity but the joint orientation angles are normal, then joint instability or incongruency is the underlying cause of the MAD.

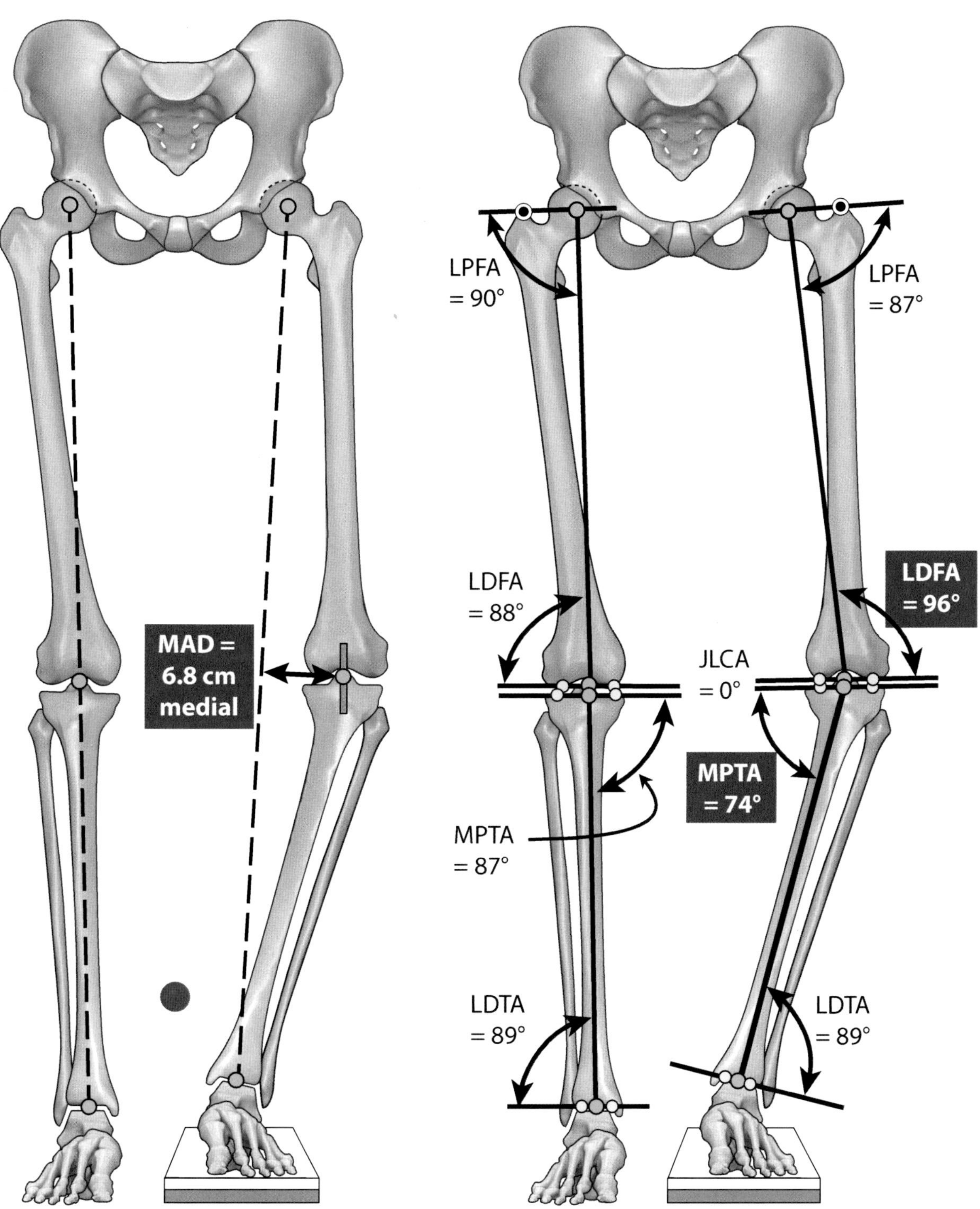


**Fig. 1:** The first step of MAP is "M", which is measuring the MAD. This example has obvious genu varum of the left lower extremity. Measuring the MAD allows you to objectively quantify and document the deformity. This patient has a medial MAD of 6.8 cm (magnification marker = 2.54 cm).

**Fig. 2:** The second step of MAP is "A", which is to analyze the joint angles. The analysis of the mechanical joint angles shows there are abnormalities of the LDFA and MPTA in the left lower extremity. This assessment points to contributing deformities from the femur and tibia.

## MAP: Analysis for Frontal Plane Case Example 1

The following example will explain each step in the MAP the ABC strategy in the frontal plane (Table 1).

### Step 1: Measure the MAD

We will begin with a full-length standing AP x-ray, and draw a mechanical axis line from the center of the femoral head to the center of the ankle. Establish the MAD by measuring the perpendicular distance between the center of the knee joint and the mechanical axis that was just drawn. A goal of corrective surgery is a mechanical axis that passes directly through the center of the knee (MAD = 0±3 mm). A value for MAD that is outside of this range is considered to be abnormal. The clinical significance of an abnormal MAD, or the need to correct the MAD, is determined by the patient's symptoms and the surgeon's clinical judgment. A person with normal limbs may have an MAD up to 17 mm medial, but this individual may be more prone to medial compartment arthritis in the future. Thus far, the following has been determined for the MAP portion of the analysis:

**MAP**

**M** = Measure the Mechanical Axis Deviation (MAD) = 6.8 cm medial

**A** = Analyze the joint angles

**P** = Pick the deformed bone

### Step 2: Analyze the joint angles

The next step in the analysis is the "A" of "MAP": analyze the joint angles (Fig. 2). This analysis will allow you to determine which limb segment is contributing to the deformity. First, draw the joint orientation lines for the proximal and distal femur and the proximal and distal tibia. Next, draw the mechanical axis of the femur and the tibia. Finally, measure the appropriate joint orientation angles and compare them with the population normal (Table 2) or the normal opposite limb. The analysis of the joint angles in Figure 2 and Table 2 shows that there are abnormalities in the LDFA and MPTA.

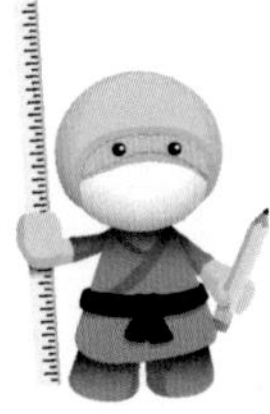

*Sensei says,*
*"Even though the proximal femoral angle is not typically relevant when there is a distal femoral deformity, it is always wise to measure all the angles."*

Students often ask whether to use the mechanical or anatomic axis when analyzing the joint angles. The mechanical axis of each bone segment is most often used during the MAP portion of the analysis because the overall goal in planning is to align the mechanical axis of the entire limb.

**MAP**

**M** = Measure the MAD = 6.8 cm medial

**A** = Analyze the joint angles: LDFA = 96°, MPTA = 74°

**P** = Pick the deformed bone

### Step 3: Pick the deformed bones

The third step is the "P" of the mnemonic, which stands for picking the bone segment that is contributing to the deformity. Bone selection is based on the above joint angle analysis and any clinically relevant factors. In this example, the joint angle analysis points to contributing factors from the femur and tibia (Fig. 2). Since both the femur and the tibia have abnormal values, we will pick both for surgical reconstruction.

In this case example, a simple initial observation would lead the surgeon to conclude that the patient has a straightforward varus deformity of the left tibia. However, by using the mnemonic MAP the ABCs, the surgeon is able to accurately determine that this deformity has multiple components. This concludes the MAP portion of the analysis.

**MAP**

**M** = Measure the Mechanical Axis Deviation (MAD) = 6.8 cm medial

**A** = Analyze the joint angles: LDFA = 96°, MPTA = 74°

**P** = Pick the deformed bones: Femur and tibia

## ABCs: An Overview

### A = Apex of deformity

The ABCs must be performed separately for each bone segment that you selected for correction. The first step of the ABCs is "A," which is to determine the apex of the deformity. The apex is the exact location of the deformity in the bone segment. The apex has previously been called the center of rotation of angulation (CORA). We now prefer the simpler term "apex."

To locate the apex of the deformity, draw the proximal and distal axes lines. The apex is located where the proximal axis and the distal axis intersect. Every bone segment, no matter how short, has an axis. The proximal axis is above the level of the deformity, and the distal axis is below the level of the deformity.

To create these lines in the femur, two different planning methodologies can be used: either anatomic axis planning or mechanical axis planning. Mechanical axis planning, although more complicated, is recommended in most cases as a direct method of realigning the mechanical axis of the limb. Anatomic axis planning is a more relevant planning strategy when intramedullary fixation is planned. We will use femoral mechanical axis planning for the illustrative example that follows. In the chapter entitled "Femoral Axis Planning: Frontal and Sagittal Planes," multiple strategies will be introduced that can be used to determine the proximal and distal axis lines of the femur.

### B = Bone cut

The next step in the ABCs is "B," which is to choose the location of the bone cut (i.e., level of the osteotomy). Ideally, the bone cut should be at the same level as the apex, which will allow the bony margins and proximal and distal axes to align perfectly. This creates an ideal correction that will have perfect mechanical and radiographic alignment. However, it is not always possible to choose a bone cute through the apex of the deformity, either from an anatomic, biologic, or mechanical stability point of view. Therefore, the surgeon needs to plan carefully and consider the amount of translation that will occur when the bone cut is not through the apex.

### C = Correction

The final step in the ABCs of the femur is "C," which is perform the bony correction. Acute correction and gradual correction use different methods to achieve the same outcome. Both correction methods require the placement of a hinge point that we call a thumbtack. In the original Ilizarov Method, a rudimentary mechanical hinge was placed onto a circular external fixation device and an osteotomy was rotated around that point. "Paper doll" planning methods of the past involved working with an outline drawing of deformed bones and cutting the paper doll at the osteotomy level. A thumbtack would be inserted at the planned hinge point and the paper doll would be angulated to mimic the operative correction. In the MAP the ABCs method, we refer to the rotational point of correction as a thumbtack, despite electronic planning applications eliminating any need for a literal and tactile tack. The thumbtack allows the distal fragment to angulate in relation to the proximal fragment.

## ABCs: Analysis for Frontal Plane Case Example 1, Femur

### Step 4: Apex of deformity (femur)

Single-level deformities have one apex in a bone segment. Complex deformities can have multiple apexes within the same bone segment. Case example 1 is a simple, single-level femoral deformity in the frontal plane.

In this example, create the proximal femoral axis (red line) by drawing the proximal femoral joint line and drawing a normal LPFA of 87° (Fig. 3A). This matches the LPFA of the normal contralateral limb. The surgeon can choose whether to use the value of the normal contralateral limb or the value that is the population normal. For more information on the proximal femoral axis, see "Identifying the Proximal Femoral Mechanical Axis in the Frontal Plane" and "Create Normal mLPFA Strategy," both in the chapter entitled "Femoral Axis Planning: Frontal and Sagittal Planes."

Create the distal femoral axis (blue line) by drawing the distal femoral joint line and then creating an LDFA of 88° from the center of the knee (Fig. 3A). The value of 88° is used because it matches the contralateral normal lower limb and is within the population normal for the LDFA. For more information on the

© 2023 Sinai Hospital of Baltimore

distal femoral axis, see "Identifying the Distal Femoral Mechanical Axis in the Frontal Plane" and "Create Normal mLDFA Strategy," both in the chapter entitled "Femoral Axis Planning: Frontal and Sagittal Planes."

The apex of the deformity is located where the proximal and distal femoral axes intersect (Fig. 3B). In this example, the distal segment that is below the level of the deformity is very short because the center of the deformity is located on the joint line. The magnitude of the deformity (8° varus) is the magnitude of the acute angle that is created by the intersection of the proximal and distal axes (Fig. 3B).

## ABCs (Femur)

**A** = Apex of deformity: Located on distal femoral joint line; Magnitude of deformity = 8° varus

**B** = Bone cut (choose the level of the osteotomy)

**C** = Correction

## Step 5: Bone cut (femur)

In this example, the apex is at the level of the joint. Obviously, an osteotomy cannot be performed at this level. The solution is to perform an osteotomy at a level that is feasible for the local anatomy and affords enough bone for mechanical fixation of the distal segment, while simultaneously being as close as possible to the apex. In this example, make the bone cut at the distal femoral metaphysis (Fig. 4). With this strategy, the osteotomy will allow for perfect alignment of the proximal and distal axes. However, the bony margins will demonstrate an obligatory translation at the osteotomy site. Translation is a linear shift in any plane. The amount of translation (7 mm in this example) is the distance between the proximal and distal axis lines at the level of the chosen osteotomy site (Fig. 4).

The amount of acceptable obligatory translation is surgeon dependent. Usually, at least 50% bone apposition is desired at the osteotomy site. Also,

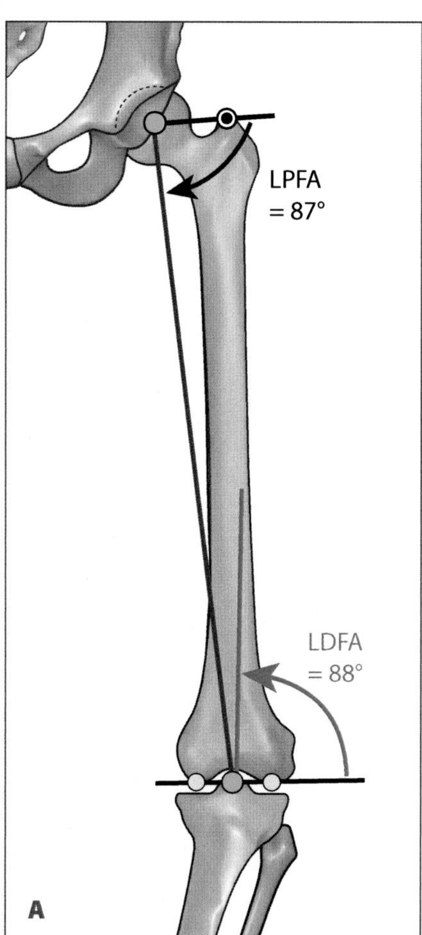


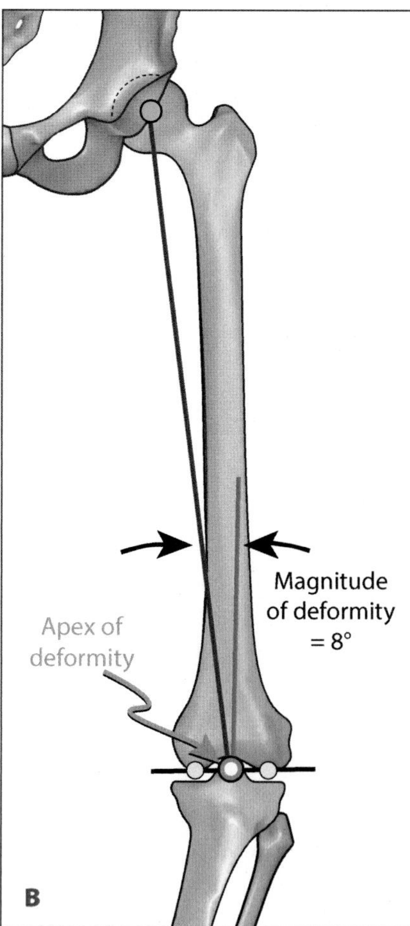


**Fig. 3: A**, The proximal femoral axis (*red line*) is created by drawing a normal LPFA (87°). The distal femoral axis (*blue line*) is created by drawing the distal femoral joint line and then forming an LDFA of 88° from the center of the knee. The value of 88° is used because it matches the contralateral normal lower limb and is within the population normal for the LDFA. **B**, The intersection of the proximal and distal axes is the apex of the deformity. Note that the apex is located on the distal femoral joint line. The magnitude of the deformity (8°) is the value of the acute angle that is formed at the apex.

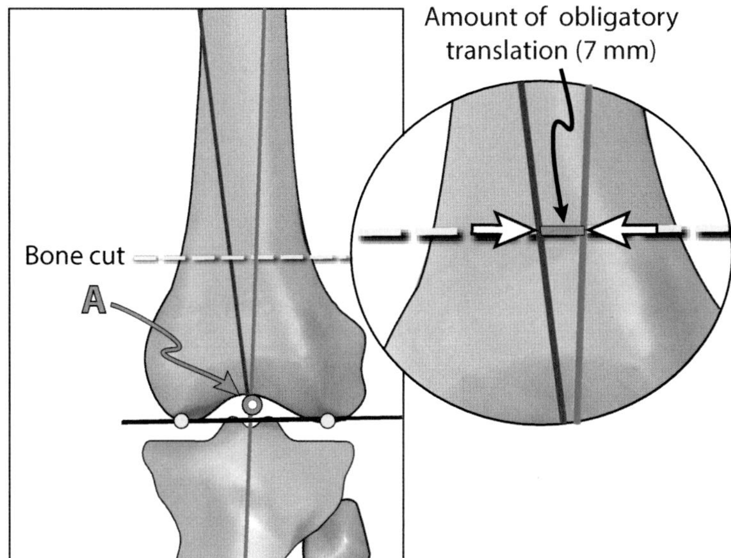


**Fig. 4:** The bone cut is placed as close as possible to the apex, but this location must be safe anatomically and afford adequate bone for stable fixation. Once the osteotomy level has been determined, the obligatory translation can be measured as the distance between the proximal and distal axis lines at the level of the bone cut (7 mm).

large translations that result in visible prominences may not be cosmetically appealing or acceptable to the patient.

### ABCs (Femur)

**A** = Apex of deformity: located on distal femoral joint line; Magnitude of deformity = 8° varus

**B** = Bone cut (choose the level of the osteotomy): Distal femoral metaphysis (not at level of apex)

**C** = Correction

### Step 6: Correction (femur)

In this example, we will demonstrate both gradual and acute correction of the femoral deformity (for brief descriptions of each strategy, see Table 1).

To determine the placement of the thumbtack, first locate the obtuse angle that is created by the intersection of the proximal and distal axes. In Figure 5A, the obtuse angle is 172°. Next, draw a line that bisects this obtuse angle and passes through the apex (Fig. 5A). This line is called the correction bisector line or correction level (C-level). The thumbtack (point of hinge rotation) must always be placed on the C-level. This will be discussed in more detail in the rules that appear later in this chapter. It is very important to note that, in this example, the thumbtack cannot be placed at the level of the bone cut. In Figure 5B, the thumbtack is placed on the C-level at the apex. The placement of the thumbtack results in a neutral wedge osteotomy with 7 mm of obligatory translation after the proximal and distal axes are aligned (Fig. 5C). Opening, closing, and neutral wedge osteotomies will be described in more detail when we perform the ABCs of the tibia.

In this particular example, an acute femoral correction would be the most common treatment approach. To acutely correct the deformity, perform a neutral wedge osteotomy. To align the proximal and distal femoral axes, translate the distal fragment medially 7 mm as planned during the analysis (Fig. 6). Then angulate the distal fragment until an LDFA of 88° is achieved (Fig. 5C). The summated motion of the acute translation and angulation is actually a single rotation about the thumbtack. It is important to plan acute corrections preoperatively and then match this pattern of translation and angulation when you are in the operating room.

Note that the convention is to consider rotation to be axial plane movement. Angulation is a coronal or sagittal plane rotation whereas translation is a linear shift in any plane. If required for acute correction, translation and/or rotation are always performed first. Angulation (if required for acute correction) is always performed last. Angulating an osteotomy will "lock" the bone fragment preventing or blocking translation or axial rotation.

© 2023 Sinai Hospital of Baltimore 

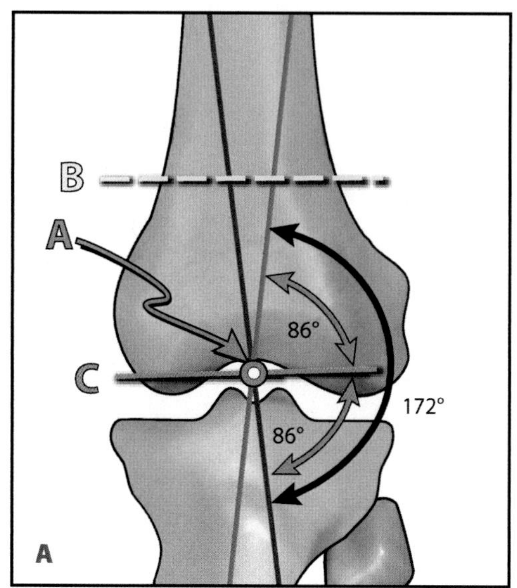


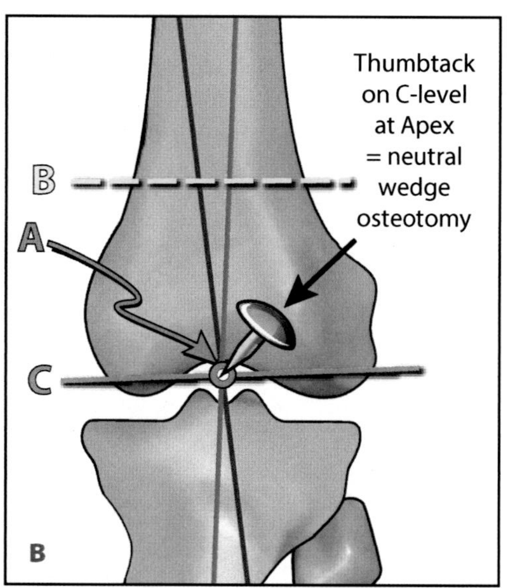


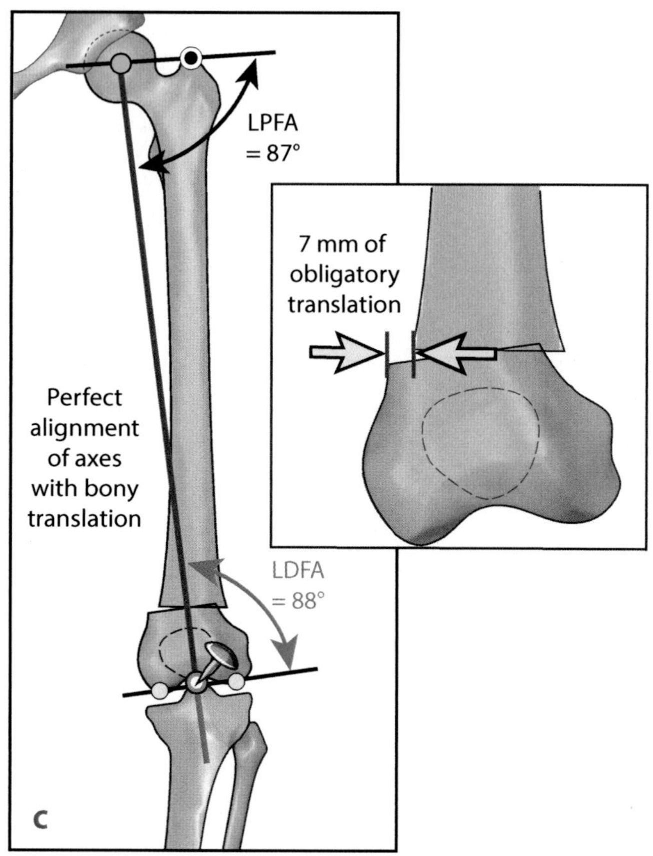


**Fig. 5: A**, To determine the placement of the thumbtack, identify the obtuse angle (172°) that is created by the intersection of the proximal and distal axes. The C-level (*orange line*) bisects this obtuse angle and passes through the apex (*A*). **B**, The thumbtack is placed on the C-level at the apex, which results in a neutral wedge osteotomy. **C**, The proximal and distal axes are aligned so that the goal of planning, a final LDFA of 88°, is achieved along with the expected obligatory translation. Note the impaction that occurs on the convex side of the deformity. B, bone cut; C, C-level.

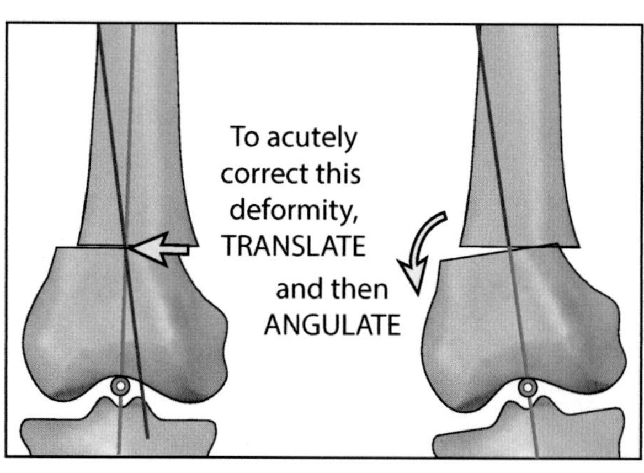


**Fig. 6:** To perform this acute correction, translate and then angulate the bone segment to match the pattern of translation and angulation that you determined during preoperative planning. Note that the net effect of this translation and angulation is that you are angulating the distal fragment around the thumbtack that you placed in Figure 5B.

To perform a gradual correction, perform an osteotomy and then gradually angulate the bone segment around the thumbtack until the proximal and distal axes are aligned (Fig. 5C). During gradual correction, the thumbtack represents the mechanical hinge of an Ilizarov or TrueLok device (Orthofix, Inc., Lewisville, TX). The thumbtack can also represent a virtual hinge that is used in a six-axis external fixation system or hexapod. For gradual correction, it is critical to place the thumbtack at the correct location.

### ABCs (Femur)

**A** = Apex of deformity: Located on distal femoral joint line; Magnitude of deformity = 8° varus

**B** = Bone cut (choose the level of the osteotomy): Distal femoral metaphysis (not at level of apex)

**C** = Correction: Gradual or acute correction with a neutral wedge osteotomy and obligatory translation (since bone cut not at level of apex)

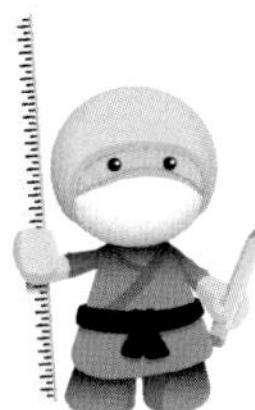

*Sensei says,*
*"The wise surgeon will place the bone cut as close as possible to the apex, but always, always place the thumbtack on the C-level."*

## ABCs: Analysis for Frontal Plane Case Example 1, Tibia

### Step 7: Apex of deformity (tibia)

Since the ABCs must be performed separately for each bone segment that was selected for correction, the tibial segment is now ready to be addressed. To locate the apex of the deformity, use the proximal and distal mechanical axis lines of the tibia. In the chapter entitled "Tibial Axis Planning: Frontal and Sagittal Planes," multiple strategies will be presented that can be used to determine the proximal and distal axis lines of the tibia.

To determine the proximal axis of the tibia, extend the normal femoral mechanical axis into the proximal tibia (Fig. 7). This strategy assumes that the knee joint lines are parallel or nearly parallel (normal JLCA) and that the LDFA is normal. This extended femoral mechanical axis is now the proximal tibial axis. For more information on the proximal axis of the tibia, see "Identifying the Proximal Tibial Axis in the Frontal Plane" and, because it was determined the LDFA is now normal in the corrected femur, we can use the "Normal Femoral Mechanical Axis Strategy," both found in the chapter entitled "Tibial Axis Planning: Frontal and Sagittal Planes."

To create the distal tibial axis, draw a simple mid-diaphyseal axis (Fig. 8). For more information

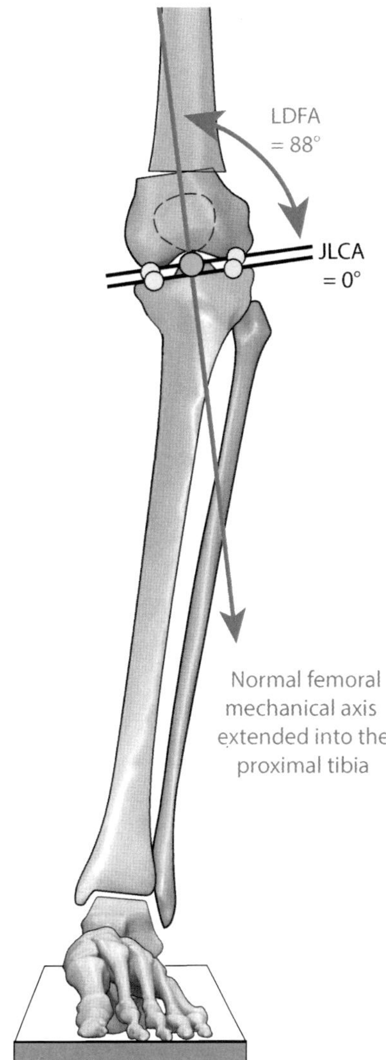


**Fig. 7:** To draw the proximal tibial axis, extend the normal femoral mechanical axis into the proximal tibia.

© 2023 Sinai Hospital of Baltimore

on the distal axis of the tibia, see "Identifying the Distal Tibial Axis in the Frontal Plane" and "Mid-diaphyseal Line Strategy," both in the chapter entitled "Tibial Axis Planning: Frontal and Sagittal Planes." To check for a hidden deformity, measure the LDTA formed by the mid-diaphyseal line. In this example, the LDTA is normal, which means that a hidden deformity does not exist near the ankle.

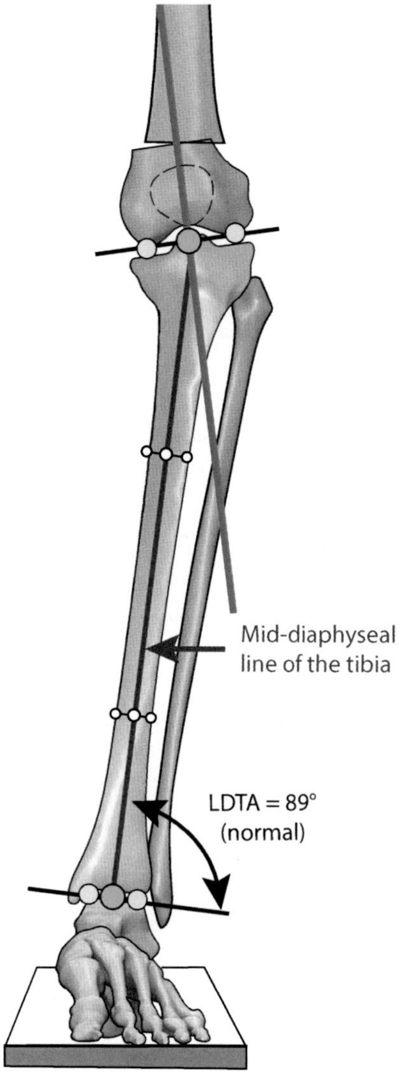

Mid-diaphyseal line of the tibia

LDTA = 89° (normal)

**Fig. 8:** To determine the distal tibial axis, use a simple mid-diaphyseal line (*red line*). When using this strategy, it is mandatory to measure the LDTA formed by the mid-diaphyseal line to ensure a hidden deformity does not exist. In this case, the LDTA is 89°, which is within the normal range. If the LDTA is abnormal, then a distal metaphyseal deformity needs to be identified and addressed.

If the LDTA was abnormal, then the tibia might have a distal metaphyseal deformity that would need to be addressed. Note that an abnormal LDTA would indicate a multiapical deformity. The distal "hidden" apex would be located by using the "Normal LDTA Strategy" (see the chapter entitled "Tibial Axis Planning: Frontal and Sagittal Planes") to identify the distal axis line.

The apex is located at the intersection of the proximal and distal tibial axes (Fig. 9). The magnitude of the acute angle that is created by the intersection of the proximal and distal axes is the magnitude of deformity, which is 14° (varus).

### ABCs (Tibia)

**A** = Apex of deformity: Located in the proximal tibia; Magnitude of deformity = 14° varus

**B** = Bone cut (choose the level of the osteotomy)

**C** = Correction

### Step 8: Bone cut (tibia)

The next step is to choose the level of the bone cut. The ideal osteotomy site is at the level of the apex. This will be discussed in more detail in the rules that appear later in this chapter. In this example, the level of the apex would not be anatomically feasible. For this example, make the bone cut in the proximal tibia, which is distal to the apex but still as close as possible to the apex to decrease the obligatory translation (Fig. 10). The amount of translation (16 mm in this example) is the distance between the proximal and distal axis lines at the level of the chosen osteotomy site. This obligatory translation is normally acceptable; however, the amount and position of the translation must be preoperatively determined by the surgeon to ensure the acceptability.

### ABCs (Tibia)

**A** = Apex of deformity: Located in the proximal tibia; Magnitude of deformity = 14° varus

**B** = Bone cut (choose the level of the osteotomy): Proximal tibia (not at level of apex)

**C** = Correction

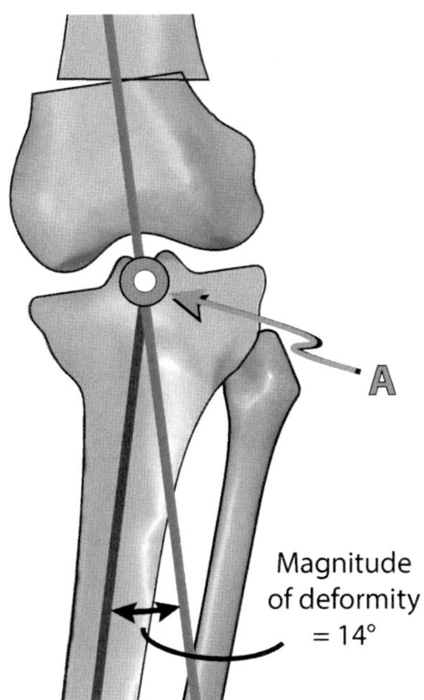


Fig. 9: The intersection of the proximal and distal tibial axes is the apex (*A*) of the deformity and the ideal correction level. The magnitude of the deformity is the value of the acute angle (14°) that is created by the intersection of the proximal and distal axes.

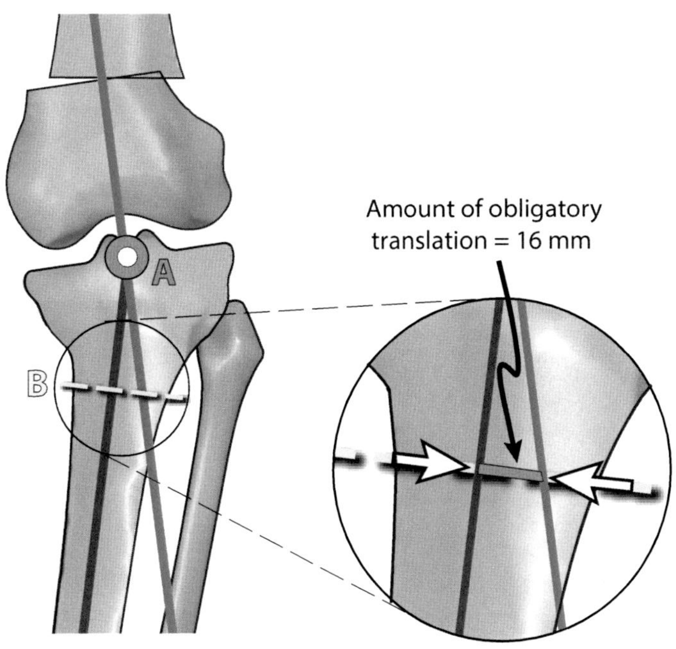


Fig. 10: Place the bone cut (*B*) as close as possible to the apex to reduce the necessary translation and yet allow enough bone for adequate fixation. A, apex.

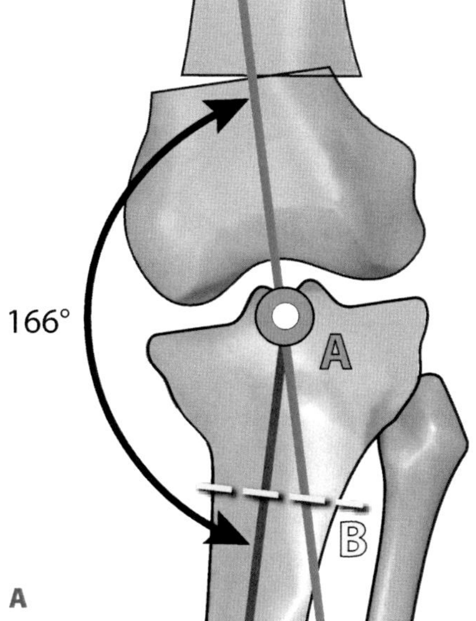


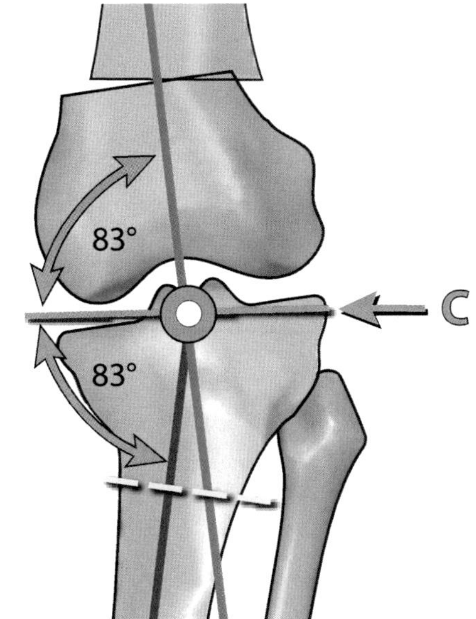


Fig. 11: A, To determine the placement of the thumbtack, identify the obtuse angle (166°) that is created by the intersection of the proximal and distal axes. B, The C-level (*orange line*) bisects this obtuse angle and passes through the apex. A, apex; B, bone cut; C, C-level.

© 2023 Sinai Hospital of Baltimore 

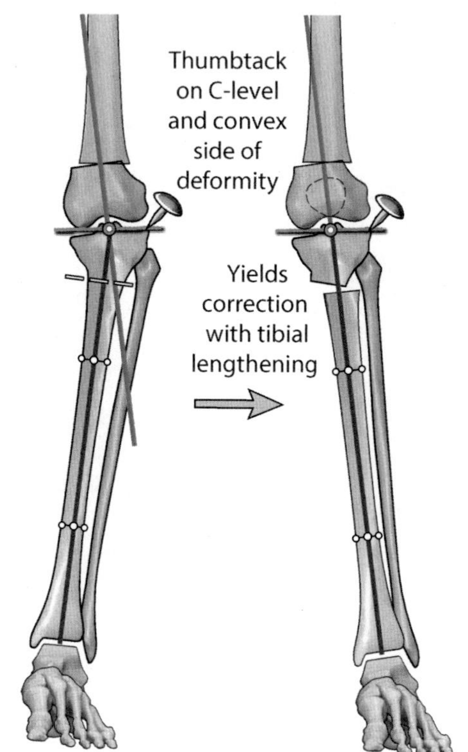


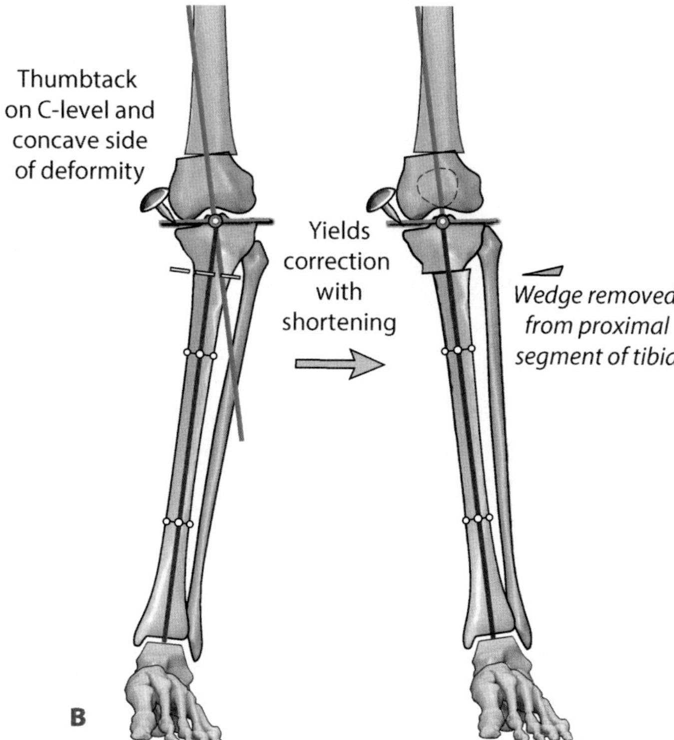


**Fig. 12:** These panels show what happens when the thumbtack is placed at various locations along the C-level. **A**, Opening wedge osteotomy. **B**, Closing wedge osteotomy. **C**, Neutral wedge osteotomy.

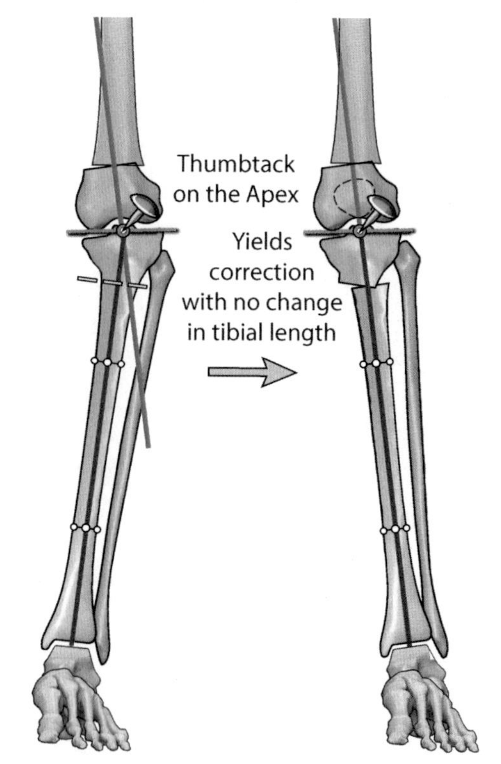


**Table 3**

**Opening Wedge Osteotomy**

- Thumbtack placed on the C-level on the convex side of the deformity (Fig. 12A)
- Results in correction with lengthening (distraction)

**Closing Wedge Osteotomy**

- Thumbtack placed on the C-level on the concave side of the deformity (Fig. 12B)
- Results in correction with shortening (compression)

**Neutral Wedge**

- Thumbtack placed on the apex (Fig. 12C)
- Results in correction with no change in bone length (distraction and compression)

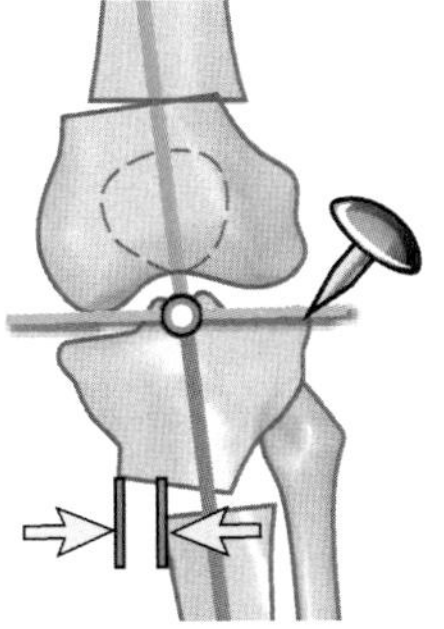
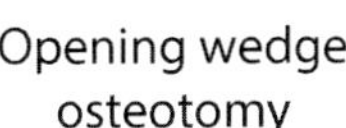
Opening wedge osteotomy

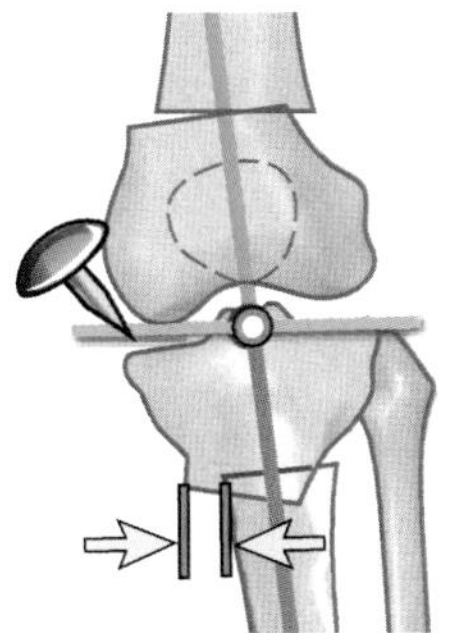
Closing wedge osteotomy

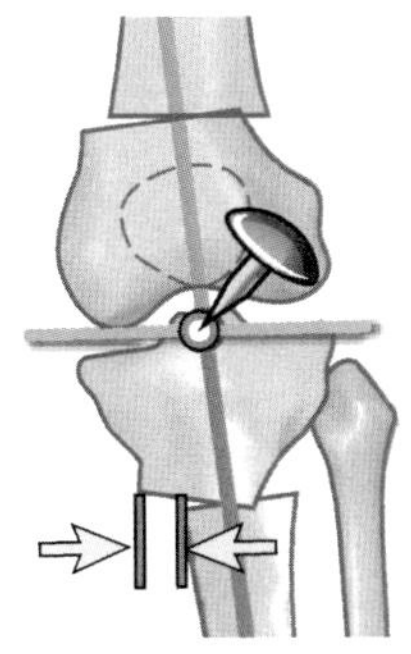
Neutral wedge osteotomy

**Fig. 13:** When the osteotomy is not on the same level as the apex, bony translation will occur (*yellow arrows*). Note the obligatory translation for all types of osteotomies in this particular example.

## Step 9: Correction (tibia)

The final step in the ABCs of the tibia is to perform the correction. In this example, we will perform a gradual correction of the tibia. To determine the placement of the thumbtack, first locate the obtuse angle that is created by the intersection of the proximal and distal axes (166°; Fig. 11A). Next, draw a C-level that bisects the obtuse angle and passes through the apex (Fig. 11B).

Place the thumbtack on the C-level. Whether you correct the deformity by performing an opening, closing, or neutral wedge osteotomy is dependent on the position of the thumbtack in relation to the deformity (Table 3). An opening wedge osteotomy (Fig. 12A) occurs when the thumbtack is placed on the C-level on the convex side of the deformity. This osteotomy results in correction with lengthening. A closing wedge osteotomy (Fig. 12B) occurs when the thumbtack is placed on the C-level on the concave side of the deformity. This osteotomy results in correction with shortening. A neutral wedge osteotomy (Fig. 12C) occurs when the thumbtack is placed on the apex. This osteotomy results in correction with no change in length. Whenever the osteotomy is not at the level of the apex, obligatory bony translation will occur (Fig. 13). The farther the thumbtack is moved along the C-level line away from the apex, the greater the lengthening or shortening is increased.

The thumbtack must always be on the C-level to ensure the proximal and distal axes will align perfectly after correction is achieved (Fig. 14). If the thumbtack is not placed on the C-level, the axis lines will be parallel and offset after correction (Fig. 15). This will result in under correction of the deformity and an abnormal MAD. In this scenario, the osteotomy will need to be overcorrected to align the mechanical axis. However, the overcorrection to align the mechanical axis will result in malaligning the ankle joint with an unacceptable LDTA of 84° (Fig. 15C). Refer to Rule #2 in the following section for more information.

© 2023 Sinai Hospital of Baltimore

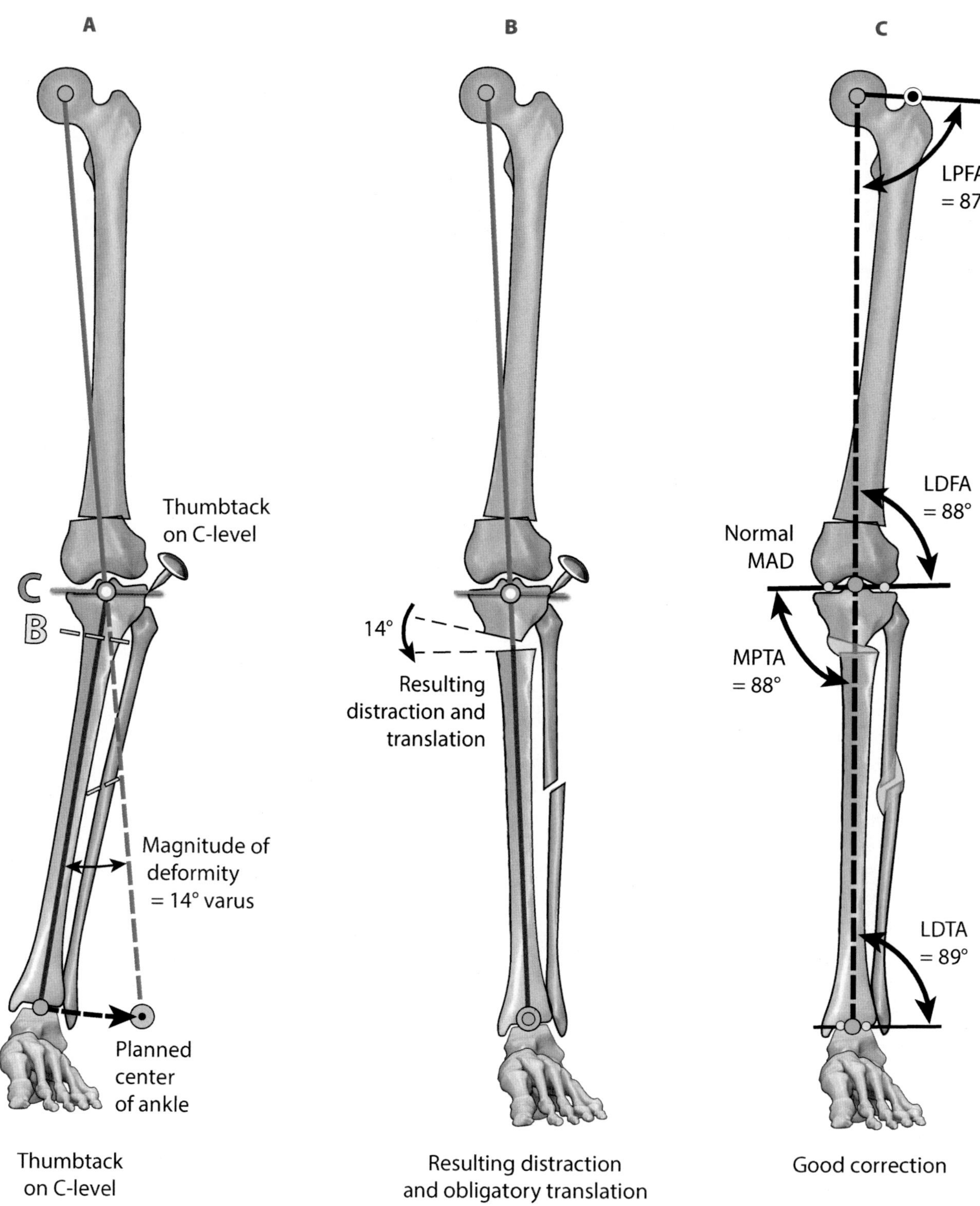


**Fig. 14: A,** The thumbtack is placed on the C-level. **B,** Correcting the deformity results in distraction and obligatory translation, but the proximal and distal axis lines are perfectly aligned. **C,** A good correction is achieved in which the mechanical axis passes through the center of the knee and all the joint orientation angles are normal. B, bone cut; C, C-level.

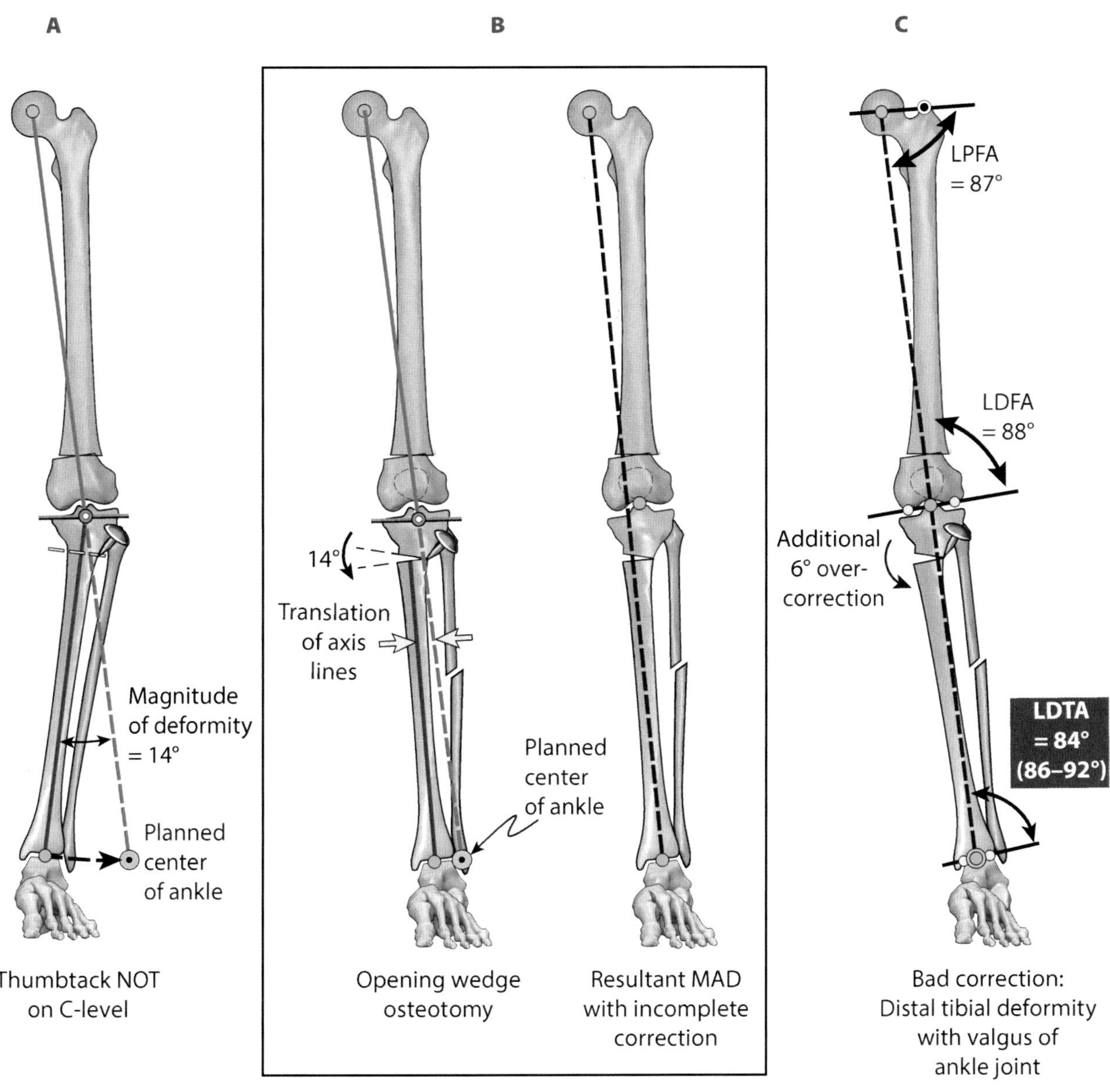


**Fig. 15: A**, The thumbtack is placed incorrectly on the bone cut instead of on the C-level. **B**, After gradual correction, this results in translation of the axis lines so that they are parallel and not aligned. This residual translational deformity is subtle, but it results in an incomplete correction of the mechanical axis. Deformity correction has not been achieved because the deformity is under corrected and an abnormal MAD still exists. **C**, Aligning the distal tibial segment to the normal mechanical axis can only be accomplished by over rotating the distal fragment around the erroneously placed thumbtack. The overcorrection of the osteotomy site allows for the center of the ankle to be aligned with the normal mechanical axis. However, this overcorrection has resulted in malalignment of the ankle joint. The ankle joint, which had a normal LDTA of 89° during the initial joint angle analysis, has now been altered to an LDTA of 84°. This change in the LDTA occurred because the thumbtack was placed incorrectly.

© 2023 Sinai Hospital of Baltimore

**Table 4. Summary of Case Example 1 (Figures 1–11, 14, 16)**

**MAP**

**M** = Measure the MAD = 6.8 cm medial

**A** = Analyze the joint angles: LDFA = 96°
MPTA = 74°

**P** = Pick the deformed bones: Femur and tibia

**ABCs (Femur)**

**A** = Apex of deformity: Located on distal femoral joint line; Magnitude of deformity = 8° varus

**B** = Bone cut (choose the level of the osteotomy): Distal femoral metaphysis (not at level of apex)

**C** = Correction: Gradual or acute correction with a neutral wedge osteotomy and obligatory translation (since bone cut not at level of apex)

**ABCs (Tibia)**

**A** = Apex of deformity: Located in the proximal tibia; Magnitude of deformity = 14° varus

**B** = Bone cut (choose the level of the osteotomy): Proximal tibia (not at level of apex)

**C** = Correction: Gradual correction with opening wedge osteotomy and obligatory translation (since bone cut not at level of apex)

Figure 16 summarizes the planning and shows the correction of the example used throughout the first part of this chapter. In the femur, the thumbtack is placed on the C-level at the apex (Fig. 16D). This thumbtack location results in a neutral wedge osteotomy with no lengthening. In the tibia, the thumbtack is placed on the C-level on the convex side of the deformity resulting in an opening wedge osteotomy with lengthening (Fig. 16G). Both the femoral and tibial correction will have obligatory translation. By following the MAP the ABCs process, we have accomplished a complete analysis of this case and have formulated a surgical strategy that will result in a normal mechanical axis and normal lower limb alignment (Table 4).

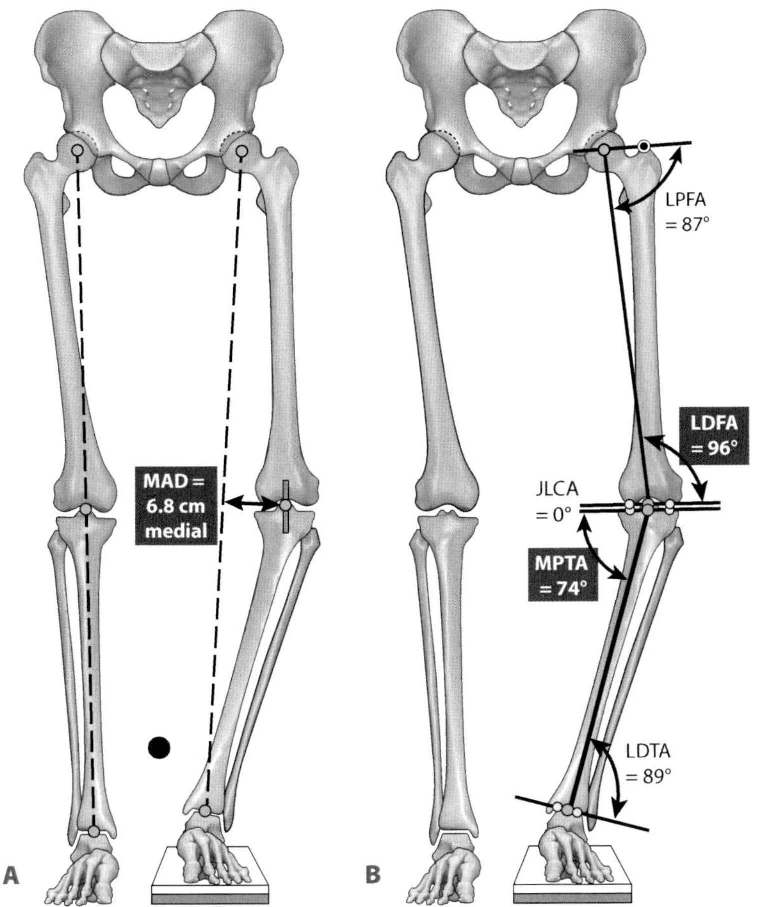


**Fig. 16:** Summary of MAP the ABCs for case example 1. **A** and **B**, The left limb had an abnormal MAD, LDFA, and MPTA. Both the femur and the tibia have deformities. **C**, The femur was corrected first. The proximal axis (*red line*) was drawn by creating a normal LPFA of 87°. The distal femoral axis (*blue line*) was drawn by creating an LDFA of 88°, matching the contralateral LDFA. The apex was at the level of the knee joint, and the magnitude of the deformity was 8°. **D** and **E**, The bone cut was made proximal to the apex, which resulted in obligatory translation. The correction level (C-level) passed through the apex and bisected the obtuse angle that was formed at the intersection of the proximal and distal axis lines. The thumbtack was placed on the C-level at the apex, which resulted in a neutral wedge osteotomy and full correction of the femur. Note the obligatory translation because the bone cut was not able to be made at the apex. B, bone cut; C, C-level.

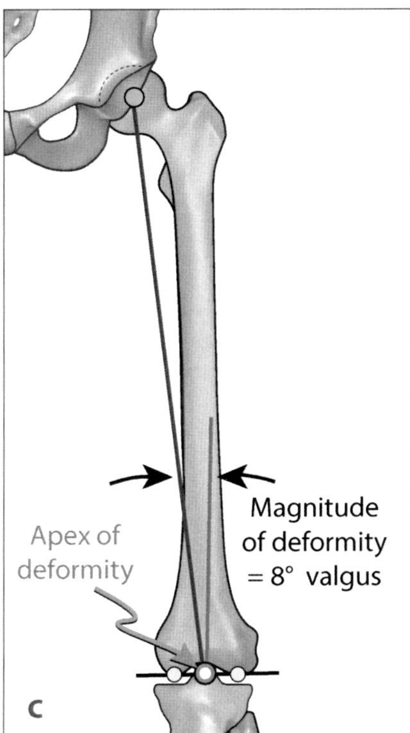


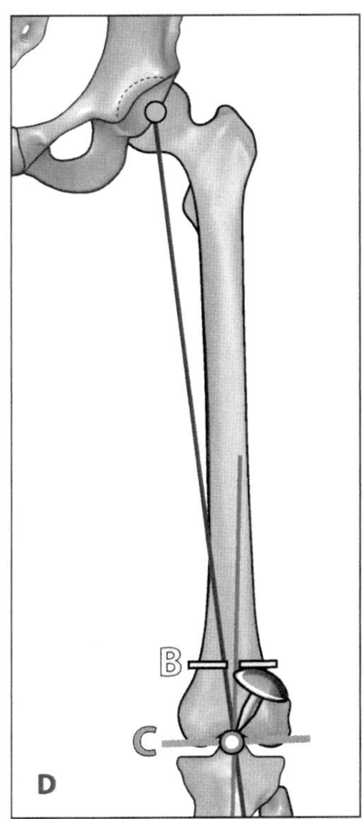


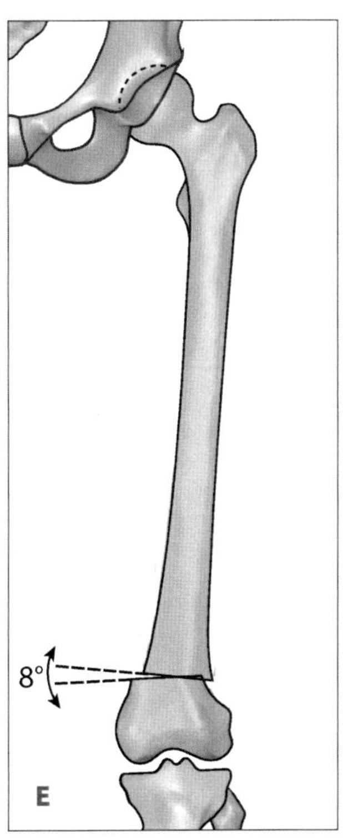


© 2023 Sinai Hospital of Baltimore

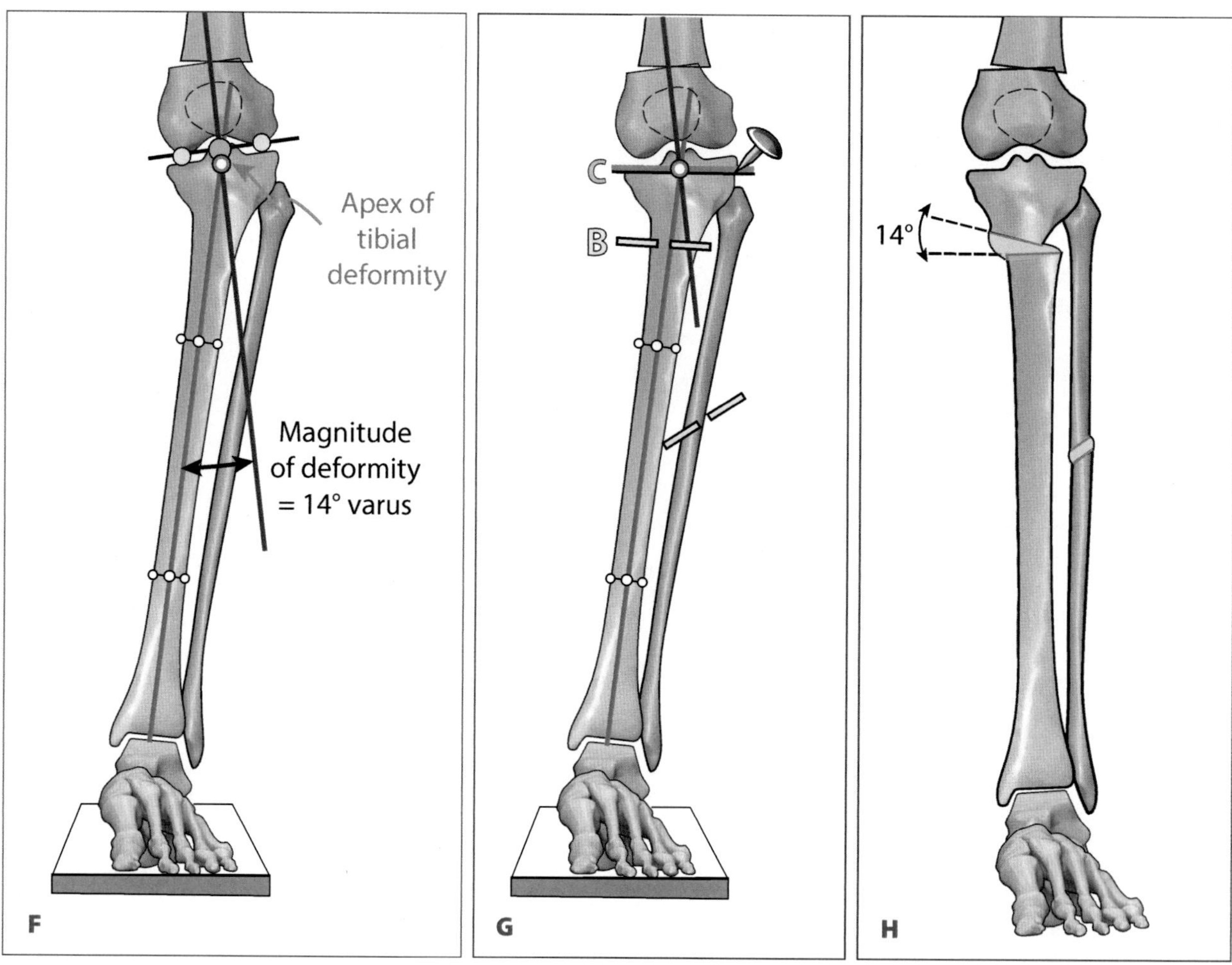


**Fig. 16 (continued): F**, Since the femoral correction resulted in a normal femur, the normal femoral mechanical axis was able to be extended into the proximal tibia to create the proximal tibial axis (*red line*). The tibial mid-diaphyseal line was used as the distal tibial axis (*blue line*). The apex was at the intersection of the proximal and distal axis lines, and the magnitude of deformity was 14°. **G** and **H**, The tibial and fibular bone cut were made distal to the apex. The C-level passed through the apex and bisected the obtuse angle that was formed at the intersection of the proximal and distal axis lines. The thumbtack was placed on the C-level on the convex side of the deformity, which resulted in an opening wedge osteotomy. Note the obligatory translation because the bone cut was not able to be made at the apex. B, bone cut; C, C-level.

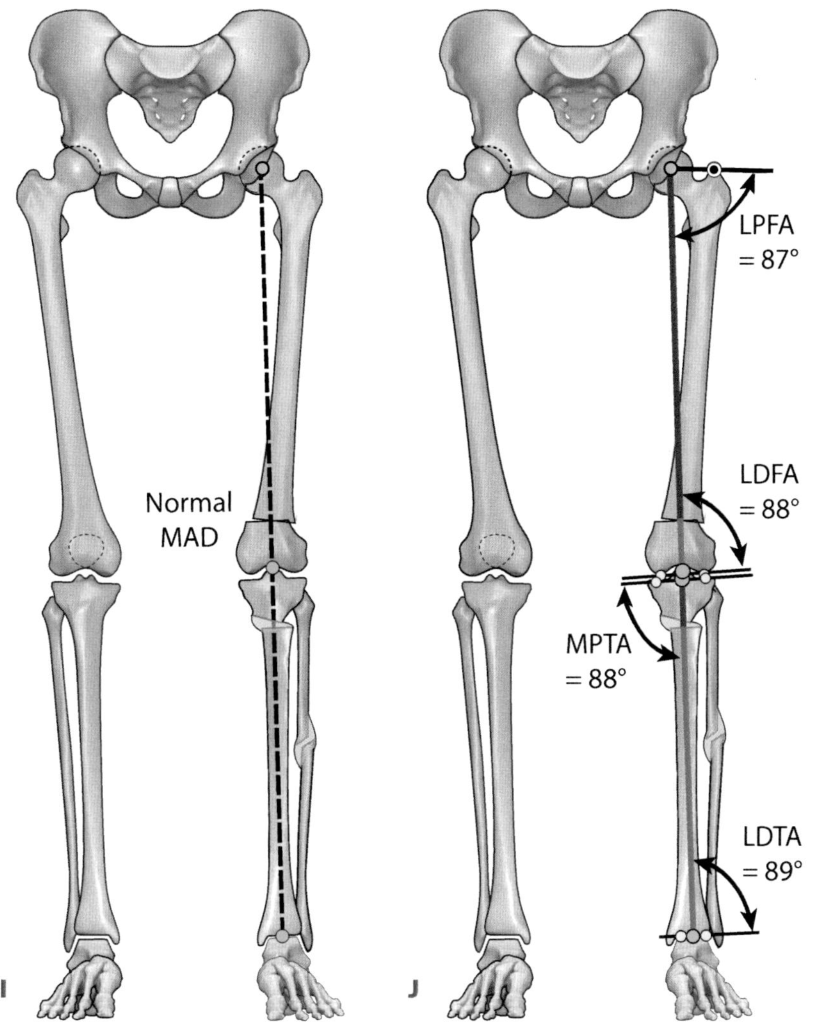


**Fig. 16 (continued): I** and **J**, The MAD, LDFA, and MPTA were corrected to normal values. The LPFA and LDTA remained normal and did not change during treatment.

## Osteotomy Rules and Considerations

After completing Example 1 in MAP the ABCs, a review of osteotomy rules and considerations is appropriate. When correcting a malaligned limb, the locations of the apex of deformity and the C-level are both out of the surgeon's control. However, the surgeon does have control over determining the location of the osteotomy as well as the placement of the hinge point of correction (thumbtack) along the C-level. The osteotomy site and thumbtack position will both affect the final osteotomy appearance and axis alignment.

### Rule 1: Place Osteotomy as Close to Apex as Possible

Because the osteotomy location and thumbtack are determined by the surgeon, osteotomy guidelines are essential to obtain axis alignment and acceptable bony alignment. The guiding principle of the osteotomy is to perform it as near to the apex of deformity as possible (Fig. 17). The farther the osteotomy is from the apex, the farther the bony margins will shift or translate. This shifting of bony margins is called obligatory translation. There are three possible osteotomy scenarios, each with their own outcomes or consequences.

#### Osteotomy Scenario #1

When the osteotomy is placed at the same location as the apex of deformity,

- The proximal and distal bone segment axes align
- The bone margins align (Fig. 18)

#### Osteotomy Scenario #2

When the osteotomy is placed at a different level than the apex of deformity,

- The proximal and distal bone segment axes align
- The bone margins do not align (Fig. 19)

### Rule 2: Place Thumbtack Along the C-level

There is only one thumbtack rule: It must always be on the C-level. The C-level is defined as the bisector of the obtuse angle formed from the intersection of the proximal and distal axes. Each deformity creates an acute and obtuse angle. The acute angle created by the proximal and distal bone segment axes is the magnitude of deformity. This acute angle has an accompanying obtuse angle. The bisector line of this obtuse angle passes through the apex and is the C-level. In osteotomy scenarios 1 and 2, the thumbtack is located on the C-level. Osteotomy scenario 3 pertains to the location of the thumbtack.

#### Osteotomy Scenario #3

When the thumbtack is placed away from the C-level,

- The proximal and distal bone segment axes do not align
- The bony margins do not align (Fig. 20)

The acceptability of the preceding osteotomy scenarios in any given situation is relative and depends on the entire clinical picture. However, the osteotomy guidelines should be viewed as follows by the novice deformity surgeon:

**Osteotomy Scenario #1: Preferred**

**Osteotomy Scenario #2: Acceptability is relative**

**Osteotomy Scenario #3: Should be avoided**

The final concept of thumbtack placement is the effect its location along the C-level line has upon the osteotomy. The C-level is technically a plane but may be easier to understand as a line within either the coronal or sagittal plane. The exact location of the thumbtack along this line/plane will result in variable osteotomy characteristics as the angular correction occurs (Fig. 21).

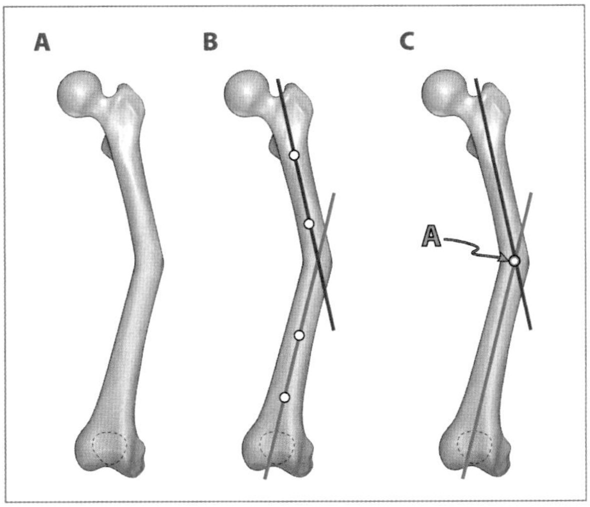

**Fig. 17:** **A**, Left femoral varus deformity. **B**, Anatomic planning. **C**, the apex at the obvious level of deformity. A, apex.

**Scenario 1: Preferred**

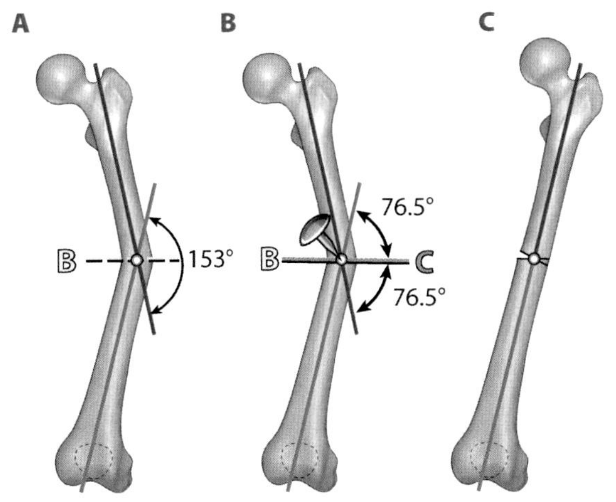


**Fig. 18:** Osteotomy scenario #1. **A**, The osteotomy (*dotted yellow line*) is placed at the same location as the apex of deformity. **B**, The thumbtack is placed on the apex on the C-level (*orange line*). **C**, The result is perfect alignment of the axis and perfect alignment of the bony margins. B, bone cut; C, C-level.

**Scenario 2: Relative Acceptability**

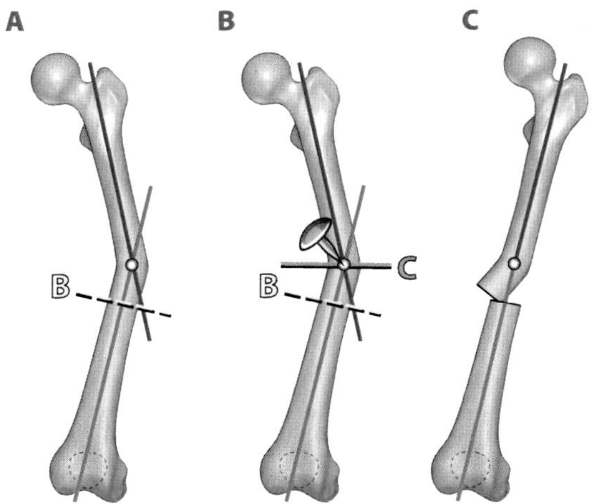


**Fig. 19:** Osteotomy scenario #2. **A**, The osteotomy (*dotted yellow line*) is placed distal to the apex. **B**, The thumbtack is placed on the apex on the C-level (*orange line*). **C**, The result is perfect alignment of the axes but bony margins are not aligned due to obligatory translation. The bony margin alignment is due to the placement of the osteotomy away from the C-level. B, bone cut; C, C-level.

**Scenario 3: Avoid**

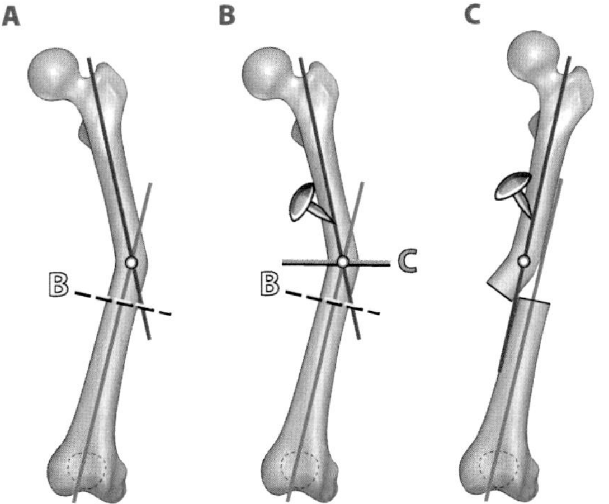


**Fig. 20:** Osteotomy scenario #3. **A**, The osteotomy (*dotted yellow line*) is placed distal to the apex. **B**, The thumbtack erroneously has been placed away from the C-level. **C**, The result is malalignment of both axes and bony margins. B, bone cut; C, C-level.

© 2023 Sinai Hospital of Baltimore

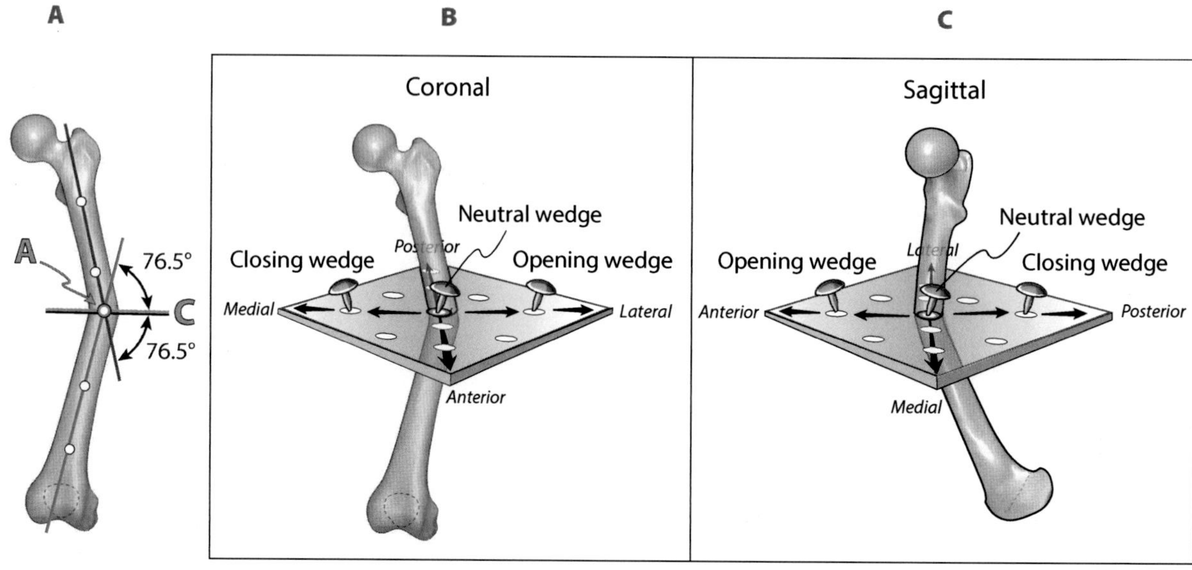


**Fig. 21: A**, The apex is along the C-level, which appears here as a line in the coronal view. **B**, The C-level is demonstrated more accurately as a plane; the thumbtack could concievably be placed anywhere within this plane. The position of potential thumbtack points for opening and closing wedge osteotomies in the coronal plane are demonstrated. **C**, The C-level is again demonstrated as a plane; the thumbtack could concievably be placed anywhere within this plane. The position of potential thumbtack points for opening and closing wedge osteotomies in the sagittal plane are demonstrated. A, apex; C, C-level.

### Thumbtack Scenario #1: On the apex of the deformity

The osteotomy will be a neutral wedge osteotomy with an opening wedge osteotomy on the concave side of the bone and a closing wedge osteotomy on the convex side of the bone. There is no change in length at the osteotomy site (Fig. 22A).

### Thumbtack Scenario #2: On the convex side of the deformity

The osteotomy will be an opening wedge osteotomy with length gain at the osteotomy site. The farther the thumbtack is placed from the apex on the convex side of the correction level, the more length is gained at the osteotomy (Figs. 22B, 22C).

### Thumbtack Scenario #3: On the concave side of the deformity

The osteotomy will be a closing wedge osteotomy with shortening/compression at the osteotomy site. The farther the thumbtack is placed from the apex on the concave side of the correction level, the more shortening or compression occurs at the osteotomy (Figs. 22D, 22E).

Although current 3D corrective devices (computer-assisted hexapod external fixators) nullify a true "hinge point," the above rules and concepts are still relative to understand how a deformity correction is occurring and how to achieve the anticipated goal of normal alignment.

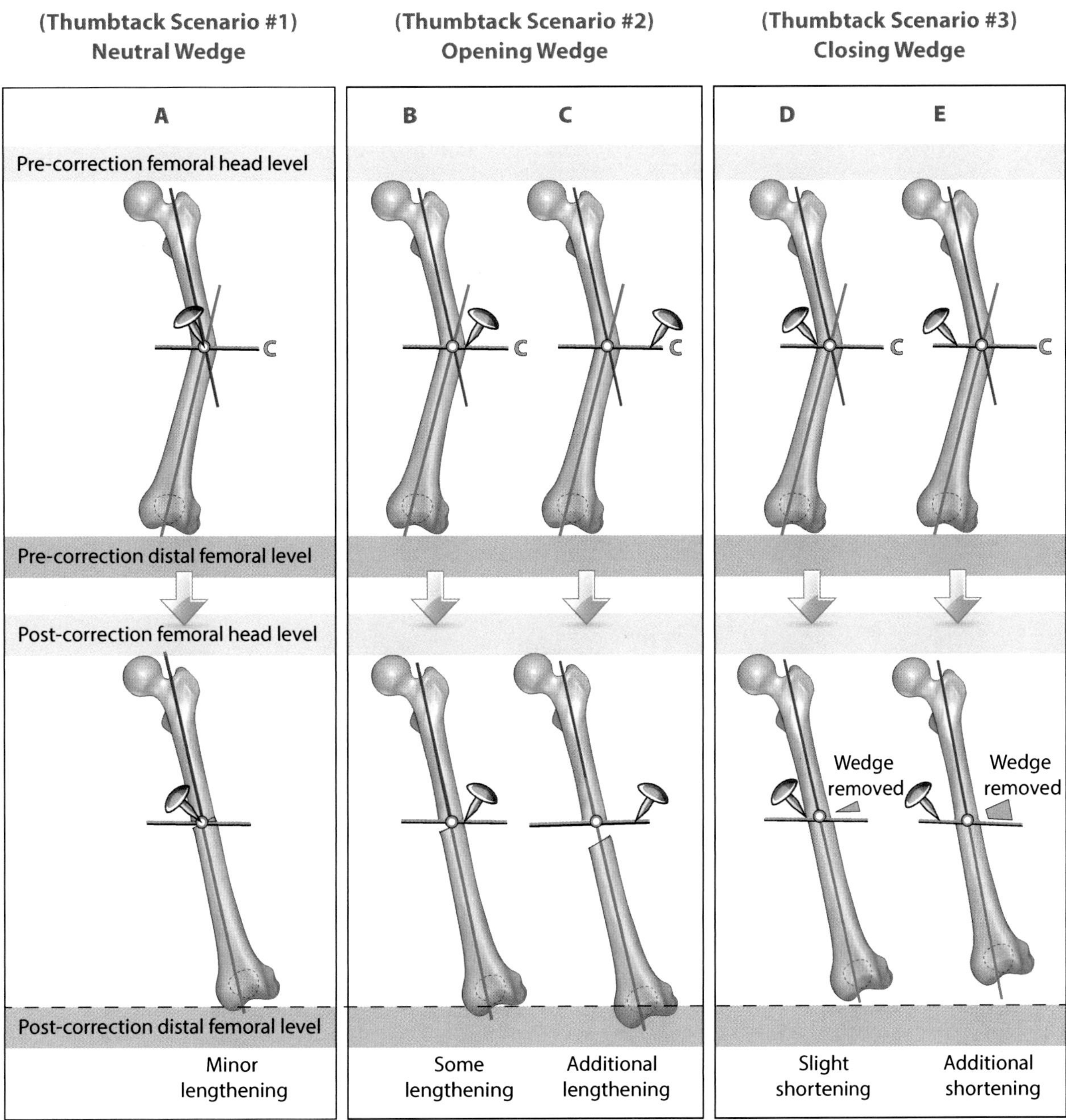


**Fig. 22: A**, The thumbtack is at the apex, resulting in a neutral wedge osteotomy after angular correction. **B**, The thumbtack is placed on the convex surface of the deformity, resulting in an opening wedge osteotomy after angular correction. The opening wedge osteotomy technique adds length to the bone segment. **C**, The thumbtack is placed along the C-level further away from the convexity of the deformity, resulting in perfect alignment of the axes and concurrent distraction/lengthening of the osteotomy site. **D**, The thumbtack is placed on the concavity of the bone deformity, which results in a closing wedge osteotomy and shortening of the limb segment. **E**, The thumbtack is along the C-level further away from the concavity of the deformity, resulting in axial alignment with angular correction and shortening/compression. C, C-level.

© 2023 Sinai Hospital of Baltimore 

## Osteotomy Considerations

Now that the concept of making the osteotomy at the level of the apex of deformity is established, what does the surgeon need to consider when deciding the exact location of an osteotomy in the "real world?"

### Osteotomy Consideration #1: Axis alignment supersedes bony alignment

The goal of limb deformity treatment is the correction of the mechanical or anatomic axis of the bone segment or limb. The bone alignment at the osteotomy site is relative; bone margins do not necessarily need to align. Successful surgery requires the re-establishment of a normal mechanical axis in the coronal and sagittal planes. The goals of bony alignment are bone healing and avoidance of unacceptable bony prominences. With the advancements of surgical implants, exact bony alignment is not needed for stability. In other words, axis alignment trumps bone margin alignment (Fig. 23A).

### Osteotomy Consideration #2: Cause no harm

The apex of deformity might occur at the level of a joint or a physis. Using this location for an osteotomy is not feasible without damaging the joint or growth plate. This is a common reason for osteotomy scenario #2. The amount of obligatory translation or bone shift can be determined preoperatively. The distance between the proximal and distal axis lines at the level of planned osteotomy is equal to the amount of obligatory translation that will occur after realignment (Figs. 23B, 23C, and 24).

**A**

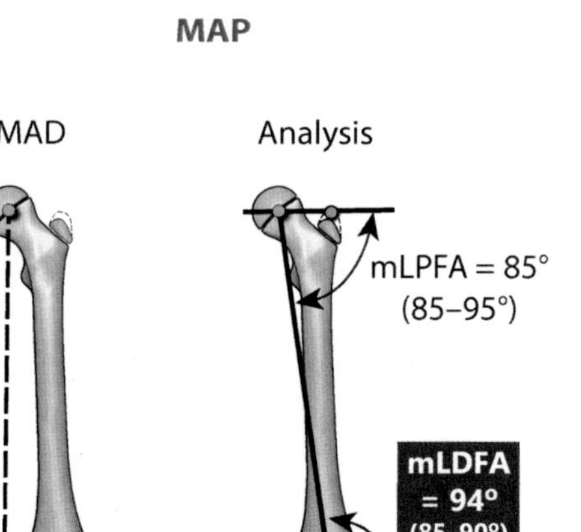


**Fig. 23: A,** Typical appearance of genu varus secondary to Blount disease with the analysis demonstrating mild deformity of the distal femur (mLDFA of 94°) and significant deformity of the proximal tibia (MPTA of 77°). JLCA, joint line convergence angle; LDTA, lateral distal tibial angle; MAD, mechanical axis deviation; mLDFA, mechanical lateral distal femoral angle; mLPFA, mechanical lateral proximal femoral angle; MPTA, medial proximal tibial angle.

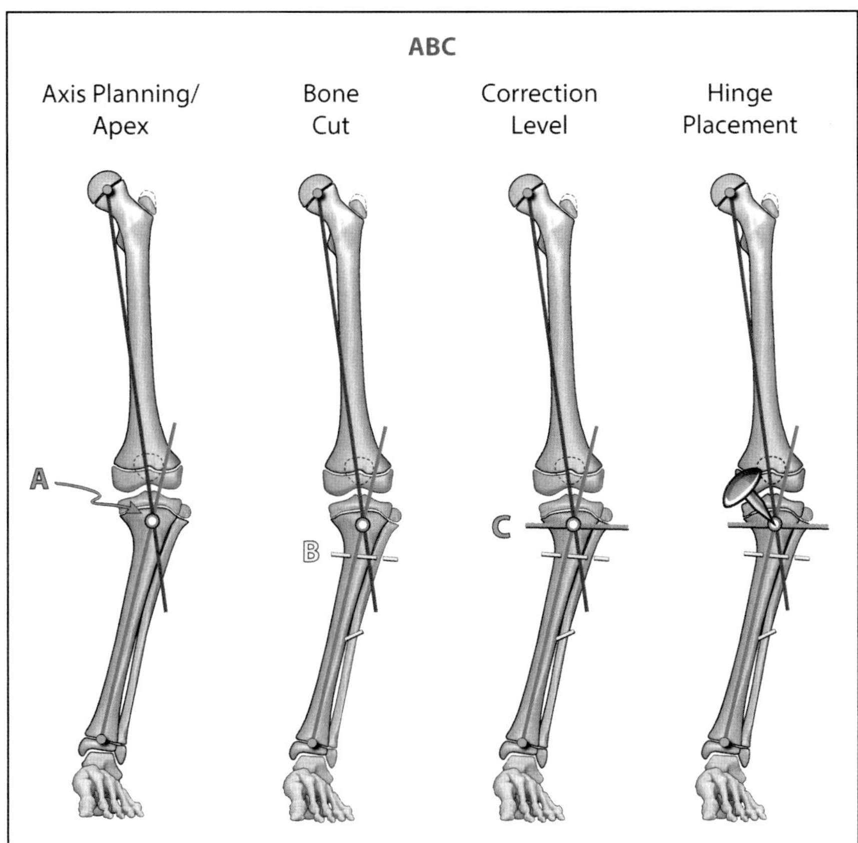


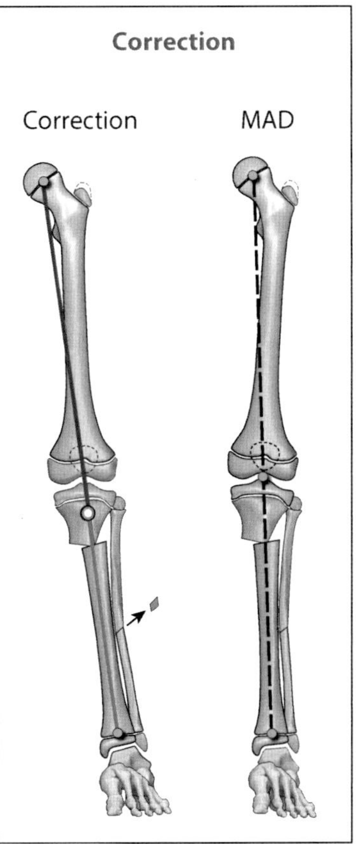


**Fig. 23 (continued): B**, ABC planning with acceptance of the mild femoral deformity demonstrates the apex of the deformity to be adjacent to proximal tibial physis. The osteotomy site was placed away from the apex to avoid injury of the physis and to afford adequate bone for stable fixation. Although the bone cut is away from the C-level, the thumbtack remains at the apex, anticipating osteotomy scenario #2. The obligatory translation can be measured as the distance between the proximal and distal axes at the level of the planned osteotomy. **C**, MAD demonstrates excellent correction of the mechanical axis and axes alignment of the tibia with acceptable bony obligatory translation.
A, apex; B, bone cut; C, C-level; MAD, mechanical axis deviation.

© 2023 Sinai Hospital of Baltimore

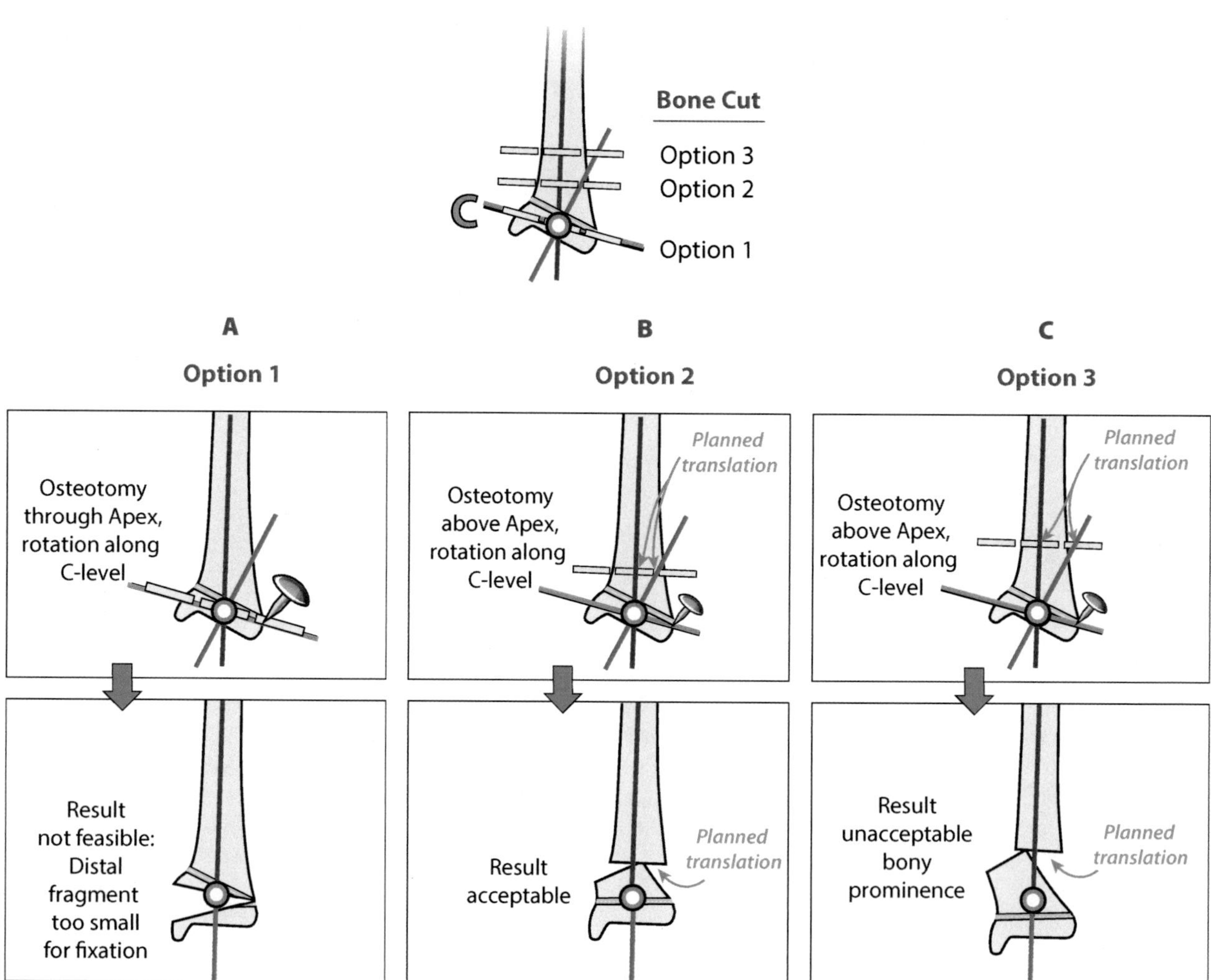


**Fig. 24:** **A**, Option 1 demonstrates a planned osteotomy site that is unacceptable due to the proximity of the joint. Additionally, the amount of bone is inadequate for fixation. **B**, Option 2 demonstrates a bone cut that is safer, and the fragment is adequate for fixation with acceptable obligatory translation. **C**, Option 3 demonstrates a safe location of the osteotomy with adequate bone for fixation, but increased obligatory translation resulting in an unacceptable bony prominence. C, C-level.

## Osteotomy Consideration #3: Bone healing

Avoiding osteotomies at locations of previous infections or unhealthy sclerotic bone is a good strategy (Fig. 25A). If the apex of deformity exists within this area of poor bone, the situation calls for osteotomy scenario #2 to be followed. However, significant obligatory translations of the bony margins might reduce the bony contact surface and jeopardize bone healing. In principle, maintaining bone contact of at least 50% is a good rule of thumb. However, this is not an absolute rule and depends on the entire clinical picture. For example, children heal with minimal bone contact in certain circumstances.

## Osteotomy Consideration #4: Stable fixation

When placing the osteotomy as close to the apex as possible, the amount of bone left for stable fixation must be taken into consideration. Each bone segment must have at least three points of stable fixation, especially when considering external fixation. With the advent of locking plate technology, smaller bone segments can be stabilized, allowing for osteotomies to be placed closer to an apex in a more optimal location (Fig. 25B). Another strategy used to place the osteotomy as close to an unfeasible apex as possible is an oblique osteotomy. The osteotomy is directed towards the apex/correction level and an opening wedge osteotomy is performed. This allows for larger bone segments with better fixation and healing and minimizes obligatory translation (Fig. 25C).

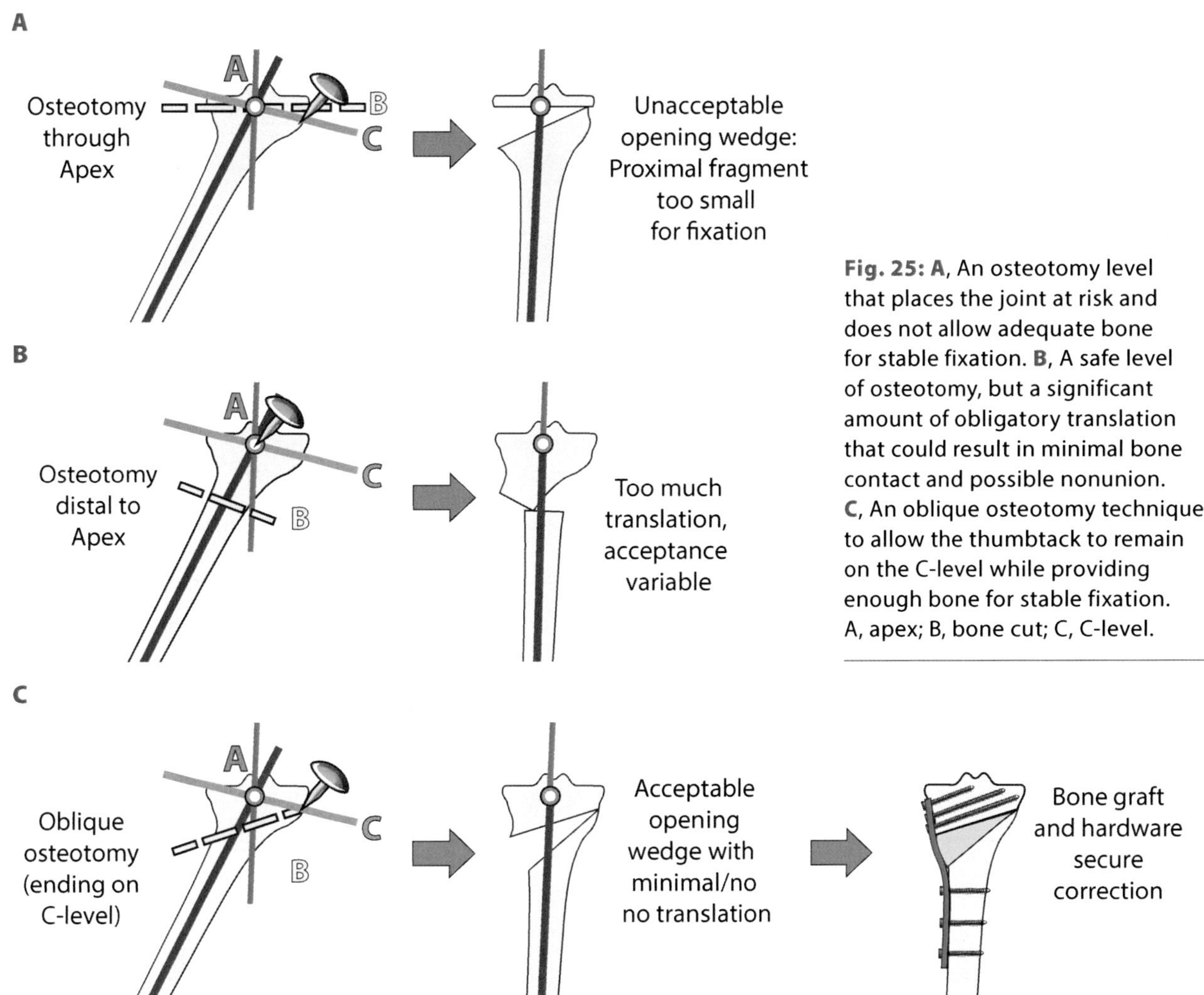


**Fig. 25: A**, An osteotomy level that places the joint at risk and does not allow adequate bone for stable fixation. **B**, A safe level of osteotomy, but a significant amount of obligatory translation that could result in minimal bone contact and possible nonunion. **C**, An oblique osteotomy technique to allow the thumbtack to remain on the C-level while providing enough bone for stable fixation. A, apex; B, bone cut; C, C-level.

© 2023 Sinai Hospital of Baltimore

## Osteotomy Consideration #5: Avoidance of unacceptable bony prominences

This occurs when there is obligatory translation of the osteotomy site in certain anatomic locations. The subcutaneous border of the tibia and the supramalleolar area of the ankle are anatomic locations at risk for this issue (Fig. 26). Other anatomic locations such as the femur are less problematic with bony translations or angulations due to the amount of soft tissue coverage (Figs. 24C, 27).

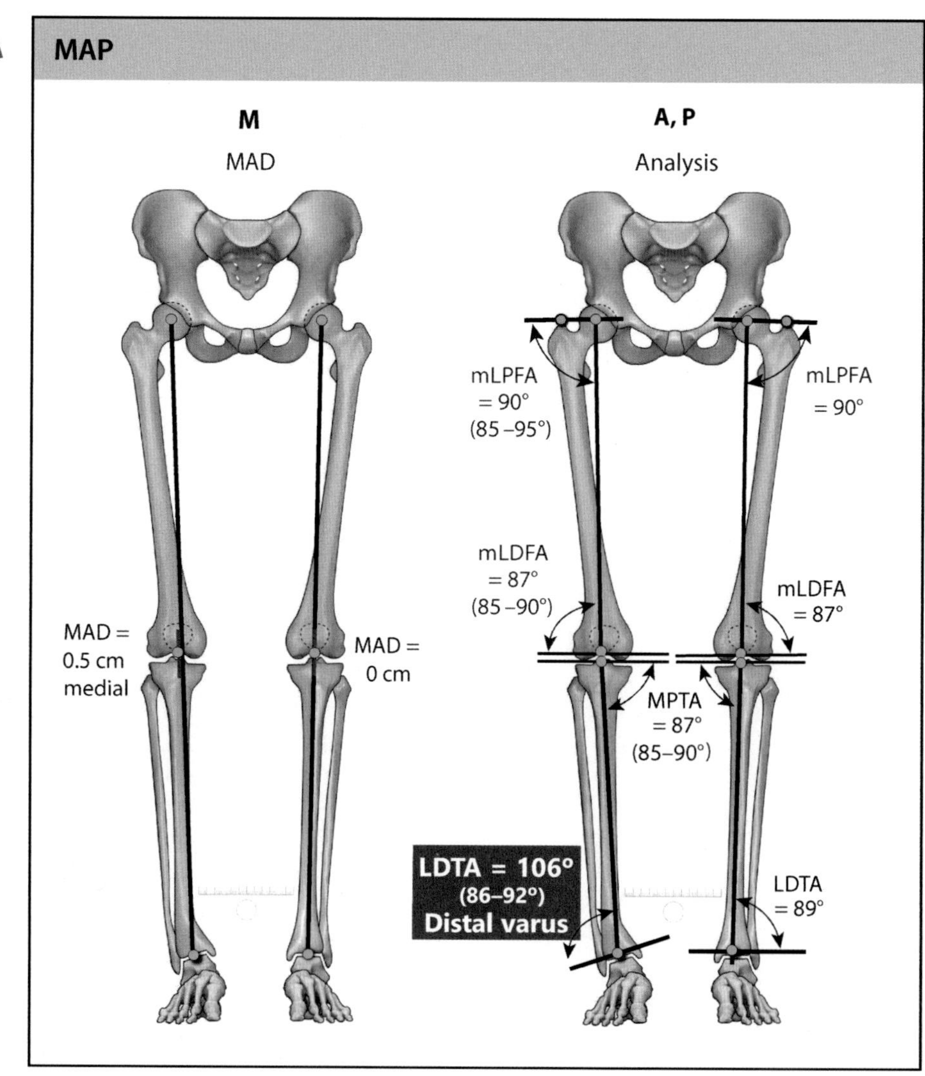


**Fig. 26: A,** The MAP analysis identifies a normal MAD. The angle analysis establishes the distal varus deformity in the right tibia. LDTA, lateral distal tibial angle; MAD, mechanical axis deviation; mLDFA, mechanical lateral distal femoral angle; mLPFA, mechanical lateral proximal femoral angle; MPTA, medial proximal tibial angle.

B

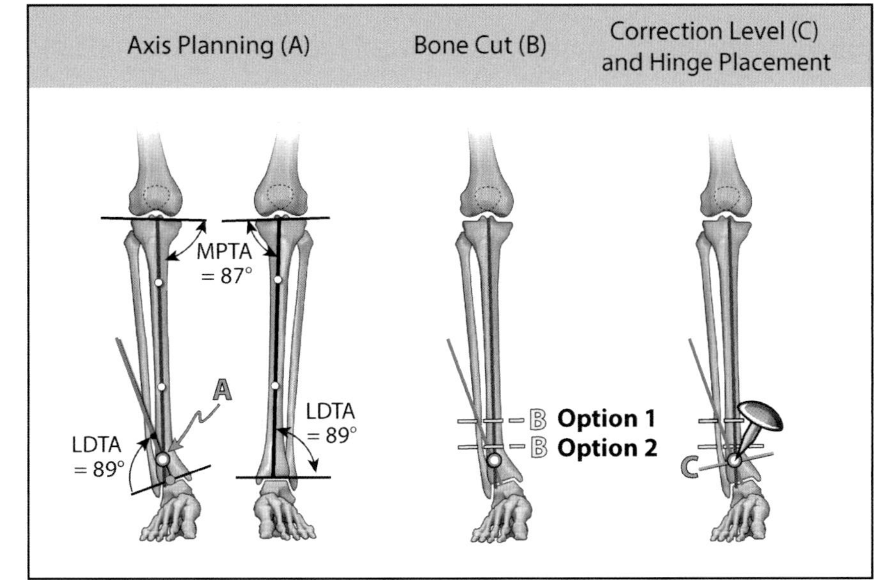


C

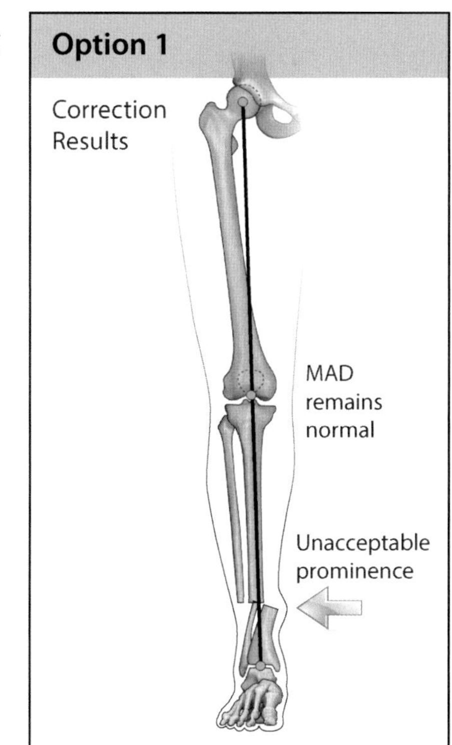


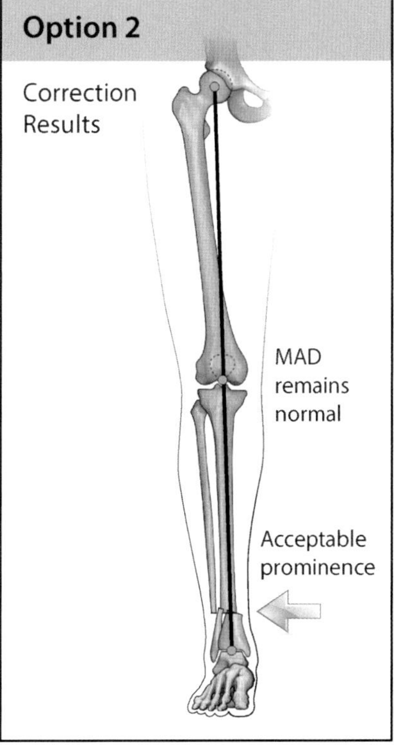


**Fig. 26 (continued): B**, The analysis determines an apex close to the ankle joint. Two osteotomy options are drawn. The thumbtack is placed on the apex for both options. **C**, In Option 1, the osteotomy is performed significantly proximal to the apex, allowing for a large distal bone segment for fixation. With correction, there is significant and unacceptable bony translation resulting in minimal bone contact and an unacceptable bony prominence. In Option 2, the correction is at a more appropriate level that is both safe to the ankle joint and allows minimal obligatory translation resulting in excellent alignment, adequate bone contact, and no significant clinical bony prominence. This demonstrates the variability of osteotomy scenario 2 which requires preoperative planning for bony translation resulting from the placement of the determined osteotomy level. A, apex; B, bone cut; C, C-level; LDTA, lateral distal tibial angle; MAD, mechanical axis deviation; MPTA, medial proximal tibial angle.

© 2023 Sinai Hospital of Baltimore 

A

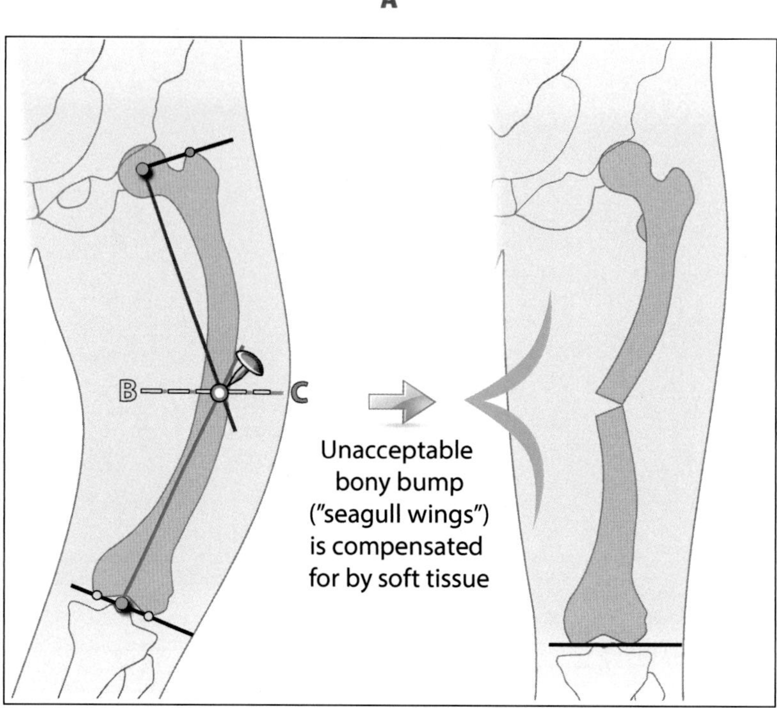


B

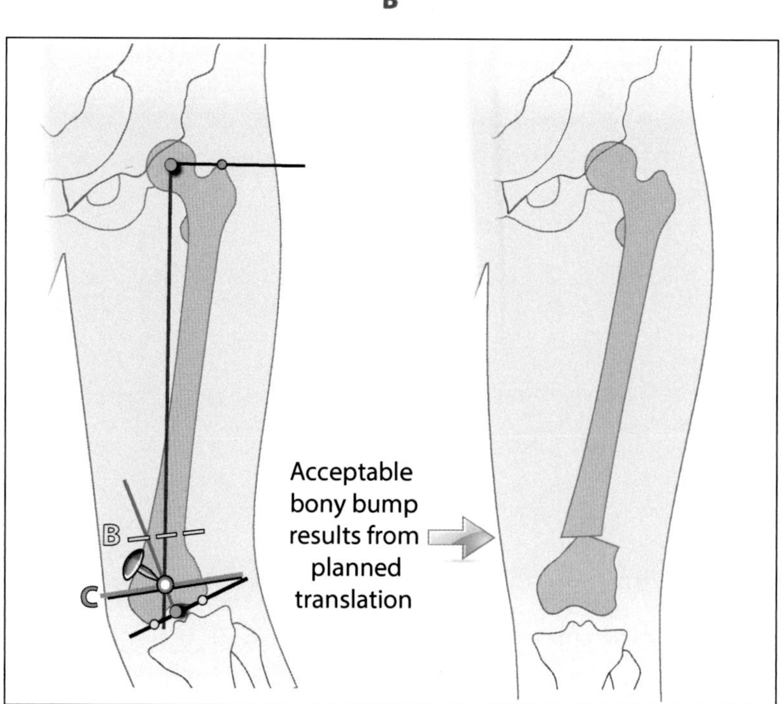


**Fig. 27: A**, Bony alignment and bony prominence has a relative acceptance depending on bone segment and soft tissue coverage. The multiple apical deformity can be corrected with a single osteotomy resulting in a "gull wing" femoral configuration. However, the clinical alignment is normal due to the surrounding soft tissue coverage. **B**, Additional example of obligatory translation in a distal femoral valgus correction with no clinical bony prominence due to soft tissue coverage. This exemplifies the variable acceptability of bony translation.

Now that the osteotomy rules, scenarios, and considerations have been explained, a second example will be used to illustrate these concepts.

## MAP the ABCs:
## Frontal Plane Case Example 2

The following example will show the MAP the ABCs process for another frontal plane deformity. Keep in mind the location of the correction level line and placement of the hinge point. What osteotomy rule was utilized? Is the osteotomy placement acceptable?

## MAP Analysis for Case Example 2

### Step 1: Measure the MAD

The MAD is 3.5 cm medial, which is abnormal (Fig. 28A).

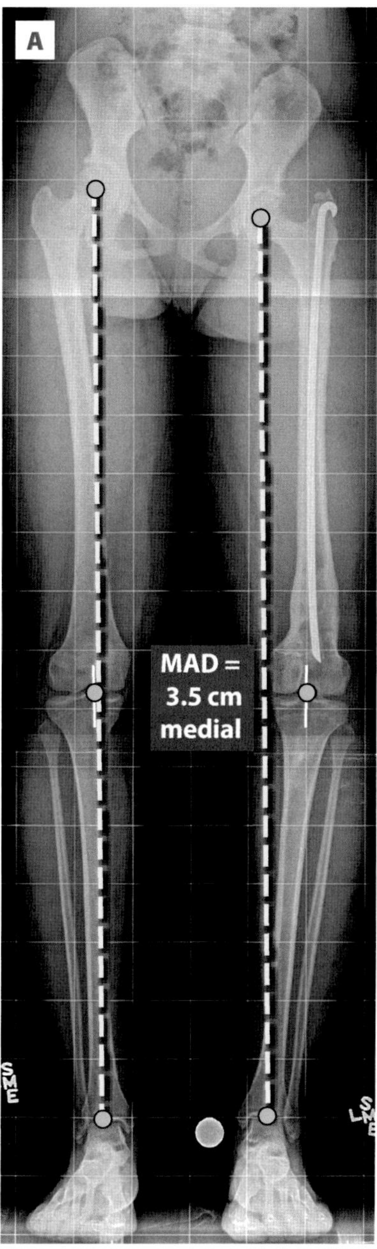


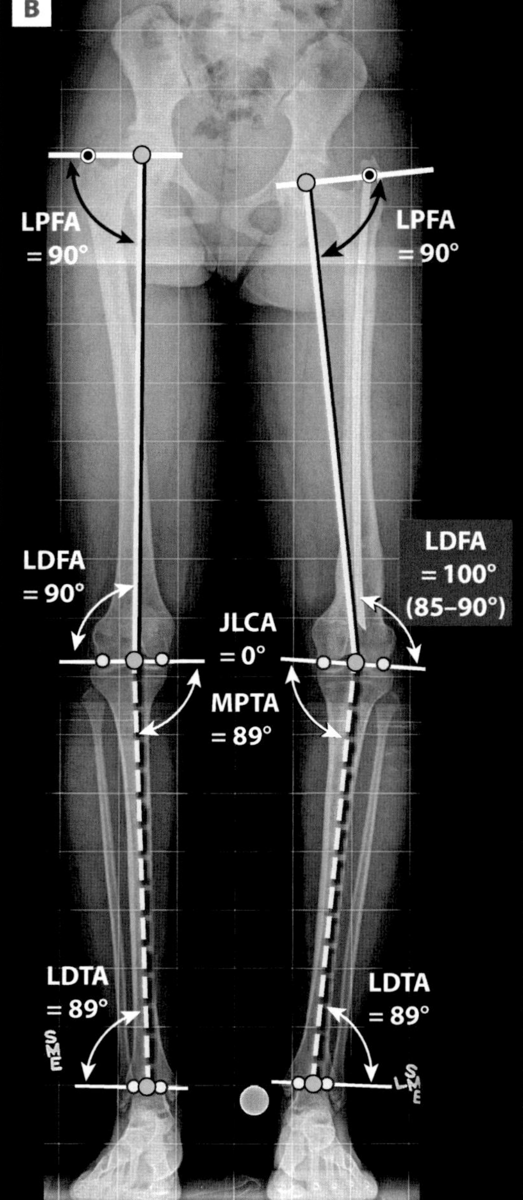


**Fig. 28: A**, The mechanical axis of the left limb is abnormal with an MAD of 3.5 cm medial. **B**, The joint angle analysis of the left limb shows that the LDFA is abnormal.

### Step 2: Analyze the joint angles

The joint angles of the right limb are normal (Fig. 28B). One joint angle in the left limb is abnormal:

LDFA = 100° (abnormal)

### Step 3: Pick the deformed bone

The analysis shows that the left femur is the bone segment of interest.

## ABCs of the Femur for Case Example 2

### Step 4: Apex of the deformity

We plan to use an intramedullary nail to correct this deformity; therefore, we will use anatomic axis planning. To draw the proximal axis, a mid-diaphyseal line is drawn (Fig. 29A). The MPFA formed by the mid-diaphyseal line is checked to see if a hidden proximal deformity exists. Since the MPFA is normal, there is no proximal metaphyseal deformity and the mid-diaphyseal line can be used. For more information, refer to "Mid-diaphyseal Line Strategy" in the chapter entitled "Tibial Axis Planning: Frontal and Sagittal Planes." To draw the distal axis, first draw the distal femoral joint line (Fig. 29B). Then draw another line that creates a normal aLDFA range. This value for the aLDFA matches the aLDFA of the normal contralateral limb (not shown). The magnitude of the deformity is the magnitude of the acute angle that is created by the intersection of the proximal and distal axis lines (Fig. 29B). Mark the apex at the intersection of the proximal and distal axis lines (Fig. 29B).

### Step 5: Bone cut

The ideal osteotomy is made at the level of the apex. In this example, the apex is located at the knee joint; therefore, it is not feasible to make a bone cut at this location. The bone cut is made proximal to the apex (Fig. 29C), which means that obligatory translation will occur during correction.

### Step 6: Correction

Plan an acute correction with an intramedullary nail. The C-level is created by drawing a line that passes through the apex and bisects the obtuse angle that is formed by the proximal and distal axis lines (Fig. 29C). The thumbtack is always placed on the C-level (Rule #2). In this case, the thumbtack is placed along the C-level on the convex side of the deformity to produce an opening wedge osteotomy (Fig. 29C). The opening wedge osteotomy will result in bone lengthening. The placement of the bone cut proximal to the level of the apex will result in obligatory translation (Rule #1).

After acute correction, the proximal and distal axis lines are collinear (Fig. 30A). The mechanical axis now falls slightly medial to the center of the knee (Fig. 30B). The LDFA has been corrected to normal (Fig. 30C). Table 5 summarizes the MAP the ABCs for Case Example 2.

The mnemonic MAP the ABCs can be used to approach and analyze any bony deformity in a simplified and consistent manner. Using the same step-by-step MAP approach will allow you to consistently delineate and understand the deformity. The ABCs will allow you to correctly identify the apex and magnitude of the deformity as well as the correction level. By adhering to the rules that the thumbtack must always be placed on the C-level and that the bone cut must be as close as possible to the apex, you will consistently obtain correction of the deformity. The same sequence of evaluation and planning is used for sagittal plane deformities, which will be explained in the chapter entitled "Deformity Analysis in the Sagittal Plane."

**Table 5. Summary of Case Example 2, Left Limb (Figures 28–30)**

**MAP**

**M** = Measure the MAD = 3.5 cm medial

**A** = Analyze the joint angles: LDFA = 100°

**P** = Pick the deformed bone: Femur

**ABCs (Femur)**

**A** = Apex of deformity: Located on distal femoral joint line; Magnitude of deformity = 11°

**B** = Bone cut (choose the level of the osteotomy): Distal femoral metaphysis (not at level of apex)

**C** = Correction: Acute correction with an opening wedge osteotomy, an intramedullary device, and obligatory translation (since bone cut not at level of apex)

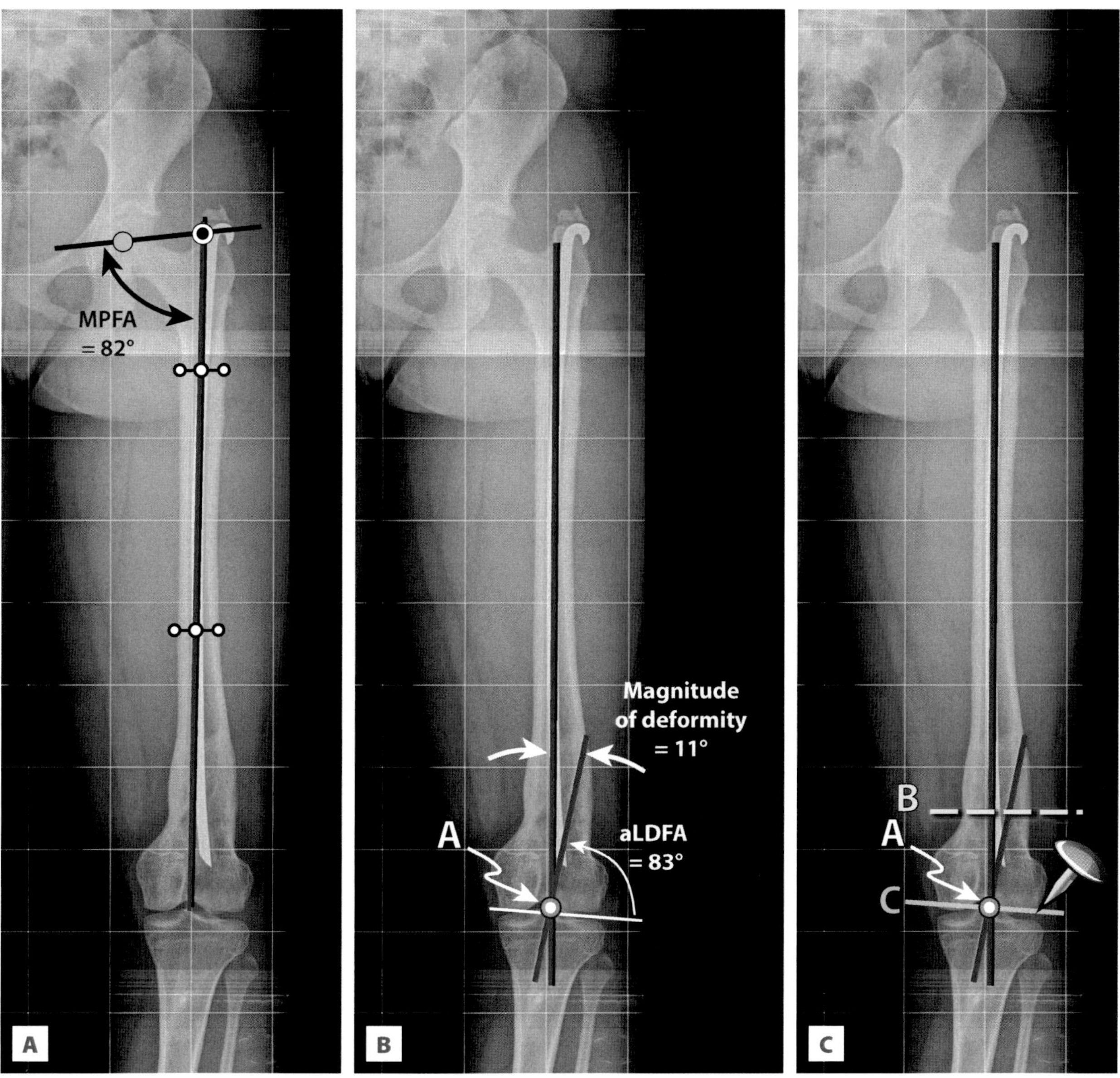


**Fig. 29:** **A**, The proximal axis is a mid-diaphyseal line (*red line*). The MPFA is normal; therefore, a hidden proximal metaphyseal deformity is not present and the mid-diaphyseal line can be used as the proximal axis. Note that the NSA can be used instead of the MPFA to see if there is a hidden proximal femoral deformity. **B**, The distal axis (*blue line*) is drawn by creating a normal aLDFA of 83°. This value for the aLDFA matches the aLDFA of the normal contralateral limb (not shown). The magnitude of the deformity is 11°. **C**, The apex is located at the intersection of the proximal and distal axis lines. The C-level passes through the apex and bisects the obtuse angle that is formed by the proximal and distal axis lines. The thumbtack is placed along the C-level on the convex side of the deformity to produce an opening wedge osteotomy, which will result in bone lengthening. Obligatory translation will occur because the bone cut was not made at the level of the apex. A, apex; B, bone cut; C, C-level.

© 2023 Sinai Hospital of Baltimore 

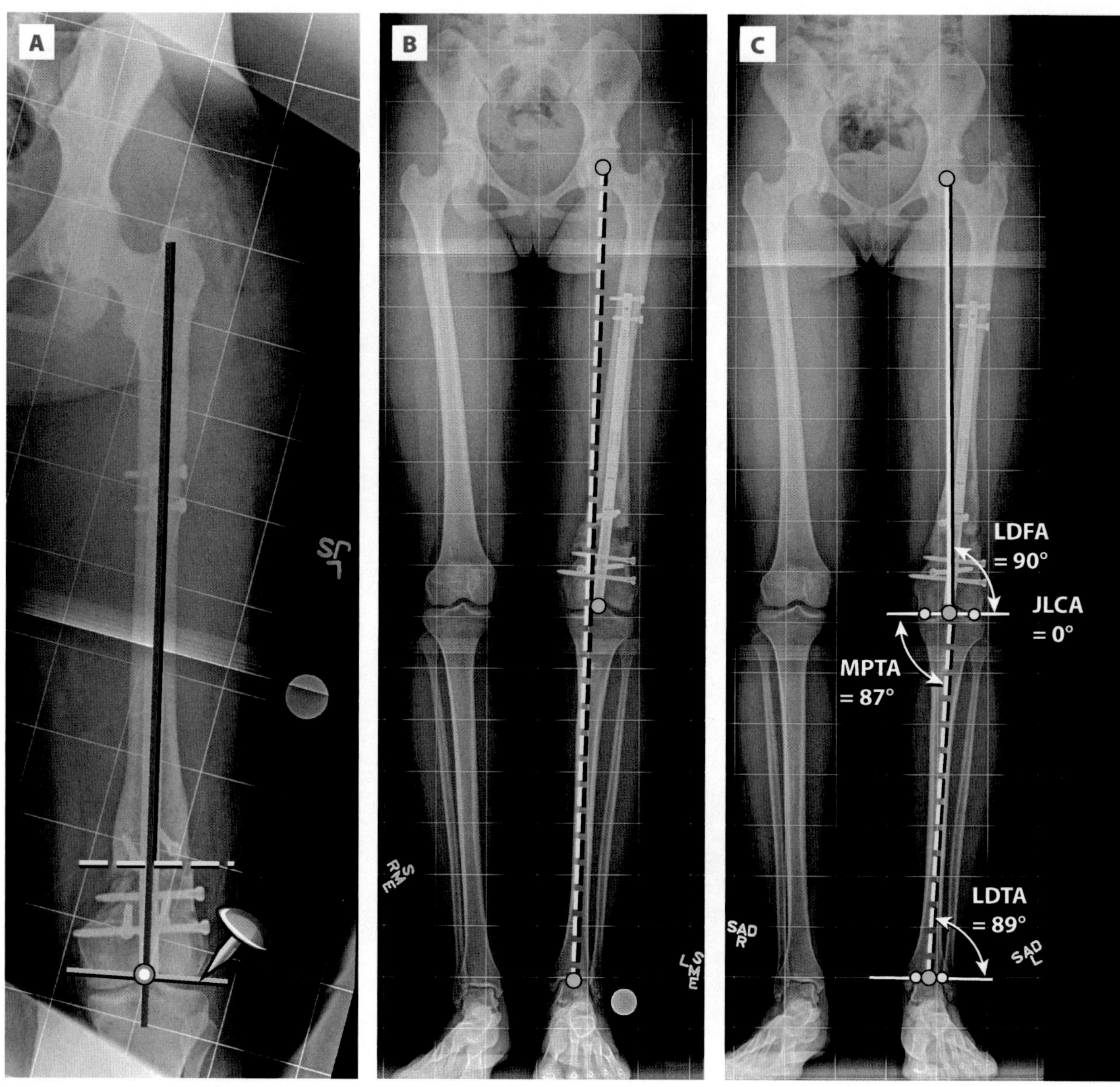


**Fig. 30:** **A**, After acute correction, the proximal and distal axis lines are collinear. **B**, The mechanical axis is slightly medial to the center of the knee. **C**, The LDFA has been normalized. The JLCA, MPTA, and LDTA remained normal and did not change during treatment.

# Chapter 7

# Deformity Analysis in the Sagittal Plane

Philip K. McClure, MD
Shawn C. Standard, MD
Michael J. Assayag, MD

The process of MAP the ABCs remains the same for the sagittal plane. Range of motion of the knee in the sagittal plane adds a level of complexity. Therefore, joint motion or lack of joint motion can contribute to or compensate for sagittal plane deformities. This soft-tissue component (i.e., joint contracture, joint hypermobility) is a variable that must be understood, quantified, and addressed during deformity analysis and correction in the sagittal plane.

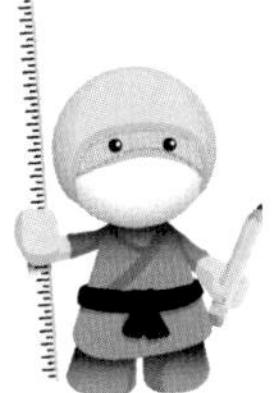

*Sensei says,*
*"The knee, with its joint motion in the sagittal plane, can compensate for significant deformities in this plane, unlike frontal plane deformities. This situation requires careful and accurate analysis of the sagittal plane."*

The MAP process begins with a full length standing lateral view x-ray with the knee positioned in maximum extension as described in the chapter entitled "Obtaining X-rays of the Lower Limbs." The MAP the ABCs process in the sagittal plane is very similar to MAP the ABCs in the frontal plane. For the "M" in MAP, the sagittal plane mechanical axis deviation (MAD) is measured. In the "A" in MAP, the sagittal plane joint angles are analyzed.

To measure the sagittal plane MAD in the "M" step of MAP, the mechanical axis of the lower extremity is drawn from the center of femoral head to the center of the ankle (Fig. 1). In the sagittal plane of the normal knee, this line should lie anterior

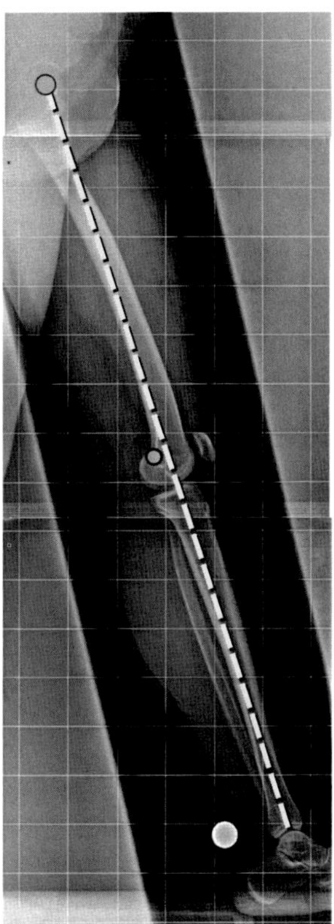

**Fig. 1:** On a full length standing lateral view x-ray, the sagittal plane mechanical axis is defined as a line from the center of the femoral head to the center of the ankle. The normal sagittal plane mechanical axis passes slightly anterior to the hinge point of the knee (*purple point*) and stays within the confines of the distal femur.

© 2023 Sinai Hospital of Baltimore

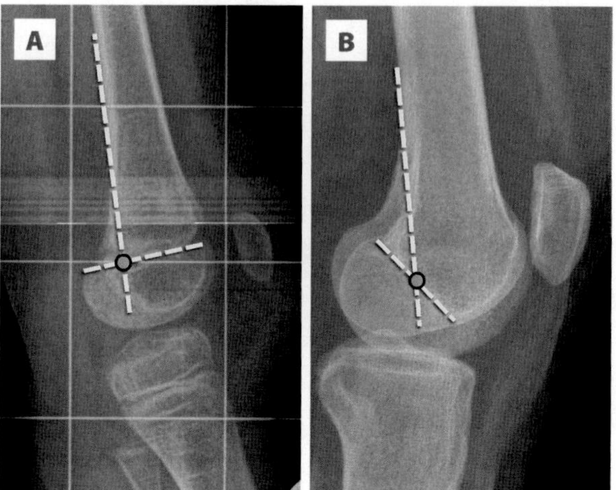


**Fig. 2: A**, In children, the hinge point of the knee is located at the intersection of the posterior femoral cortex and the distal femoral physis/physeal scar. **B**, In individuals who are skeletally mature, the hinge point of the knee is located at the intersection of the posterior femoral cortex and the Blumensaat line.

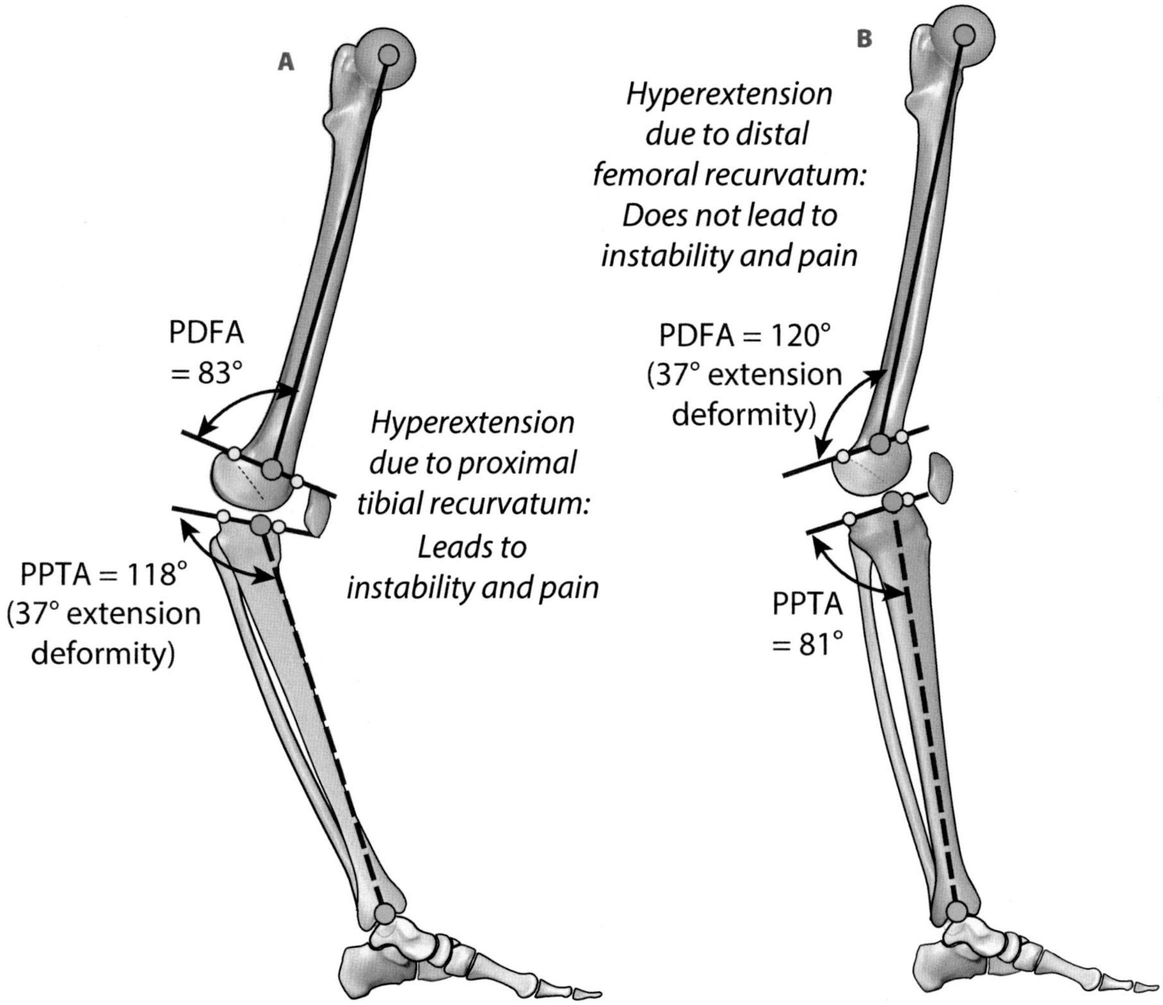

A

PDFA = 83°

PPTA = 118° (37° extension deformity)

*Hyperextension due to proximal tibial recurvatum: Leads to instability and pain*

B

*Hyperextension due to distal femoral recurvatum: Does not lead to instability and pain*

PDFA = 120° (37° extension deformity)

PPTA = 81°

**Fig. 3: A**, Hyperextension due to a significantly increased slope of the tibia can result in instability and pain even though the patient will not demonstrate clinical hyperextension or "back kneeing" during gait. This bony configuration can result from anterior tibial growth arrest or asymmetric growth in bony dysplasias. **B**, Hyperextension due to distal femoral recurvatum does not cause joint instability or pain. This bony configuration is common in patients with achondroplasia.

to the hinge point of the knee (Fig. 2) and stay within the confines of the distal femur. With the mechanical axis anterior to the hinge point of the knee, the knee joint is able to lock in full extension allowing the quadriceps muscle to relax and prevent muscle fatigue. However, if the mechanical axis lies anterior to the hinge point of the knee but outside the confines of the distal femur, then a hyperextension deformity of the knee exists (Fig. 3). Although hyperextension might be noted on a full length standing lateral view x-ray with the patient maximally extending his/her knees, a neurologically normal patient (e.g., no poliomyelitis, muscular dystrophy, spasticity) typically will not hyperextend his or her legs during gait. With severe hyperextension deformities of the proximal tibia, increased slope and posterior positioning of the tibia on the femur are present, which can lead to subjective instability and pain (Fig. 3).

If the sagittal plane mechanical axis indicates a deformity, then the next step in the MAP process is performed. This next step is the "A" in MAP and involves analyzing five sagittal plane joint angles. Three of the five sagittal plane joint angles (PDFA, PPTA, and ADTA) determine the amount of bony deformity present in each bone segment (Fig. 4). For a description of how to draw these joint angles, please see Chapter 1. Note that the anticipated contribution of a bony sagittal deformity to the apparent knee deformity can also be calculated with basic trigonometry (see Appendix); however, basic deformity analysis is a simpler process.

During the "A" step of the MAP process, two additional angles are also measured: the sagittal mechanical axes angle (SMAA) and the sagittal joint line angle (SJLA). These angles help to analyze the confounding factor of knee motion in the sagittal plane.

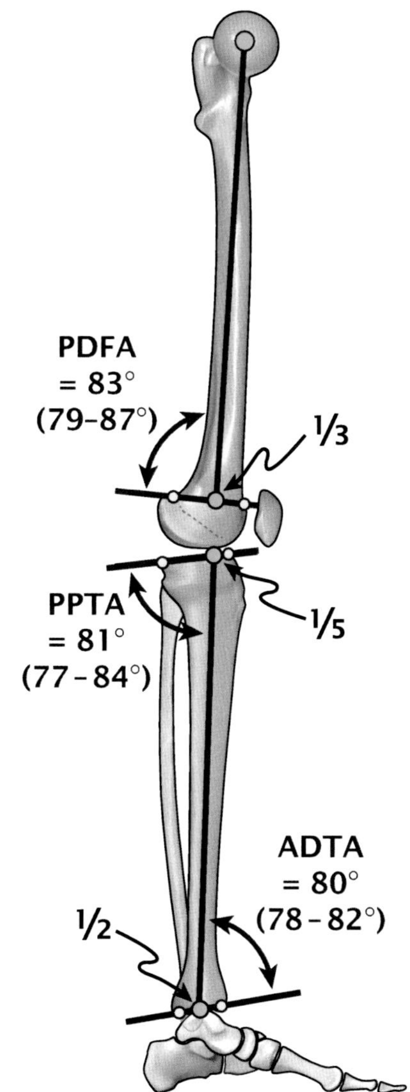


**Fig. 4:** Normal posterior distal femoral angle (PDFA), posterior proximal tibial angle (PPTA), and anterior distal tibial angle (ADTA).

© 2023 Sinai Hospital of Baltimore

The SMAA is the angle formed by the modified mechanical axis of the femur and the modified mechanical axis of the tibia (Fig. 5A). These two axes also can be called segmental mechanical axes. The SMAA represents the overall position of the knee joint and will determine if the knee joint is in a neutral position (Fig. 5A), a flexion position (Fig. 5B), or a hyperextended position (Fig. 5C). In a normal limb, the sagittal mechanical axes of the femur and tibia will be collinear (Fig. 6) and the SMAA will be 0° (± 2°). If a deformity is present, the intersection of the tibial and femoral sagittal mechanical axes will create an SMAA that quantifies the total amount of flexion or hyperextension apparent at the knee (Fig. 5B and 5C).

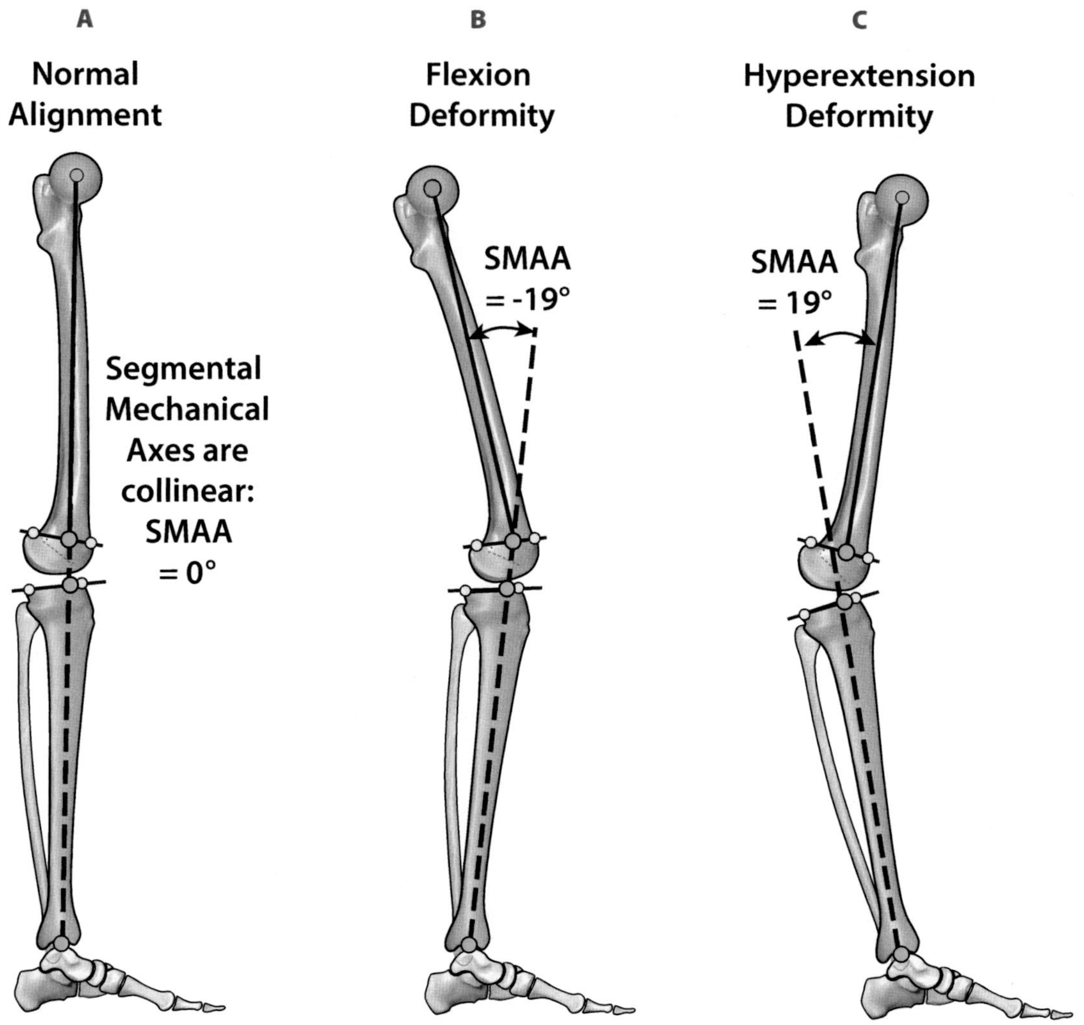


**Fig. 5:** Maximum extension views. **A**, Collinear segmental mechanical axes of the femur and the tibia show that the sagittal mechanical axes angle (SMAA) is 0° and the limb has normal sagittal plane alignment. **B**, SMAA shows that a flexion deformity is present (SMAA = -19° flexion). **C**, SMAA shows that a hyperextension deformity is present (SMAA = 19° hyperextension).

The sagittal joint line angle (SJLA) is the angle formed by the distal femoral joint line and the proximal tibial joint line (Fig. 7). The sagittal joint line angle of the knee correlates with the frontal plane JLCA. While the average normal value of the frontal plane JLCA is 0° (indicating no varus or valgus laxity in the knee ligaments), the average normal value of the SJLA is 16° ± 3° (Fig. 7). The normal value for the SJLA was determined by conducting a review of 130 normal full length standing lateral view x-rays (normal PDFA and PPTA, collinear tibial and femoral mechanical axes). An SJLA less than 16° indicates flexion, while an SJLA greater than 16° indicates extension (Fig. 8). We will be using the SJLA as a final step to verify or check the soft-tissue contribution to the deformity.

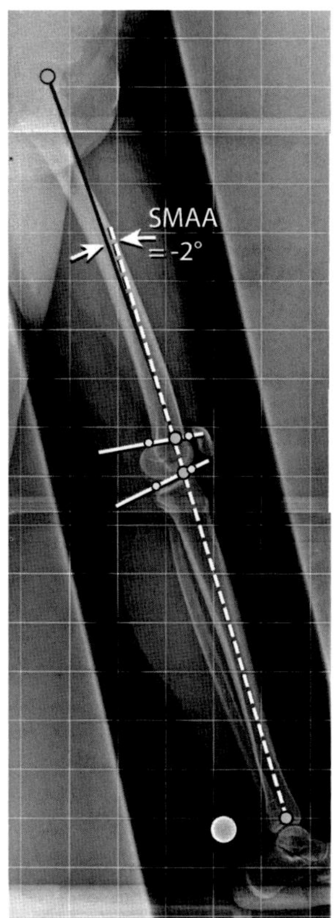


**Fig. 6:** In a normal limb, the segmental mechanical axes of the femur and tibia are collinear when the lower extremity is fully extended. Note that the sagittal mechanical axes angle (SMAA) of -2° (flexion) is within normal limits.

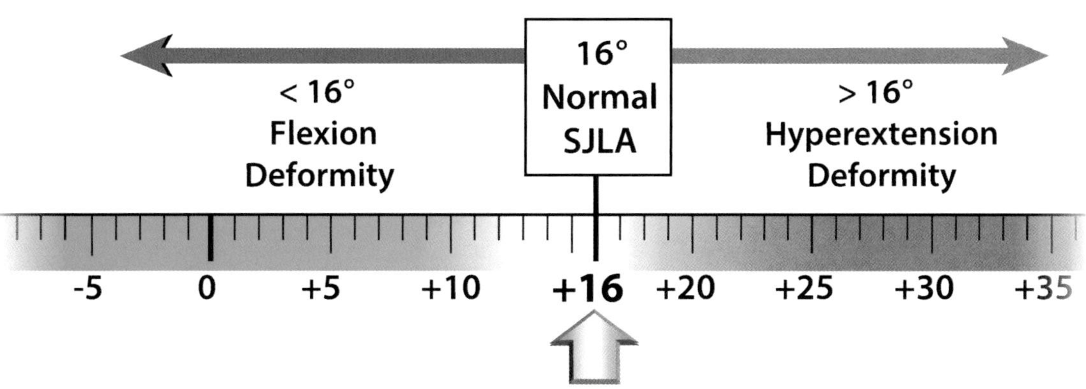


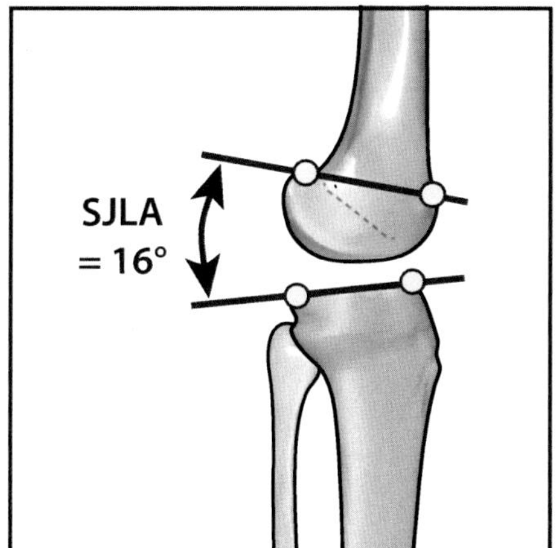


**Fig. 7:** The average normal value of the sagittal joint line angle (SJLA) is 16°. An SJLA less than 16° indicates flexion, while an SJLA greater than 16° indicates hyperextension.

© 2023 Sinai Hospital of Baltimore

To determine the soft-tissue component of the deformity around the knee joint, the bony deformity analysis of the angles about the knee (PDFA and PPTA) is compared to the results of the segmental analysis (SMAA). The SMAA quantifies the total amount of soft-tissue and bony deformity that is present around the knee joint (flexion contracture or hyperextension). The PDFA determines the amount of bony deformity present in the femoral segment. The PPTA determines the amount of bony deformity present in the tibial segment. The apparent knee deformity (SMAA) and the bony contributions (PDFA and PPTA) can then be reconciled to reveal the soft-tissue contribution.

You may remember that the sagittal plane analysis in previous versions of this textbook have focused on the anterior cortical line (ACL) measurement to

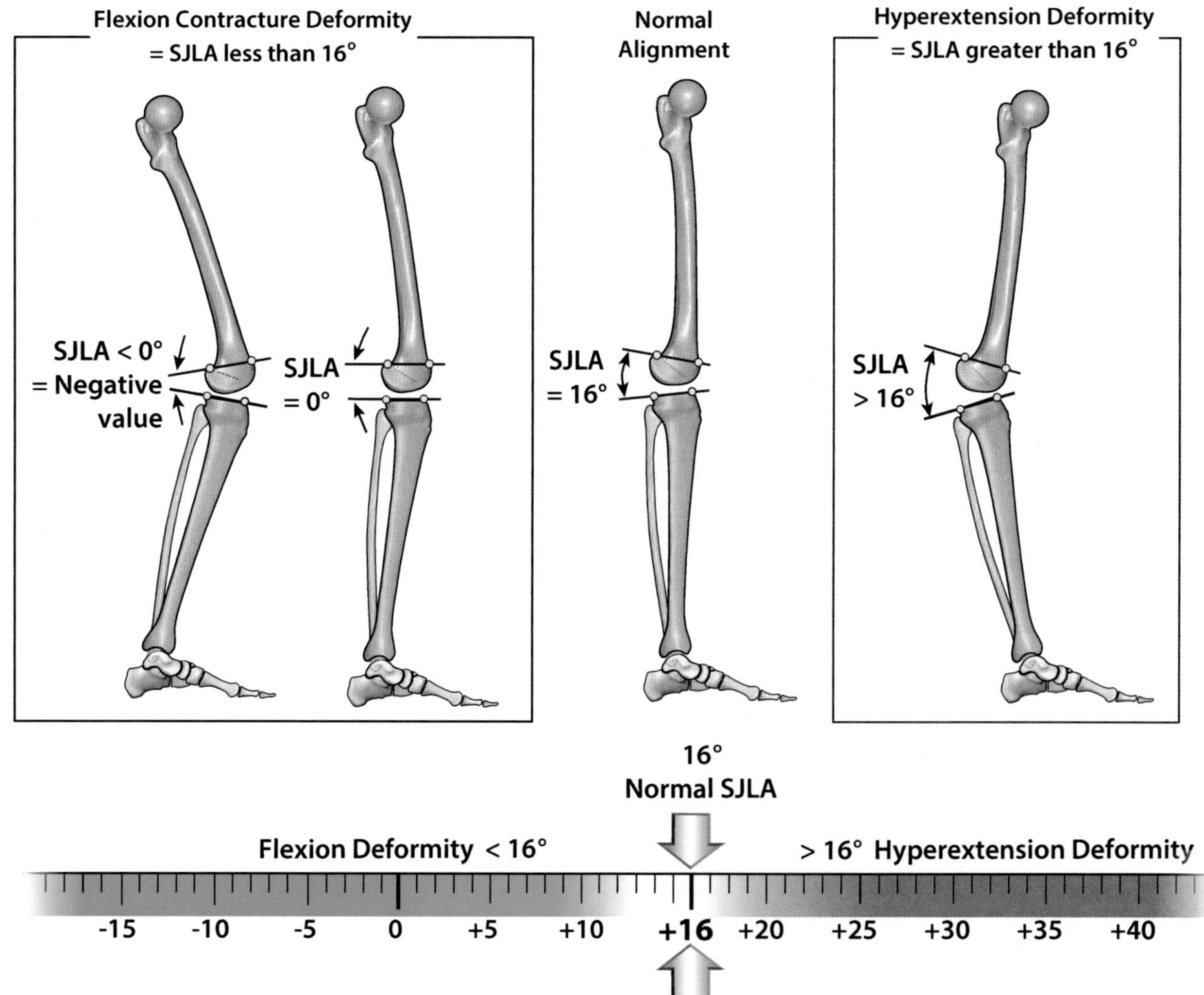


**Fig. 8:** A sagittal joint line angle (SJLA) less than 16° indicates flexion deformity while an SJLA greater than 16° indicates hyperextension deformity.

determine the soft-tissue contribution, but this has been replaced with the SMAA. The anterior cortical line measurement is an accurate representation of sagittal deformity as manifested at the knee in only a subset of deformities that are epiphyseal or physeal in nature. Deformities that are in the meta-diaphyseal or diaphyseal regions of the bone will not be represented by the anterior cortical line measurement but still need to be considered as they may generate apparent contraction of the knee and compensatory differences in the soft tissue. In many of these cases, drawing consistent anterior cortical lines can be difficult (Fig. 9). Since the ACL measurement can be used only in a subset of sagittal deformities and it can be challenging to draw consistent anterior cortical lines, we will focus on the SMAA in this chapter.

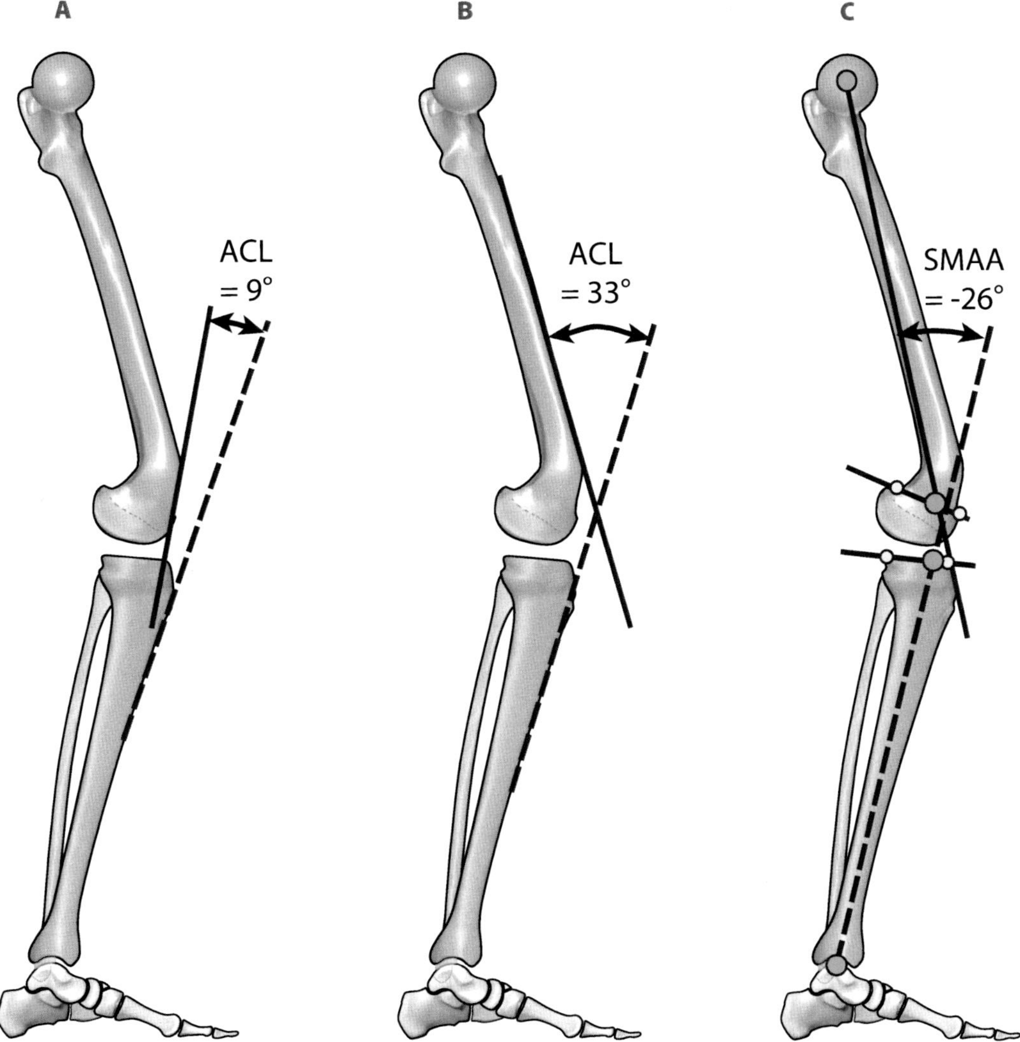


**Fig. 9: A** and **B**, A consistent anterior cortical line (ACL) measurement can be difficult to define. Even through each panel shows the same deformity, the ACL measurement may vary depending on how one draws each anterior cortical line. This is particularly evident in metabolic bone disease. **C**, The sagittal mechanical axes angle (SMAA) uses anatomic landmarks so that it can be drawn consistently.

© 2023 Sinai Hospital of Baltimore

## Soft-tissue Contribution Resolution

The soft-tissue contribution (i.e., flexion contracture, hyperextension) in the sagittal plane can be calculated by using the Seesaw Method, Formula Method, or Table Method. Once readers are familiar with each method, they will find that each is a variation on a theme and they may choose the method that feels the most sensible to them. After using one of the three methods, the SJLA can be utilized to check that the calculation of the soft-tissue contribution is correct.

### Sagittal Seesaw Method

To understand deformity in the sagittal plane on a conceptual level, it is helpful to think of a seesaw or balance (Fig. 10). In the first step of each method, the PDFA and PPTA should be measured and the difference from the normal value of that angle should be calculated. The SMAA should also be determined. With the values for SMAA and the total bony deformity, the soft-tissue contribution can be obtained. In Figure 10A, the total bony deformity is 33° flexion (13° flexion [femur] + 20° flexion [tibia] = 33° flexion). The soft-tissue and bony deformities together (Fig. 10B, left side) must balance against

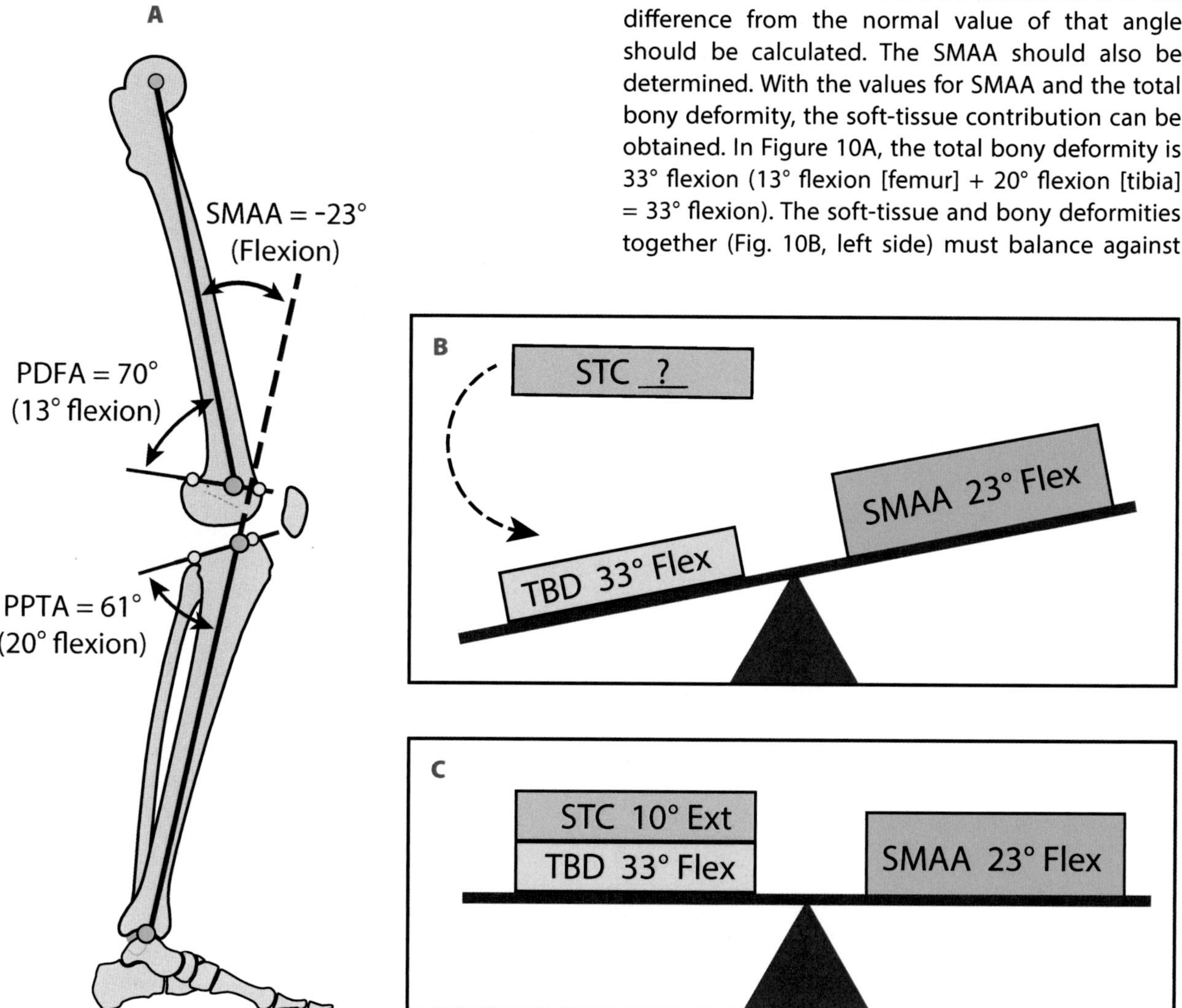


**Fig. 10: Seesaw Method. A**, Example of sagittal plane bony and soft-tissue deformities. The total bony deformity is 33° flexion (13° flexion [femur] + 20° flexion [tibia] = 33° flexion). **B** and **C**, After determining the sagittal mechanical axes angle (SMAA) and the total bony deformity (TBD), the concept of a seesaw or balance can be used to obtain the soft-tissue contribution (STC). The soft-tissue contribution and total bony deformity (*left side*) must balance against the SMAA (*right side*). In this example, adding 10° extension from the soft-tissue contribution to the left side of the seesaw balances the SMAA (23° flexion) on the right side of the seesaw (STC 10° extension + TBD 33° flexion = SMAA 23° flexion). Ext, extension; Flex, flexion; PDFA, posterior distal femoral angle; PPTA, posterior proximal tibial angle.

the SMAA (Fig. 10B, right side). If the total bony deformity does not equal the SMAA, soft-tissue contribution always makes up the difference. For example, an SMAA of 23° flexion (Fig. 10B, right side) must be balanced against the total bony deformity and the soft-tissue contribution (Fig. 10B, left side). The soft-tissue contribution (either flexion or extension) is added to the total bony deformity (Fig. 10B, left side) to balance the scale and account for all components of the deformity. In this example, adding 10° extension to the left side of the seesaw (Fig. 10C, left side) as the soft-tissue contribution balances the SMAA (23° flexion) on the right side of the seesaw (STC 10° extension + TBD 33° flexion = SMAA 23° flexion).

Increasing SMAA must be accounted for in either total bony deformity or soft-tissue contribution. One degree of extension can be seen as "neutralizing" one degree of flexion, while an additional degree of flexion "increases" the load. As always, it is essential to ensure that adequate maximum extension images have been obtained; calculations that are based on poor or improperly positioned x-rays will be misleading.

## Sagittal Formula Method

A formula can also be used to calculate the soft-tissue contribution:

SMAA = (Femoral Bony Deformity +
Tibial Bony Deformity) +
Soft-tissue Contribution About the Knee

Then solve for the soft-tissue contribution using basic algebra:

Soft-tissue Contribution About the Knee =
SMAA – (Femoral Bony Deformity +
Tibial Bony Deformity)

Figure 11 shows how the Formula Method can be used along with the SMAA, femoral bony deformity, and tibial bony deformity to find the soft-tissue contribution. In the formula, negative values denote flexion and positive values denote extension. This convention is chosen because flexion is associated with a decrease in the posterior joint angles as well as a decreasing joint line angle. If you consider the normal values to be your starting ("zero") point, the value of this convention is evident.

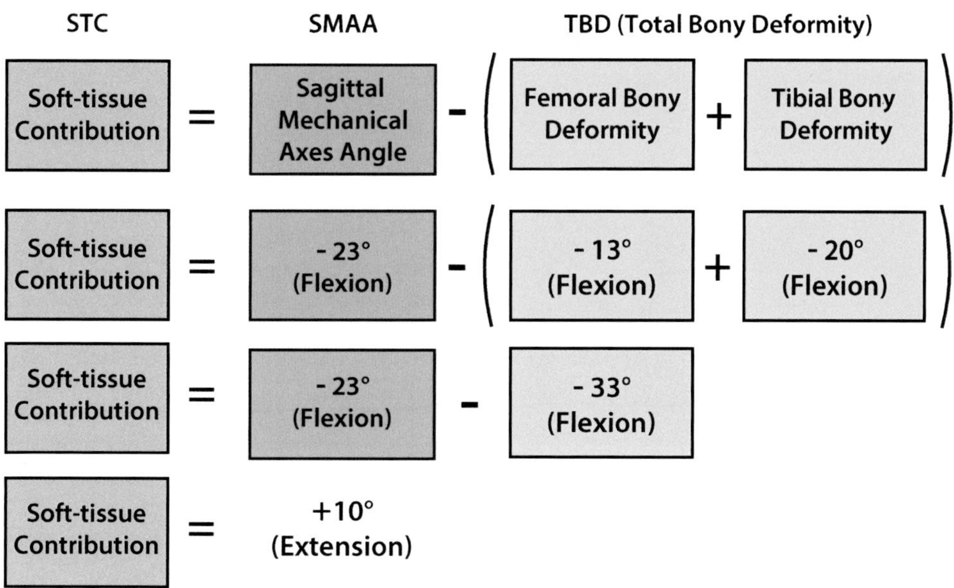


**Fig. 11: Formula Method** using the deformity shown in Figure 10A. Note that negative values denote flexion and positive values denote extension. The total bony deformity is made up of the distal femoral bony deformity and the proximal tibial bony deformity.

## Sagittal Table Method

The second method to reconcile soft-tissue contribution is the Table Method. This is a non-algebraic, visual method to analyze the soft-tissue contribution. In constructing the table (Fig. 12), PDFA less than 83° is recorded in the flexion column, while PDFA greater than 83° is recorded as extension; the magnitude is recorded next to it. The PPTA is treated similarly (around the "zero point" of 81°).

The soft-tissue contribution of a sagittal deformity is the difference between the bony deformity and the overall position of the lower extremity in the sagittal plane. Record each value (SMAA, PDFA, PPTA) in the table (Fig. 12), with flexion in the negative column and extension in the positive column. PDFA and PPTA (Fig. 12, Line 1) are then combined to determine the total bony deformity (Fig. 12, Line 2). Be careful, as the bony contributions of the tibia and femur may be in opposite directions. The total bony deformity (Fig. 12, Line 2) is then reconciled with the SMAA (Fig. 12, Line 3) to show the soft-tissue component (Fig. 12, Line 4).

## Checking Your Results: Sagittal Joint Line Angle

An additional technique for checking the calculated soft-tissue contribution (STC) is to evaluate the SJLA. Remember that a neutral SJLA (16°) indicates a knee with normal alignment with no flexion or hyperextension. SJLA values less than 16° indicate flexion, while SJLA values greater than 16° indicate extension (Figs. 7 and 8). In order to check your results from the Seesaw, Formula, or Table Methods, take the value that was calculated for the soft-tissue contribution and add 16° (with flexion as a negative and extension as a positive soft-tissue contribution). The answer should equal the SJLA that was measured on the x-ray:

SJLA = 16° + STC

Research is underway to determine the validity of the SJLA method to evaluate soft-tissue contribution to the overall knee position. With further validation, the SJLA method will evolve into a stand-alone method.

# Sagittal Plane Examples

To show the complexity of the sagittal plane, let's look at an example in which the SMAA denotes a 26° flexion deformity of the knee joint (Fig. 13A). However, after joint angle analysis, it is determined that the distal femur has a bony deformity of 20° (flexion) and that the proximal tibia is normal. This joint angle analysis must be examined along with the SMAA to obtain a complete picture of the deformity. The soft-tissue contribution can be determined by using the Formula (Fig. 13B), Seesaw, or Table Method (Fig. 13C). Remember that in the Formula and the Table Methods, negative values are used for flexion and positive values are used for extension.

In Figure 13C, the Table Method is used and the PDFA, PPTA, and SMAA are recorded in the table (Fig. 13C, Lines 1 and 3). PDFA and PPTA (Fig. 13C, Line 1) are then combined to determine the total bony deformity (Fig. 13C, Line 2). The total bony deformity (Fig. 13C, Line 2) is then reconciled

| | | | Flexion (Negative Value) | | Extension (Positive value) | |
|---|---|---|---|---|---|---|
| | 1 | Femur (PDFA) | ___ (≤ 83°) | (-) ___ | Δ(+)___ | ___ (≥83°) |
| | | Tibia (PPTA) | ___ (≤ 81°) | (-) ___ | Δ(+)___ | ___ (≥81°) |
| TBD | 2 | TBD (Total Bony Deformity) | | (-) ___ | (+) ___ | |
| + STC | 4 | STC (Soft-tissue Contribution)* | | (-) ___ | (+) ___ | |
| SMAA | 3 | SMAA (Sag. Mechanical Axes Angle) | | (-) ___ | (+) ___ | |

*Soft-tissue contribution of < 5° degrees flexion or < 5° hyperextension is most likely insignificant.

**Fig. 12: Table Method.** PDFA, posterior distal femoral angle; PPTA, posterior proximal tibial angle.

A

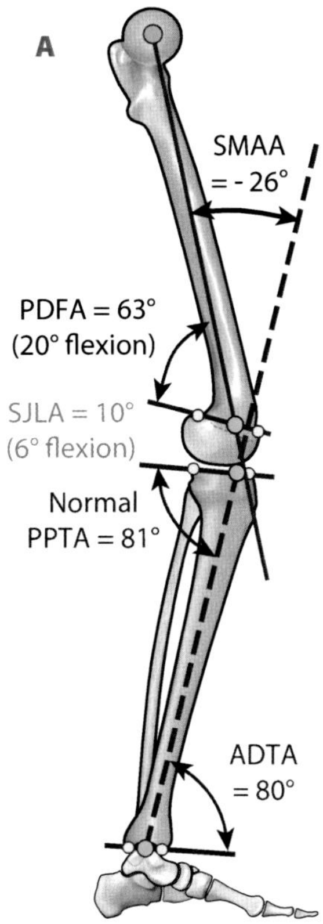

SMAA = - 26°

PDFA = 63° (20° flexion)

SJLA = 10° (6° flexion)

Normal PPTA = 81°

ADTA = 80°

B

| STC | | SMAA | | TBD (Total Bony Deformity) | | |
|---|---|---|---|---|---|---|
| Soft-tissue Contribution | = | Sagittal Mechanical Axes Angle | - ( | Femoral Bony Deformity | + | Tibial Bony Deformity ) |
| Soft-tissue Contribution | = | - 26° (Flexion) | - ( | - 20 (Flexion) | + | 0° ) |
| Soft-tissue Contribution | = | - 26° (Flexion) | - | - 20° (Flexion) | | |
| Soft-tissue Contribution | = | - 6° (Flexion) | | | | |

C

| | | | | Flexion (Negative Value) | Extension (Positive value) |
|---|---|---|---|---|---|
| | 1 | Femur (PDFA) | 63° (≤ 83°) | (-) 20°Δ(+)___ | ___ (≥83°) |
| | | Tibia (PPTA) | 81° (≤ 81°) | (-) 0°Δ(+)___ | ___ (≥81°) |
| TBD | 2 | TBD (Total Bony Deformity) | | (-) 20° (+) ___ | |
| + STC | 4 | STC (Soft-tissue Contribution)* | | (-) 6° (+) ___ | |
| SMAA | 3 | SMAA (Sag. Mechanical Axes Angle) | | (-) 26° (+) ___ | |

*Soft-tissue contribution of < 5° degrees flexion or < 5° hyperextension is most likely insignificant.

D

Check Sagittal Joint Line Angle:

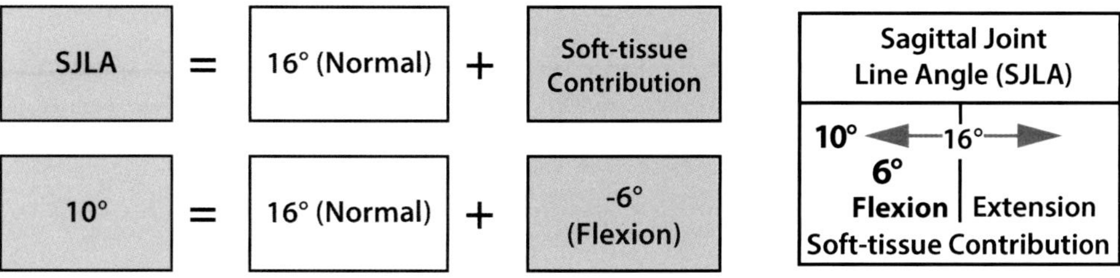


**Fig. 13:** This figure demonstrates the need for careful analysis in the sagittal plane. **A**, Example of sagittal plane bony and soft-tissue deformities. The measurement of the SMAA shows that there is a flexion deformity of 26° that is caused by a distal femoral deformity of 20° flexion with an additional soft-tissue contribution. The tibia is normal (PPTA = 81° and ADTA = 80°), and the patient does not have any ankle complaints. **B**, Formula Method is used to determine the soft-tissue contribution. **C**, Table Method is used to determine the soft-tissue contribution. **D**, Sagittal joint line angle is used to check the calculated soft-tissue contribution.

with the SMAA (Fig. 13C, Line 3) to show the soft-tissue component (Fig. 13C, Line 4). Since a negative value denotes flexion, the patient has a 6° soft-tissue flexion contracture. To double check our analysis, the calculated soft-tissue contribution can be compared to the sagittal joint line angle (normal 16°) (Fig. 13D).

For the same deformity (Fig. 14A), if only the distal femur is normalized by performing a 20° opening wedge osteotomy (Figs. 14B and 14C), a 6° soft-tissue flexion contracture deformity will still be present (Fig. 14D). However, full correction could possibly be achieved through physical therapy, a bony overcorrection of 6°, or a soft-tissue release to gain 6° of additional extension (Fig. 14E).

Multiple combinations of bony deformities and soft-tissue contributions around the knee can result in a similar clinical deformity (Fig. 15). Bony deformity and soft-tissue abnormalities can contribute to or compensate for the deformity. This is complex and requires careful analysis to formulate the correct treatment strategy.

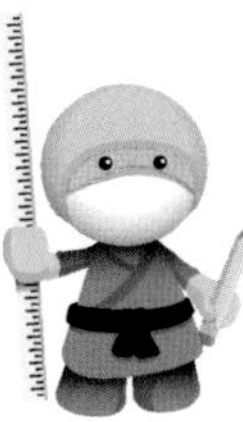

*Sensei says,*

*"Multiple combinations of bony deformities and soft-tissue contributions can result in the same deformity in the sagittal plane. The SMAA must be compared to the results of the joint angle analysis to determine how much of the total distal femoral and proximal tibial deformity is comprised of bony deformity and how much is comprised of soft-tissue deformity."*

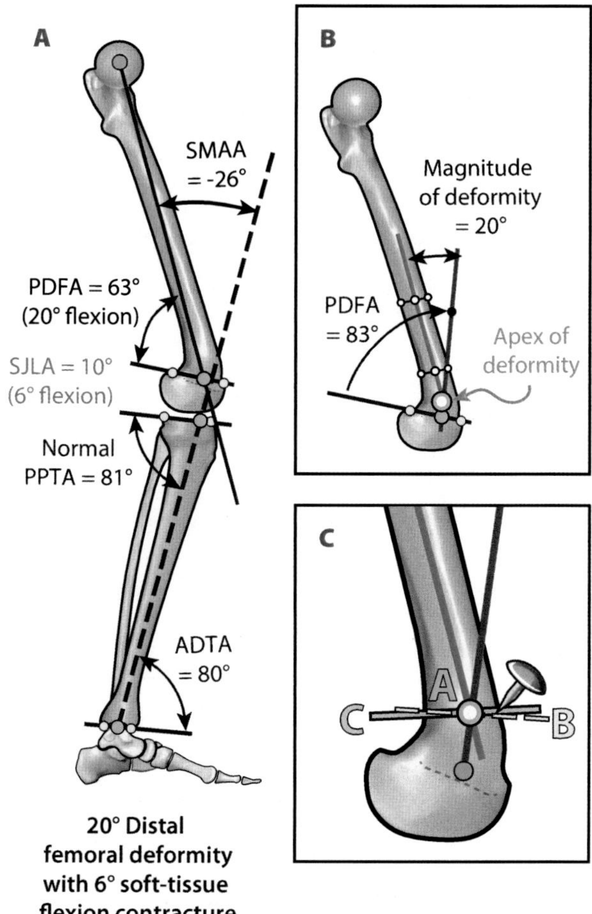


**Fig. 14:** Same deformity depicted in Fig. 13. **A**, The SMAA shows that there is a flexion deformity of 26° that is caused by a distal femoral deformity of 20° with an additional soft-tissue flexion contracture of 6°. **B** and **C**, Only the distal femur is normalized by performing a 20° opening wedge osteotomy.

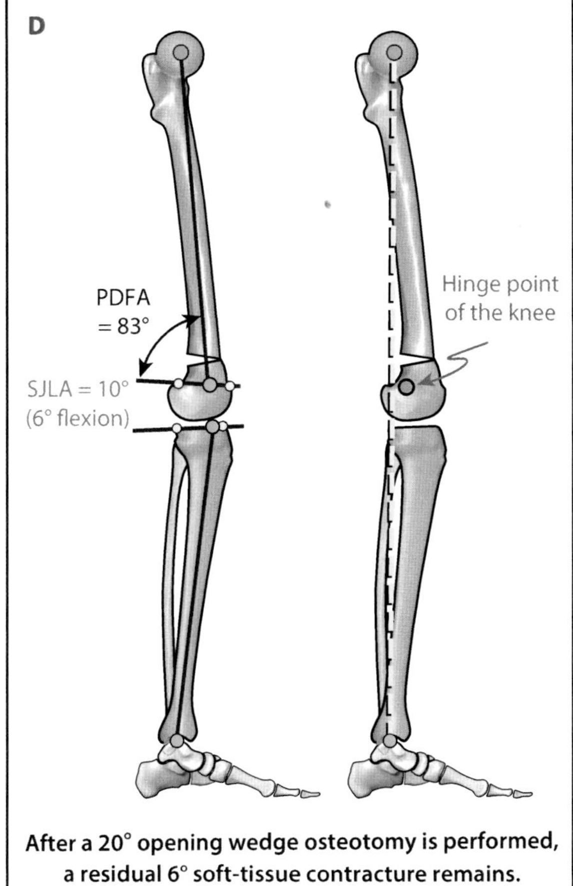


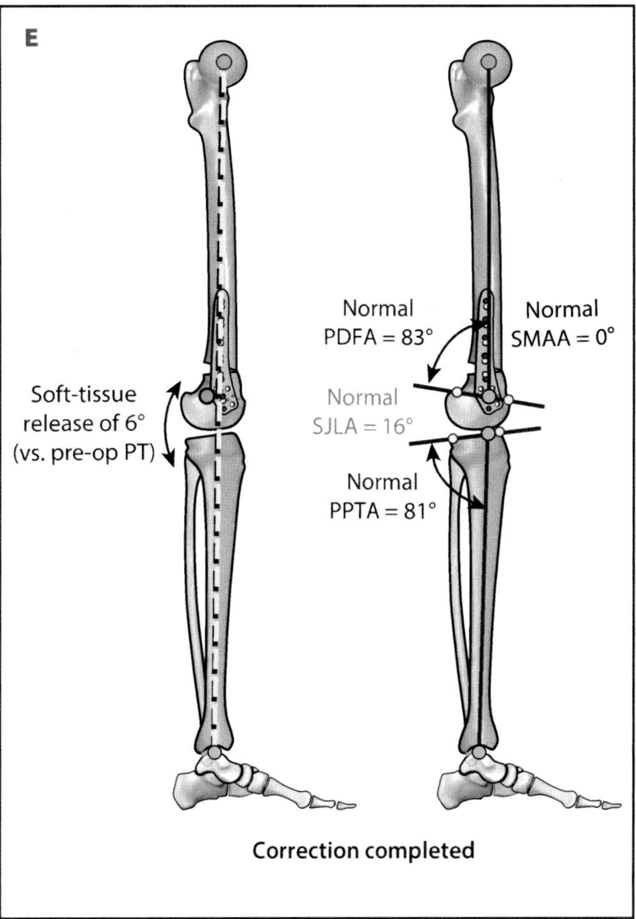


**Fig. 14 (continued): D**, After bony correction, a 6° soft-tissue flexion contracture deformity will still be present. **E**, Performing a 6° soft-tissue release results in full correction. A, apex; ADTA, anterior distal tibial angle; B, bone cut; C, C-level; PDFA, posterior distal femoral angle; PPTA, posterior proximal tibial angle; PT, physical therapy; SJLA, sagittal joint line angle; SMAA, sagittal mechanical axes angle.

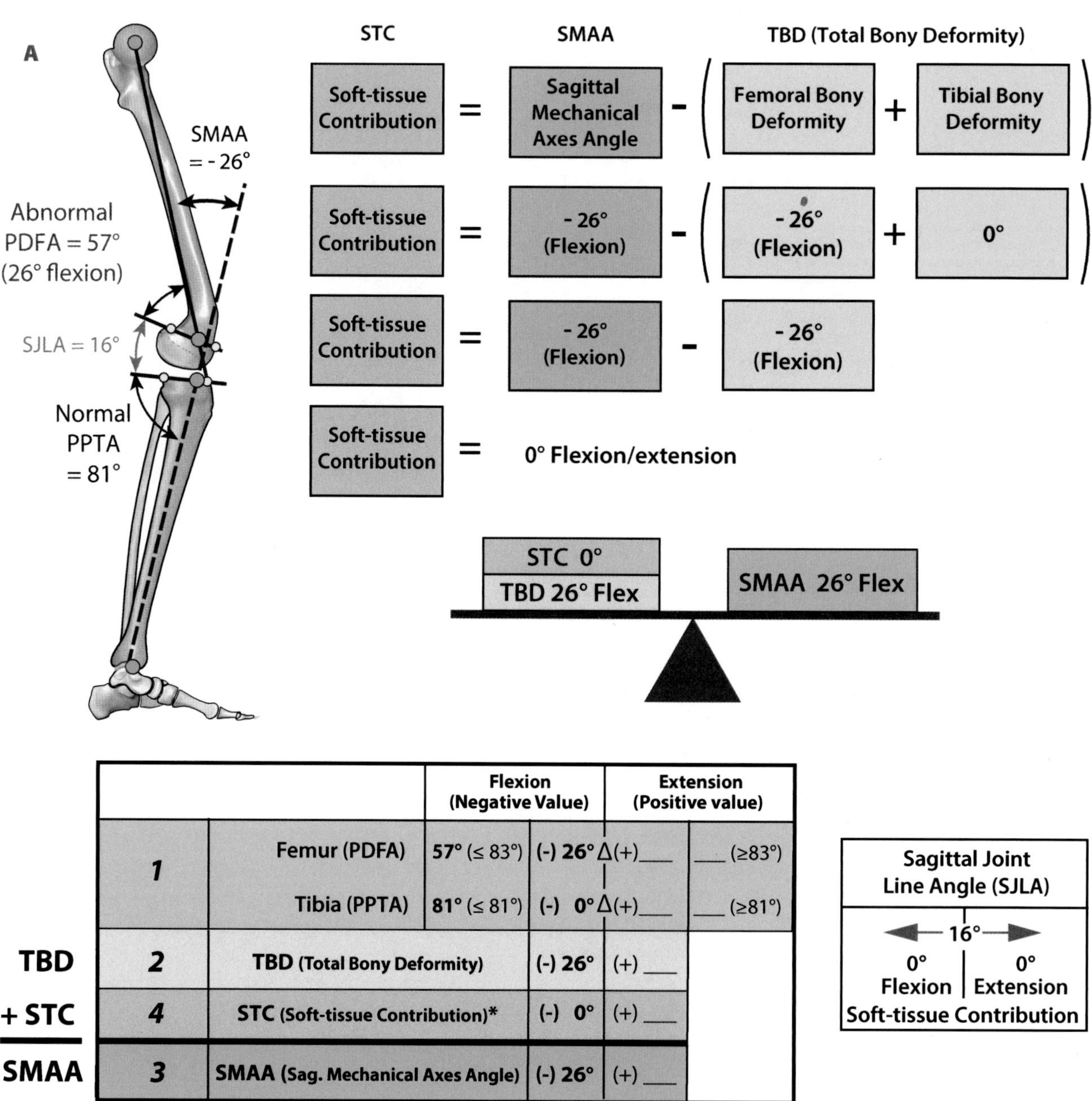


| | | | Flexion (Negative Value) | Extension (Positive value) | |
|---|---|---|---|---|---|
| 1 | Femur (PDFA) | 57° (≤ 83°) | (-) 26° Δ(+)___ | | ___(≥83°) |
| | Tibia (PPTA) | 81° (≤ 81°) | (-) 0° Δ(+)___ | | ___(≥81°) |
| 2 | TBD (Total Bony Deformity) | | (-) 26° | (+) ___ | |
| 4 | STC (Soft-tissue Contribution)* | | (-) 0° | (+) ___ | |
| 3 | SMAA (Sag. Mechanical Axes Angle) | | (-) 26° | (+) ___ | |

***Soft-tissue contribution of < 5° degrees flexion or < 5° hyperextension is most likely insignificant.**

**Fig. 15:** This set of figures illustrates the need to perform a careful analysis and compare the magnitude of the SMAA to the magnitude of the bony deformity found during joint analysis. Note that all these deformities occur in the distal femur or proximal tibia; therefore, the SMAA represents the total amount of soft-tissue and bony deformity about the knee. Each panel shows a similar knee flexion deformity measured by the SMAA. However, a careful analysis of the joint angles shows different etiologies for each of the knee flexion deformities. In each example, the anterior distal tibial angle is normal and/or the patient does not have any ankle complaints. The Formula, Seesaw, and Table Methods are included for each panel as well as checking the soft-tissue contribution analysis using the SJLA. Remember that in the Formula and Table Methods, negative values denote flexion and positive values denote extension. Ext, extension; Flex, flexion; PDFA, posterior distal femoral angle; PPTA, posterior proximal tibial angle; SJLA, sagittal joint line angle; SMAA, sagittal mechanical axes angle; STC, soft-tissue contribution; TBD, total bony deformity.

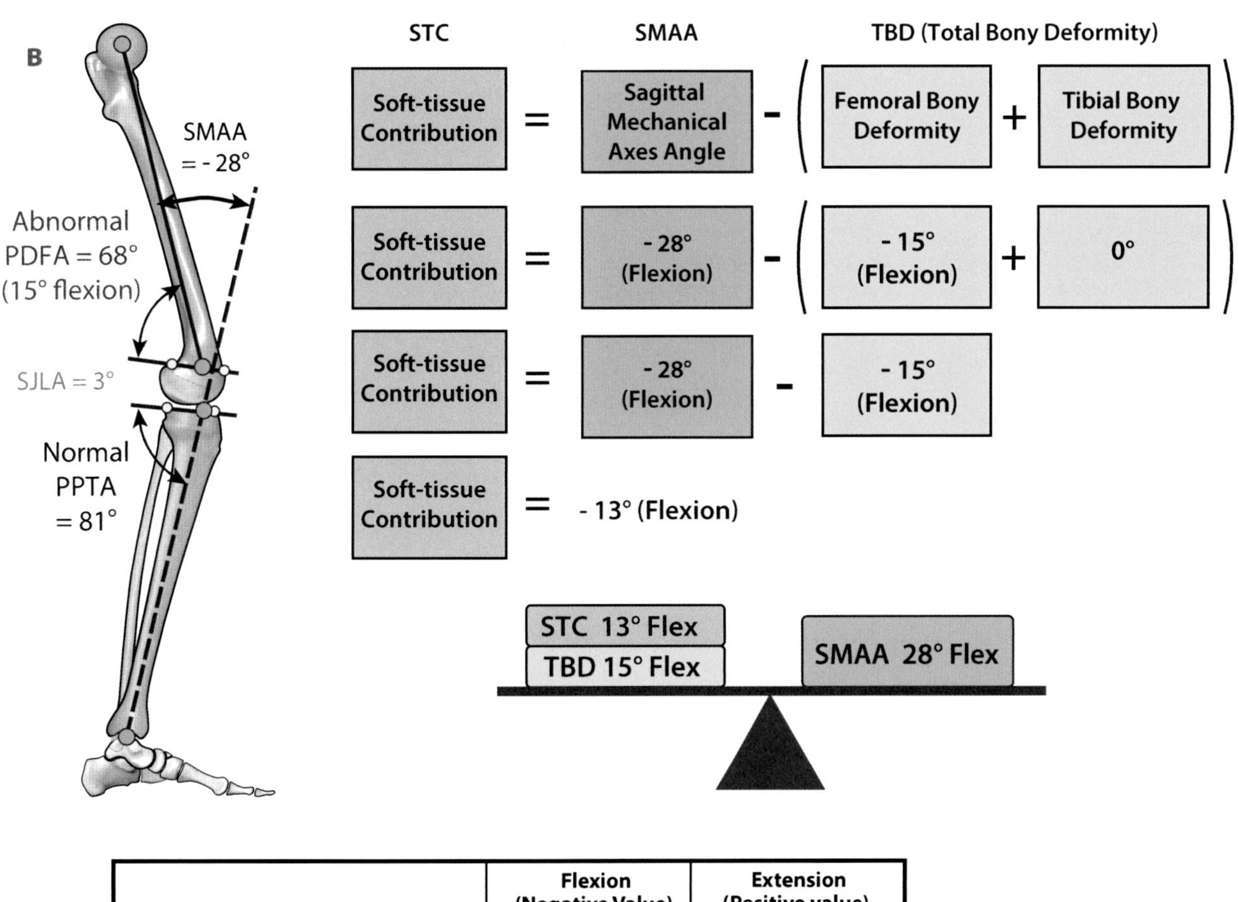


| | | | Flexion (Negative Value) | | Extension (Positive value) | |
|---|---|---|---|---|---|---|
| | 1 | Femur (PDFA) | 68° (≤ 83°) | (-) 26° | Δ(+)___ | ___ (≥83°) |
| | | Tibia (PPTA) | 81° (≤ 81°) | (-) 0° | Δ(+)___ | ___ (≥81°) |
| **TBD** | 2 | **TBD (Total Bony Deformity)** | | (-) 15° | (+) ___ | |
| **+ STC** | 4 | **STC (Soft-tissue Contribution)*** | | (-) 13° | (+) ___ | |
| **SMAA** | 3 | **SMAA (Sag. Mechanical Axes Angle)** | | (-) 28° | (+) ___ | |

*Soft-tissue contribution of < 5° degrees flexion or < 5° hyperextension is most likely insignificant.

| Sagittal Joint Line Angle (SJLA) |
|---|
| 3° ◄— 16° —► <br> 13° <br> Flexion \| Extension <br> Soft-tissue Contribution |

**Fig. 15 (continued).**

© 2023 Sinai Hospital of Baltimore

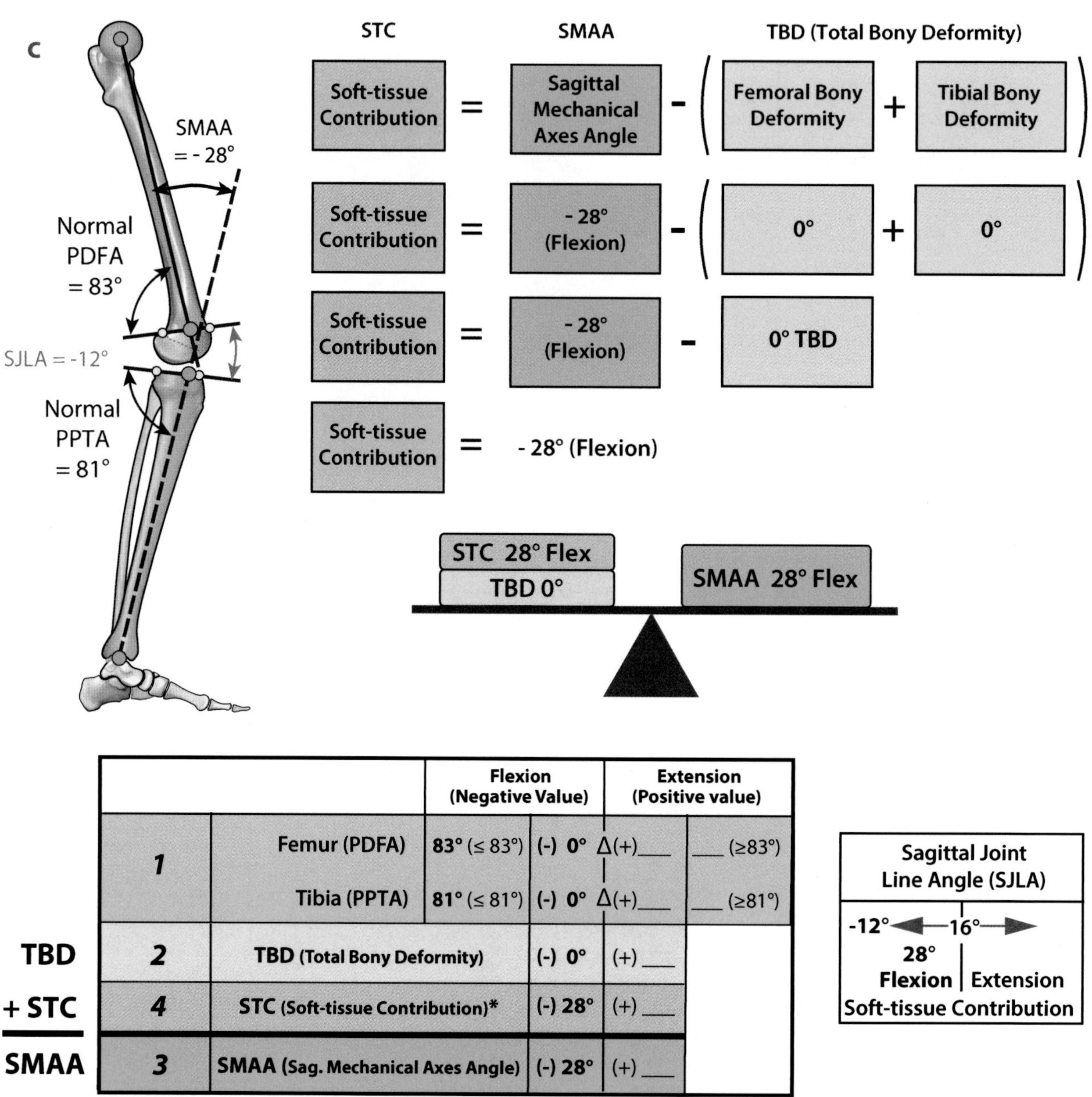


| | | | | Flexion (Negative Value) | Extension (Positive value) | |
|---|---|---|---|---|---|---|
| | 1 | Femur (PDFA) | 83° (≤ 83°) | (-) 0° | Δ(+)___ | ___ (≥83°) |
| | | Tibia (PPTA) | 81° (≤ 81°) | (-) 0° | Δ(+)___ | ___ (≥81°) |
| TBD | 2 | TBD (Total Bony Deformity) | | (-) 0° | (+) ___ | |
| + STC | 4 | STC (Soft-tissue Contribution)* | | (-) 28° | (+) ___ | |
| SMAA | 3 | SMAA (Sag. Mechanical Axes Angle) | | (-) 28° | (+) ___ | |

*Soft-tissue contribution of < 5° degrees flexion or < 5° hyperextension is most likely insignificant.

**Fig. 15 (continued).**

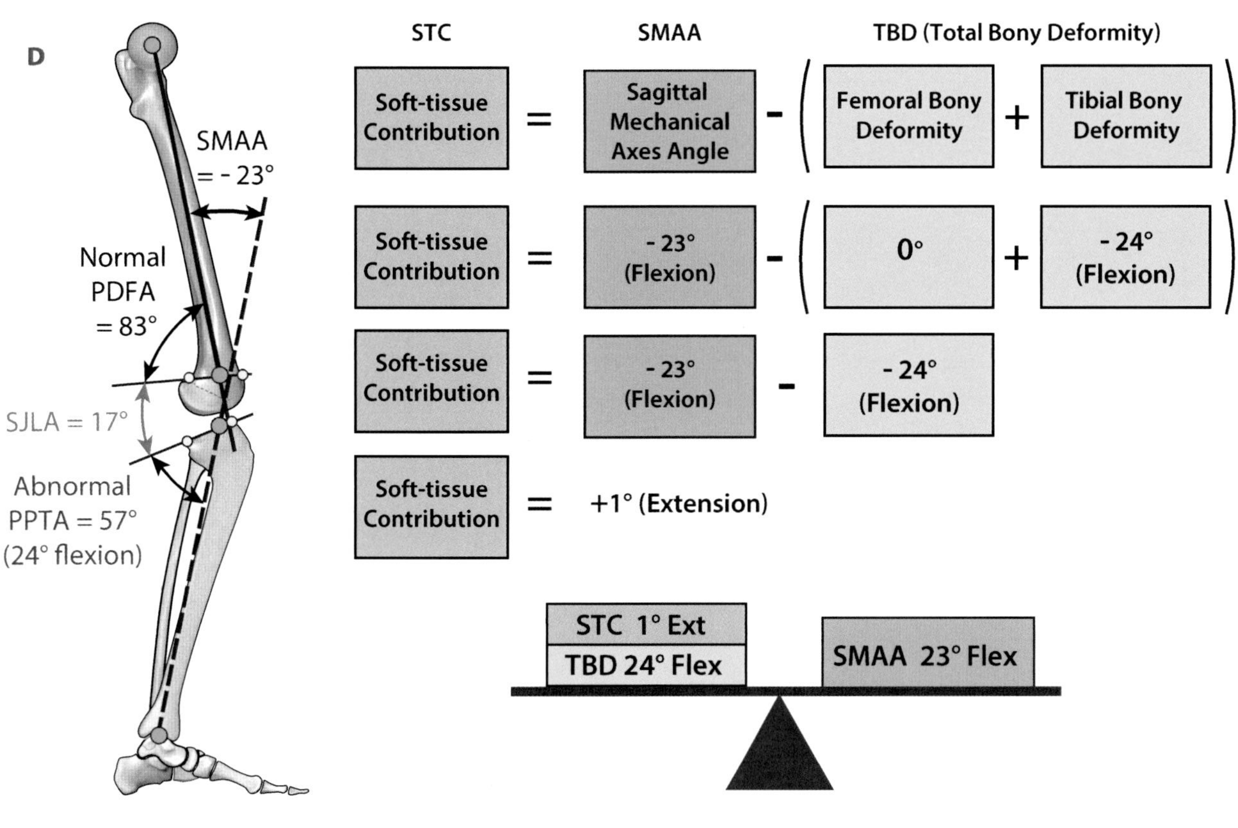


| | | | Flexion (Negative Value) | | Extension (Positive value) | |
|---|---|---|---|---|---|---|
| | 1 | Femur (PDFA) | 83° (≤ 83°) | (-) 0° | Δ(+)___ | ___ (≥83°) |
| | | Tibia (PPTA) | 57° (≤ 81°) | (-) 24° | Δ(+)___ | ___ (≥81°) |
| **TBD** | 2 | **TBD** (Total Bony Deformity) | | (-) 24° | (+) ___ | |
| **+ STC** | 4 | **STC** (Soft-tissue Contribution)* | | (-)___ | (+) 1° | |
| **SMAA** | 3 | **SMAA** (Sag. Mechanical Axes Angle) | | (-) 23° | (+) ___ | |

*Soft-tissue contribution of < 5° degrees flexion or < 5° hyperextension is most likely insignificant.

| Sagittal Joint Line Angle (SJLA) | |
|---|---|
| 16° | 17° |
| 0 Flexion | 1° **Extension** |
| Soft-tissue Contribution | |

**Fig. 15 (continued).**

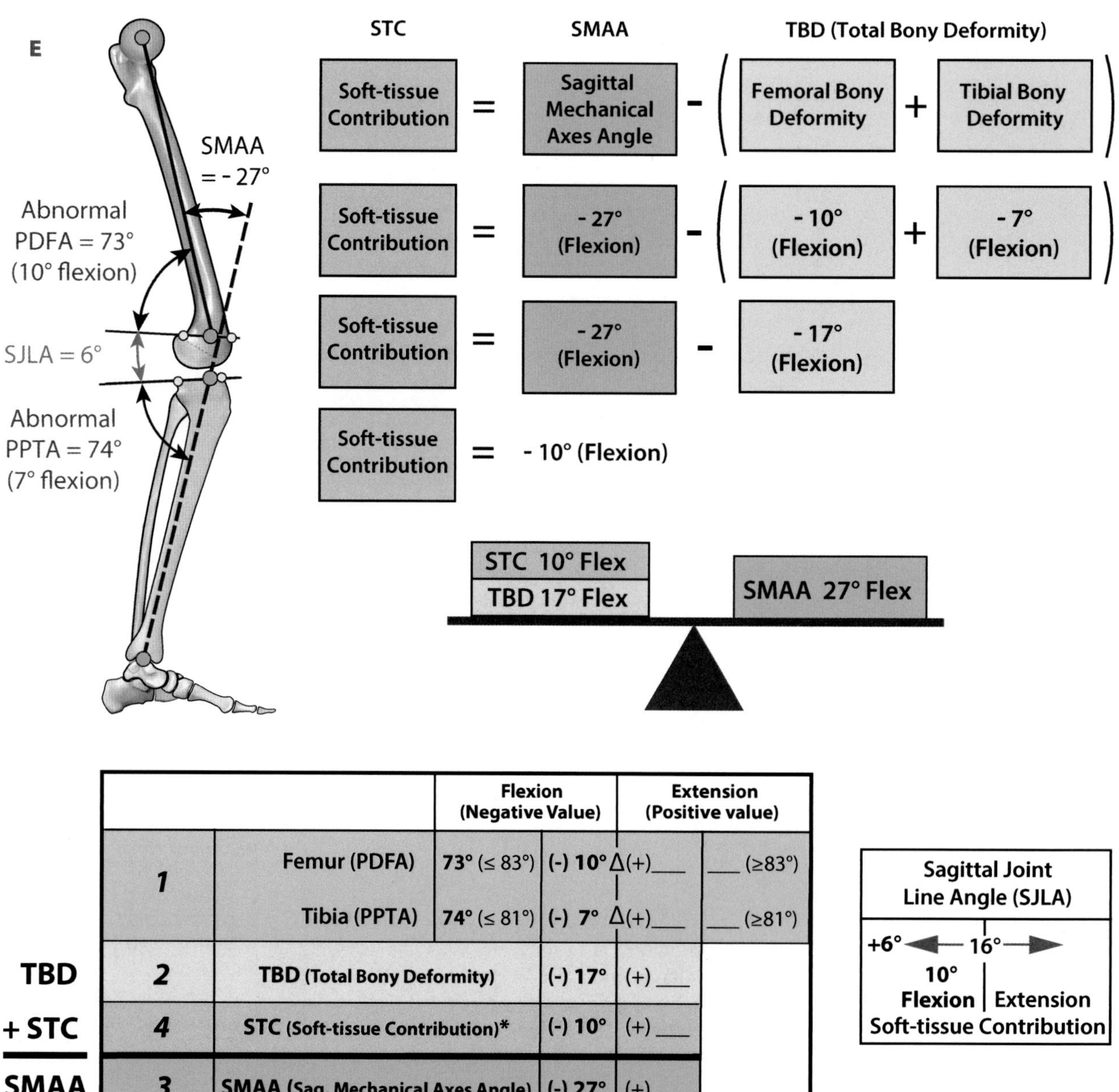


| | | | | Flexion (Negative Value) | | Extension (Positive value) |
|---|---|---|---|---|---|---|
| | 1 | Femur (PDFA) | 73° (≤ 83°) | (-) 10° Δ | (+)___ | ___ (≥83°) |
| | | Tibia (PPTA) | 74° (≤ 81°) | (-) 7° Δ | (+)___ | ___ (≥81°) |
| TBD | 2 | TBD (Total Bony Deformity) | | (-) 17° | (+) ___ | |
| + STC | 4 | STC (Soft-tissue Contribution)* | | (-) 10° | (+) ___ | |
| SMAA | 3 | SMAA (Sag. Mechanical Axes Angle) | | (-) 27° | (+) ___ | |

*Soft-tissue contribution of < 5° degrees flexion or < 5° hyperextension is most likely insignificant.

**Fig. 15 (continued).**

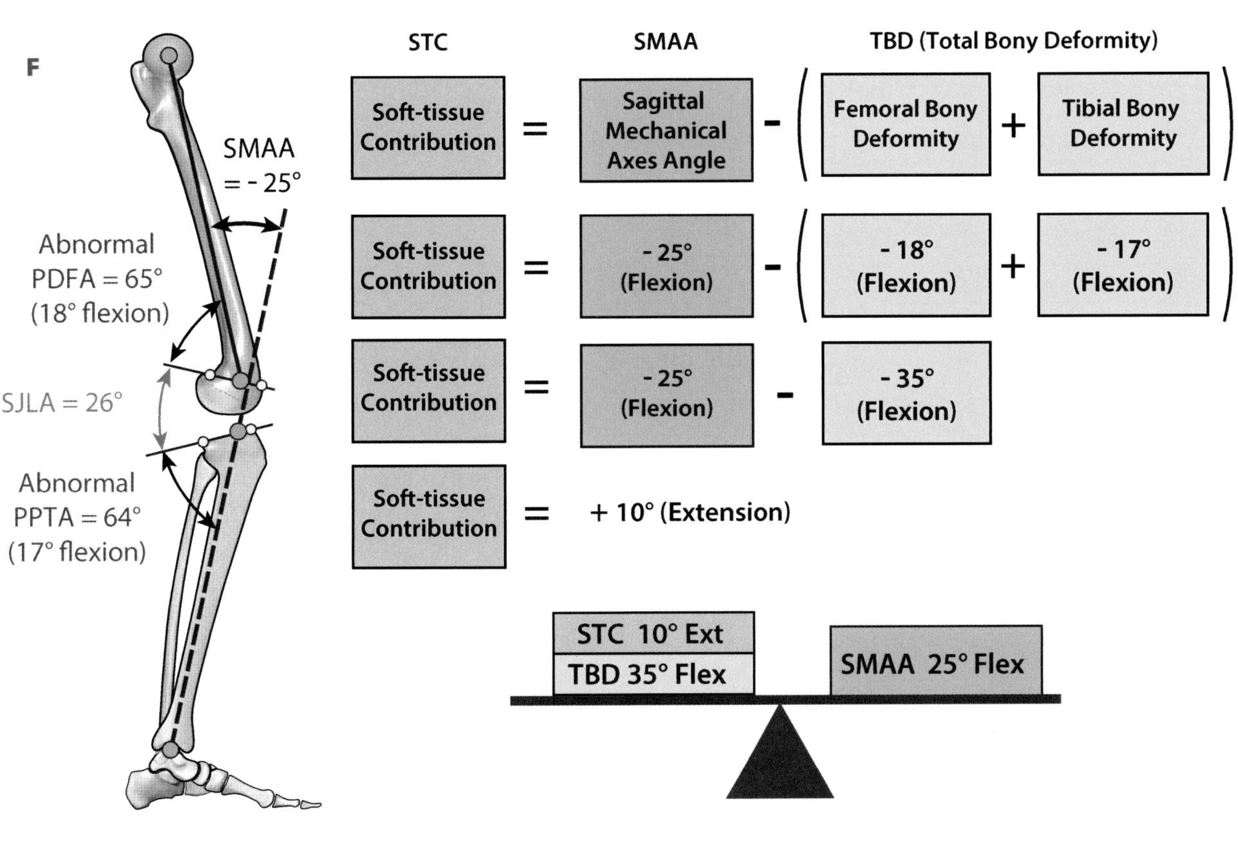


| | | | | Flexion (Negative Value) | Extension (Positive value) | |
|---|---|---|---|---|---|---|
| | 1 | Femur (PDFA) | 65° (≤ 83°) | (-) 18° Δ | (+)___ | ___ (≥83°) |
| | | Tibia (PPTA) | 64° (≤ 81°) | (-) 17° Δ | (+)___ | ___ (≥81°) |
| **TBD** | 2 | **TBD** (Total Bony Deformity) | | (-) 35° | (+) ___ | |
| **+ STC** | 4 | **STC** (Soft-tissue Contribution)* | | (-) __ | (+) 10° | |
| **SMAA** | 3 | **SMAA** (Sag. Mechanical Axes Angle) | | (-) 25° | (+) ___ | |

*Soft-tissue contribution of < 5° degrees flexion or < 5° hyperextension is most likely insignificant.

| Sagittal Joint Line Angle (SJLA) | |
|---|---|
| ◄— 16° | —► 26° |
| | 10° |
| Flexion | Extension |
| Soft-tissue Contribution | |

**Fig. 15 (continued).**

© 2023 Sinai Hospital of Baltimore

## MAP the ABCs: Sagittal Plane Case Example

The following example will show the MAP the ABCs process in the sagittal plane (Table 1). A 17-year-old male with history of previous hip reconstruction (e.g., femoral head osteotomy secondary to Perthes disease) presents with complaints of right knee pain during prolonged walking.

### MAP Analysis

#### Step 1: Measure the MAD

The sagittal plane mechanical axis deviation is obvious in the right lower extremity when compared with the left lower extremity (Fig. 16). The mechanical axis of the left limb is slightly anterior to the hinge point of the knee and within the confines of the distal femur, which is normal alignment. The mechanical axis of the right limb is significantly anterior to the hinge point of the knee and lies outside the confines of the distal femur, which shows that a significant deformity is present.

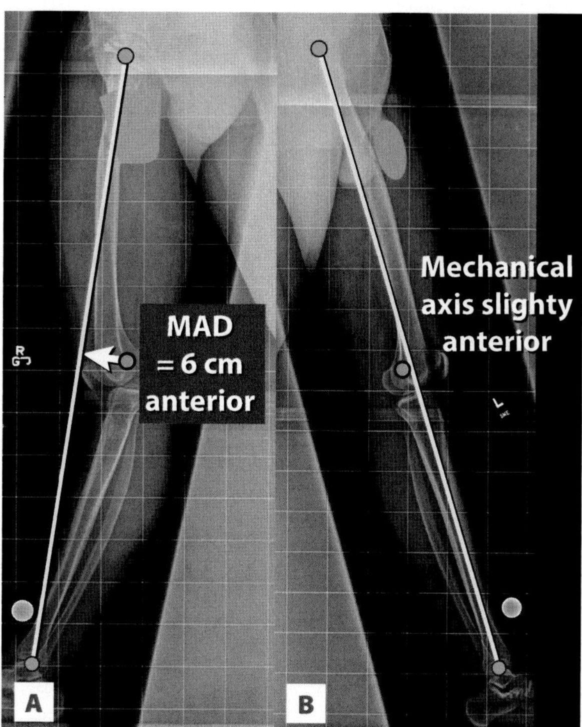


**Fig. 16:** Sagittal plane mechanical axis deviation (MAD) of the right (**A**) and left (**B**) limb.

**Table 1. Summary of MAP the ABCs in the Sagittal Plane**

**MAP**

**M** = Measure the MAD
**A** = Analyze the joint angles
**P** = Pick the deformed bone

**ABC**

**A** = Apex of deformity
**B** = Bone cut (choose the level of the osteotomy)
**C** = Correction

#### Step 2: Analyze the joint angles

The joint angles of the right limb are (Figs. 17 and 18):

- SMAA = 16° (hyperextension)
- PDFA = 82° (slightly abnormal)
- PPTA = 104° (abnormal extension)
- ADTA = 84° (slightly abnormal but accepted because the patient is not symptomatic – record as flexion)
- SJLA= 10° (abnormal)

The patient has a hyperextension deformity of the right proximal tibia of 23° (104° - 81° = 23° extension). A slight femoral flexion deformity is also present (83° – 82° = 1° flexion). The 10° SJLA is also abnormal.

The Formula, Seesaw, or Table Methods can be used to determine that the soft-tissue contribution is 6° flexion (Fig. 19). Note that the SJLA in this example is 10°, indicating 6° of soft-tissue compensation (Fig. 19D). This patient will likely respond to preoperative physical therapy.

#### Step 3: Pick the deformed bone

The analysis shows that the right proximal tibia is the bone segment of interest and the general area of deformity.

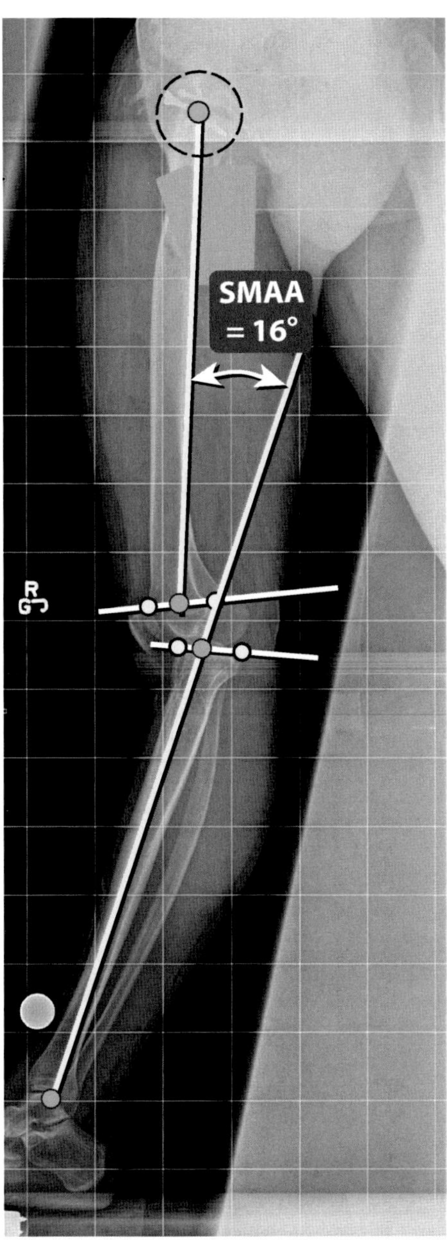


Fig. 17: The segmental mechanical axes of the right limb are not collinear and show that the limb has a 16° hyperextension deformity.

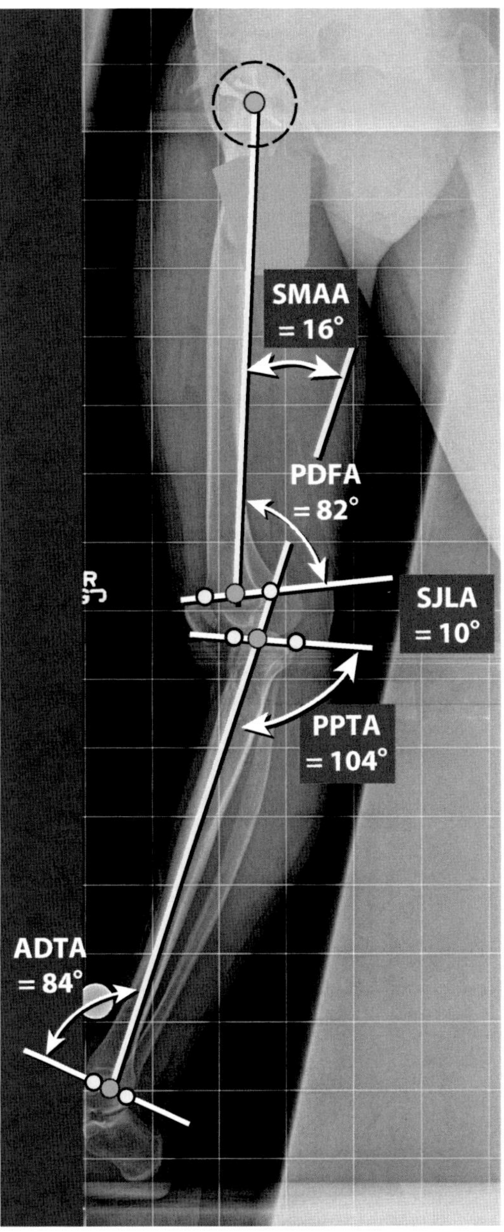


Fig. 18: Joint angle analysis of the right limb. Note that the PPTA, SJLA, and SMAA are abnormal. The patient's ankle was not symptomatic; therefore, the slight deformity represented by the ADTA of 84° is accepted. ADTA, anterior distal tibial angle; PDFA, posterior distal femoral angle; PPTA, posterior proximal tibial angle; SJLA, sagittal joint line angle; SMAA, sagittal mechanical axes angle.

© 2023 Sinai Hospital of Baltimore

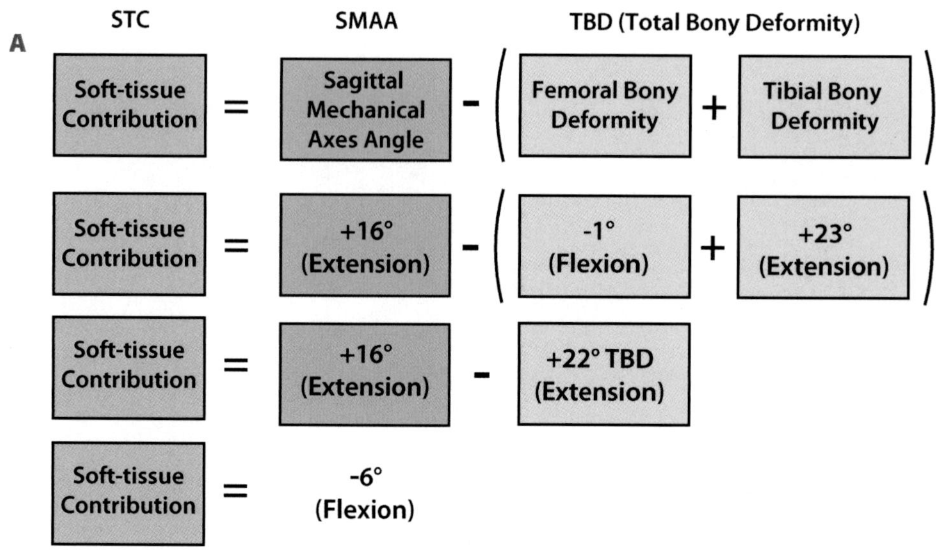


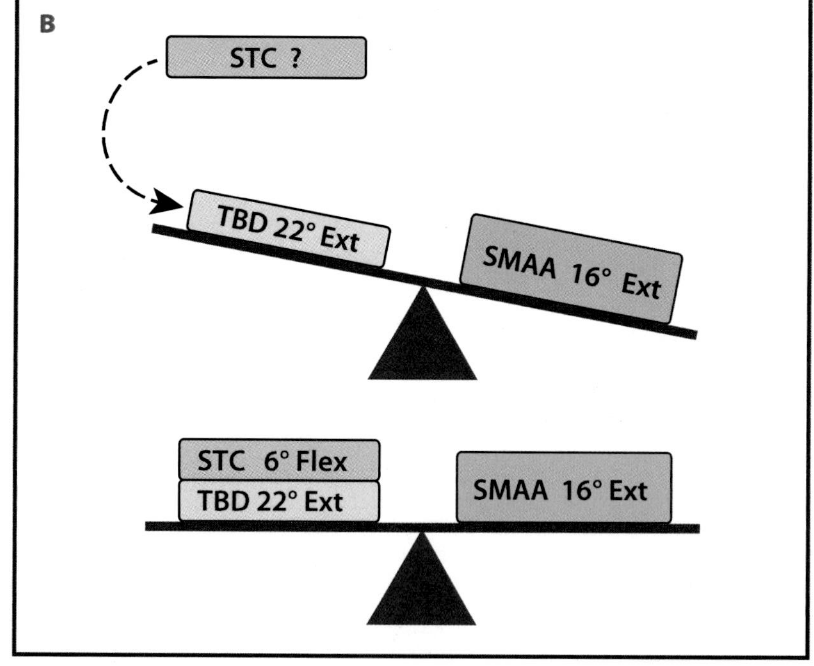


**Fig. 19: A**, Formula Method of determining soft-tissue contribution. **B**, Seesaw Method. **C**, Table Method. **D**, Check the soft-tissue contribution result by using the SJLA. Ext, extension; Flex, flexion; PDFA, posterior distal femoral angle; PPTA, posterior proximal tibial angle; SJLA, sagittal joint line angle; SMAA, sagittal mechanical axes angle; STC, soft-tissue contribution; TBD, total bony deformity.

C

| | | | Flexion (Negative Value) | | Extension (Positive value) | |
|---|---|---|---|---|---|---|
| | 1 | Femur (PDFA) | 82° (≤ 83°) | (-) 1° | Δ(+)___ | ___ (≥83°) |
| | | Tibia (PPTA) | ___ (≤ 81°) | (-)___ | Δ(+) 23° | 104° (≥81°) |
| TBD | 2 | TBD (Total Bony Deformity) | | (-)___ | (+) 22° | |
| + STC | 4 | STC (Soft-tissue Contribution)* | | (-) 6° | (+)___ | |
| SMAA | 3 | SMAA (Sag. Mechanical Axes Angle) | | (-)___ | (+) 16° | |

*Soft-tissue contribution of < 5° degrees flexion or < 5° hyperextension is most likely insignificant.

D

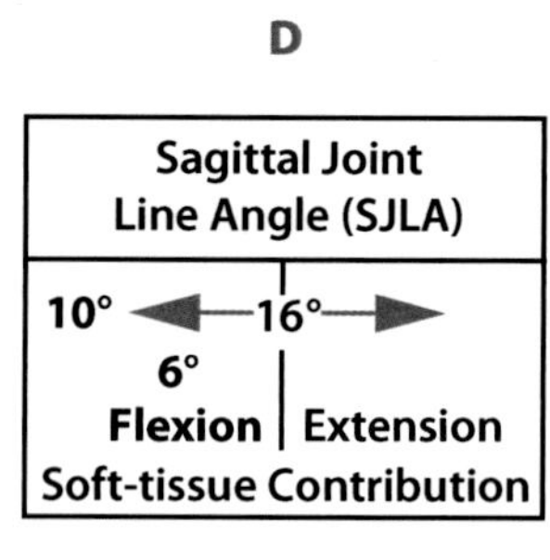

## ABCs of the Tibia

### Step 4: Apex of the deformity (tibia)

To draw the proximal axis, first draw the proximal tibial joint line (Fig. 20A). Draw another line (red line) that starts at a point 1/5 of the total length of the joint line from the anterior cortex and creates a PPTA of 81°.

The distal axis (yellow line) is drawn as a mid-diaphyseal line (Fig. 20B). Since the mid-diaphyseal line is used for the distal axis, the ADTA formed by the mid-diaphyseal line must be checked to see if it is normal. The ADTA is slightly abnormal, but this value is accepted as normal because the patient did not report any ankle problems. If the ADTA was significantly abnormal, a distal metaphyseal deformity may exist and would need to be addressed.

Mark the apex at the intersection of the proximal and distal tibial axes (Fig. 20C). The magnitude of the acute angle that is created by the intersection of the proximal and distal axes is the magnitude of the deformity.

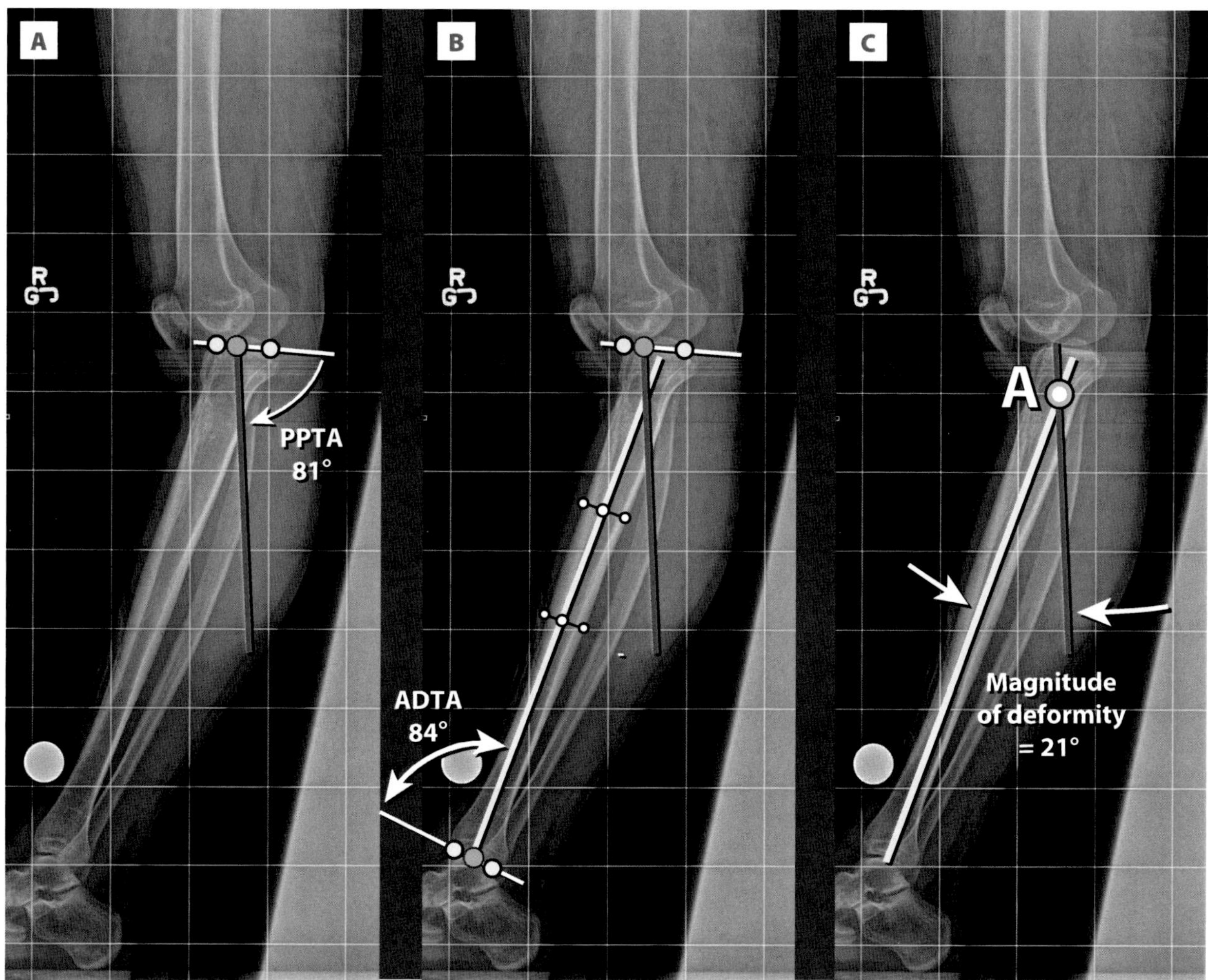


**Fig. 20: A**, The proximal axis line (*red line*) is determined by drawing the proximal tibial joint line and creating a normal PPTA of 81°. **B**, The distal axis (*yellow line*) is a mid-diaphyseal line. Since the mid-diaphyseal line is used for the distal axis, the ADTA must be checked for a hidden distal metaphyseal deformity. **C**, The apex is located at the intersection of the proximal and distal axes. The magnitude of deformity (21°) is the acute angle formed by the intersection of the proximal and distal axes. A, apex; ADTA, anterior distal tibial angle; PPTA, posterior proximal tibial angle.

© 2023 Sinai Hospital of Baltimore

### Step 5: Bone cut (tibia)

Ideally, the bone cut should be at the same level as the apex. In this example, the bone cut is made distal to the level of the apex, which will result in obligatory translation (Fig. 21A). The amount of translation is the distance between the proximal and distal axis lines at the level of the chosen osteotomy site.

**Table 2. Summary of Case Example 1 (Figures 16–21)**

**MAP**

**M** = Measure the MAD = 6 cm anterior

**A** = Analyze the joint angles:

- PPTA = 104°
- SMAA = 16°
- SJLA = 10°

**P** = Pick the deformed bone: Tibia

**ABCs (Tibia)**

**A** = Apex of deformity: Located in the proximal tibia; Magnitude of deformity = 21°

**B** = Bone cut (choose the level of the osteotomy): Proximal tibia

**C** = Correction: Gradual correction with opening wedge osteotomy and obligatory translation

### Step 6: Correction (tibia) (Table 2)

Plan a gradual correction with an external fixation device. The C-level is determined by drawing a line that passes through the apex and bisects the obtuse angle that is formed by the proximal and distal axes (Fig. 21B). The thumbtack (point of hinge rotation) is always placed on the C-level. In this case, the thumbtack is placed along the C-level on the convex side of the deformity to produce an opening wedge osteotomy (Fig. 21B). Perform an opening wedge osteotomy and then gradually rotate the bone segment around the thumbtack until the proximal and distal axes are aligned (Fig. 21C). In this case, we chose to use external fixation to correct the deformity and perform concurrent lengthening to correct the LLD. Check the alignment by drawing a sagittal plane mechanical axis and compare its location to the hinge point of the knee (Fig. 21D). The mechanical axis is slightly anterior to the hinge point of the knee and falls within the confines of the distal femur, which is considered to be normal alignment. The PDFA, PPTA, and ADTA are now normal (Fig. 21E).

MAP the ABCs is the same process for the sagittal plane as it is for the frontal plane. The joint motion in the sagittal plane creates an additional variable that must be taken into account during the MAP phase of the process. However, with careful evaluation and analysis, the MAP the ABCs procedure yields an accurate assessment that allows for the creation of a successful treatment strategy.

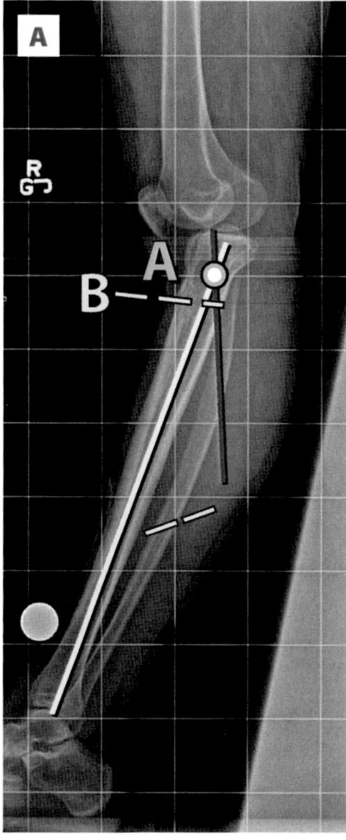


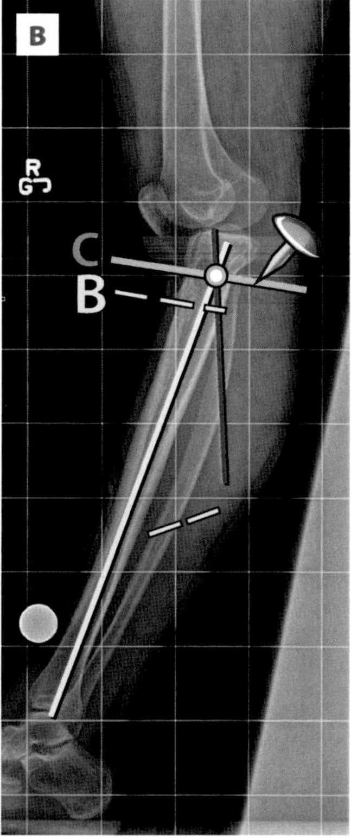


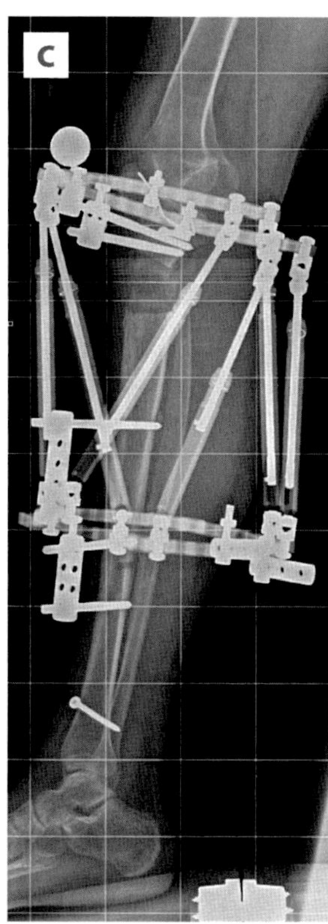


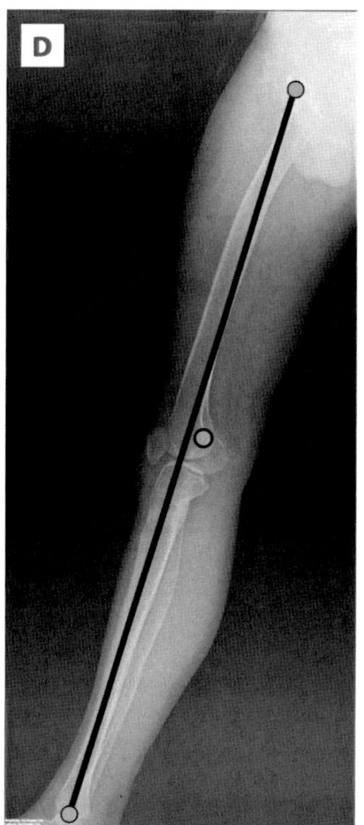


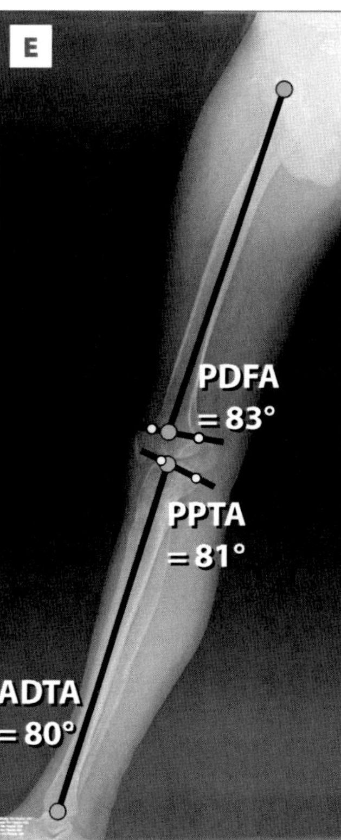


**Fig. 21: A**, The bone cut (*yellow dashed line*) is made distal to the apex. **B**, The C-level (*orange line*) is determined by drawing a line that passes through the apex and bisects the obtuse angle that is formed by the proximal and distal axes. The thumbtack (*point of hinge rotation*) is always placed on the C-level. Since there is limb length discrepancy, the thumbtack is placed along the C-level on the convex side of the deformity to produce an opening wedge osteotomy. Opening wedge osteotomies add length. A circular frame with six-axis deformity correction was used. **C**, X-ray obtained during healing phase. **D**, Final x-ray shows the sagittal plane mechanical axis line, which now passes anterior to the hinge point of the knee and within the confines of the distal femur. **E**, Normal alignment was achieved. A, Apex; ADTA, anterior distal tibial angle; B, bone cut; C, C-level; PPTA, posterior proximal tibial angle; PDFA, posterior distal femoral angle.

# Chapter 8

# Tibial Axis Planning: Frontal and Sagittal Planes

Philip K. McClure, MD

Shawn C. Standard, MD

Axis planning is defined as the ability to identify the axis of a given bone or bone segment. A deformed tibia can be divided into a proximal segment above the deformity and a distal segment below the deformity. All bony segments, no matter how short, have an axis. A tibial deformity results in the angulation of both the bone and the bone axis (both the anatomic and the mechanical axis lines).

Axis planning identifies the proximal and distal axis lines of the deformed bone or bone segment. The intersection of the proximal and distal axis lines shows the location of the deformity, which is called the apex of the deformity. A single-level deformity creates a single apex; a double-level deformity creates two apexes. Complex cases with multiple-level deformities may have three or more apexes. Multiple-level deformities may even be in different planes.

Each bony deformity must be evaluated in the frontal plane, the sagittal plane, and the axial plane (rotational profile). The frontal and sagittal planes of a bone are evaluated by axis planning analysis of the AP and lateral view x-rays. The axial plane (rotation profile) is evaluated by clinical rotational profile or computed tomography scan.

The mnemonic MAP the ABCs has been explained in previous chapters ("Deformity Analysis and Osteotomy Strategies: Frontal Plane" and "Deformity Analysis in the Sagittal Plane"). This process allows the surgeon to analyze the limb deformity, identify the apex of the deformity, and formulate a plan for correction. This chapter will describe strategies that can be used to draw the proximal and distal axes and identify the apex (the "A" of the ABCs). The bone cut/osteotomy level (the "B" in the ABCs) and correction (the "C" of the ABCs) will also be shown in each example.

For every example in this chapter, at least one deformity was found in the tibia during the MAP analysis in the frontal and sagittal planes. When performing the MAP analysis in the sagittal plane, it is essential to remember to evaluate the SMAA (the angle formed by the femoral and tibial segmental mechanical axes). The comparison of the SMAA and the bony deformity analysis of the angles about the knee (PDFA and PPTA) will provide valuable information about how the soft-tissue and bony deformities contribute to the overall sagittal plane deformity around the knee.

This chapter will begin with axis planning of simple, single-level tibial deformities in the frontal plane and progress to multiple-level deformities in the frontal plane. Then sagittal plane axis planning for single-level deformities and multiple-level deformities will be presented.

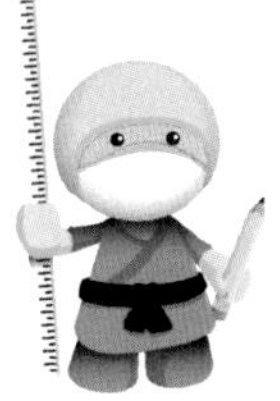

*Sensei says,*
*"In a normal tibia, the anatomic and mechanical axes of the tibia are essentially the same."*

© 2023 Sinai Hospital of Baltimore

## Tibial Axis Planning: Frontal Plane

### Identifying the Proximal Tibial Axis in the Frontal Plane

Three strategies can be used to identify the axis of the proximal tibial segment:

#### Normal Femoral Mechanical Axis Strategy:

Extend the normal femoral mechanical axis into the proximal tibia (Fig. 1). To use this strategy, the knee joint lines must be parallel or nearly parallel (normal JLCA) and the mLDFA must be normal.

#### Mid-diaphyseal Line Strategy:

Use the mid-diaphyseal line of the proximal tibial segment (Fig. 1). This strategy assumes that the proximal tibia has a straight segment that is long enough to define a line. If you use this strategy, you must measure the MPTA (normal range, 85–90°) formed by the proximal axis (i.e., the anatomic axis of the proximal bone segment) to check for a hidden deformity in the proximal tibia. If the MPTA is significantly abnormal, then the limb might have a single-level proximal metaphyseal deformity or a double-level deformity (proximal metaphyseal plus another deformity) that needs to be addressed.

#### Create Normal MPTA Strategy:

Use the proximal joint line to create a normal MPTA (85°–90°) from the center of the knee (Fig. 1). You may use the average normal value for MPTA or use the MPTA value of the contralateral normal limb.

### Identifying the Distal Tibial Axis in the Frontal Plane

Two strategies can be used to identify the axis of the distal tibial segment:

#### Mid-diaphyseal Line Strategy:

Use the distal tibial segment's mid-diaphyseal line (Fig. 2). This strategy assumes that the distal tibia has a straight segment that is long enough to define a line. If you use this strategy, you must measure the LDTA (normal range, 86–92°) formed by the distal axis (i.e., the anatomic axis of the distal bone segment) to check for a hidden deformity in the distal tibia. If the LDTA is significantly abnormal, then the limb might have a single-level distal metaphyseal deformity or a double-level deformity (distal metaphyseal plus another deformity) that needs to be addressed.

#### Create Normal LDTA Strategy:

If the LDTA is abnormal, use the distal joint line to create a normal LDTA from the center of the ankle joint (Fig. 2). You may use the average normal value for the LDTA (89°) or use the LDTA value of the contralateral normal limb.

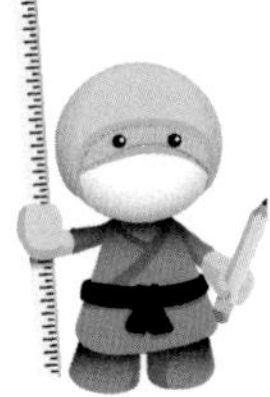

*Sensei says,*
*"If the mid-diaphyseal line is being used to identify the proximal tibial axis or the distal tibial axis, the associated proximal (MPTA) or distal (LDTA) angle must be checked to look for a hidden metaphyseal deformity."*

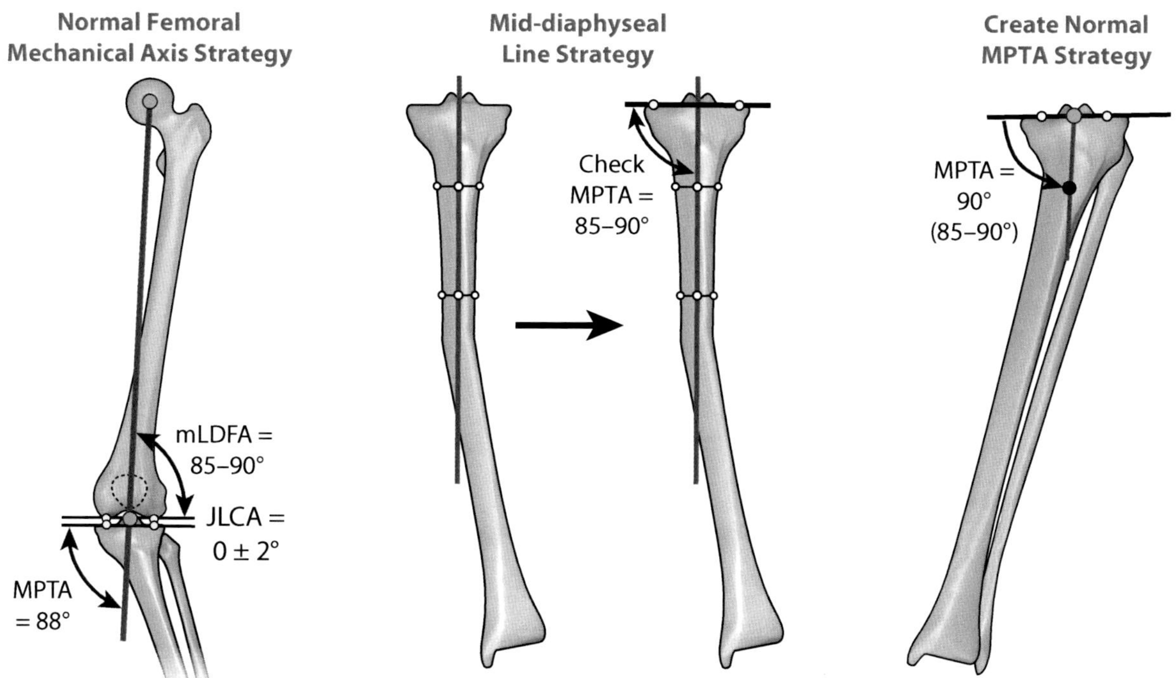


**Fig. 1:** Three strategies can be used to identify the axis of the proximal tibial segment in the frontal plane. **Normal Femoral Mechanical Axis Strategy:** Extend the normal femoral mechanical axis into the proximal tibia. The limb must have a normal JLCA and mLDFA. As long as the JLCA is normal, the resulting MPTA will equal the normal mLDFA. **Mid-diaphyseal Line Strategy:** Use the mid-diaphyseal line of the proximal tibial segment. You must measure the MPTA (normal range, 85–90°) formed by the proximal axis (i.e., the anatomic axis of the proximal bone segment) to check for a hidden deformity in the proximal tibia. If the MPTA is significantly abnormal, then a proximal hidden deformity exists. **Create Normal MPTA Strategy:** If the MPTA is abnormal, use the proximal joint line to create a normal MPTA (normal range, 85–90°) from the center of the knee.

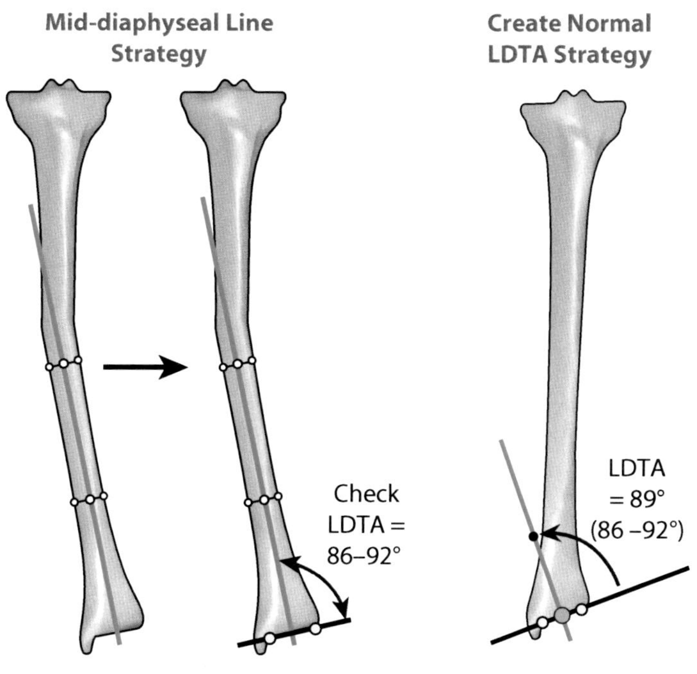


**Fig. 2:** Two strategies can be used to identify the axis of the distal tibial segment in the frontal plane. **Mid-diaphyseal Line Strategy:** Use the distal tibial segment's mid-diaphyseal line. You must measure the LDTA (normal range, 86–92°) formed by the distal axis (i.e., the anatomic axis of the distal bone segment) to check for a hidden deformity in the distal tibia. If the LDTA is significantly abnormal, then a distal hidden deformity exists. **Create Normal LDTA Strategy:** If the LDTA is abnormal, use the distal joint line to create a normal LDTA (normal range, 86–92°) from the center of the ankle joint.

© 2023 Sinai Hospital of Baltimore

## Diaphyseal Deformity (Fig. 3)

This type of deformity allows for easy identification of the proximal and distal axes.

**Angle Analysis:**

During the MAP analysis, we drew the mechanical axis of the bone segment and determined that the MPTA and the LDTA were both abnormal.

**Step 1:** Draw the mid-diaphyseal axis of the proximal segment and the mid-diaphyseal axis of the distal segment. These are the proximal and distal axes.

**Step 2:** Since mid-diaphyseal lines were used for both axes, the knee and ankle joint angles must be checked to look for a hidden deformity near the joints. The MPTA formed by the proximal axis (i.e., the anatomic axis of the proximal bone segment) is 90°, and the LDTA formed by the distal axis (i.e., the anatomic axis of the distal bone segment) is 90°. Both are within the range of normal; therefore, the bone does not have a hidden proximal or distal metaphyseal deformity.

**Step 3:** Mark the apex of the deformity at the intersection of the proximal and distal axes.

**Step 4:** Measure the magnitude of the deformity by measuring the magnitude of the acute angle (not the obtuse angle) created by the intersection of the proximal and distal axes. The magnitude is 10° (valgus).

**Step 5:** Bone Cut: Place the osteotomy as close to the apex as possible. In this example, the osteotomy can be performed at the level of the apex because this level is feasible anatomically. Also, the resulting proximal and distal bony fragments are large enough for stable fixation.

**Step 6:** Correction (part 1): Draw the C-level. The C-level passes through the apex and bisects the obtuse angle that is created by the intersection of the proximal and distal axes. The bone segments are always angulated about a hinge point or "thumbtack" placed on the C-level. In this example, the thumbtack is on the apex, which is a point that is located on the C-level.

**Step 7:** Correction (part 2): Angulating the bone segments around the thumbtack results in a neutral wedge osteotomy with complete alignment of the bone and both axes. The neutral wedge correction occurs because the thumbtack was placed on the apex in the center of the bone. No obligatory translation occurs because the bone cut was at the level of the apex. The bone on the medial cortex (medial to the thumbtack) is compressed during correction. Measure the MPTA and LDTA to confirm that they are now within the range of normal.

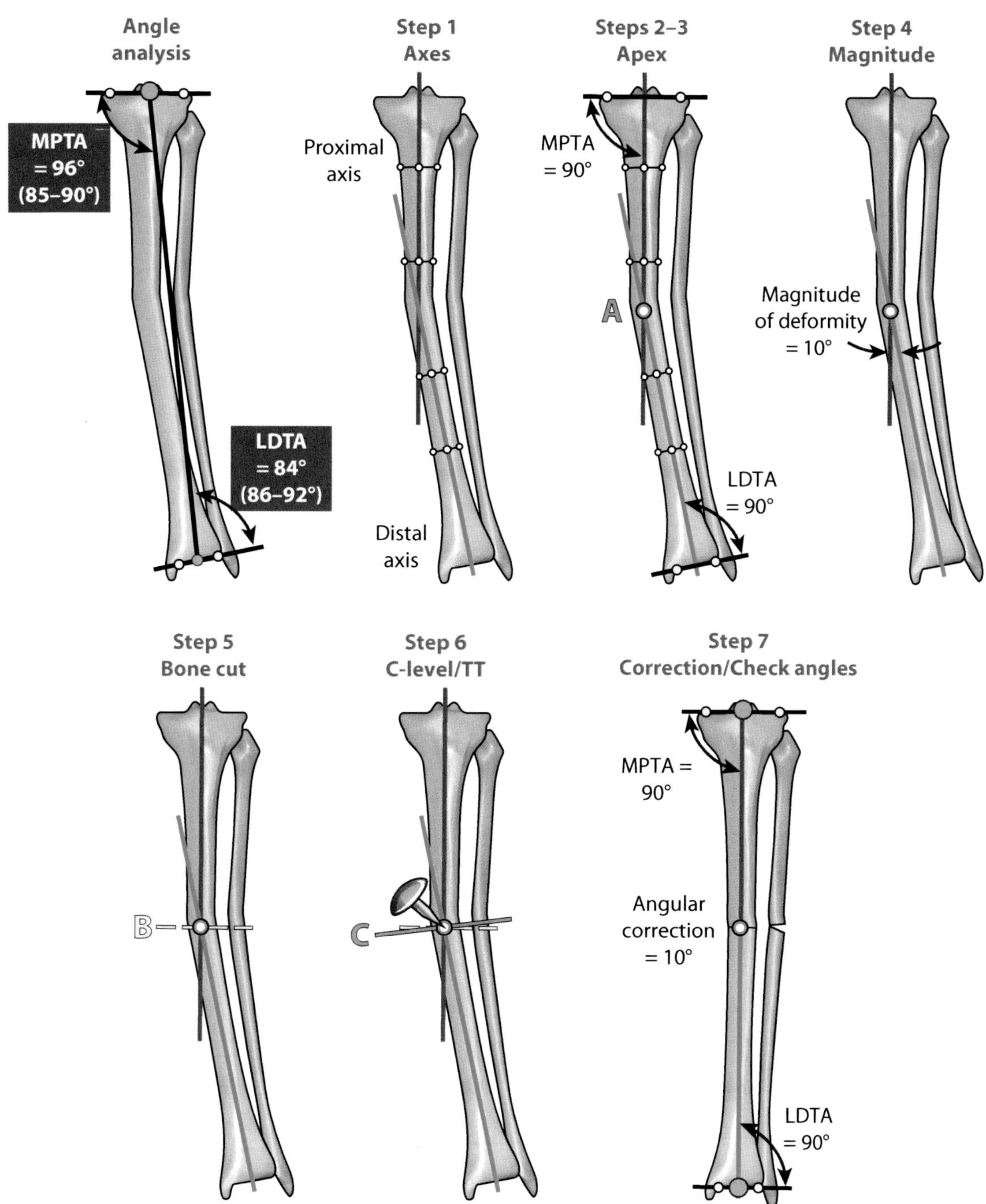


**Fig. 3:** Analysis of frontal plane tibial diaphyseal deformity. The MPTA and LDTA are both abnormal. The proximal and distal axes are drawn using the mid-diaphyseal lines of the proximal and distal bone segments. Since mid-diaphyseal lines were used for both axes, the knee and ankle joint angles must be checked to look for a hidden deformity near the joints. The MPTA and LDTA formed by the proximal and distal axis lines (i.e., the anatomic axis lines of the proximal and distal bone segments) are both normal; therefore, the bone does not have a proximal or distal metaphyseal deformity. The bone cut is made at the level of the apex. The bone segments are angulated around a thumbtack placed on the apex, which creates a neutral wedge osteotomy. A neutral wedge osteotomy results in perfect alignment of both the axes and bony margins. No obligatory translation occurs because the bone cut was at the level of the apex. A, apex; B, bone cut; C, C-level; TT, thumbtack.

© 2023 Sinai Hospital of Baltimore

## Metaphyseal Deformity: Creating a Normal Joint Angle and Using It as an Axis Line (Fig. 4)

Metaphyseal deformities of the tibia present a challenge because one of the bony segments is very short. This means that a simple mid-diaphyseal line cannot be drawn for the deformed proximal or distal metaphyseal bone segment. One strategy to find the short segment's axis is to draw a line from the center of the joint line to create a normal joint angle.

**Angle Analysis:** During the MAP analysis, we drew the mechanical axis of the bone segment and determined that the MPTA and the LDTA were both abnormal.

**Step 1:** Draw the joint line of the proximal tibia (short bone segment), and mark the center of the knee. To draw the short segment's axis, create an angle from the center of the knee that equals a normal MPTA (87°). This is the proximal axis.

**Step 2:** Draw the mid-diaphyseal line of the tibia. This is the distal axis. Since a mid-diaphyseal line was used for the distal axis, the distal joint angle must be checked to look for a hidden metaphyseal deformity. The LDTA formed by the distal axis (i.e., the anatomic axis of the distal bone segment) is 90° (normal); therefore, the bone does not have a distal metaphyseal deformity.

**Step 3:** Mark the apex of the deformity at the intersection of the proximal and distal axes.

**Step 4:** Measure the magnitude of the deformity by measuring the magnitude of the acute angle created by the intersection of the proximal and distal axes. The magnitude is 14° varus.

**Step 5:** Bone Cut: Place the osteotomy as close to the apex as possible. The tibial osteotomy is performed distal to the apex because it is not feasible to perform an osteotomy at the level of the apex from an anatomic stability point of view. The placement of the osteotomy must provide a proximal fragment that is large enough for bony fixation. The fibular osteotomy is performed at a more distal location to avoid the peroneal nerve and its branches. Since the tibial osteotomy is not performed at the level of the apex, bony translation will occur during the correction. The amount of translation is the distance between the proximal and distal axis lines at the level of the osteotomy site.

**Step 6:** Correction (part 1): Draw the C-level. The C-level passes through the apex and bisects the obtuse angle that is created by the intersection of the proximal and distal axes. The bone segments are always angulated about a thumbtack placed on the C-level. This example shows the thumbtack on the apex, which is located on the C-level.

**Step 7:** Correction (part 2): Angulating the bone segments around the thumbtack results in a neutral wedge osteotomy with complete alignment of the axes. Note the slight obligatory translation of the tibial bony margins due to the placement of the tibial osteotomy away from the level of the apex. Measure the MPTA and LDTA to confirm that they are now within the range of normal.

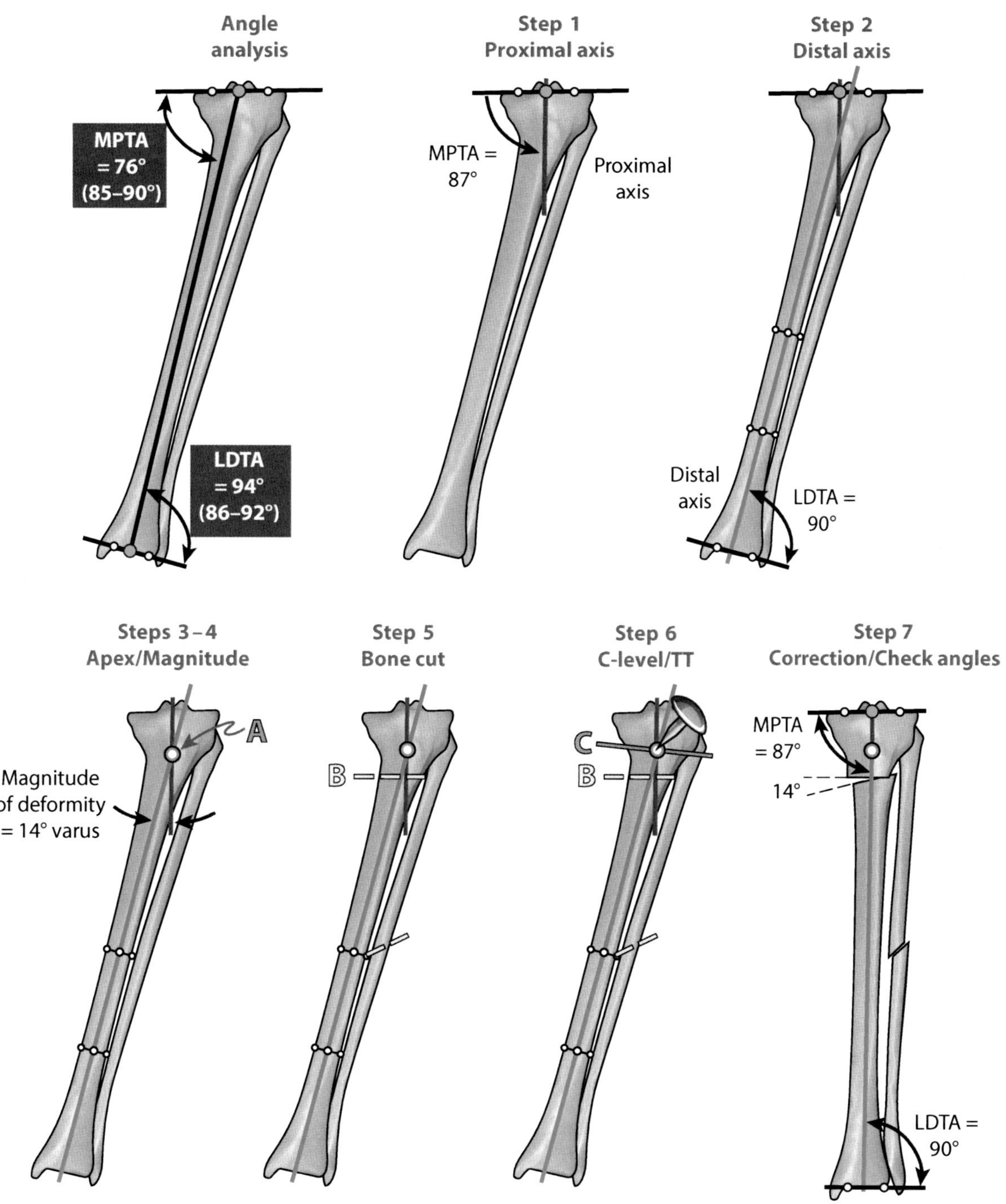


**Fig. 4:** Analysis of frontal plane proximal tibial metaphyseal deformity. The MPTA and LDTA are both abnormal. In this example, the proximal bone segment is very short; therefore, a mid-diaphyseal line cannot be used for the proximal axis. Draw the axis of the short proximal segment by creating an angle from the center of the knee that equals a normal MPTA (87°). The distal axis is created by using a mid-diaphyseal line and checking the ankle joint angle formed by the anatomic axis line of the distal bone segment. The LDTA formed by the distal axis is normal; therefore, the bone does not have a distal metaphyseal deformity. The tibial bone cut is made distal to the apex. Note that the fibular osteotomy is performed at a more distal location to avoid the peroneal nerve. The bone segments are angulated around a thumbtack placed on the apex. This results in a neutral wedge osteotomy with perfect axis alignment but slight bony translation because the bone cut was not made at the apex. A, apex; B, bone cut; C, C-level; TT, thumbtack.

© 2023 Sinai Hospital of Baltimore

## Metaphyseal Deformity: Using the Normal Femoral Mechanical Axis as a Proximal Tibial Axis (Fig. 5)

The other strategy for identifying the proximal tibial segment axis in a metaphyseal deformity is to use the mechanical axis from the normal ipsilateral femur.

**Angle Analysis:**
During the MAP analysis, we drew the femoral and tibial mechanical axes and determined that the MPTA was abnormal. The LDFA, JLCA, and LDTA were all normal.

**Step 1:** Draw the ipsilateral mechanical axis of the femur.

**Step 2:** Since the LDFA and JLCA are normal, the mechanical axis of the femur can be used as the proximal tibial axis. To do this, extend the femoral mechanical axis into the proximal tibia. As long as the JLCA is normal, the resulting MPTA will equal the normal LDFA.

**Step 3:** Draw the mid-diaphyseal line of the tibia. This is the distal axis. Since a mid-diaphyseal line was used for the distal axis, the distal joint angle must be checked to look for a hidden metaphyseal deformity. The LDTA formed by the distal axis (i.e., the anatomic axis of the distal bone segment) is 90° (normal); therefore, the bone does not have a distal metaphyseal deformity.

**Step 4:** Mark the apex at the intersection of the proximal and distal axes. Measure the magnitude of the deformity by measuring the magnitude of the acute angle created by the intersection of the proximal and distal axes. The magnitude is 20° valgus.

**Step 5:** Bone Cut: Place the osteotomy as close to the apex as possible. In this example, the tibial osteotomy is placed distal to the apex because it is not feasible to perform an osteotomy at the level of the apex from an anatomic point of view. Also, the distal placement of the osteotomy ensures that the resulting proximal fragment is large enough for stable fixation. Since the tibial osteotomy is not performed at the level of the apex, translation of the bony margins will occur during the correction. The amount of translation is the distance between the proximal and distal axis lines at the level of the osteotomy site. The fibular osteotomy is performed at a more distal location to avoid peroneal nerve injury.

**Step 6:** Correction (part 1): Draw the C-level. The C-level passes through the apex and bisects the obtuse angle that is created by the intersection of the proximal and distal axes. The bone segment is always angulated about a thumbtack placed on the C-level. This example shows the thumbtack on the apex, which is located on the C-level.

**Step 7:** Correction (part 2): Angulating the bone segments around the thumbtack results in a neutral wedge osteotomy with complete alignment of the axes. Note the obligatory translation of bone due to the placement of the tibial osteotomy away from the level of the apex. Measure the MPTA and LDTA to confirm that they are within the range of normal.

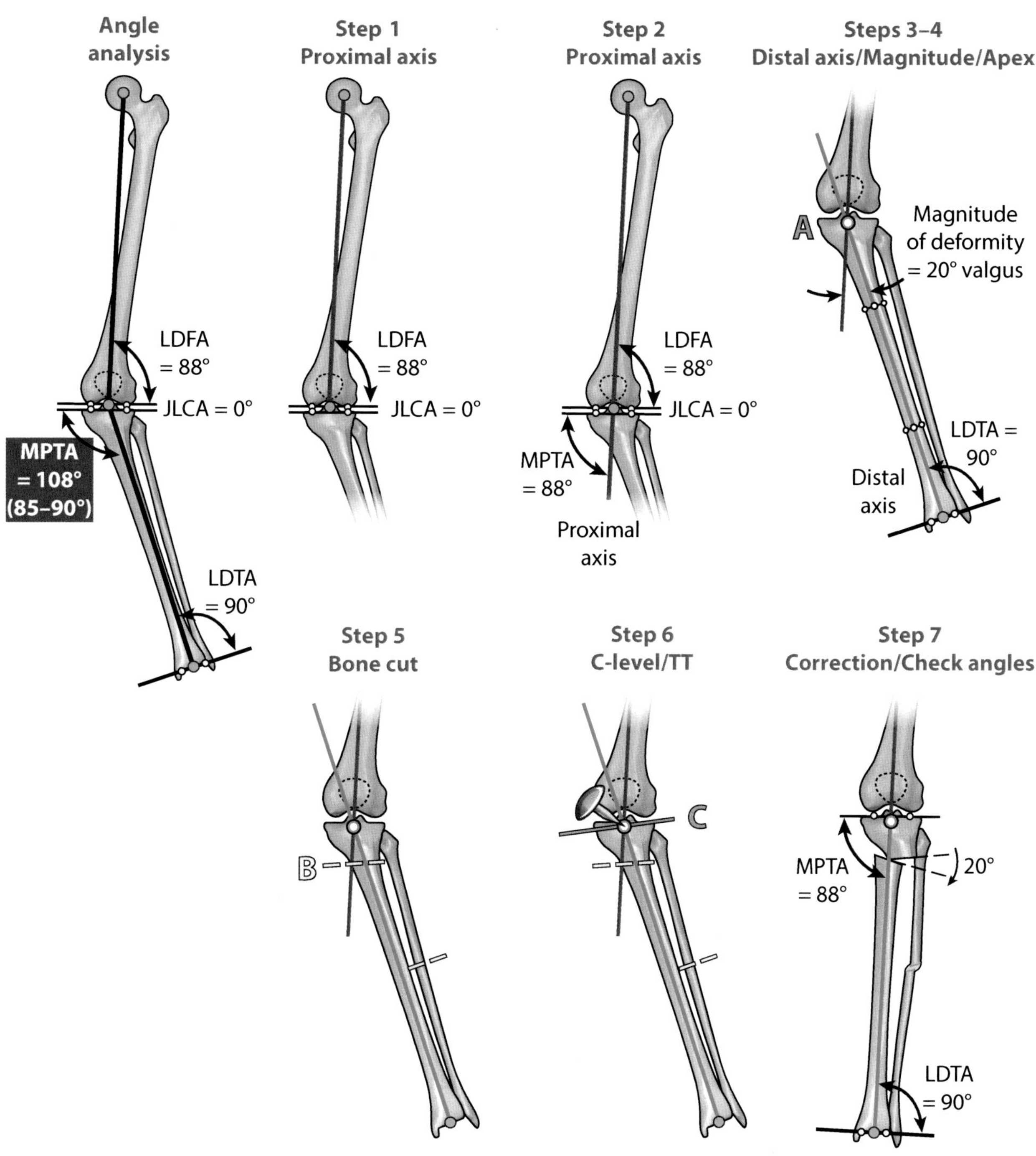


**Fig. 5:** Analysis of frontal plane proximal tibial metaphyseal deformity. The MPTA is abnormal. In this example, the proximal bone segment is very short; therefore, a mid-diaphyseal line cannot be used for the proximal axis. Draw the mechanical axis of the femur. If the LDFA and JLCA are normal, then extend the femoral mechanical axis into the proximal tibia and use this as the proximal axis. The distal axis is created by drawing a mid-diaphyseal line. The LDTA formed by the distal axis is normal; therefore, the bone does not have a distal metaphyseal deformity. The bone cut is made distal to the apex. Note that the fibular osteotomy is performed at a more distal location to avoid the peroneal nerve. The bone segments are angulated around a thumbtack placed on the apex. This results in a neutral wedge osteotomy with perfect axis alignment but bony translation because the bone cut was not made at the apex. This translation is not only desirable but necessary for correct alignment of the axes. A, apex; B, bone cut; C, C-level; TT, thumbtack.

## Frontal Plane: Multiple-level Deformity

A secondary, hidden deformity in the metaphyseal region can be missed if a more obvious mid-shaft deformity is present. This is why the proximal or distal joint angles should be assessed when the mid-diaphyseal planning lines are used to draw the proximal or distal axis lines.

The following situations indicate that a multiple-level or hidden translational deformity is present:

- The apex created by the intersection of the proximal and distal axis lines does not match the obvious deformity (Fig. 6A).
- The bone has a long, curving bow (such as long bone deformities from rickets or osteogenesis imperfecta) (Fig. 6B).
- The proximal and distal axis lines intersect at a location that is outside of the bone (medial or lateral to the bone) and correcting the deformity using this apex is not the ideal approach (e.g., correcting at this apex will create an unacceptable cosmetic appearance) (Fig. 6C).
- The proximal and distal axis lines intersect at a location that is proximal or distal to the entire bone segment (Fig. 6D).
- The bone segment has an obvious deformity plus the MPTA formed by the mid-diaphyseal line (proximal axis) is abnormal (Fig. 6E) or the LDTA formed by the mid-diaphyseal line (distal axis) is abnormal (Fig. 6F).

## Identifying Multiple Apexes in the Frontal Plane

If a multiple-level deformity is present, multiple apexes must be identified. For a double-level deformity, two apexes must be identified. This means that three axis lines need to be drawn instead of only two axis lines.

When you use a mid-diaphyseal line as the proximal or distal axis, you must measure the associated proximal or distal joint angle formed by this mid-diaphyseal axis to check for a hidden secondary deformity. Whether these joint angles are normal or abnormal can help you determine how to draw the third axis line for double-level deformity:

- If the MPTA formed by the mid-diaphyseal axis of the proximal bone segment is abnormal, then you can use the proximal joint line to create a normal MPTA. This normal MPTA axis line becomes a new proximal axis line (third axis line).
- If the LDTA formed by the mid-diaphyseal axis of the distal bone segment is abnormal, you can use the distal joint line to create a normal LDTA. This normal LDTA axis line becomes a new distal axis line (third axis line) (Fig. 7).
- If the MPTA and LDTA formed by the proximal and distal mid-diaphyseal axis lines are both normal, then draw a mid-diaphyseal line in the apparent middle segment to create a third axis (Fig. 8).

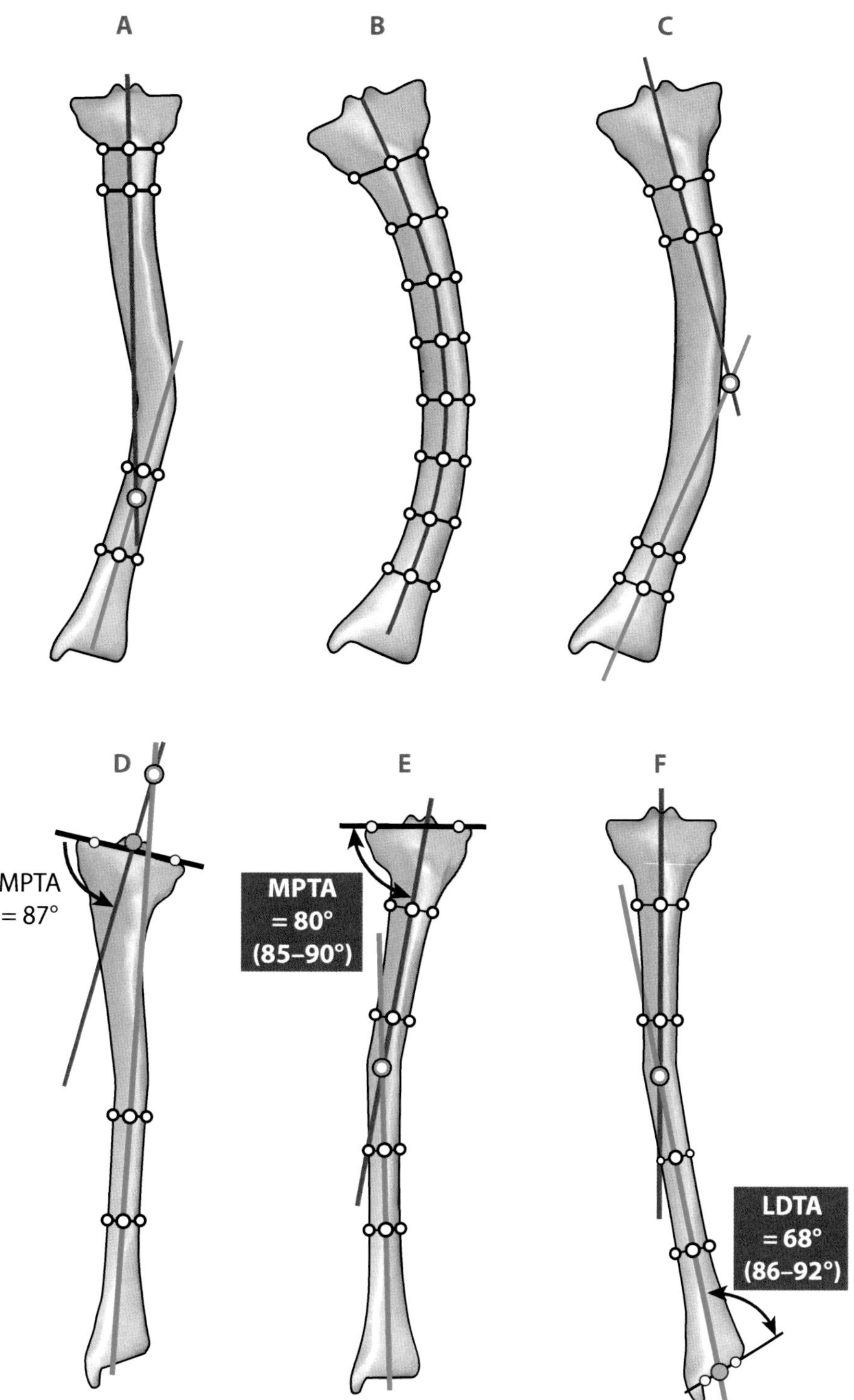


**Fig. 6:** Indicators of multiple-level deformities in the frontal plane. **A**, The apex created by the intersection of the proximal and distal axis lines does not match the obvious deformity. **B**, The bone has a long, curving bow. **C**, The proximal and distal axis lines intersect at a location that is outside of the bone (medial or lateral to the bone). **D**, The proximal and distal axis lines intersect at a location that is proximal or distal to the entire bone segment. **E**, The bone segment has an obvious deformity plus an abnormal MPTA formed by the mid-diaphyseal line (proximal axis). **F**, The bone segment has an obvious deformity plus an abnormal LDTA formed by the mid-diaphyseal line (distal axis).

*© 2023 Sinai Hospital of Baltimore*

## When the Joint Angle Formed by the Mid-diaphyseal Axis Is Abnormal (Fig. 7)

**Angle Analysis:**

During the MAP analysis, we drew the tibial mechanical axis and determined that the LDTA was abnormal.

**Step 1:** Draw the mid-diaphyseal axis of the proximal segment and the mid-diaphyseal axis of the distal segment. These are the proximal and distal axes.

**Step 2:** Since mid-diaphyseal lines were used for both axes, the knee and ankle joint angles must be checked for a second deformity near the joints. The MPTA formed by the proximal axis (i.e., the anatomic axis of the proximal bone segment) is normal (90°), but the LDTA formed by the distal axis (i.e., the anatomic axis of the distal bone segment) is 76° (abnormal). This abnormal LDTA means that a second deformity exists near the ankle.

**Step 3:** A second deformity exists near the ankle (abnormal LDTA), which means that a second apex must be identified. A third axis line needs to be drawn to identify the second apex. Create a normal LDTA from the center of the distal joint line. This third line will intersect with the mid-diaphyseal line in the metaphyseal region and identify the second apex of the multiapical deformity.

**Step 4:** Three axis lines axis lines have been drawn: a proximal axis (red line), a middle axis (green line), and a distal axis (blue line). Mark Apex$^1$ at the intersection of the proximal (red) and middle (green) axis lines. The magnitude of the deformity at Apex$^1$ is 9°. Mark Apex$^2$ at the intersection of the middle (green) and distal (blue) axis lines. The magnitude of the deformity at Apex$^2$ is 13°.

**Step 5:** Bone Cuts: Perform two osteotomies as close to each apex as possible. The proximal tibial osteotomy can be performed at the level of Apex$^1$ because this level is feasible from an anatomic point of view. Also, the resulting bony fragments are large enough for stable fixation. The distal tibial osteotomy is placed slightly proximal to Apex$^2$ because it is not feasible to perform an osteotomy at this level and achieve stable bony fixation. Since the distal tibial osteotomy is not performed at the level of Apex$^2$, a small amount of bony translation will occur in the distal segment during the correction. One fibular osteotomy is performed at a more distal location to Apex$^1$ to avoid the peroneal nerve. The second fibular osteotomy is at the same level as the distal osteotomy.

**Step 6:** Correction (part 1): Draw the two C-levels. The C-levels pass through each apex and bisect the obtuse angle that is created by the intersection of the axes. The bone segments are always angulated about thumbtacks placed on each C-level. This example shows that one thumbtack is placed on Apex$^1$ and the other thumbtack is placed along the C-level of Apex$^2$ on the convex side of the deformity.

**Step 7:** Correction (part 2): Angulating the bone segments around the thumbtacks results in a proximal neutral wedge osteotomy and a distal opening wedge osteotomy. Note that complete alignment of the bone and the axes occurs at Apex$^1$. Slight obligatory bony translation occurs in the distal fragment because the distal osteotomy was not placed at the level of Apex$^2$. However, despite the slight bony translation, the axis lines are perfectly aligned. Measure the MPTA and LDTA to confirm that they are within the range of normal.

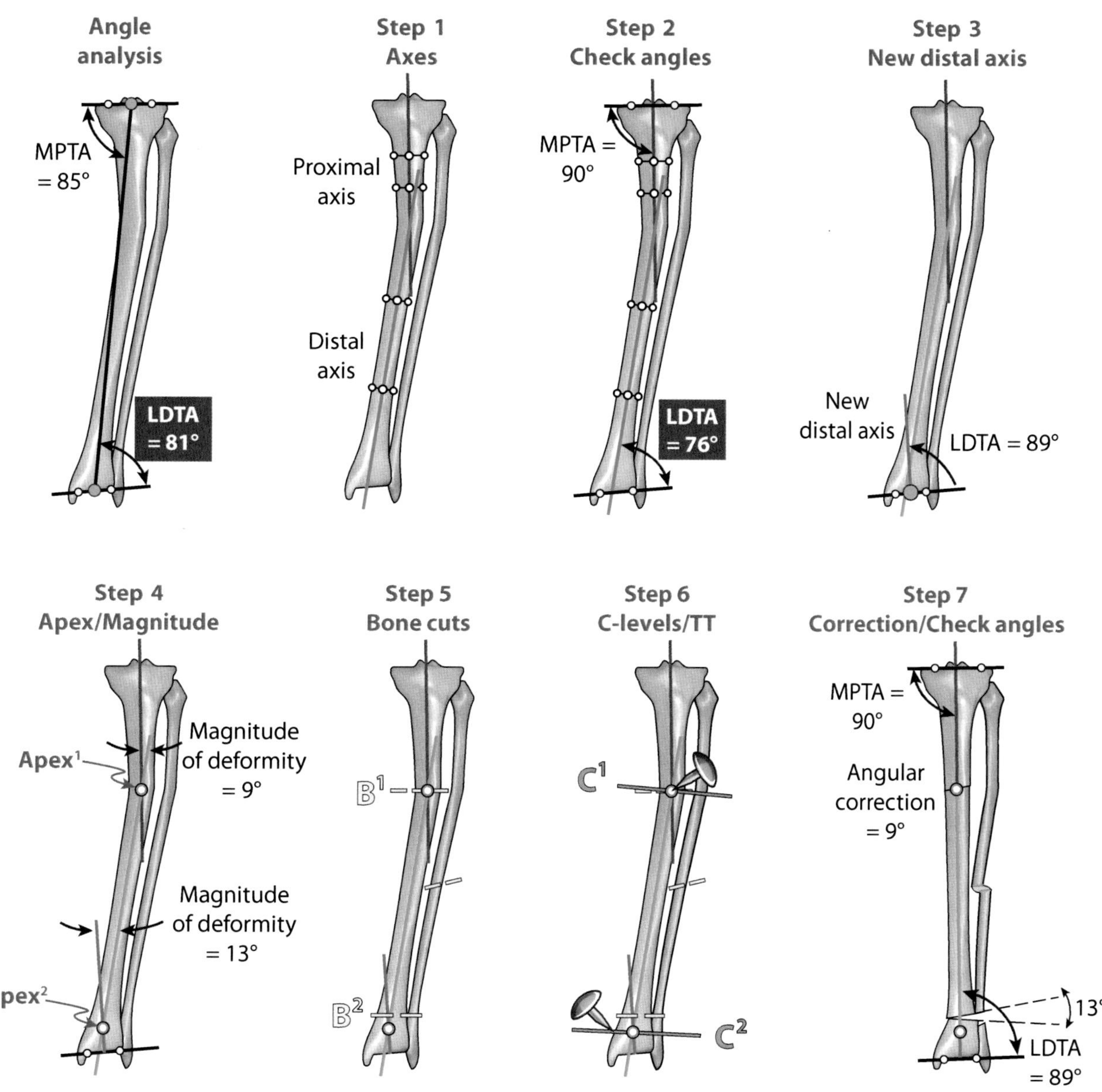


**Fig. 7:** Analysis of frontal plane multiapical tibial deformity. When you use a mid-diaphyseal line as the proximal or distal axis, you must measure the associated proximal or distal joint angle formed by the mid-diaphyseal axis to check for a hidden deformity. In this case, the LDTA created by the mid-diaphyseal axis is abnormal (Step 2). This abnormal LDTA means that a second deformity exists near the ankle and that a second apex must be identified. In Step 3, a new distal axis line (*blue line*) is drawn to identify the second apex by creating a normal LDTA. The proximal bone cut is made at the level of $Apex^1$ and the distal bone cut is made proximal to $Apex^2$, resulting in slight bony translation. Note that one fibular osteotomy is performed distal to $Apex^1$ to avoid the peroneal nerve. The second fibular osteotomy is performed at the level of the distal tibial bone cut. The bone segment is angulated around a proximal thumbtack placed on the apex and a distal thumbtack placed along the C-level on the convex side of the deformity. A proximal neutral wedge osteotomy and a distal opening wedge osteotomy are performed. A, apex; B, bone cut; C, C-level; TT, thumbtack.

© 2023 Sinai Hospital of Baltimore

## When the Joint Angles Formed by Both Mid-diaphyseal Axis Lines Are Normal (Fig. 8)

**Angle Analysis:**

During the MAP analysis, we drew the tibial mechanical axis and determined that the MPTA and LDTA were both abnormal.

**Step 1:** Draw the mid-diaphyseal axis of the proximal segment and the mid-diaphyseal axis of the distal segment. These are the proximal and distal axis lines.

**Step 2:** Mark the apex at the intersection of the proximal and distal axis lines. The apex is located outside and lateral to the tibia, which denotes a multiple-level deformity. We call this apex a Summated Apex. In this case, we need to find a way to represent the multiple apexes of the deformity so that we can develop a better treatment option.

**Step 3:** Since mid-diaphyseal lines were used for both axis lines, check the proximal and distal tibial joint angles. The MPTA formed by the proximal axis (i.e., the anatomic axis of the proximal bone segment) is normal (89°), and the LDTA formed by the distal axis (i.e., the anatomic axis of the distal bone segment) is also normal (88°).

**Step 4:** If the joint angles are normal, then draw a mid-diaphyseal line in the apparent middle segment (green line). This will be a "best fit" line in most circumstances.

**Step 5:** Mark the intersection of the proximal and middle axis lines. Then mark the intersection of the middle and distal axis lines. These two apexes are the Component Apexes. When the deformities represented by the two Component Apexes are combined, they are equivalent to the deformity that is represented by the Summated Apex.

**Step 6:** Measure the magnitude of deformity at Component Apex[1] (20°) and Component Apex[2] (17°).

**Step 7:** Bone Cuts: Perform two osteotomies as close to each apex as possible. The proximal osteotomy is at the level of Component Apex[1] and the distal osteotomy is at the level of Component Apex[2].

**Step 8:** Correction (part 1): Draw the two C-levels. The bone segments are always angulated about thumbtacks placed on each C-level. This example shows that the two thumbtacks are placed along the C-levels on the convex side of the deformities.

**Steps 9–10:**

Correction (part 2): Angulating the bone segments around the thumbtacks results in a proximal opening wedge osteotomy and a distal opening wedge osteotomy. Note the complete alignment of the bone and the axes. Bony translation does not occur because the bone cuts were made at the level of each Component Apex. Measure the MPTA and LDTA to confirm that they are within the range of normal.

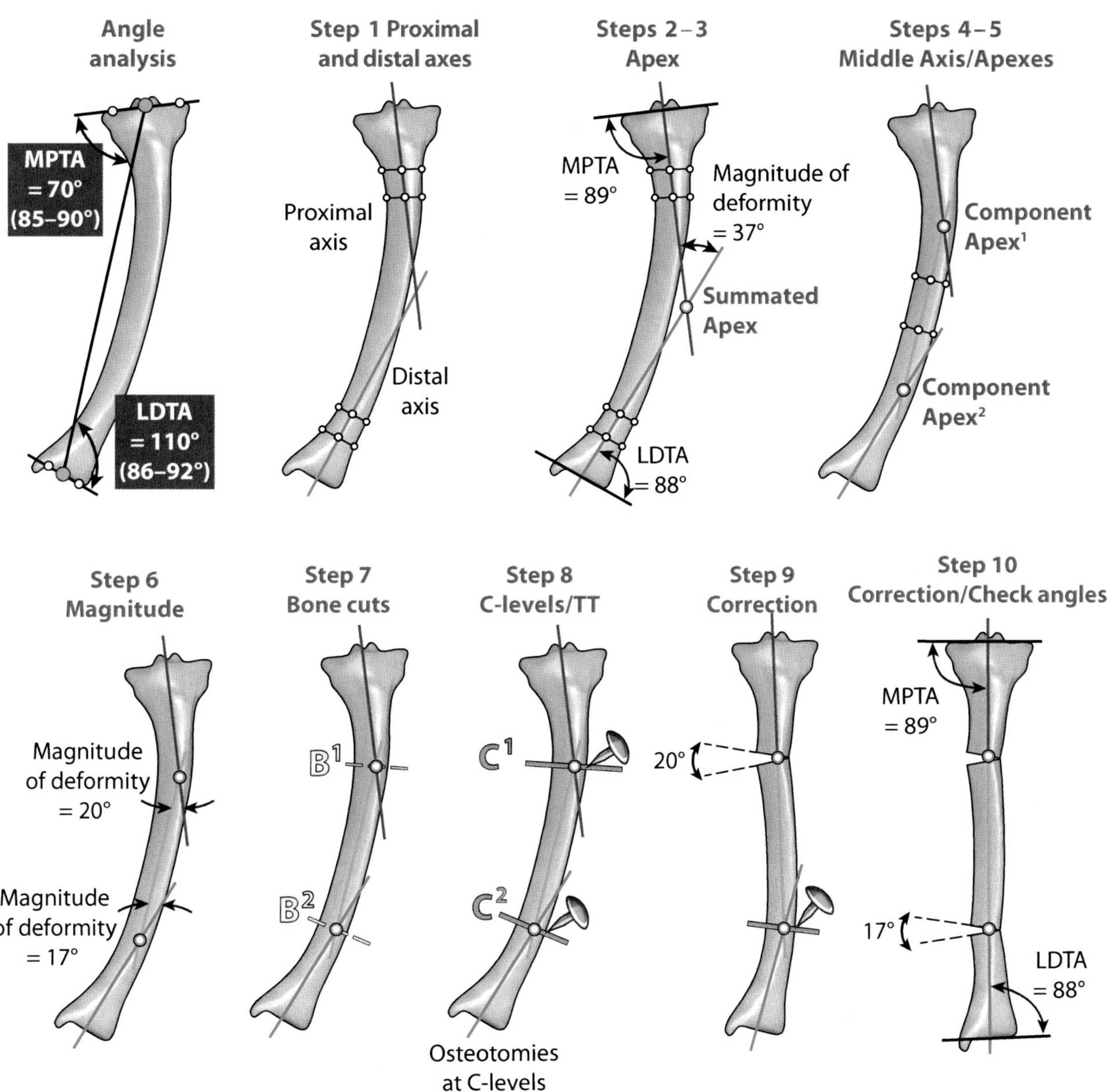


**Fig. 8:** Frontal plane analysis of a bowed tibia. The mid-diaphyseal axis of the proximal segment and the mid-diaphyseal axis of the distal segment are used as the proximal and distal axis lines, respectively. The apex in Step 2 falls outside and lateral to the bone, which denotes a multiple-level deformity. This apex is a Summated Apex. Since the MPTA formed by the proximal axis and the LDTA formed by the distal axis are both normal, we need to find another way to create a third axis line. A mid-diaphyseal line is drawn in the apparent middle segment (*green line*). The intersection of the proximal and middle axis lines is Component Apex[1], and the intersection of the middle and distal axis lines is Component Apex[2]. When the deformities represented by the two Component Apexes are combined, they are equivalent to the deformity that is represented by the Summated Apex. Bone cuts are made through the apexes, and the bone segments are angulated around proximal and distal thumbtacks placed along the C-levels on the convex side of each deformity. Proximal and distal opening wedge osteotomies are performed at the level of Component Apex[1] and Component Apex[2]. A, apex; B, bone cut; C, C-level; TT, thumbtack.

© 2023 Sinai Hospital of Baltimore 

## Tibial Axis Planning: Sagittal Plane

Before you can find the apex in the sagittal plane, you must perform the MAP analysis. To determine the soft-tissue component of the deformity around the knee joint, the bony deformity analysis of the angles about the knee (PDFA and PPTA) is compared to the SMAA. The SMAA quantifies the total amount of soft-tissue and bony deformity that is present around the knee joint (flexion contracture or hyperextension). This comparison of the SMAA to the bony deformity will provide valuable information about how the soft-tissue and bony deformities contribute to the overall deformity around the knee and will be essential to develop an effective treatment strategy.

### Identifying the Proximal Tibial Axis in the Sagittal Plane

Two strategies can be used to identify the axis of the proximal tibial segment in the sagittal plane:

#### Mid-diaphyseal Line Strategy:

Use the proximal tibial segment's mid-diaphyseal line (Fig. 9). This strategy assumes that the proximal tibia has a straight segment that is long enough to define a line. If you use this strategy, you must measure the PPTA (normal range, 77–84°) formed by the proximal axis (i.e., the anatomic axis of the proximal bone segment) to check for a hidden deformity in the proximal tibia. If the PPTA is significantly abnormal, then the limb might have a single-level proximal metaphyseal deformity or a double-level deformity (proximal metaphyseal plus another deformity) that needs to be addressed.

#### Create Normal PPTA Strategy:

Use the proximal tibial joint line to create a normal PPTA from a point 1/5 of the total length of the joint line from the anterior cortex (Fig. 9). You may use the average normal value for the PPTA (81°) or use the PPTA value of the contralateral normal limb.

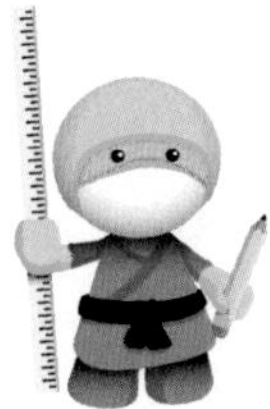

*Sensei says,*

*"The posterior proximal tibial angle (PPTA) is created by drawing a line starting at a point 1/5 of the total length of the joint line from the anterior cortex."*

### Identifying the Distal Tibial Axis in the Sagittal Plane

Two strategies can be used to identify the axis of the distal tibial segment in the sagittal plane:

#### Mid-diaphyseal Line Strategy:

Use the distal tibial segment's mid-diaphyseal line (Fig. 10). This strategy assumes that the distal tibia has a straight segment that is long enough to define a line. If you use this strategy, you must measure the ADTA (normal range, 78–82°) formed by the distal axis (i.e., the anatomic axis of the distal bone segment) to check for a hidden deformity in the distal tibia. If the ADTA is significantly abnormal, then the limb might have a single-level distal metaphyseal deformity or a double-level deformity (distal metaphyseal plus another deformity) that needs to be addressed.

#### Create Normal ADTA Strategy:

Use the distal joint line to create a normal ADTA from the center of the ankle joint (Fig. 10). You may use the average normal value for the ADTA (80°) or use the ADTA value of the contralateral normal limb.

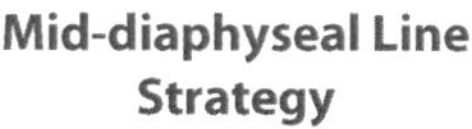


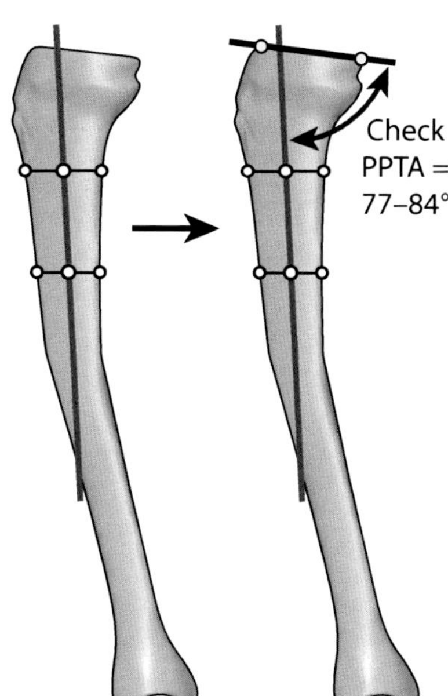


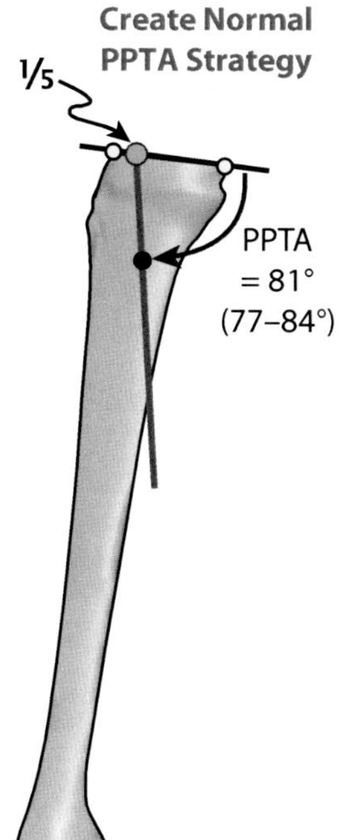


**Fig. 9:** Two strategies can be used to identify the axis of the proximal tibial segment in the sagittal plane. **Mid-diaphyseal Line Strategy:** Use the mid-diaphyseal line of the proximal tibial segment. You must measure the PPTA (normal range, 77–84°) formed by the proximal axis (i.e., the anatomic axis of the proximal bone segment) to check for a hidden deformity in the proximal tibia. If the PPTA is significantly abnormal, then a hidden proximal deformity is present. **Create Normal PPTA Strategy:** If the PPTA is abnormal, use the proximal joint line to create a normal PPTA (normal range, 77–84°) from a point 1/5 of the total length of the joint line from the anterior cortex.

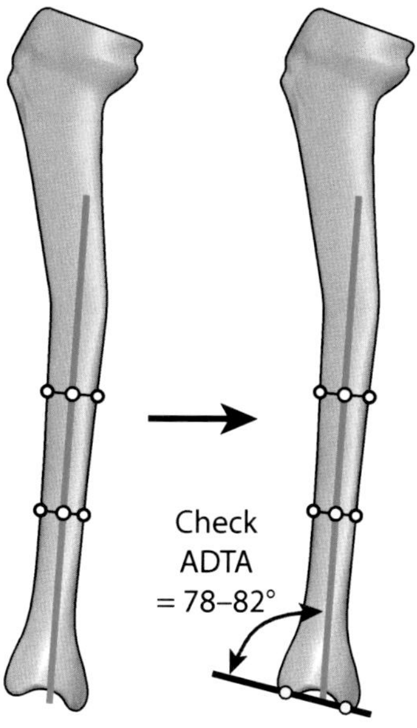


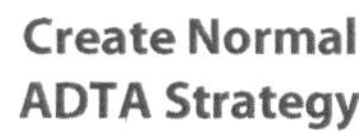


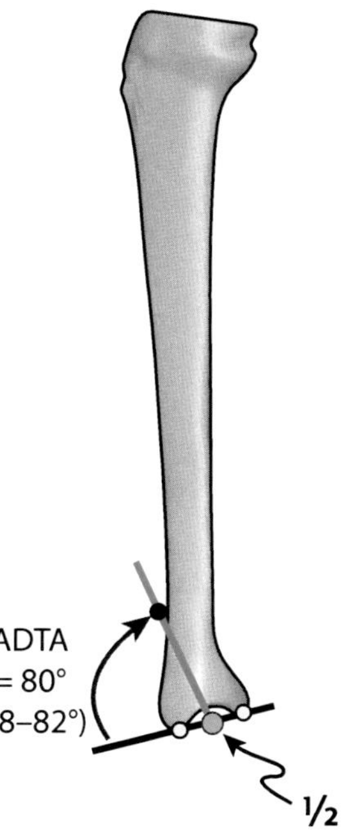


**Fig. 10:** Two strategies can be used to identify the axis of the distal tibial segment in the sagittal plane. **Mid-diaphyseal Line Strategy:** Use the distal tibial segment's mid-diaphyseal line. You must measure the ADTA (normal range, 78–82°) formed by the distal axis (i.e., the anatomic axis of the distal bone segment) to check for a hidden deformity in the distal tibia. If the ADTA is significantly abnormal, then a hidden distal deformity is present. **Create Normal ADTA Strategy:** If the ADTA is abnormal, use the distal joint line to create a normal ADTA (normal range, 78–82°) from the center of the ankle joint.

© 2023 Sinai Hospital of Baltimore

## Diaphyseal Deformity (Fig. 11)

This type of deformity allows for easy identification of the proximal and distal axes.

**Angle Analysis:**

During the MAP analysis, we drew the modified mechanical axis and determined that the PPTA and ADTA were both abnormal. After comparing the SMAA to the bony deformity analysis, we determined that there was no soft-tissue component to the deformity around the knee.

**Step 1:** Draw the mid-diaphyseal axis of the proximal segment and the mid-diaphyseal axis of the distal segment. These are the proximal and distal axes.

**Step 2:** Since mid-diaphyseal lines were used for both axes, the knee and ankle joint angles must be checked to look for a metaphyseal deformity near the joints. The PPTA formed by the proximal axis (i.e., the anatomic axis of the proximal bone segment) is 80°, and the ADTA formed by the distal axis (i.e., the anatomic axis of the distal bone segment) is 80°. Both are within the range of normal; therefore, the bone does not have a proximal or distal metaphyseal deformity.

**Step 3:** Mark the apex of the deformity at the intersection of the proximal and distal axes.

**Step 4:** Measure the magnitude of the acute angle created by the intersection of the proximal and distal axes. The magnitude of the deformity is 11°.

**Step 5:** Bone Cut: Place the osteotomy as close to the apex as possible. In this example, the osteotomy can be performed at the level of the apex because this level is feasible anatomically. Also, the resulting bony fragments are large enough for bony fixation.

**Step 6:** Correction (part 1): Draw the C-level by bisecting the obtuse angle created by the proximal and distal axes. The bone segment is always angulated about a thumbtack placed on the C-level. This example shows the thumbtack placed along the C-level on the convex side of the deformity.

**Step 7:** Correction (part 2): Angulating the bone segments around the thumbtack results in an opening wedge osteotomy with complete alignment of the bone and the axes. Measure the PPTA and ADTA to confirm that they are now within the range of normal.

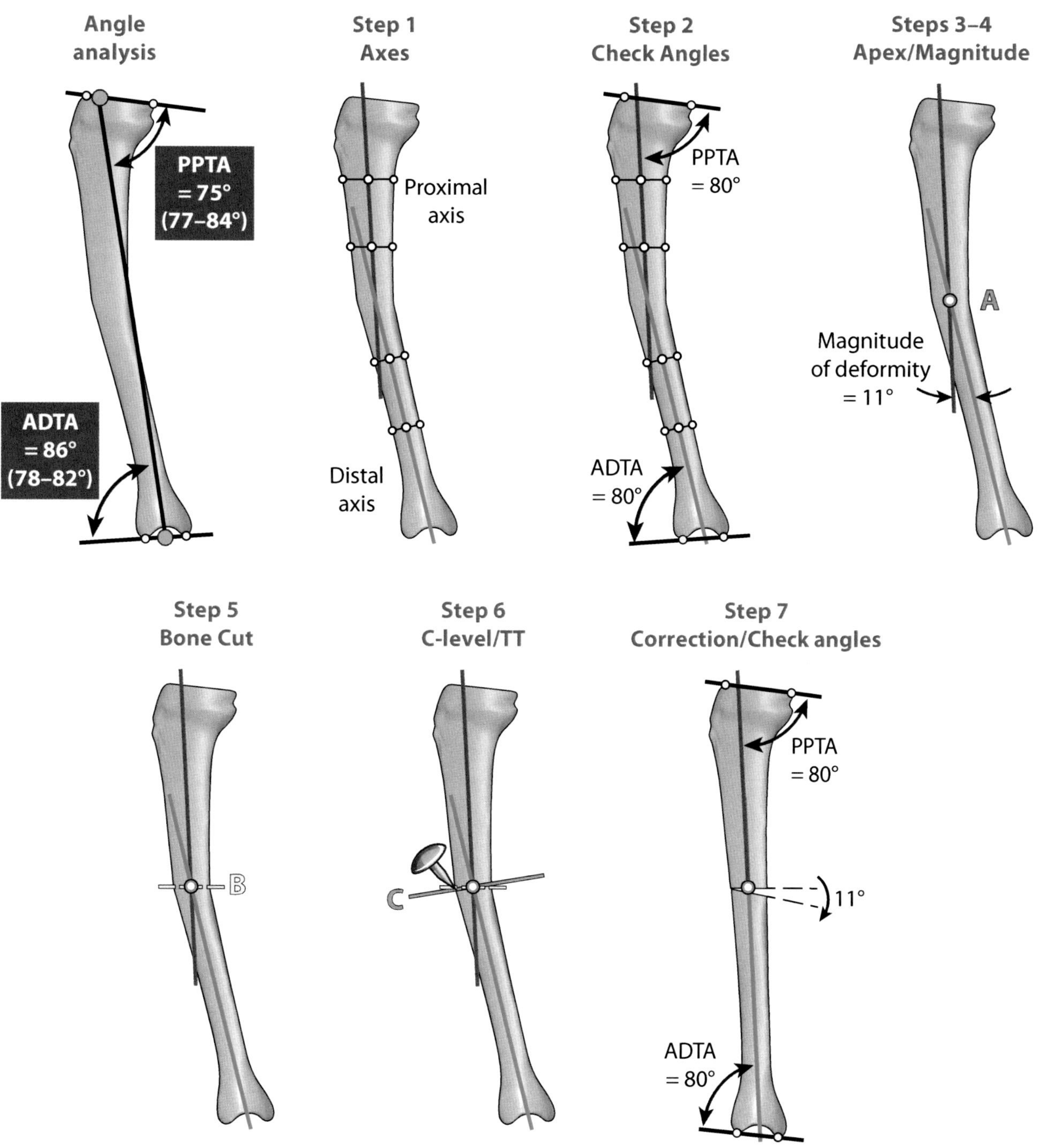


**Fig. 11:** Analysis of sagittal plane tibial diaphyseal deformity. The proximal and distal axes are drawn using the mid-diaphyseal lines of the proximal and distal segments. Since mid-diaphyseal lines are used for both axes, the knee and ankle joint angles must be checked to look for deformities near the joints. The PPTA and ADTA formed by the proximal and distal axis lines are both normal; therefore, the bone does not have a proximal or distal metaphyseal deformity. The bone cut is at the level of the apex. The bone segment is angulated around a thumbtack placed along the C-level on the convex side of the deformity. This results in an opening wedge osteotomy and perfect alignment of the bone margins and axis lines. A, apex; B, bone cut; C, C-level; TT, thumbtack.

© 2023 Sinai Hospital of Baltimore

## Metaphyseal Deformity

Metaphyseal deformities of the tibia present an analytical challenge because one of the bony segments is very short. A simple mid-diaphyseal line cannot be drawn accurately for the small segment. Often, this type of deformity is subtle and can be missed. To find the short segment's axis, draw a line from the appropriate point on the joint line to create a normal joint angle.

### Metaphyseal Deformity: Creating a Normal Joint Angle and Using It as an Axis Line (Fig. 12)

**Angle Analysis:** During the MAP analysis, we drew the modified mechanical axis and determined that the ADTA was abnormal. After comparing the SMAA to the bony deformity analysis, we determined that no soft-tissue or bony deformities exist around the knee.

**Step 1:** Draw the mid-diaphyseal line of the tibia. This is the proximal axis. The PPTA formed by the proximal axis (i.e., the anatomic axis of the proximal bone segment) is normal; therefore, the bone does not have a proximal metaphyseal deformity.

**Step 2:** Since the distal tibia is the short segment, use the distal tibial joint line to create a normal ADTA (80°) from the center of the ankle. This line is the distal axis.

**Step 3:** Mark the apex of the deformity at the intersection of the proximal and distal axis lines.

**Step 4:** The magnitude of deformity is 23°.

**Step 5:** Bone Cut: Place the osteotomy as close to the apex as possible. The osteotomy is performed proximal to the apex because it is not feasible to perform an osteotomy at the level of the apex from an anatomic or mechanical stability point of view. Since the osteotomy is not performed at the level of the apex, bony translation will occur during the correction. The amount of translation is the distance between the proximal and distal axis lines at the level of the osteotomy site.

**Step 6:** Correction (part 1): Draw the C-level. The bone segment is always angulated about a thumbtack placed on the C-level. This example shows the thumbtack placed on the C-level on the convex side of the deformity.

**Step 7:** Correction (part 2): Angulating the bone segments around the thumbtack results in an opening wedge osteotomy with complete alignment of the axes. Note the obligatory translation of bone due to the placement of the osteotomy away from the level of the apex. Despite the bony translation, the proximal and distal axes are perfectly aligned. Measure the PPTA and ADTA to confirm that they are within the range of normal.

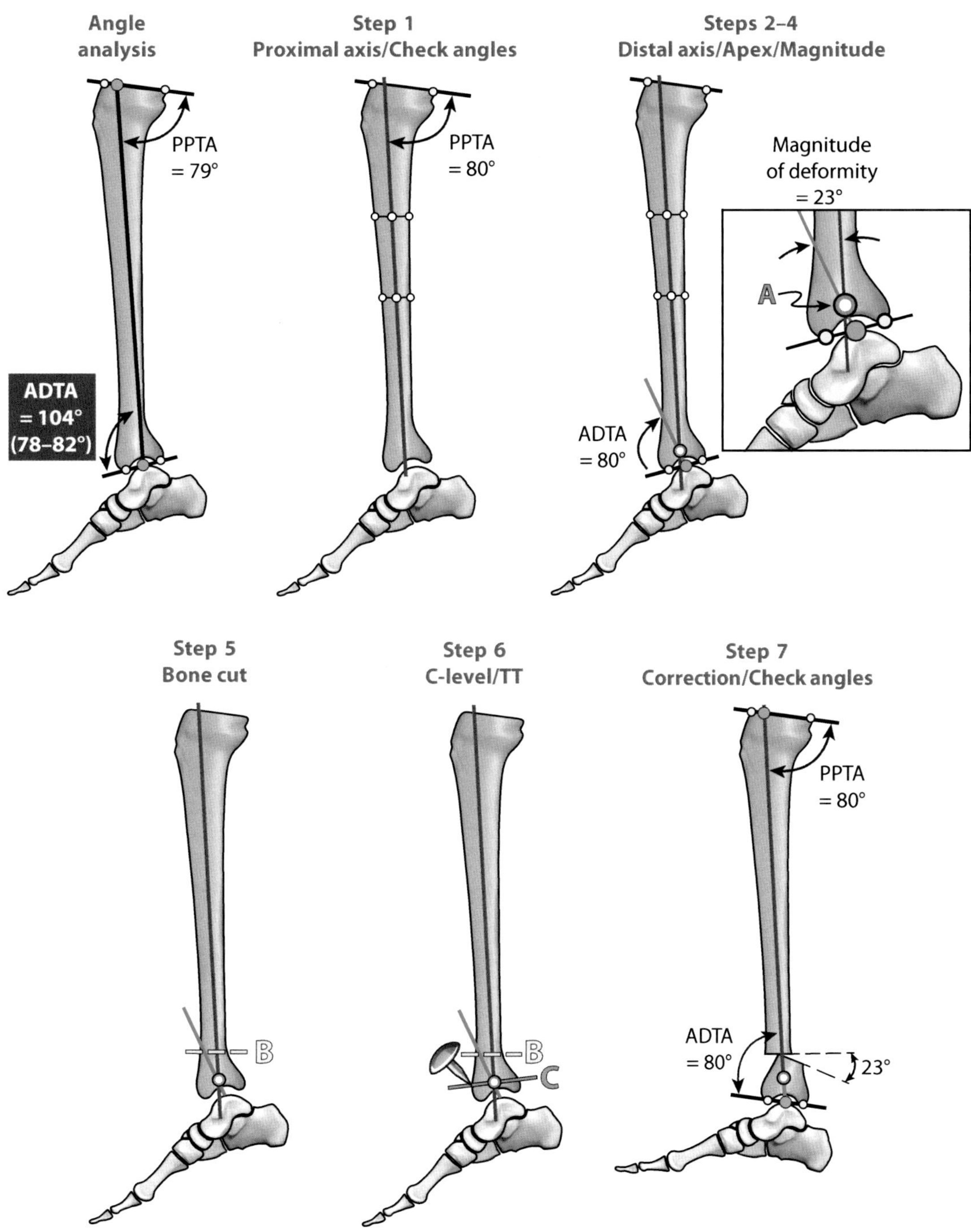


**Fig. 12:** Sagittal plane analysis of distal tibial metaphyseal deformity. Since the mid-diaphyseal line is used for the proximal axis, the proximal joint angle must be checked to look for a second deformity near the knee. The PPTA formed by the proximal axis line is normal (80°); therefore, the bone does not have a proximal metaphyseal deformity. The distal tibial segment is the short segment, which means that a mid-diaphyseal line cannot be used as the distal axis. To draw the distal axis, use the distal tibial joint line to create a normal ADTA (80°) from the center of the ankle. The bone cut is made proximal to the apex. The bone segments are corrected around a thumbtack placed along the C-level on the convex side of the deformity. An opening wedge osteotomy is performed proximal to the level of the apex, resulting in obligatory bony translation. Although the bony margins must translate, the axes are perfectly aligned. A, apex; B, bone cut; C, C-level; TT, thumbtack.

© 2023 Sinai Hospital of Baltimore

## Sagittal Plane: Multiple-Level Deformity

If a multiple-level deformity is present, multiple apexes must be identified. A secondary deformity can exist in the metaphyseal region that can be subtle and may be missed if an obvious mid-shaft deformity is present. This is why the joint angles should be assessed when the mid-diaphyseal planning lines are used to draw the proximal or distal axis lines. A multiple-level or hidden translational deformity is present when:

- The apex does not match the obvious deformity (Fig. 13A).
- The bone has a long, curving bow (e.g., rickets, osteogenesis imperfecta) (Fig. 13B).
- The proximal and distal axis lines intersect at a location that is outside of the bone (anterior or posterior to the bone) and correcting the deformity using this apex is not the ideal approach (e.g., correcting at this apex will create an unacceptable cosmetic appearance) (Fig. 13C).
- The proximal and distal axes intersect at a location that is proximal or distal to the entire bone segment (Fig. 13D).
- The bone segment has an obvious deformity plus an abnormal proximal or distal joint angle (Fig. 13E).
- The proximal and distal axes are parallel and do not intersect because of a translational deformity (Fig. 13F).

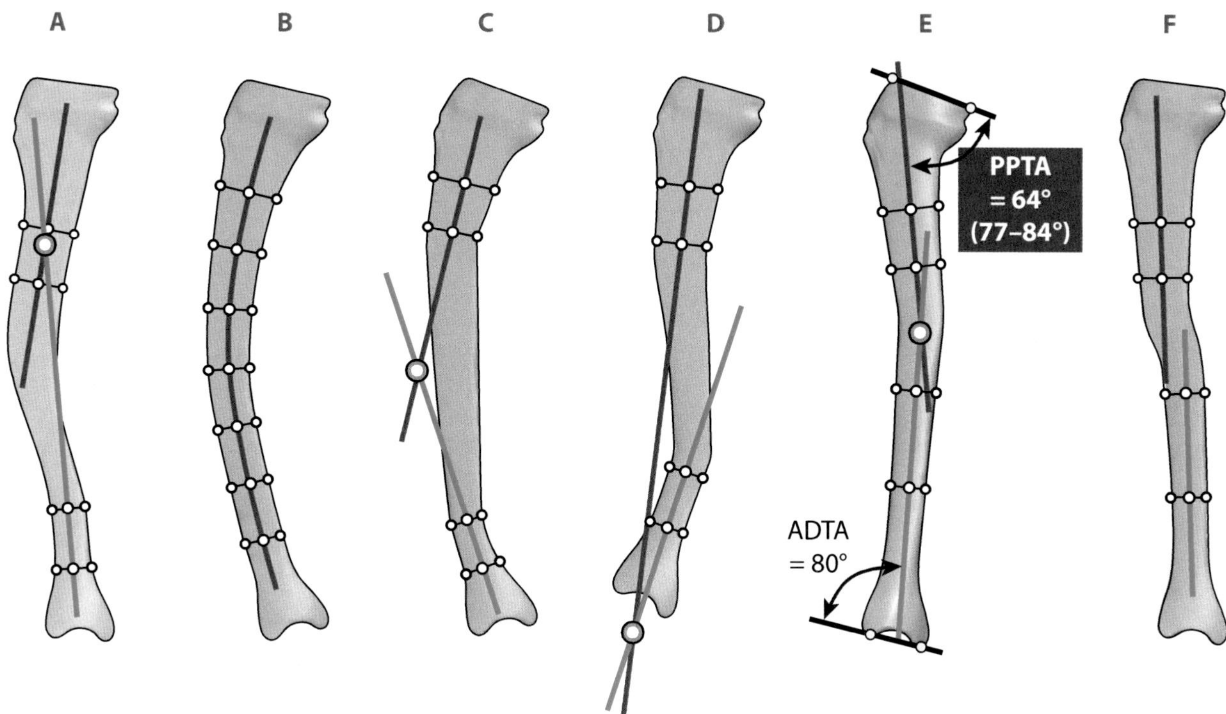


**Fig. 13:** Indicators of multiple level deformities in the sagittal plane. **A**, The apex created by the intersection of the proximal and distal axis lines does not match the obvious deformity. **B**, The bone has a long, curving bow. **C**, The proximal and distal axis lines intersect at a location that is outside of the bone (anterior or posterior to the bone). **D**, The proximal and distal axis lines intersect at a location that is proximal or distal to the entire bone segment. **E**, The bone segment has an obvious deformity plus an abnormal PPTA (shown) or ADTA (not shown) formed by the mid-diaphyseal lines. **F**, The proximal and distal axis lines are parallel and do not intersect (translational deformity).

*© 2023 Sinai Hospital of Baltimore*

## Identifying Multiple Apexes in the Sagittal Plane (Fig. 14)

**Angle Analysis:**

During the MAP analysis, we drew the modified mechanical axis and determined that the PPTA and ADTA were abnormal. After comparing the SMAA to the bony deformity analysis, we determined that there was no soft-tissue component to the deformity around the knee.

**Step 1:** Draw the mid-diaphyseal axis of the proximal segment and the mid-diaphyseal axis of the distal segment. These are the proximal and distal axes.

**Step 2:** Since mid-diaphyseal lines were used for both axes, the knee and ankle joint angles must be checked for a deformity near the joints. The ADTA formed by the distal axis is normal; however, the PPTA formed by the proximal axis is abnormal. The abnormal PPTA means that in addition to the obvious deformity in the mid-diaphysis, a second deformity exists in the proximal metaphysis.

**Step 3:** A second deformity exists near the knee (abnormal PPTA), which means that a second apex must be identified. A new proximal axis line needs to be drawn to identify the second apex. To draw this new proximal axis (red line), create a normal PPTA of 80° from a point 1/5 of the total length of the joint line from the anterior cortex. This third line will intersect with the mid-diaphyseal line (green line) in the metaphyseal region and identify the second apex of the multiapical deformity.

**Step 4:** Three axis lines have been drawn: a proximal axis (red line), a middle axis (green line), and a distal axis (blue line). Mark Apex[1] at the intersection of the proximal (red) and middle (green) axis lines. The magnitude of the deformity at Apex[1] is 15°. Mark Apex[2] at the intersection of the middle (green) and distal (blue) axis lines. The magnitude of the deformity at Apex[2] is 9°.

**Step 5:** Bone Cut: Perform two osteotomies as close to each apex as possible. The proximal osteotomy is distal to Apex[1] due to anatomic and bony fixation considerations. Since the osteotomy is not performed at the level of Apex[1], bony translation will occur during the correction. The distal osteotomy is performed at the level of Apex[2] because this level is feasible from an anatomic and mechanical stability point of view.

**Step 6:** Correction (part 1): Draw the C-levels. The bone segment is always angulated about thumbtacks placed on the C-levels. This example shows that the proximal and distal thumbtacks are placed along the C-levels on the convex sides of the deformities.

**Step 7:** Correction (part 2): Angulating the bone segments around the thumbtacks results in two opening wedge osteotomies with complete alignment of the axes. Note the obligatory translation of the proximal bone fragment due to the placement of the osteotomy away from the level of Apex[1]. Measure the PPTA and ADTA to confirm that they are now within the range of normal.

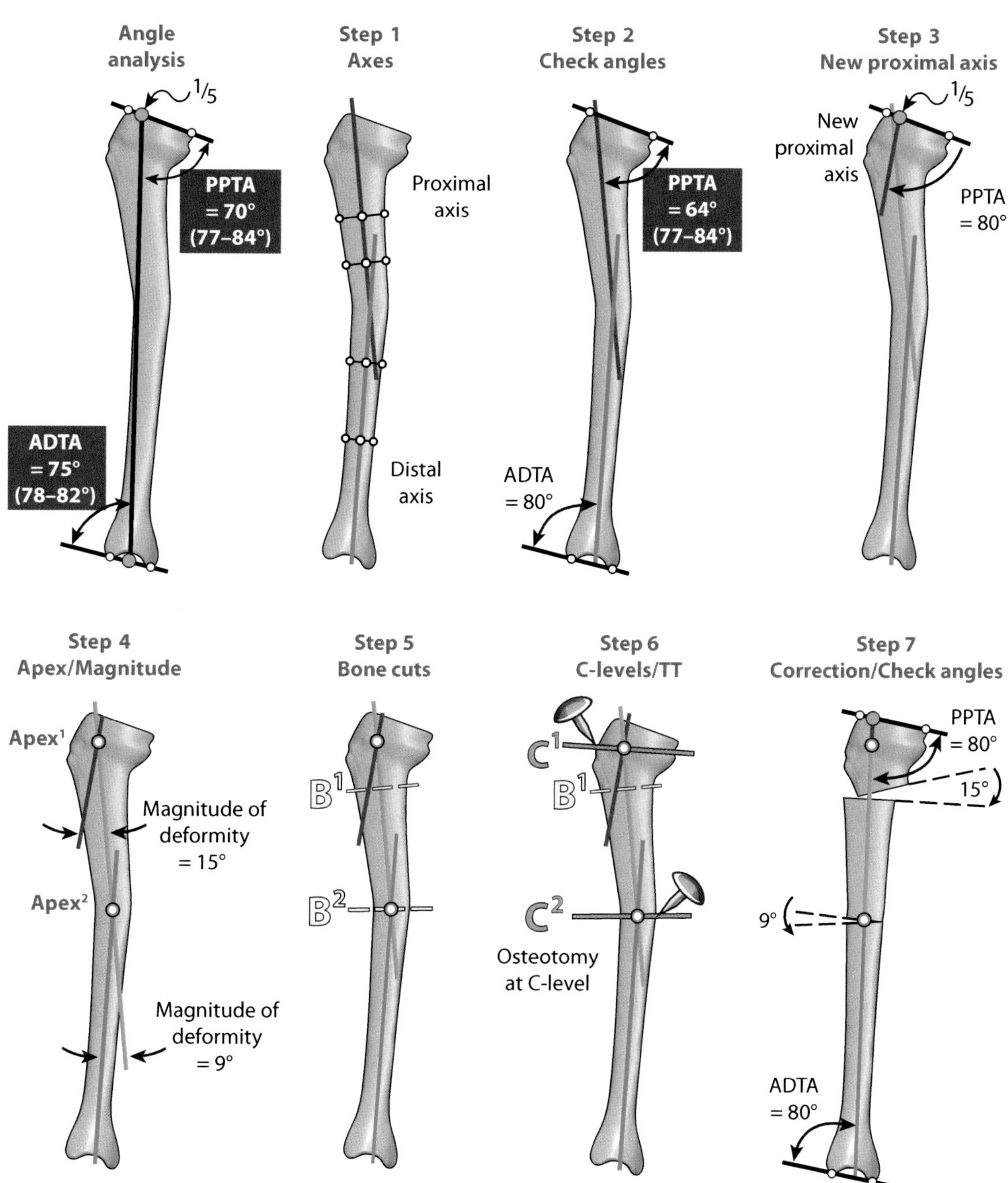


**Fig. 14:** Sagittal plane analysis of multiapical tibial deformity. The mid-diaphyseal axis of the proximal segment and the mid-diaphyseal axis of the distal segment are initially drawn as the proximal and distal axes. Since mid-diaphyseal lines were used for both axes, the knee and ankle joint angles must be checked for a metaphyseal deformity near the joints. The abnormal PPTA (64°) formed by the proximal axis means that a second deformity exists near the knee and that a second apex must be identified. A third axis line needs to be drawn to identify the second apex. To draw this third line, which will be a new proximal axis line, a normal PPTA of 80° is drawn. This new proximal axis line will intersect with the mid-diaphyseal line in the metaphyseal region and identify the second apex of the multiapical deformity. The bone segment is angulated around proximal and distal thumbtacks placed along the C-levels on the convex sides of the deformities. A proximal opening wedge osteotomy is performed distal to Apex[1], resulting in bony translation. A distal opening wedge osteotomy is performed at the level of Apex[2]. Although the bony margins at the proximal osteotomy site must translate, perfect alignment of the axis lines is achieved. A, apex; B, bone cut; C, C-level; TT, thumbtack.

© 2023 Sinai Hospital of Baltimore

## Summary

Axis planning identifies the apex or apexes of the deformity. After the surgeon has mastered axis planning, then any bone segment or deformity can be analyzed and simplified into axis lines and apexes. This analysis will allow the surgeon to confidently choose the appropriate level of the osteotomy and accurately correct the deformity.

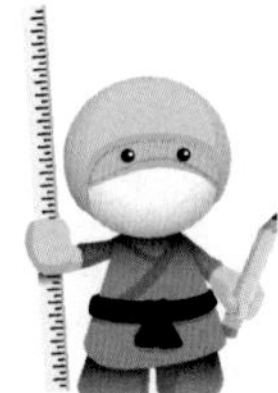

***Sensei says,***
*"The surgeon who masters axis planning will soon master the Art of Limb Alignment."*

# Chapter 9

# Femoral Axis Planning: Frontal and Sagittal Planes

Shawn C. Standard, MD

Philip K. McClure, MD

The underlying concepts for axis planning in the femur are the same as described for the tibia. However, femoral axis planning has distinct differences that must be noted. The femoral anatomic and mechanical axes are different lines, whereas the tibia's anatomic and mechanical axes are essentially the same. This important distinction results in two different planning methodologies for the femur: either anatomic axis planning or mechanical axis planning. Many consider anatomic axis planning to be more intuitive and straightforward. However, the ultimate goal is to re-align the mechanical axis of the lower limb. The more simplistic anatomic axis planning method is an indirect method of realigning the overall mechanical axis of the limb. Therefore, even though mechanical axis planning is more complicated, it is recommended in most cases because it is a direct method of realigning the overall mechanical axis of the limb. An exception to this strategy is when intramedullary fixation will be used. In this scenario, anatomic axis planning is beneficial since the intramedullary device will mimic the anatomic axis.

It is important to remember that in the frontal plane, the mechanical axis extends from the center of the femoral head to the center of the knee joint. In the sagittal plane, the modified mechanical axis connects the center of the femoral head to a point on the distal femoral joint line that is 1/3 the total length of the joint line from the anterior cortex.

For every example in this chapter, at least one deformity was found in the femur during the MAP analysis in the frontal and sagittal planes. When performing the MAP analysis in the sagittal plane, it is essential to remember to perform a complete analysis by comparing the SMAA and the bony deformity about the knee (PDFA and PPTA). This comparison will provide valuable information about how the soft-tissue and bony deformities contribute to the overall deformity around the knee.

A femoral deformity results in angulation of both the bone and the bone axes (both anatomic and mechanical axes). A deformed femur has a proximal bone segment above the deformity and a distal bone segment below the deformity. All bony segments, no matter how short, have an axis. During axis planning, the goal is to determine the proximal axis and the distal axis of the femur. The intersection of the proximal axis and the distal axis is the apex of the deformity.

This chapter will describe the axis planning strategies that can be used to draw the proximal and distal femoral axes. The goal of axis planning is to identify the apex of the deformity (the "A" of the ABCs). The bone cut/osteotomy level (the "B" in the ABCs) and correction (the "C" of the ABCs) will also be shown in each example.

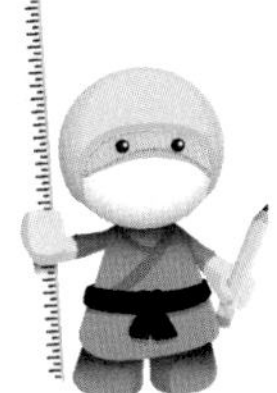

***Sensei says,***
*"Axis planning of the femur in the frontal plane can be accomplished by using anatomic axis planning or mechanical axis planning."*

© 2023 Sinai Hospital of Baltimore

## Femoral Mechanical Axis Planning: Frontal Plane

### Identifying the Proximal Femoral Mechanical Axis in the Frontal Plane

Two strategies can be used to identify the mechanical axis of the proximal femoral segment:

#### Frontal Plane Proximal Mechanical Axis–Three-line Method:

Use the three-line method to identify the proximal mechanical axis. The three-line method utilizes the anatomic-mechanical angle (AMA) that was introduced in Chapter 1 (Fig. 1). To use the three-line method, perform these three steps (Fig. 2):

**Step 1:** Draw the mid-diaphyseal line (blue line) of the proximal femur and confirm that the proximal joint angle is normal.

**Step 2:** Draw a second line (blue line) that starts at the center of the femoral head and is parallel to the mid-diaphyseal line.

**Step 3:** Draw a third line (red line) that starts at the center of the femoral head and creates an angle of 7° (average normal value of the AMA) with the second line. This third line should converge towards the anatomic axis of the proximal femur. This third line is the proximal mechanical axis of the femur.

#### Frontal Plane Proximal Mechanical Axis–Create Normal mLPFA Strategy:

Use the proximal joint line to create a normal mLPFA (85–95°) from the center of the femoral head (Fig. 2). You may use the average normal value for the mLPFA or use the mLPFA value of the contralateral normal limb. This strategy should not be used when a concurrent deformity of the femoral neck or greater trochanter is present or in children (the greater trochanter is unossified).

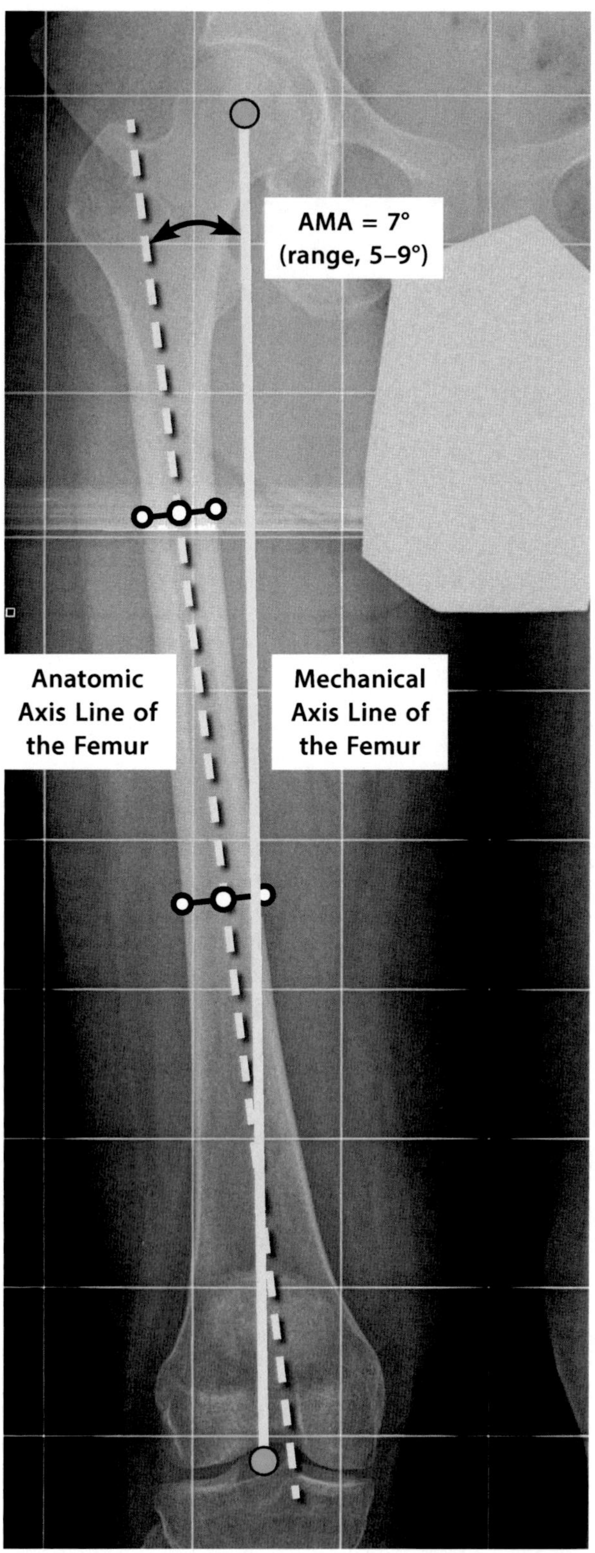


**Fig. 1:** The anatomic-mechanical angle is the angle created between the anatomic and mechanical axis lines of the femur (average, 7°; range, 5–9°).

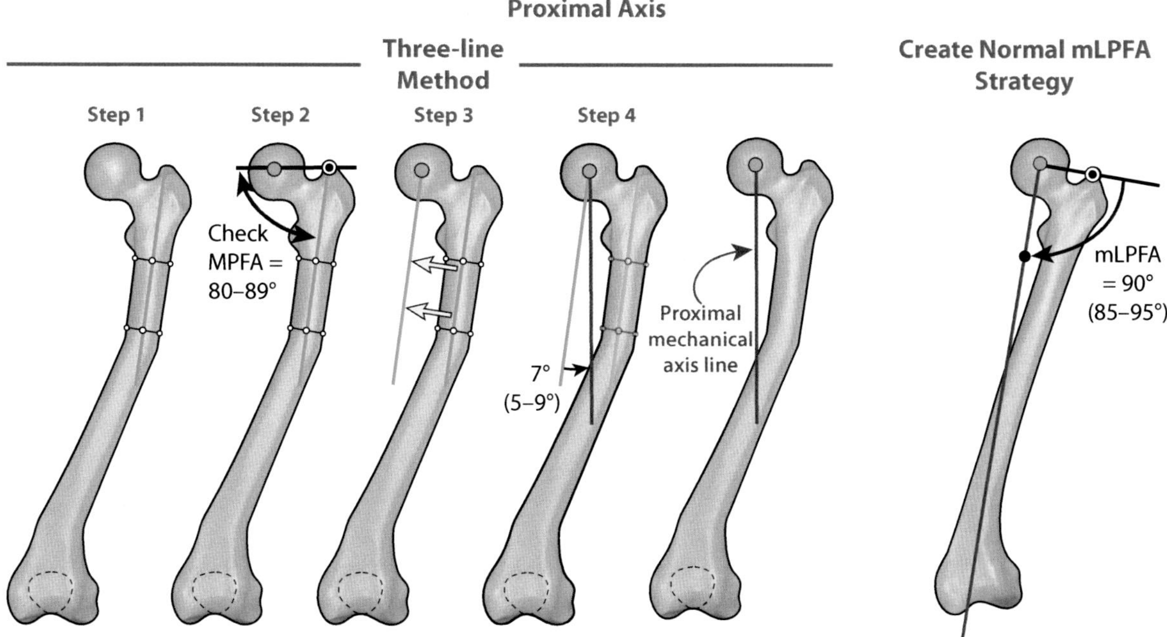


**Fig. 2:** Two strategies can be used to identify the mechanical axis of the proximal femoral segment in the frontal plane. **Three-line Method:** Use the three-line method. **Create Normal mLPFA Strategy:** Use the proximal joint line to create a normal mLPFA (normal range, 85–95°) from the center of the femoral head.

## Identifying the Distal Femoral Mechanical Axis in the Frontal Plane

Two strategies can be used to identify the mechanical axis of the distal femoral segment:

### Frontal Plane Distal Mechanical Axis–Normal Mechanical Axis Strategy:

Extend the normal tibial mechanical axis into the distal femur (Fig. 3). To use this strategy, the knee joint lines must be parallel or nearly parallel (normal JLCA) and the MPTA must be normal (85–90°).

### Frontal Plane Distal Mechanical Axis–Create Normal mLDFA Strategy:

Use the distal joint line to create a normal mLDFA (85–90°) from the center of the knee (Fig. 3). You may use the average normal value for the mLDFA or use the mLDFA value of the contralateral normal limb.

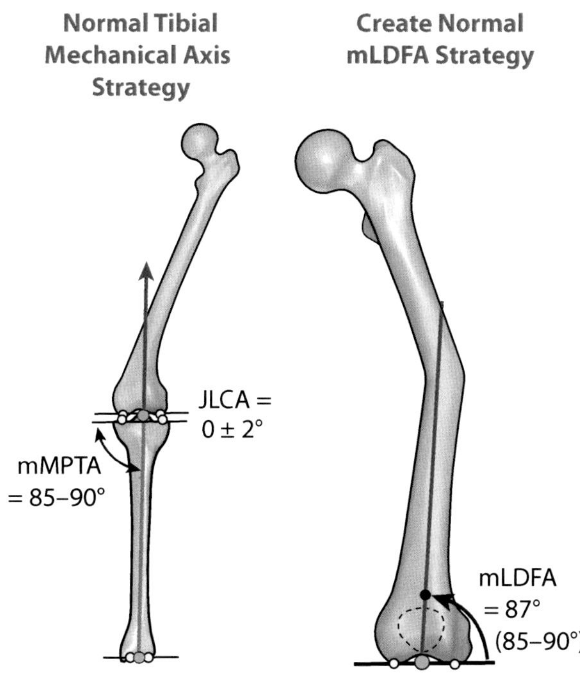


**Fig. 3:** Two strategies can be used to identify the mechanical axis of the distal femoral segment in the frontal plane. **Normal Tibial Mechanical Axis Strategy:** Extend the normal tibial mechanical axis into the distal femur. The limb must have a normal JLCA and MPTA. **Create Normal mLDFA Strategy:** Use the distal joint line to create a normal mLDFA (normal range, 85–90°) from the center of the knee.

© 2023 Sinai Hospital of Baltimore

## Frontal Plane Mechanical Axis Planning: Diaphyseal Deformity (Fig. 4)

**Angle Analysis:**

During the MAP analysis, we drew the mechanical axis of the femur and determined that the LDFA was abnormal.

### Three-line Method:

**Step 1:** Draw the mid-diaphyseal line (blue line) of the proximal femur and confirm that the proximal joint angle is normal.

**Step 2:** Draw a second line (blue line) that starts at the center of the femoral head and is parallel to the mid-diaphyseal line.

**Step 3:** Draw a third line (red line) that starts at the center of the femoral head and creates an angle of 7° (average normal value of the AMA) with the second line. This third line should converge towards the anatomic axis of the proximal femur. This third line is the proximal mechanical axis of the femur.

*Sensei says,*

*"When using the three-line method, the magnitude for the anatomic-mechanical angle (AMA) can be the population normal of 7° (range, 5–9°) or the measured AMA of the normal contralateral limb."*

### Create a Normal mLDFA:

**Step 4:** Draw the joint line of the distal femur, and mark the center of the knee. Create an angle from the center of the knee that equals a normal mLDFA (87°). This is the distal mechanical axis.

### Determine the Apex, Magnitude, Bone Cut, and Correction:

**Step 5:** Mark the apex of the deformity at the intersection of the proximal (red line) and distal (blue line) axes.

**Step 6:** Measure the magnitude of the deformity by measuring the magnitude of the acute angle created by the intersection of the proximal and distal axes. The magnitude is 30° (varus).

**Step 7:** Bone Cut: Place the osteotomy as close to the apex as possible. In this example, the osteotomy can be performed at the level of the apex because this level is feasible anatomically. Also, the resulting bony fragments are large enough for stable fixation.

**Step 8:** Correction (part 1): Draw the C-level. The C-level passes through the apex and bisects the obtuse angle that is created by the intersection of the proximal and distal axes. To achieve correction, the bone segment is angulated about a thumbtack placed on the C-level. This example shows the thumbtack placed along the C-level on the convex side of the deformity.

**Step 9:** Correction (part 2): Angulating the bone segment around the thumbtack results in an opening wedge osteotomy with complete alignment of the bone and both axes. Since the bone cut was placed at the level of the apex, bony translation does not occur. Check the LPFA and LDFA to confirm that they are within the range of normal.

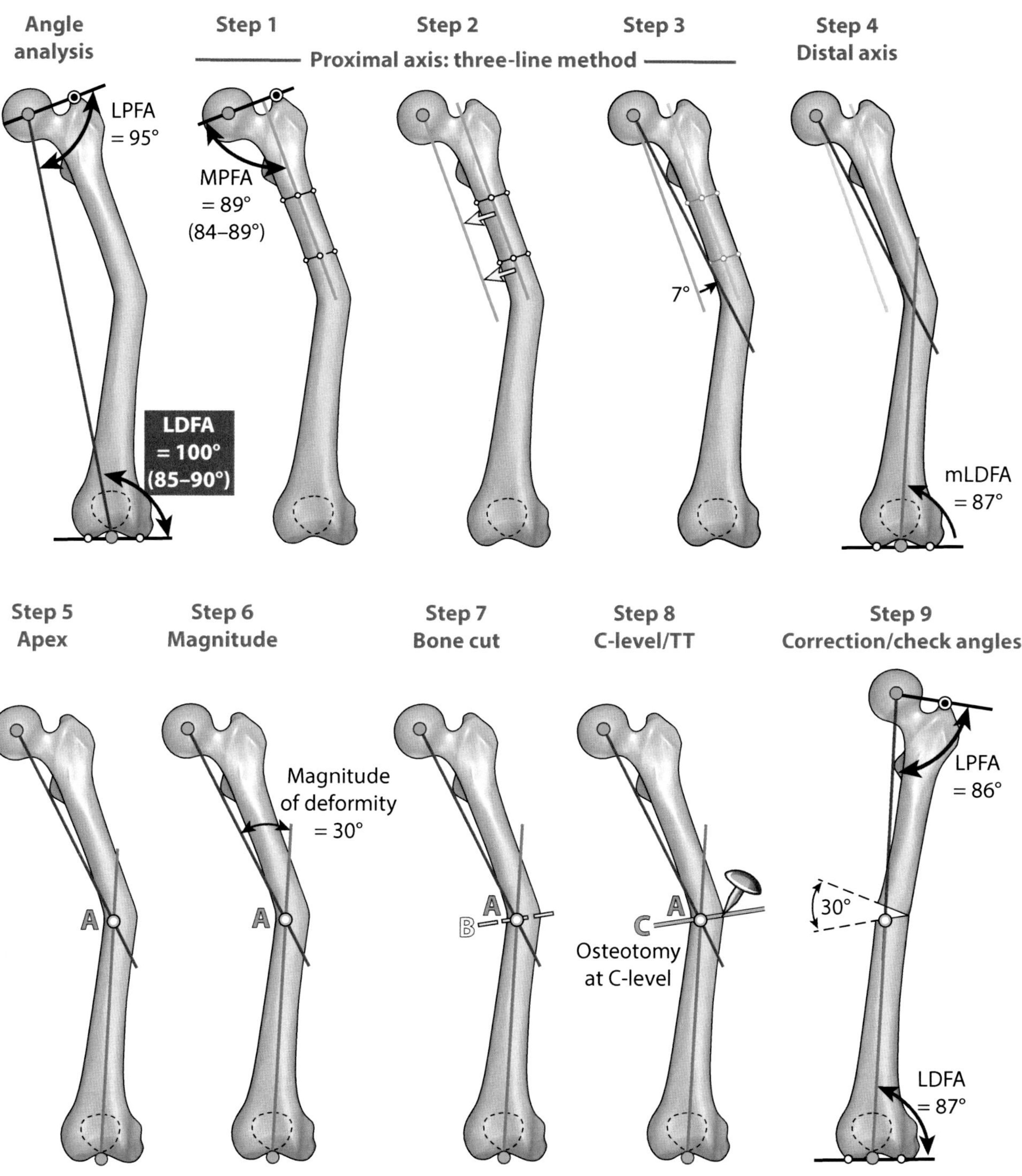


**Fig. 4:** Frontal plane analysis of a femoral diaphyseal deformity using the mechanical axis method. The LDFA is abnormal. The three-line method is used to determine the proximal axis, and a normal mLDFA is created to determine the distal axis. The bone cut is made at the level of the apex, and the thumbtack is placed along the C-level on the convex side of the deformity. Angulating the bone segment around the thumbtack results in an opening wedge osteotomy with complete alignment of the bone and both axes. A, apex; B, bone cut; C, C-level; TT, thumbtack.

© 2023 Sinai Hospital of Baltimore

## Frontal Plane Mechanical Axis Planning: Metaphyseal Deformity (Fig. 5)

**Angle Analysis:**

During the MAP analysis, we drew the mechanical axis of the femur and determined that the LDFA was abnormal.

### Create a Normal LPFA:

**Step 1:** Draw the joint line of the proximal femur from the tip of the greater trochanter to the center of the femoral head. This strategy can be used because the proximal femur has been determined to be normal during the MAP analysis. Create an angle from the center of the femoral head that equals a normal LPFA (90°). This is the proximal axis (red line).

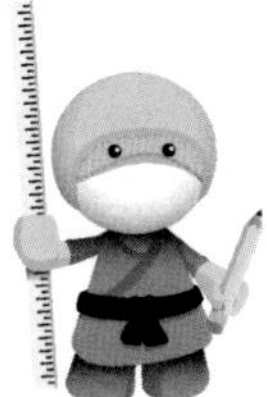

*Sensei says,*
*"Creating a normal LPFA to determine the proximal axis can only be used when the greater trochanter is ossified and the limb does not have a concurrent deformity of the femoral neck or greater trochanter."*

### Extend Normal Tibial Mechanical Axis:

**Step 2:** Draw the ipsilateral mechanical axis of the tibia and measure the MPTA. The MPTA is 89°, which is within the normal range. Also, the JLCA is within the normal range. Since the MPTA and JLCA are normal, the mechanical axis of the tibia can be used as the distal femoral axis. To do this, extend the tibial mechanical axis into the distal femur. This extended axis line is the distal femoral mechanical axis (blue line).

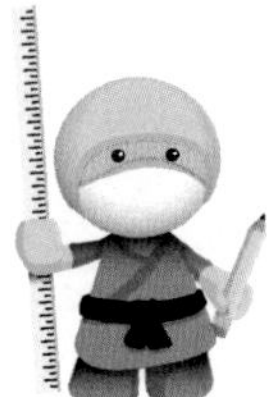

*Sensei says,*
*"The MPTA and the JLCA must both be normal in order to use the tibial mechanical axis to identify the distal femoral axis."*

### Determine the Apex, Magnitude, Bone Cut, and Correction:

**Step 3:** Mark the apex of the deformity at the intersection of the proximal (red line) and distal (blue line) axes.

**Step 4:** Measure the magnitude of the deformity by measuring the magnitude of the acute angle created by the intersection of the proximal and distal axes. The magnitude is 14° (valgus).

**Step 5:** Bone Cut: Place the osteotomy as close to the apex as possible. In this example, the osteotomy can be performed at the level of the apex because this level is feasible anatomically. Also, the resulting bony fragments are large enough for stable fixation.

**Step 6:** Correction (part 1): Draw the C-level. To achieve correction, the bone segment is always angulated about a thumbtack placed on the C-level. This example shows the thumbtack on the apex.

**Step 7:** Correction (part 2): Angulating the bone segment around the thumbtack results in a neutral wedge osteotomy with complete alignment of the bone and both axes. Since the bone cut was placed at the level of the apex, bony translation does not occur.

**Step 8:** Check the LPFA and LDFA to confirm that they are within the range of normal.

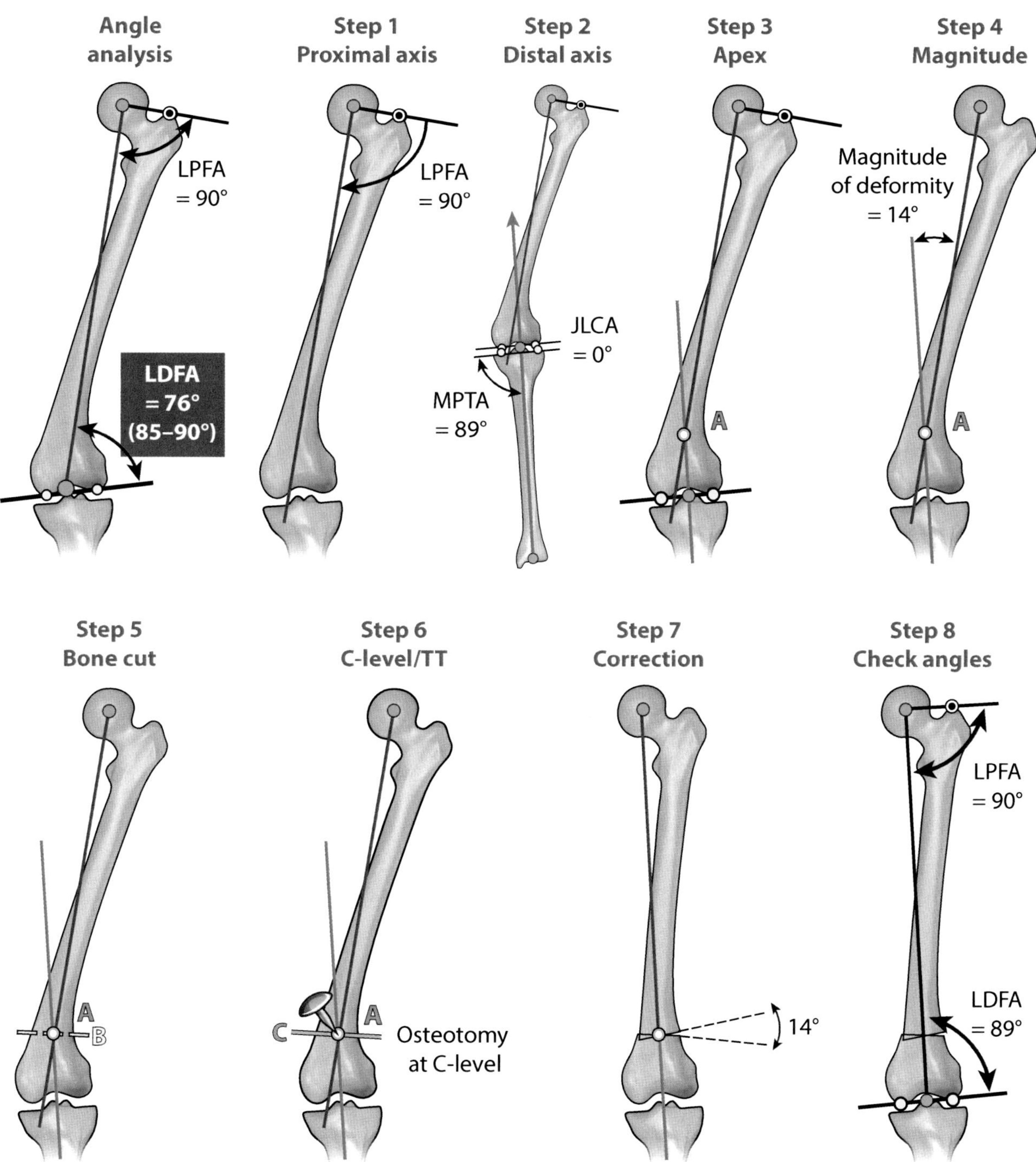


**Fig. 5:** Frontal plane analysis of a distal femoral metaphyseal deformity using the mechanical axis method. The LDFA is abnormal. A normal LPFA is created to determine the proximal axis, and the tibial mechanical axis is used to determine the distal axis. The bone cut is made at the level of the apex, and the thumbtack is placed at the apex. Angulating the bone segment around the thumbtack results in a neutral wedge osteotomy with complete alignment of the bone and both axes. A, apex; B, bone cut; C, C-level; TT, thumbtack.

© 2023 Sinai Hospital of Baltimore 

## Frontal Plane: Multiple-Level Deformity

A multiple-level deformity or hidden translational deformity is present when:

- The apex created by the intersection of the proximal and distal axis lines does not match the obvious deformity (Fig. 6A).
- The bone has a long, curving bow (e.g., rickets, osteogenesis imperfecta) (Fig. 6B).
- The proximal and distal axis lines intersect at a location that is outside of the bone (medial or lateral to the bone) (Fig. 6C).
- The proximal and distal axes do not intersect at all or intersect at a location that is proximal or distal to the entire bone segment (Fig. 6D).
- The bone segment has an obvious deformity plus an abnormal proximal or distal joint angle (Fig. 6E).

## Frontal Plane Mechanical Axis Planning: Multiple-Level Deformity (Fig. 7)

Mechanical axis planning of a femur with multiple apexes appears complicated at first glance. However, the strategy is straightforward and consists of identifying the proximal and distal mechanical axes by using the three-line method proximally and the joint angle distally. Once the proximal and distal mechanical axes are identified, then the axis of the middle segment (middle axis) is drawn using a modified three-line method.

**Angle Analysis:**

During the MAP analysis, we drew the mechanical axis of the femur and determined that the LPFA and LDFA were both abnormal.

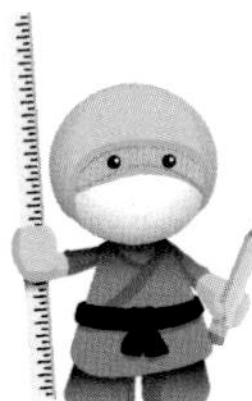

*Sensei says,*

*"If the bony deformity is obvious, the apex of the deformity should correlate with this level. If the apex is not associated with the obvious deformity, then a more complex deformity is present. The surgeon must understand this warning sign and investigate the possibility of a second hidden angular or translational deformity in the same bone segment."*

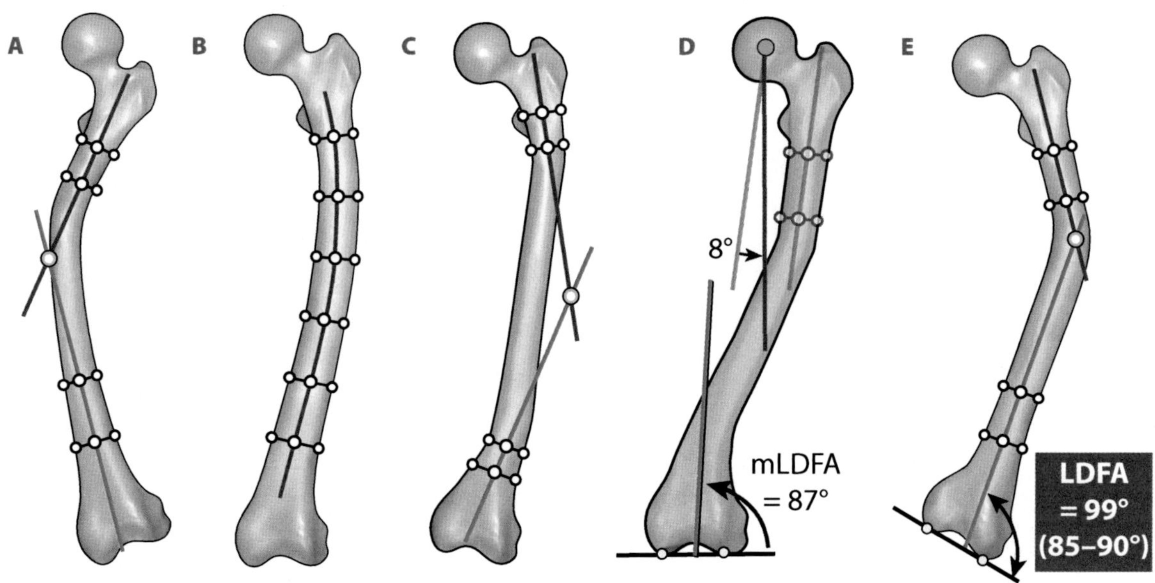


**Fig. 6:** Examples of multiple-level deformities. **A**, Apex does not match the obvious deformity. **B**, Bone has a curving bow. **C**, Proximal and distal axis lines intersect medial or lateral to the bone. **D**, The proximal and distal axis lines do not intersect or intersect at a location that is proximal or distal to the entire bone segment. **E**, The bone has an obvious deformity plus an abnormal proximal or distal joint angle.

**Use the Three-line Method:**

**Step 1:** Draw the mid-diaphyseal line of the proximal femur and confirm that the proximal joint angle is normal.

**Step 2:** Draw a second line that starts at the center of the femoral head and is parallel to the mid-diaphyseal line.

**Step 3:** Draw a third line (red line) that starts at the center of the femoral head and creates an angle of 8° (value of the AMA of the contralateral limb that is within the normal range) with the second line. This third line should converge towards the anatomic axis of the proximal femur. This third line (red line) is the proximal mechanical axis of the femur.

**Create a Normal LDFA:**

**Step 4:** Draw the joint line of the distal femur and mark the center of the knee. Create an angle from the center of the knee that equals a normal LDFA (87°). This is the distal mechanical axis (blue line).

**Step 5:** The proximal and distal axes do not intersect, which means that you are unable to mark the apex of the deformity and that this is a multiple-level deformity. The axis of the middle segment needs to be drawn in order to find the locations of the multiple apexes.

**Axis of the Middle Segment:**
**Use the Modified Three-line Method:**

**Step 6:** Draw the mid-diaphyseal line (α) of the middle segment.

**Step 7:** Draw a second line (β) that starts at the intersection of the proximal axis and the medial cortex of the femur. This β line should be parallel to the α line (mid-diaphyseal line of the middle segment).

**Step 8:** Draw a third line (dashed green line) that starts at the intersection of the proximal axis and the β line. This third line should

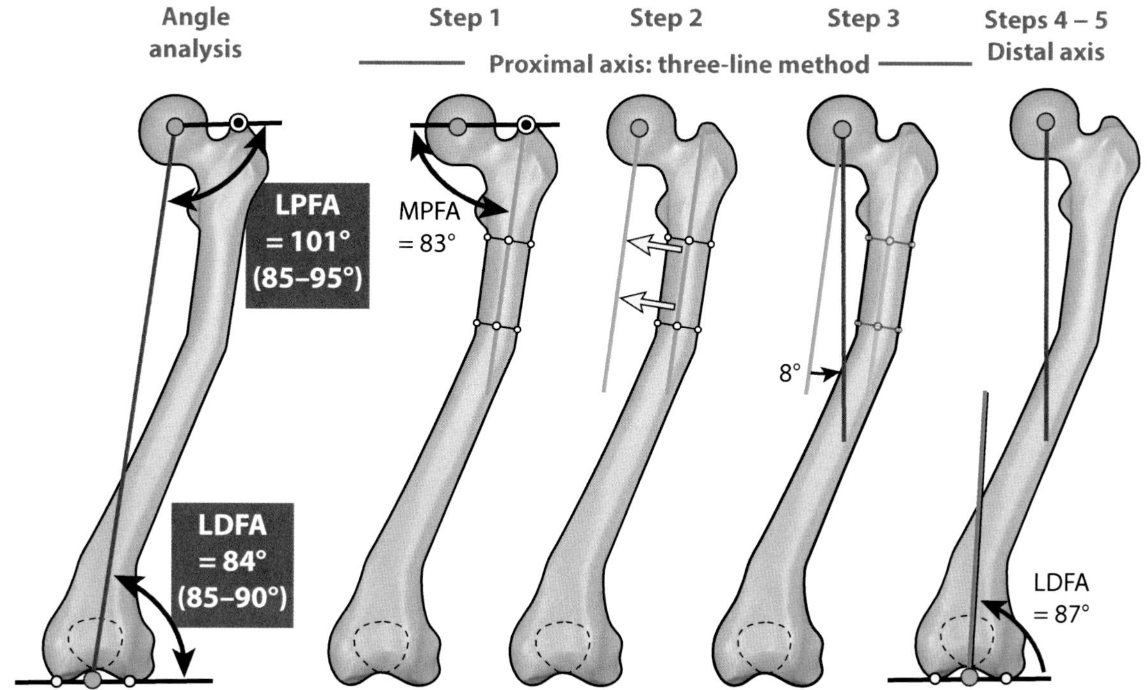


**Fig. 7:** Frontal plane analysis of a multiple-level femoral deformity using the mechanical axis method. The LPFA and LDFA are both abnormal. The three-line method is used to determine the proximal axis, and a normal LDFA is used to determine the distal axis.

© 2023 Sinai Hospital of Baltimore

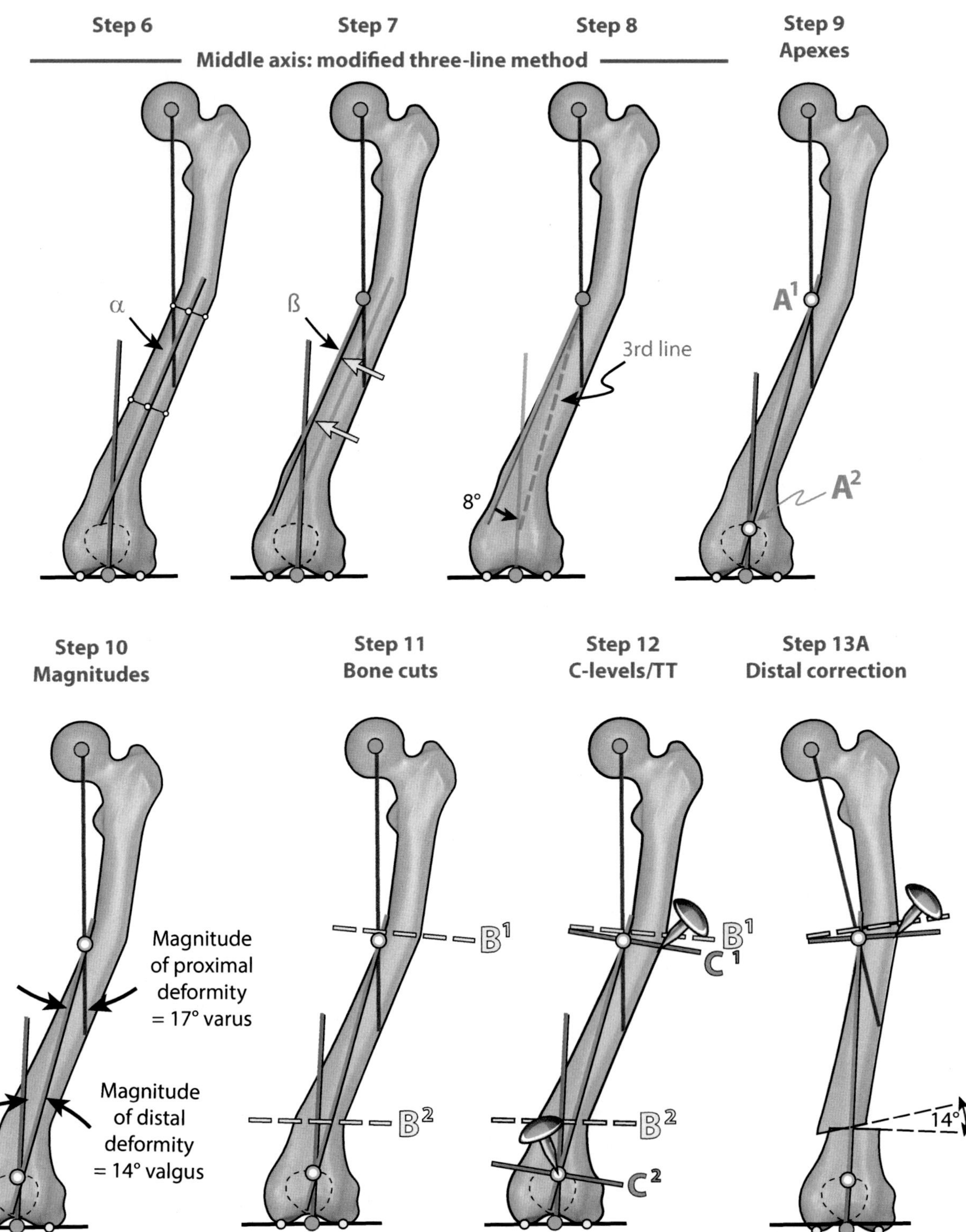


**Fig. 7 (continued):** Since these two axes do not intersect, a middle axis is drawn using a modified three-line method and two apexes are identified. Both bone cuts are made slightly proximal to the two apexes. The proximal thumbtack is placed on the convex side of the deformity, and the distal thumbtack is placed on the apex. Angulating the bone segment around the distal thumbtack results in a distal neutral wedge osteotomy. A, apex; B, bone cut; C, C-level; TT, thumbtacks.

create an angle of 8° (value of the AMA of the contralateral limb that is within the normal range) with the β line and should converge towards the anatomic axis of the middle segment. The third line (dashed green line) is the mechanical axis of the middle segment. Note that this line can be slightly translated medially and laterally (not shown) until it intersects the proximal and distal axis lines at the obvious level of the proximal and distal diaphyseal deformity. The placement that we chose for the mechanical axis of the middle segment in this example is appropriate for external fixation or plating. Translating the middle axis slightly medially or laterally will change the location of each apex and may decrease translation, which would be a better option if we were to use an intramedullary device for correction.

### Determine the Apex, Magnitude, Bone Cut, and Correction:

**Step 9:** Mark the apexes of the deformity at the intersections of the middle axis with both the proximal and with the distal axis. This femur has two apexes.

**Step 10:** Measure the magnitude of the deformity by measuring the magnitude of the acute angle created by the intersection of the proximal and distal axes with the middle axis. Apex[1] has a magnitude of deformity of 17° (varus), and Apex[2] has a magnitude of 14° (valgus).

**Step 11:** Bone Cuts: Place the osteotomies as close to the apexes as possible. One osteotomy is performed slightly proximal to Apex[1] and the other osteotomy is performed proximal to Apex[2] due to the surgeon's preference and the fixation method. Since the osteotomies are not performed at the level of the apexes, bony translation will occur during the correction. The amount of translation at osteotomy site 1 is the distance between the proximal axis and the middle axis at the level of osteotomy site 1. The amount of translation at osteotomy site 2 is the distance between the middle axis and the distal axis at the level of osteotomy site 2.

**Step 12:** Correction (part 1): Draw the two C-levels. To achieve correction, the bone segments are angulated about two thumbtacks placed on the C-levels. The proximal thumbtack is placed along the C-level on the convex side of the deformity and the distal thumbtack is placed at Apex[2].

**Step 13:** Correction (part 2): Angulating the bone segments around the thumbtacks results in a proximal opening wedge osteotomy and a distal neutral wedge osteotomy. Although complete alignment of the proximal, middle, and distal axes is achieved, obligatory bony translation occurs at both osteotomy sites. Check the LPFA and the LDFA to confirm that they are within the range of normal.

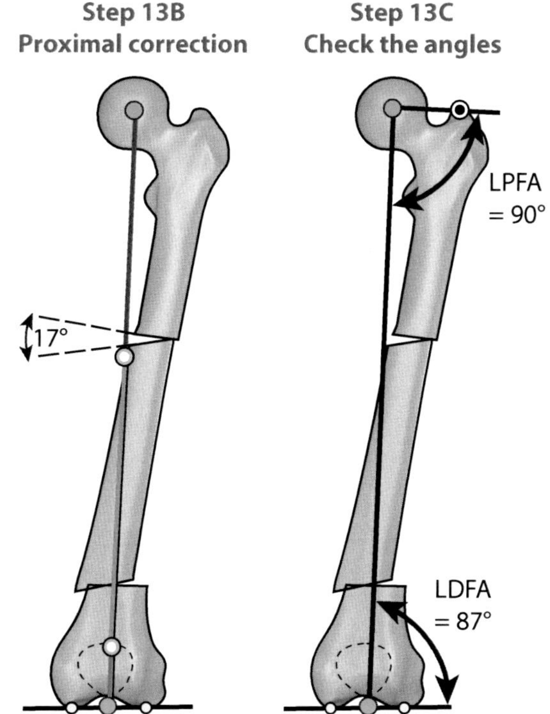


**Fig. 7 (continued):** Angulating the bone segment around the proximal thumbtack results in a proximal opening wedge osteotomy. Complete alignment of both axes is achieved, but bony translation occurs at both osteotomy sites because the osteotomies were not performed at the level of each apex.

© 2023 Sinai Hospital of Baltimore

## Femoral Anatomic Axis Planning: Frontal Plane

Anatomic axis planning utilizes the mid-line of the femoral diaphysis. Alignment of the anatomic axis is an indirect measurement to determine whether the final goal of correction has been met, which is a mechanical axis that passes through the center of the knee. Anatomic axis planning is the method of choice when full length standing x-rays are not available or when planning treatment with intramedullary nails.

### Identifying the Proximal Femoral Anatomic Axis in the Frontal Plane

Two strategies can be used to identify the anatomic axis of the proximal femoral segment:

### Frontal Plane Proximal Anatomic Axis–Mid-diaphyseal Line Strategy:

Use the mid-diaphyseal line of the proximal femoral segment (Fig. 8). This strategy assumes that the proximal femur has a straight segment that is long enough to define a line. If you use this strategy, you must measure the aMPFA (normal range, 80–89°) to check for a hidden deformity in the proximal femur. If the aMPFA is significantly abnormal, then the femur might have a single-level proximal metaphyseal deformity or a double-level deformity (proximal metaphyseal deformity plus another deformity) that needs to be addressed.

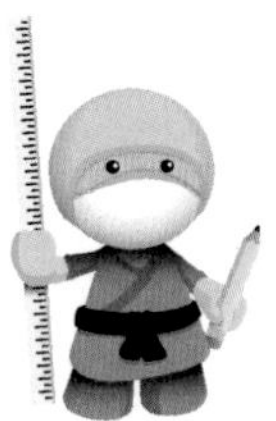

*Sensei says,*
*"In a normal femur, the mid-diaphyseal line (anatomic axis) of the proximal femoral segment will exit the bone proximally through (or near) the piriformis fossa."*

### Frontal Plane Proximal Anatomic Axis–Create Normal aMPFA Strategy:

Use the proximal joint line to create a normal aMPFA from the piriformis fossa (Fig. 8). You may use the average normal value for the aMPFA (84°) or use the aMPFA value of the contralateral normal limb. A severe proximal femoral deformity or an unossified greater trochanter would preclude this strategy because the joint line would be inaccurate.

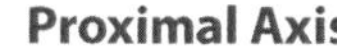


Mid-diaphyseal Line Strategy

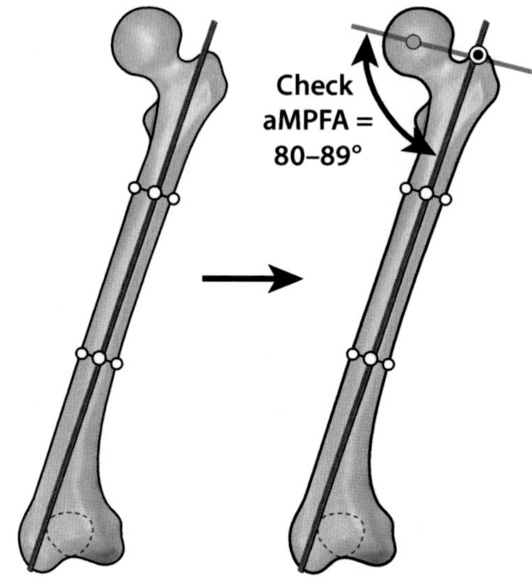


Create Normal aMPFA Strategy

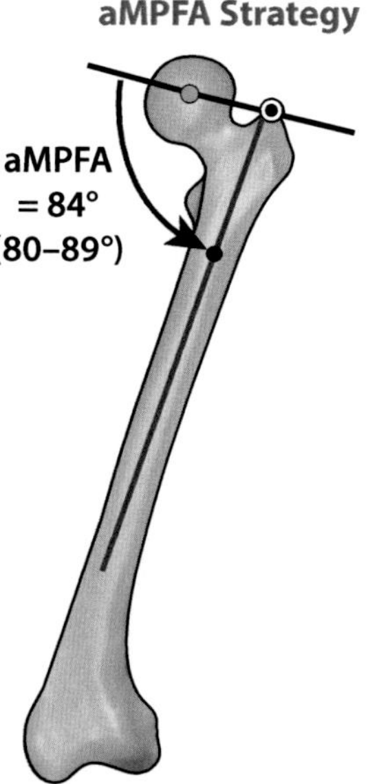


**Fig. 8:** Two strategies can be used to identify the anatomic axis of the proximal femoral segment in the frontal plane. **Mid-diaphyseal Line Strategy:** Use the mid-diaphyseal line of the proximal femoral segment. You must measure the aMPFA (normal range, 80–89°) formed by the proximal axis to check for a hidden deformity in the proximal femur. If the aMPFA is significantly abnormal, then a proximal hidden deformity exists. **Create Normal aMPFA Strategy:** Use the proximal joint line to create a normal aMPFA (normal range, 80–89°).

## Identifying the Distal Femoral Anatomic Axis in the Frontal Plane

Two strategies can be used to identify the anatomic axis of the distal femoral segment:

### Frontal Plane Distal Anatomic Axis–Mid-diaphyseal Line Strategy:

Use the mid-diaphyseal line of the distal femoral segment (Fig. 9). If you use this strategy, you must measure the aLDFA (normal range, 79–83°) to check for a hidden deformity in the distal femur. If the aLDFA is significantly abnormal, then the femur might have a single-level distal metaphyseal deformity or a double-level deformity (distal metaphyseal deformity plus another deformity) that needs to be addressed.

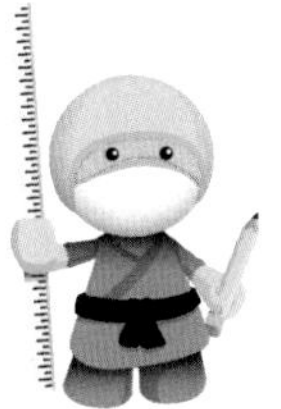

*Sensei says,*
*"In a normal femur, the mid-diaphyseal line (anatomic axis) of the distal femoral segment will exit the bone slightly medial to the center of the femoral groove."*

### Frontal Plane Distal Anatomic Axis–Create Normal aLDFA Strategy:

Use the distal joint line to create a normal aLDFA from a point on the joint line that is slightly medial to the center of the femoral groove (Fig. 9). This is the anatomic center of the knee. You may use the average normal value for the aLDFA (81°) or use the aLDFA value of the contralateral normal limb.

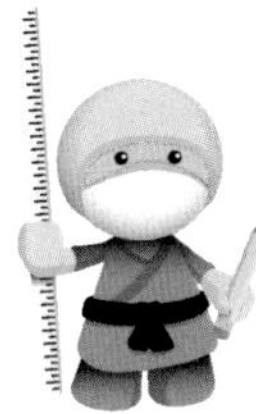

*Sensei says,*
*"If the mid-diaphyseal line strategy is being used to identify the proximal or distal femoral anatomic axis, the associated proximal or distal joint angle (aMPFA or aLDFA) must also be checked to look for a hidden metaphyseal deformity."*

**Distal Axis**

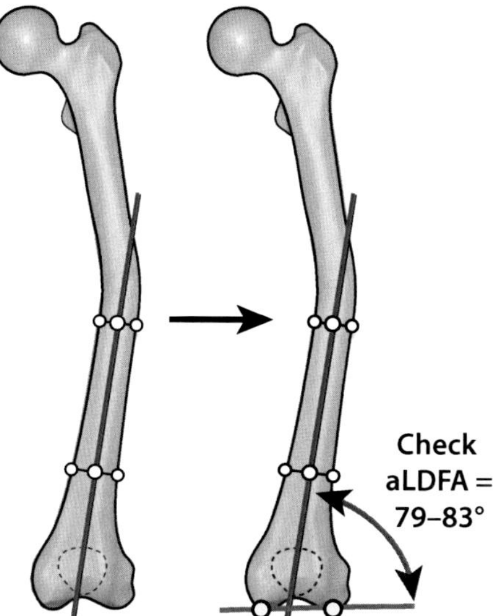


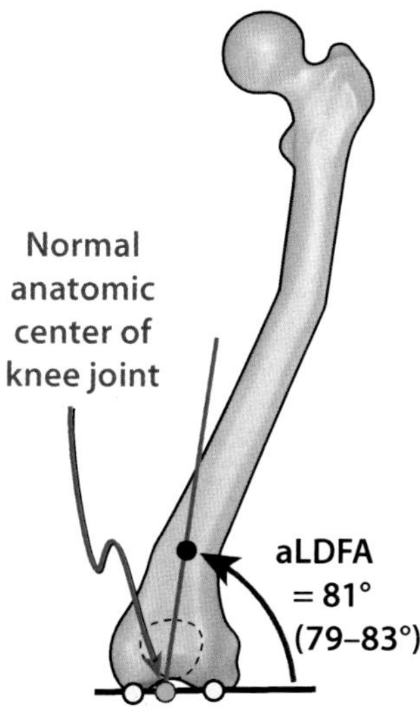


**Fig. 9:** Two strategies can be used to identify the anatomic axis of the distal femoral segment in the frontal plane. **Mid-diaphyseal Line Strategy:** Use the mid-diaphyseal line of the distal femoral segment. You must measure the aLDFA (normal range, 79–83°) formed by the distal axis to check for a hidden deformity in the distal femur. If the aLDFA is significantly abnormal, then a distal hidden deformity exists. **Create Normal aLDFA Strategy:** Use the distal joint line to create a normal aLDFA (normal range, 79–83°).

© 2023 Sinai Hospital of Baltimore

## Frontal Plane Anatomic Axis Planning: Diaphyseal Deformity (Fig. 10)

**Angle Analysis:**

During the MAP analysis, we drew the mechanical axis of the femur and determined that the LPFA and LDFA were both abnormal.

**Step 1:** Draw the mid-diaphyseal line of the proximal segment and the mid-diaphyseal line of the distal segment. These are the proximal (red line) and distal (blue line) axes.

**Step 2:** Since mid-diaphyseal lines were used for both axes, the proximal and distal joint angles must be checked to look for hidden deformities near the joints. The MPFA is 84°, and the aLDFA is 81°. Both are within the range of normal; therefore, the femur does not have a metaphyseal deformity.

**Step 3:** Mark the apex of the deformity at the intersection of the proximal and distal axes.

**Step 4:** Measure the magnitude of the deformity. The magnitude is 18° (varus).

**Step 5:** Bone Cut: Place the osteotomy as close to the apex as possible. The osteotomy can be performed at the level of the apex because this level is feasible anatomically. Also, the resulting bony fragments are large enough for stable fixation.

**Step 6:** Correction (part 1): Draw the C-level. To achieve correction, the bone segment is angulated about a thumbtack placed on the C-level. This example shows the thumbtack on the apex.

**Step 7:** Correction (part 2): Angulating the bone segment around the thumbtack results in a neutral wedge osteotomy with complete alignment of the bone and both axes.

**Step 8:** Measure the MPFA and aLDFA to confirm that they are within the range of normal.

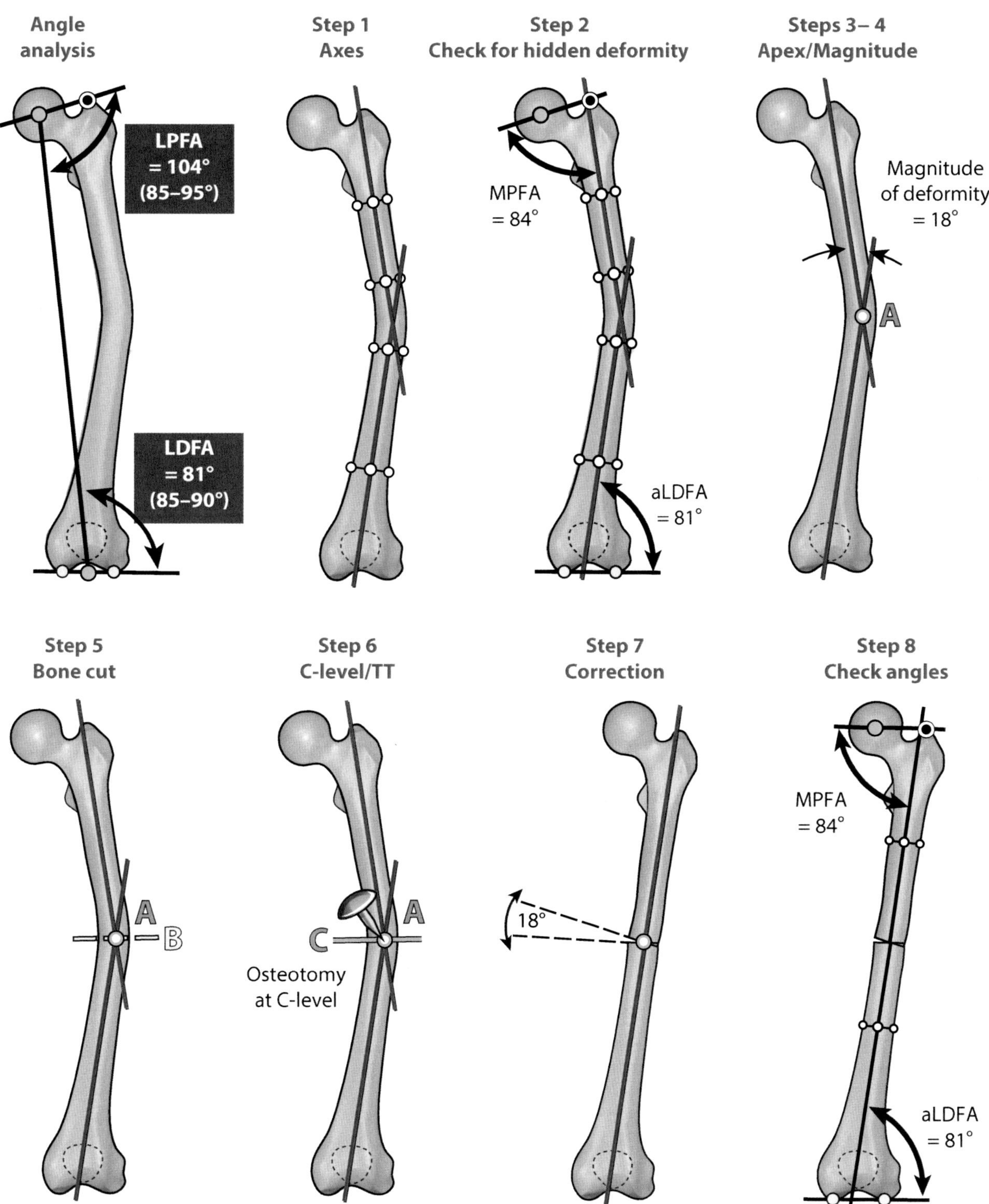


**Fig. 10:** Frontal plane analysis of a single-level, diaphyseal femoral deformity using the anatomic axis method. The LPFA and LDFA are both abnormal. The mid-diaphyseal lines of the proximal and distal segments are used to determine the proximal and distal axis lines. The bone cut is made at the level of the apex, and the thumbtack is placed on the apex. Angulating the bone segment around the thumbtack results in a neutral wedge osteotomy. Complete alignment of the bone and both axes is achieved. A, apex; B, bone cut; C, C-level; TT, thumbtack.

© 2023 Sinai Hospital of Baltimore

## Frontal Plane Anatomic Axis Planning: Metaphyseal Deformity (Fig. 11)

**Angle Analysis:**

During the MAP analysis, we drew the mechanical axis of the femur and determined that the LDFA was abnormal.

**Step 1:** Draw the mid-diaphyseal line of the proximal femur. This is the proximal anatomic axis (red line). If the deformity is located in the metaphyseal or juxta-articular region, then there will be only one obvious anatomic axis.

**Step 2:** Since the mid-diaphyseal line was used for the proximal anatomic axis, the proximal joint angle must be checked to look for a hidden deformity near the hip. The MPFA is 82°. This is within the range of normal; therefore, the femur does not have a proximal metaphyseal deformity.

**Step 3:** Since the distal femur is obviously abnormal, draw the distal axis by creating a normal joint angle. To do this, draw the joint line of the distal femur, and mark a point on the joint line that is slightly medial to the center of the femoral notch (normal anatomic center of the knee joint). Create an angle from this point that equals a normal aLDFA (81°). This is the distal anatomic axis (blue line).

**Step 4:** Mark the apex of the deformity at the intersection of the proximal and distal axes.

**Step 5:** Measure the magnitude of the deformity. The magnitude is 15° (valgus).

**Step 6:** Bone Cut: The osteotomy can be performed at the level of the apex because this level is feasible anatomically. Also, the resulting bony fragments are large enough for stable fixation.

**Step 7:** Correction (part 1): Draw the C-level. To achieve correction, the bone segment is always angulated about a thumbtack placed on the C-level. This example shows the thumbtack on the apex.

**Step 8:** Correction (part 2): Angulating the bone segment around the thumbtack results in a neutral wedge osteotomy with complete alignment of the bone and both axes.

**Step 9:** Measure the MPFA and aLDFA to confirm that they are within the range of normal.

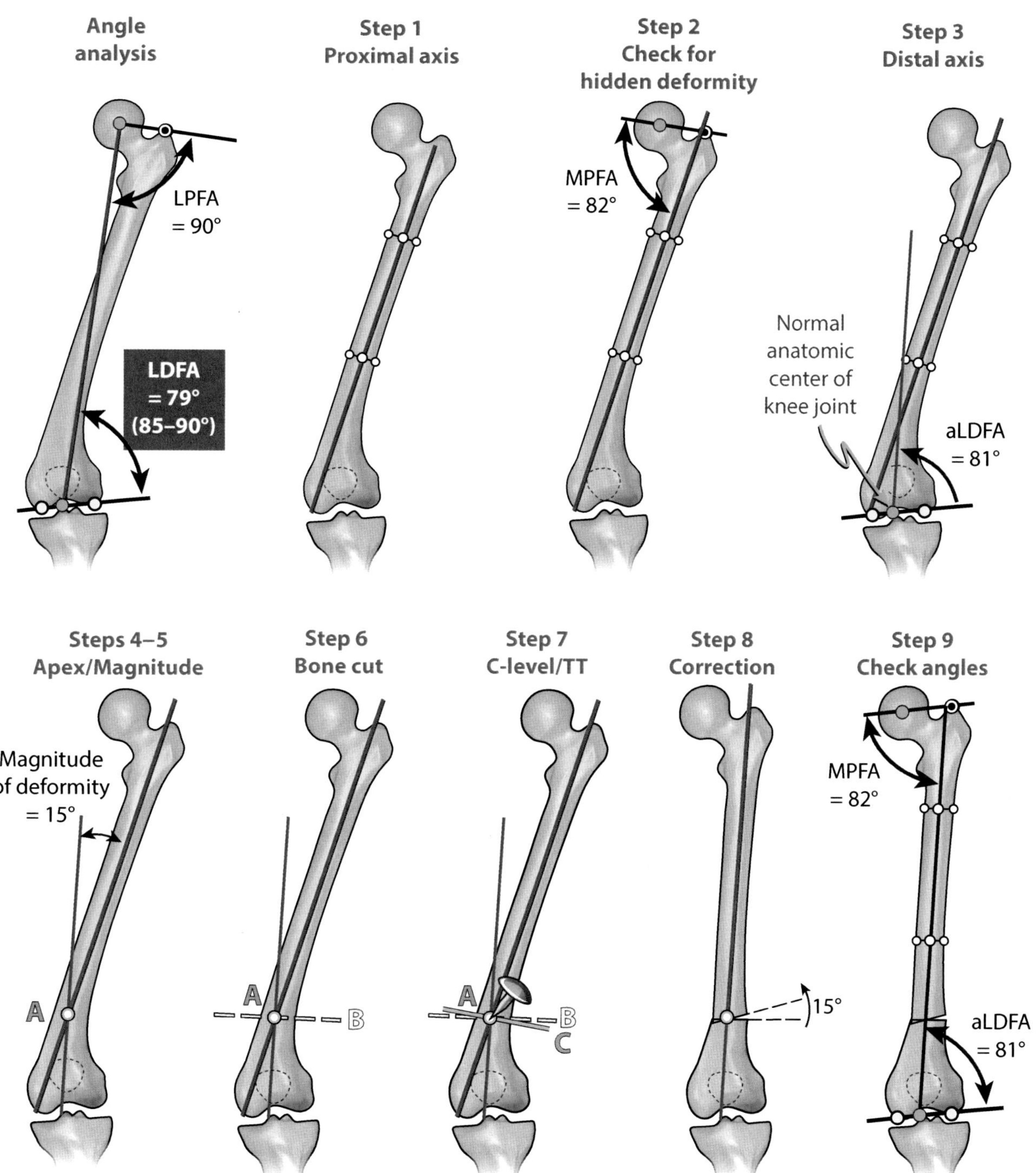


**Fig. 11:** Frontal plane analysis of a single-level metaphyseal femoral deformity using the anatomic axis method. The LDFA is abnormal. The mid-diaphyseal line of the proximal femur is used to determine the proximal axis (*red line*), and a normal aLDFA is created to determine the distal axis (*blue line*). The bone cut is made at the level of the apex, and the thumbtack is placed on the apex. Angulating the bone segment around the thumbtack results in a neutral wedge osteotomy. Complete alignment of the bone and both axes is achieved. A, apex; B, bone cut; C, C-level; TT, thumbtack.

© 2023 Sinai Hospital of Baltimore

## Frontal Plane Anatomic Axis Planning: Multiple-Level Deformity (Fig. 12)

**Angle Analysis:** During the MAP analysis, we drew the mechanical axis of the femur and determined that the LPFA and LDFA were both normal. However, the femur has an obvious deformity.

**Step 1:** Draw the mid-diaphyseal line of the proximal femur. This is the proximal anatomic axis (red line). Since the mid-diaphyseal line was used for the proximal anatomic axis, the proximal joint angle must be checked to look for a hidden proximal deformity. The MPFA is 84° (normal); therefore, the femur does not have a proximal metaphyseal deformity.

**Step 2:** Draw the joint line of the distal femur, and mark a point on the joint line that is slightly medial to the center of the femoral groove. This is the normal anatomic center of the knee joint. Create an angle from this point that equals a normal aLDFA (81°). This is the distal anatomic axis (blue line). Note that the proximal and distal axis lines do not intersect, which means that this is a multiple-level deformity.

**Step 3:** Draw a mid-diaphyseal line of the apparent middle segment. This is the middle axis (green line).

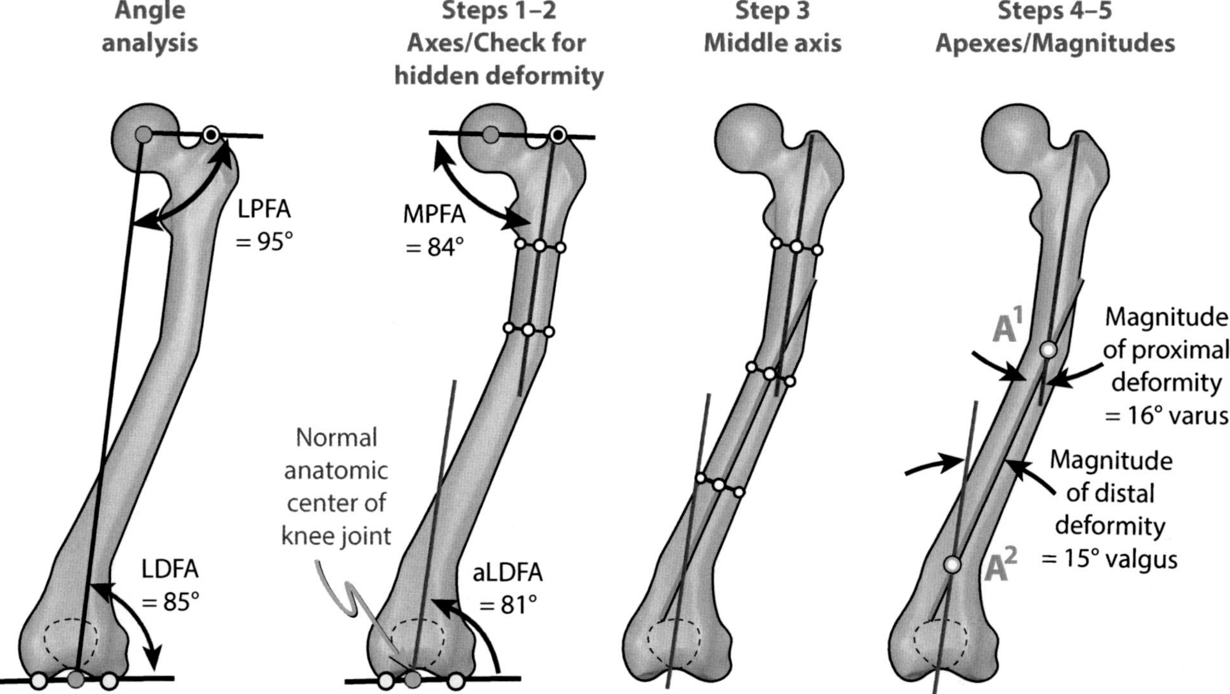


**Fig. 12:** Frontal plane analysis of a double-level femoral deformity using the anatomic axis method. The mid-diaphyseal line of the proximal femur is used to determine the proximal axis (*red line*); therefore, the MPFA is measured to check for a metaphyseal deformity. Since the MPFA is normal, the femur does not have a metaphyseal deformity. A normal aLDFA is created to determine the distal axis (*blue line*). Since these axis lines do not intersect, the middle axis is drawn (mid-diaphyseal line of the apparent middle segment) (*green line*). A, apex.

**Step 4:** Mark the intersection of the proximal and middle axes as Apex[1]. Mark the intersection of the middle and distal axes as Apex[2]. These are the apexes of the multiple deformities.

**Step 5:** The magnitude of the deformity at Apex[1] is 16° (varus) and Apex[2] is 15° (valgus).

**Step 6:** Bone Cuts: Place the osteotomies as close to each apex as possible. An osteotomy is performed at the level of Apex[1] and at the level of Apex[2].

**Step 7:** Correction (part 1): Draw the C-levels. To achieve correction, the bone segments are angulated about thumbtacks placed on the C-levels. This example shows the proximal thumbtack placed along the C-level on the convex side of the proximal deformity and the distal thumbtack placed along the C-level on the convex side of the distal deformity.

**Step 8:** Correction (part 2): Angulating the bone segments around the thumbtacks results in two opening wedge osteotomies with complete alignment of the bone and the axes.

**Step 9:** Check the MPFA and aLDFA to confirm that they are within the range of normal.

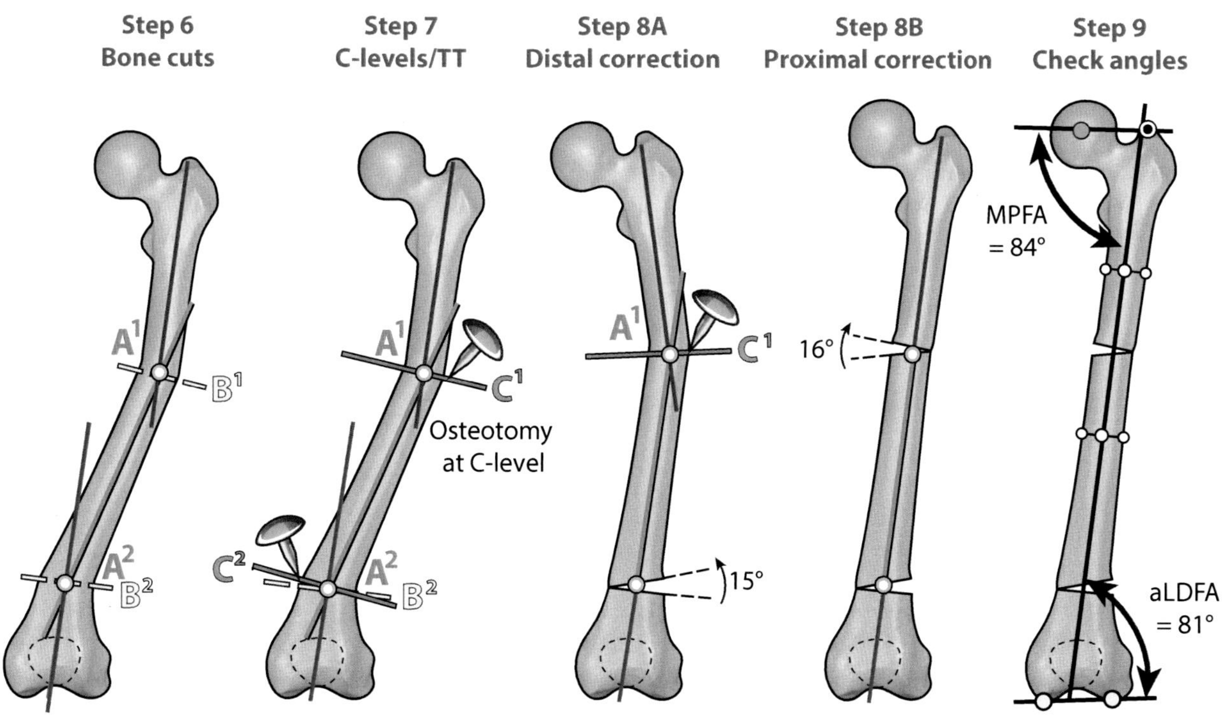


**Fig. 12 (continued):** The bone cuts are made at the level of the apexes. The proximal thumbtack is placed along the C-level on the convex side of the proximal deformity, and the distal thumbtack is placed along the C-level on the convex side of the distal deformity. Angulating the bone segments around the thumbtacks results in two opening wedge osteotomies. Complete alignment of the bone and the axes is achieved. A, apex; B, bone cut; C, C-level; TT, thumbtacks.

© 2023 Sinai Hospital of Baltimore

## Femoral Axis Planning: Sagittal Plane

The sagittal plane is more complex because the knee joint also moves in the sagittal plane. A sagittal plane deformity of the femur can result in an apparent fixed flexion deformity of the knee or a hyperextension deformity of the knee. The three components that can influence a sagittal deformity of the knee are:

1. Bony deformities of the distal femur
2. Bony deformities of the proximal tibia
3. Soft-tissue characteristics:
   - Soft-tissue laxity resulting in hyperextension of the knee joint
   - Soft-tissue contracture resulting in fixed flexion deformity of the knee

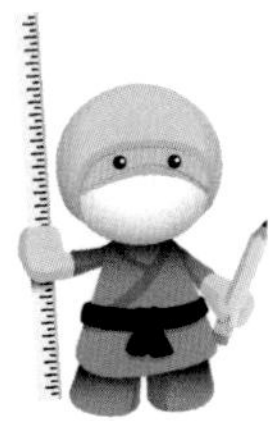

*Sensei says,*

*"The knee, with its joint motion in the sagittal plane, can compensate for significant deformities in this plane, unlike frontal plane deformities. This situation requires careful and accurate analysis of the sagittal plane."*

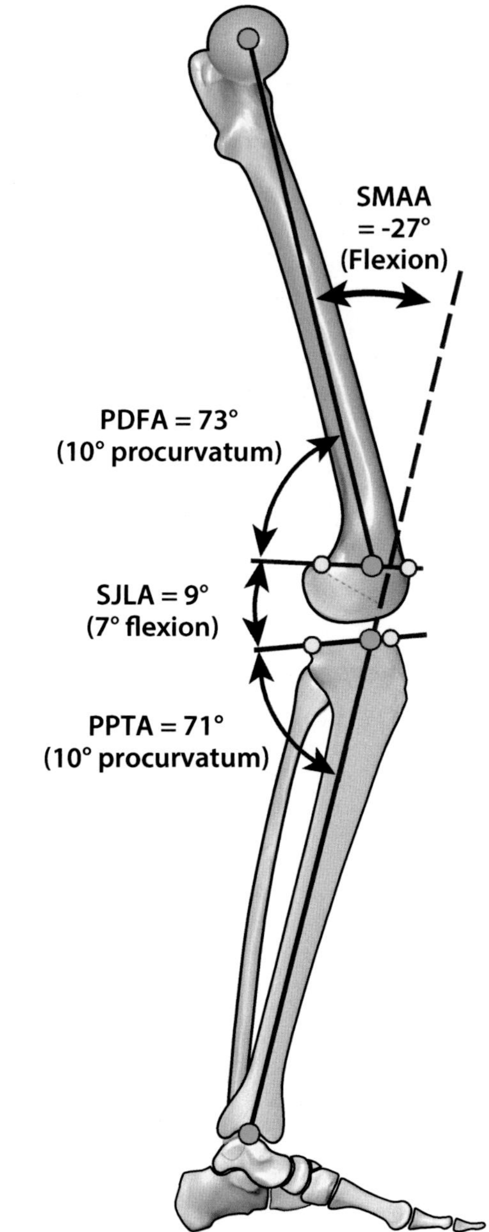


**RESULTS:**
**10° Femoral flexion deformity**
**10° Tibial flexion deformity**
**7° Soft-tissue contracture deformity**

**Fig. 13:** The sagittal mechanical axes angle (SMAA) helps you determine how much of the deformity around the knee is from distal femoral and proximal tibial bony deformities and how much is caused by soft-tissue problems (refer to the chapter entitled "Deformity Analysis in the Sagittal Plane").

Before you can find the apex in the sagittal plane, you must perform the MAP analysis. An essential part of this analysis is evaluating the segmental mechanical axes of the femur and tibia, which demonstrate whether the knee joint is in a neutral position, fixed flexion position, or hyperextended position (refer to the chapter entitled "Deformity Analysis in the Sagittal Plane" for examples of sagittal plane analysis using the SMAA). The SMAA gives you valuable information about how the soft-tissue and bony deformities contribute to the overall deformity around the knee and is essential to develop an effective treatment strategy (Fig. 13).

When MAP is done for the sagittal plane, the modified mechanical axis of the femur is used to analyze the PDFA (Fig. 14A) (see Chapter 1 for a refresher on how to draw the modified mechanical axis in the sagittal plane). If a sagittal plane x-ray of the whole femur is not able to be obtained, the anatomic axis of the distal one-third of the femur can be used to perform the MAP. If an x-ray of the whole femur is not available when performing the ABCs, the anatomic axis of the distal one-third of the femur can be used as the proximal axis (only in cases in which no other deformity is proximal). In the sagittal plane, the femur has a natural apex due to its gradual anterior bow (Fig. 14B), which is approximately 10° in a normal femur. To be more precise in determining the normal femoral anterior bow, one can measure the anterior bow on a lateral view x-ray of the contralateral normal limb. The anterior bow should always be measured during femoral axis planning. When finding apexes for deformity correction, it is important to make sure that you find the abnormal apexes, not the apex formed by the normal femoral anterior bow. If some cases, it may be appropriate to correct the femur so that no anterior femoral bow remains (e.g., when treating with an intramedullary device).

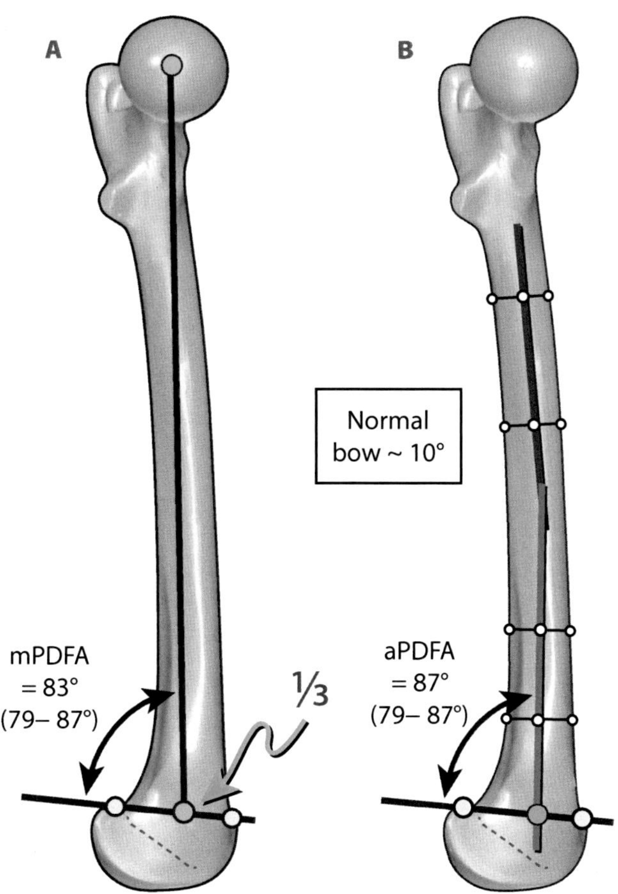


**Fig. 14:** **A**, When MAP is performed in the sagittal plane, the modified mechanical axis of the femur is used to analyze the mPDFA. **B**, In the sagittal plane, the femur has a natural apex due to its gradual anterior bow. Note that we can use the distal anatomic axis to determine the anatomic posterior distal femoral angle (aPDFA). Although in many cases the value of the aPDFA will be different from the mPDFA, we accept this slight difference and consider them to be equivalent for analysis and planning purposes.

© 2023 Sinai Hospital of Baltimore

## Identifying the Proximal Femoral Axis in the Sagittal Plane

### Sagittal Plane Proximal Axis–Mid-diaphyseal Line Strategy:

Use the proximal femoral segment's mid-diaphyseal line (Fig. 15). This strategy assumes that the proximal femur has a straight segment that is long enough to define a line. If you use this strategy, you must perform a thorough clinical examination to ensure that a proximal metaphyseal deformity does not exist (i.e., hip flexion deformity or limited hip flexion).

## Identifying the Distal Femoral Axis in the Sagittal Plane

### Sagittal Plane Distal Axis–Mid-diaphyseal Line Strategy:

In most cases, it is best to start with this strategy to determine the distal axis. Use the distal femoral segment's mid-diaphyseal line (Fig. 16). This strategy assumes that the distal femur has a straight segment that is long enough to define a line. If you use this strategy, you must measure the PDFA (normal range, 79–87°) formed by the distal axis (i.e., the anatomic axis of the distal bone segment) to check for a hidden metaphyseal deformity in the distal femur. If the PDFA is significantly abnormal, then the femur might have a single-level distal metaphyseal deformity or a double-level deformity (distal metaphyseal plus another deformity) that needs to be addressed.

### Sagittal Plane Distal Axis–Create Normal PDFA Strategy:

If there is no obvious distal mid-diaphyseal line or if the PDFA was found to be abnormal during the MAP analysis, create a distal axis using a normal PDFA (Fig. 16). Use the distal joint line to create a normal PDFA starting at a point one-third the length of the joint line from the anterior cortex. You may use the average normal value for the PDFA (83°) or use the PDFA value of the contralateral normal limb.

**Proximal Axis**
**Mid-diaphyseal Line Strategy**

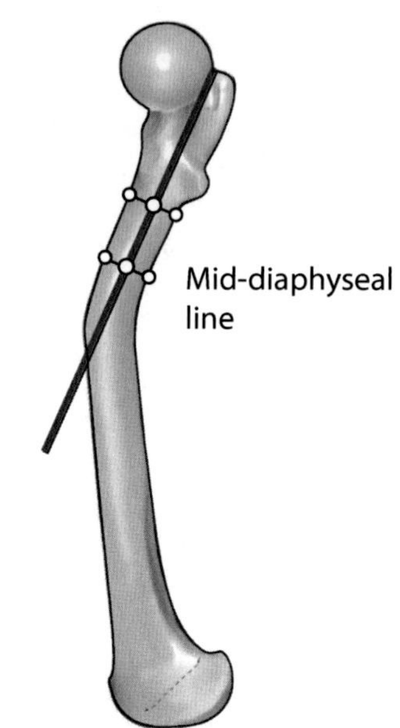


**Fig. 15:** To determine the proximal axis in the sagittal plane, draw a mid-diaphyseal line. To use this strategy, you must check for a proximal metaphyseal deformity during the clinical examination.

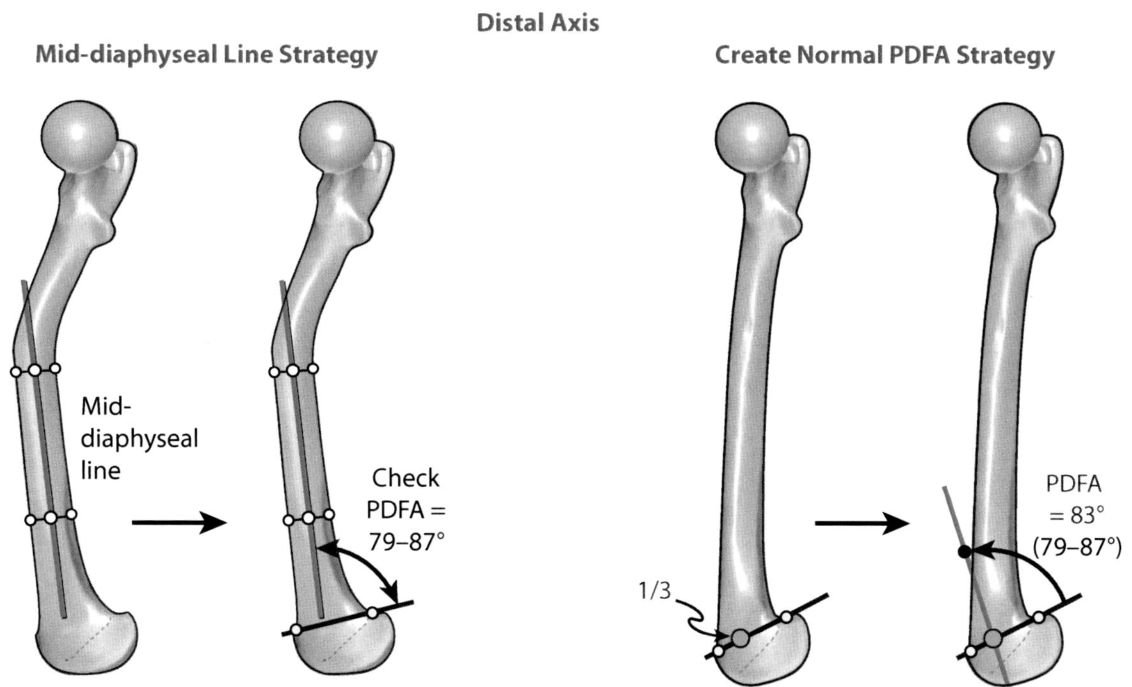


**Fig. 16:** Two strategies can be used to identify the distal axis in the sagittal plane.
**Mid-diaphyseal Line Strategy:** Draw the mid-diaphyseal line of the distal segment and confirm that the PDFA is normal.
**Create Normal PDFA Strategy:** Use the distal joint line to create a normal PDFA (normal range, 79–87°).

*© 2023 Sinai Hospital of Baltimore*

## Sagittal Plane Axis Planning: Diaphyseal Deformity (Fig. 17)

**MAD and Angle Analysis:**

During the MAP analysis, we drew the mechanical axis and determined that it was abnormal. We also drew the modified mechanical axis of the femur and determined that the PDFA was abnormal. After comparing the SMAA to the bony deformity analysis, we determined that there was no soft-tissue component to the deformity around the knee.

**Step 1:** Draw the mid-diaphyseal line of the proximal segment (red line) and the mid-diaphyseal line of the distal segment (blue line). These are the proximal and distal axis lines.

**Step 2:** Since the mid-diaphyseal line was used for the distal axis, the PDFA formed by the distal axis (i.e., the anatomic axis of the distal bone segment) must be measured. The PDFA is normal; therefore, the femur does not have a distal metaphyseal deformity. Since the mid-diaphyseal line was used for the proximal axis, a thorough clinical examination was performed and a hip deformity in the sagittal plane was not found. Also, the bow of the femur needs to be checked when analyzing a sagittal plane deformity. In this case, the anterior bow is abnormal (30°).

**Step 3:** Mark the apex of the deformity at the intersection of the axis lines.

**Step 4:** Measure the magnitude of the deformity (30°).

**Step 5:** Bone Cut: The osteotomy can be performed at the level of the apex because this level is feasible anatomically and the resulting bony fragments are large enough for stable fixation.

**Step 6:** Correction (part 1): Draw the C-level. To achieve correction, the bone segment is angulated about a thumbtack placed on the C-level. This example shows the thumbtack placed along the C-level on the convex side of the deformity.

**Step 7:** Correction (part 2): Angulating the bone segment around the thumbtack results in an opening wedge osteotomy with complete alignment of the bone and both axes.

**Step 8:** Check the joint angles to confirm that correction was achieved.

**Step 9:** Check the alignment to confirm that correction was achieved.

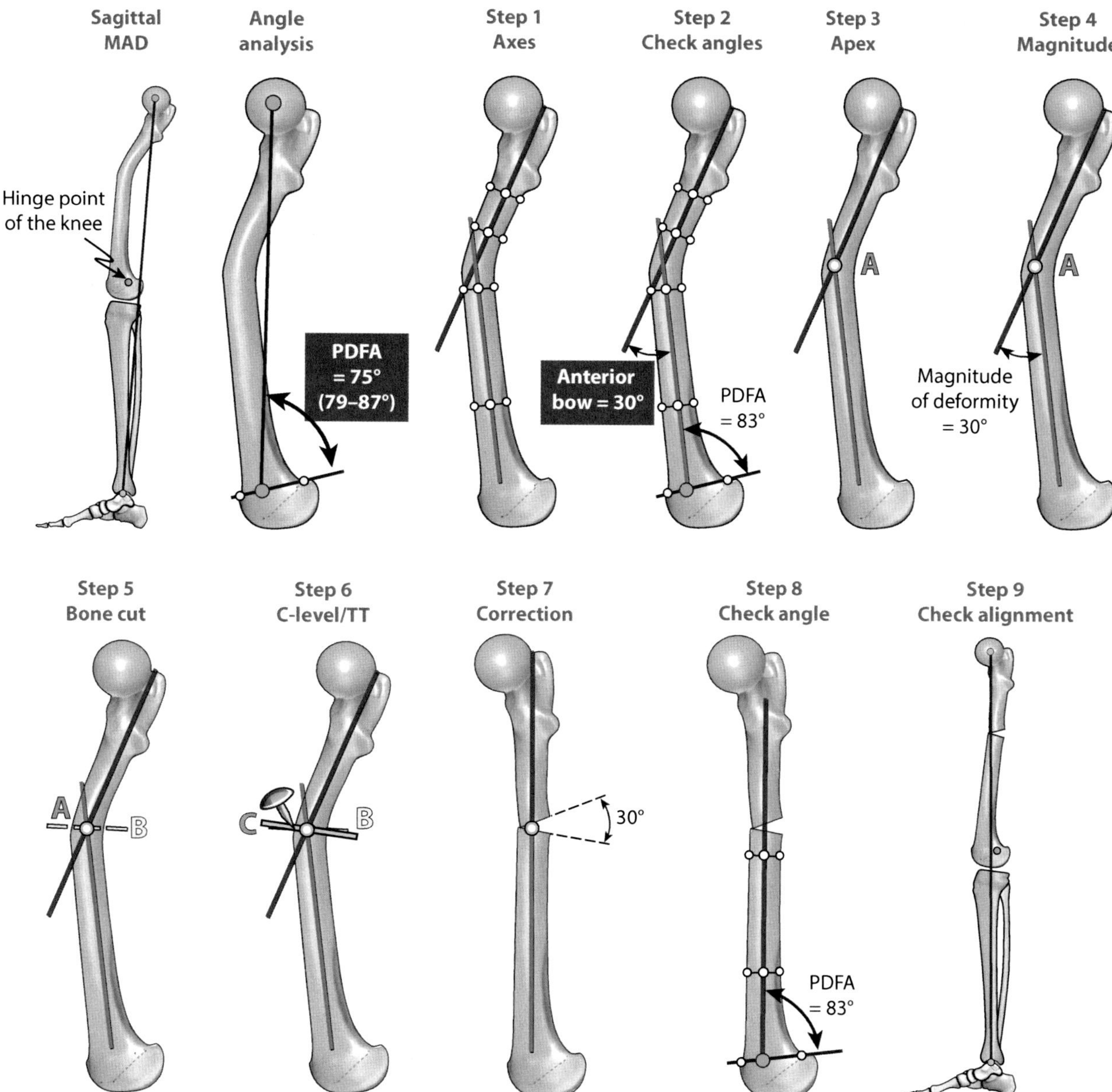


**Fig. 17:** Sagittal plane analysis of a single-level femoral diaphyseal deformity. The PDFA and mechanical axis were found to be abnormal during the MAP analysis, and comparing the SMAA to the bony deformity about the knee showed that the deformity did not have a soft-tissue component. The mid-diaphyseal lines of the proximal (*red line*) and distal (*blue line*) femur are used to determine the axes. Since mid-diaphyseal lines were used to create the axes, the bone must be examined for metaphyseal deformities. The PDFA formed by the distal axis is normal; therefore, a distal metaphyseal deformity does not exist. A proximal metaphyseal deformity was not found during clinical examination. The femoral anterior bow is abnormal. The bone cut is made at the level of the apex. The thumbtack is placed along the C-level on the convex side of the deformity. Angulating the bone segment around the thumbtack results in an opening wedge osteotomy. The axes and bony margins are completely aligned. A, apex; B, bone cut; C, C-level; TT, thumbtack.

© 2023 Sinai Hospital of Baltimore

## Sagittal Plane Axis Planning: Metaphyseal Deformity (Fig. 18)

**MAD and Angle Analysis:**

During the MAP analysis, we drew the mechanical axis and determined that it was abnormal. We also drew the modified mechanical axis of the femur and determined that the PDFA was abnormal. After comparing the SMAA to the bony deformity analysis, we determined that there was no soft-tissue component to the deformity around the knee.

**Step 1:** Draw the mid-diaphyseal line of the proximal segment (blue line) and the mid-diaphyseal line of the distal segment (red line).

**Step 2:** Since the mid-diaphyseal line was used for the proximal axis, a thorough clinical examination was performed and a proximal metaphyseal deformity/hip deformity was not found. Since the mid-diaphyseal line was used for the distal

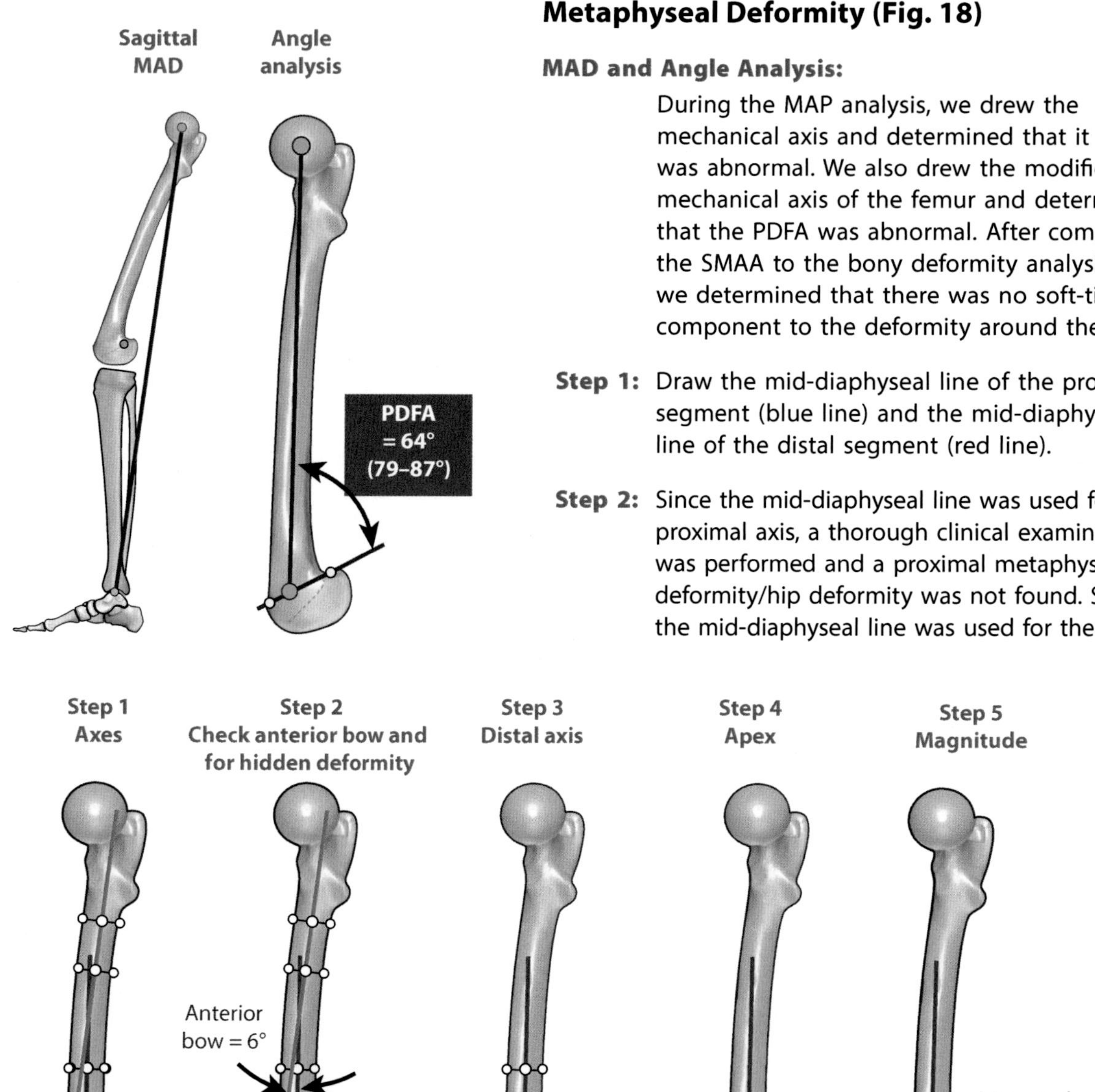


**Fig. 18:** Sagittal plane analysis of a single-level femoral metaphyseal deformity. The PDFA and mechanical axis were found to be abnormal during the MAP analysis, and comparing the SMAA to the bony deformity about the knee showed that the deformity did not have a soft-tissue component. The femur has a normal anterior bow. The mid-diaphyseal lines of the proximal and distal femur are used to determine the axes. Since mid-diaphyseal lines were used to create the axes, the bone must be examined for metaphyseal deformities. A proximal metaphyseal deformity was not found during clinical examination. The PDFA formed by the distal axis is abnormal; therefore, the femur has a distal metaphyseal deformity that needs to be identified by drawing a new distal axis. To create a new distal axis, a normal PDFA of 83° is drawn. A, apex.

axis, the PDFA formed by the distal axis (i.e., the anatomic axis of the distal bone segment) must be measured. The PDFA is abnormal; therefore, the femur has a distal metaphyseal deformity and this deformity needs to be identified. The bow of the femur also needs to be checked when analyzing a sagittal plane deformity. In this case, the anterior bow is normal (6°); therefore, the femur does not have a diaphyseal deformity.

**Step 3:** To find the metaphyseal deformity, a new distal axis must be drawn (blue line). Draw the distal joint line and create a normal PDFA (83°) starting at a point one-third the length of the joint line from the anterior cortex. The original proximal axis is not used, and the original distal axis (red line) has become the proximal axis.

**Step 4:** Mark the apex at the intersection of the proximal axis and the new distal axis.

**Step 5:** Measure the magnitude of deformity (19°).

**Step 6:** Bone Cut: The osteotomy is made proximal to the apex for anatomic consideration and to ensure that the resulting fragment is large enough for stable fixation. Since the osteotomy is not performed at the level of the apex, obligatory bony translation will occur during the correction. The amount of translation is the distance between the proximal and distal axis lines at the level of the osteotomy site.

**Step 7:** Correction (part 1): Draw the C-level. The thumbtack is placed on the apex.

**Step 8:** Correction (part 2): Angulating the bone segment around the thumbtack results in a neutral wedge osteotomy. Although complete alignment of both axes is achieved, obligatory bony translation occurs at the osteotomy site.

**Step 9:** Check the PDFA.

**Step 10:** Check the alignment to confirm that correction was achieved.

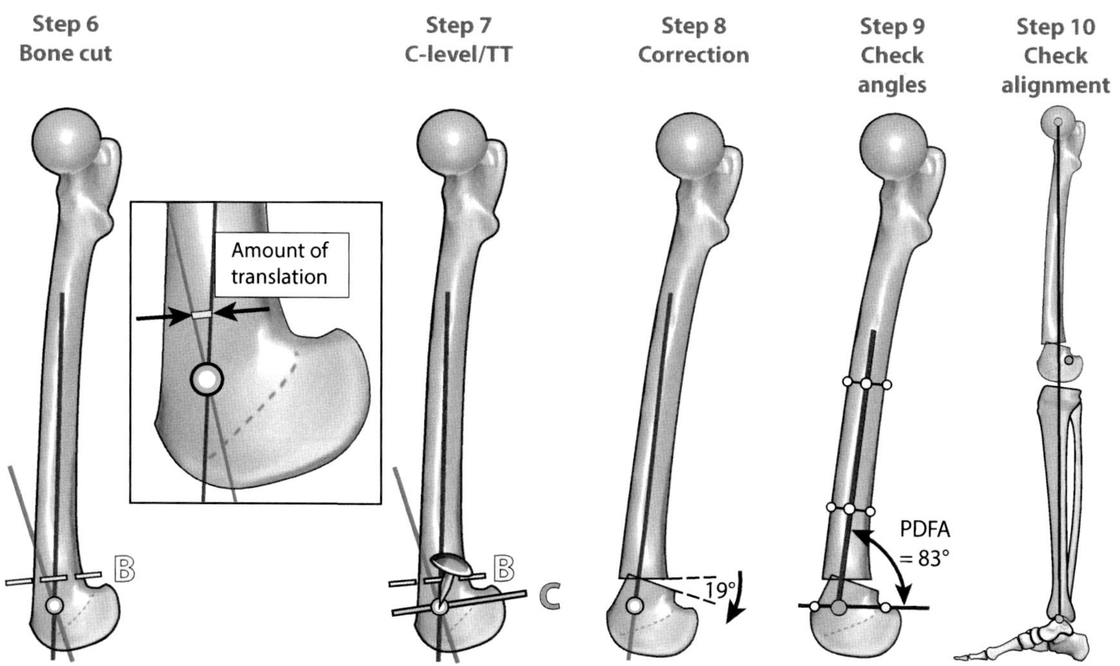


**Fig. 18 (continued):** The bone cut is made proximal to the apex, and the thumbtack is placed on the apex. Angulating the bone segment around the thumbtack results in a neutral wedge osteotomy. Complete alignment of the axes is achieved, but obligatory bony translation occurs at the osteotomy site because the osteotomy was not performed at the level of the apex. B, bone cut; C, C-level; TT, thumbtack.

© 2023 Sinai Hospital of Baltimore

## Sagittal Plane: Identifying the Axis Lines in Multiple-Level Deformities

Two strategies can be used to identify the three axis lines of a multiple-level deformity:

### Sagittal Plane Multiple-Level Deformity–Strategy 1 (Fig. 19):

Draw the mid-diaphyseal lines of the proximal segment (red line) and distal segment (blue line). Since a proximal mid-diaphyseal line was used, a thorough clinical examination should be performed to determine if a proximal metaphyseal deformity/hip deformity exists. In this example, there is no proximal deformity. Since a distal mid-diaphyseal line was used, the PDFA formed by the distal axis must be measured. The PDFA in this example is abnormal, which means that there is a distal metaphyseal deformity.

Because there is a distal metaphyseal deformity, the third axis is drawn by creating a normal PDFA starting at a point one-third of the length of the joint line from the anterior cortex. This line becomes the new distal axis (third axis).

### Sagittal Plane Multiple-Level Deformity–Strategy 2 (Fig. 19):

Draw the mid-diaphyseal lines of the proximal segment (red line) and distal segment (blue line). Since a proximal mid-diaphyseal line was used, a thorough clinical examination should be performed to determine if a proximal metaphyseal deformity/hip deformity exists. In this example, there is no proximal deformity. Since a distal mid-diaphyseal line was used, the PDFA formed by the distal axis must be measured. The PDFA in this example is normal. To create the third axis, draw the axis of the middle segment (best fit line).

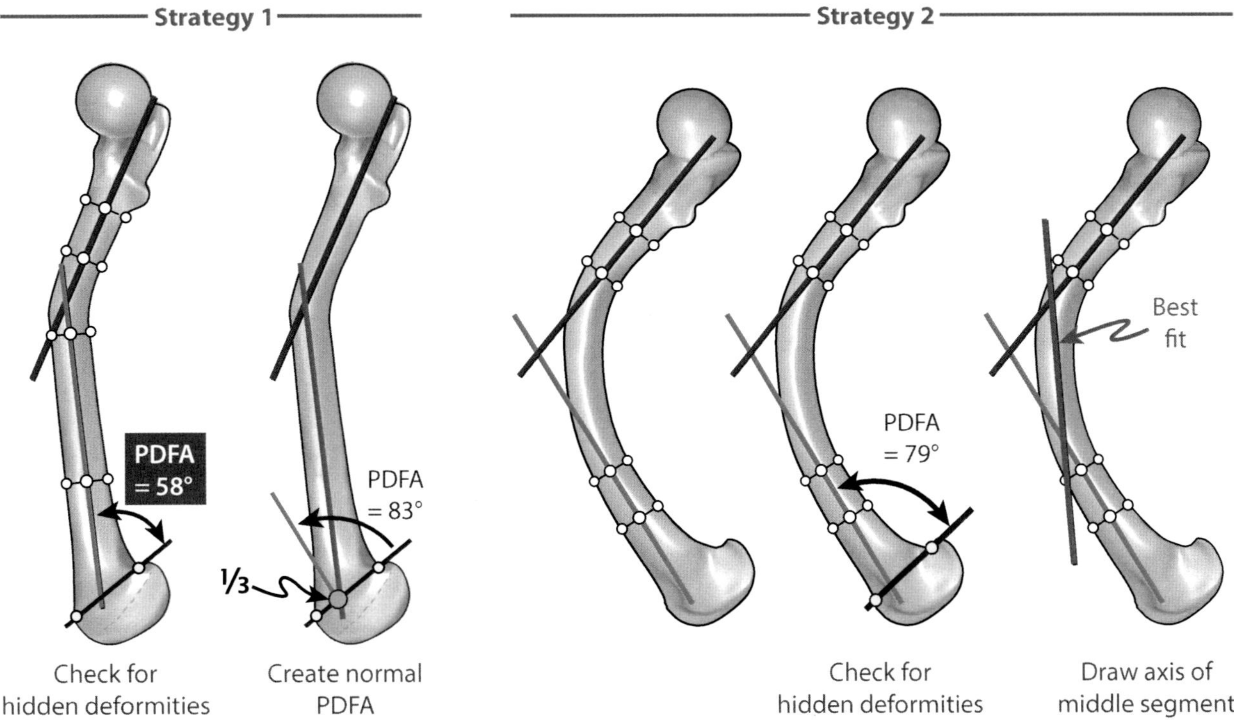


**Fig. 19:** Two strategies can be used to identify the three axis lines of a multiple-level deformity in the sagittal plane. **Strategy 1:** Draw the mid-diaphyseal lines of the proximal and distal segments. If the PDFA is abnormal, use the distal joint line to create a normal PDFA (normal range, 79–87°). This line becomes the new distal axis (third axis). **Strategy 2:** Draw the mid-diaphyseal lines of the proximal and distal segments. If the PDFA is normal, draw the axis of the middle segment (best fit line).

© 2023 Sinai Hospital of Baltimore

## Sagittal Plane Axis Planning: Multiple-Level Deformity (Fig. 20)

**MAD and Angle Analysis:**

During the MAP analysis, we drew the mechanical axis and determined that it was normal. We also drew the modified mechanical axis of the femur and determined that the PDFA was abnormal. After comparing the SMAA to the bony deformity analysis, we determined that there was no soft-tissue component to the deformity around the knee.

**Step 1:** Draw the mid-diaphyseal line of the proximal segment (red line) and the mid-diaphyseal line of the distal segment (blue line).

**Step 2:** Since the mid-diaphyseal line was used for the proximal axis, a thorough clinical examination was performed and a proximal metaphyseal deformity/hip deformity was not found. Since the mid-diaphyseal line was used for the distal axis, the PDFA formed by the distal axis (i.e., the anatomic axis of the distal bone segment) must be measured. The PDFA is abnormal; therefore, the femur has a distal metaphyseal deformity and this deformity needs to be identified. The bow of the femur also needs to be checked when analyzing a sagittal plane deformity. In this case, the posterior femoral bow is abnormal (13° recurvatum). This means that femur

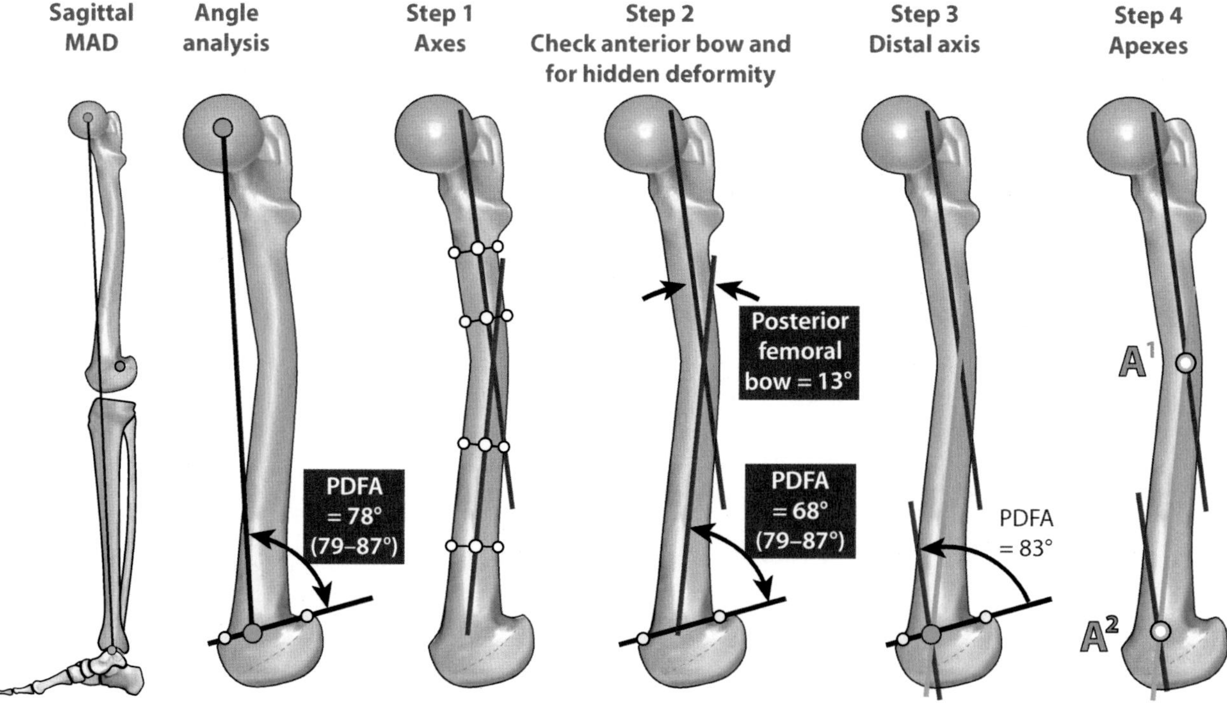


**Fig. 20:** Sagittal plane analysis of a multiple-level femoral deformity. The mechanical axis was normal, and the PDFA was found to be abnormal during the MAP analysis. Comparing the SMAA to the bony deformity about the knee showed that the deformity did not have a soft-tissue component. The mid-diaphyseal lines of the proximal and distal femur were used to determine the axes. Since mid-diaphyseal lines were used to create the axes, the bone must be examined for metaphyseal deformities. A proximal metaphyseal deformity was not found during clinical examination. The PDFA formed by the distal axis is abnormal; therefore, the femur has a distal metaphyseal deformity that needs to be identified by drawing a new distal axis. The posterior femoral bow is abnormal, which means that the bone has a diaphyseal deformity as well. Apexes will need to be identified in the diaphysis and metaphysis. The original distal axis will become the axis of the middle segment (*green line*). A normal PDFA is used to create a new distal axis (*blue line*). The apexes are identified where the proximal and middle axis lines intersect and where the middle and distal axis lines intersect. A, apex.

has a diaphyseal deformity as well as a metaphyseal deformity.

**Step 3:** The original distal axis will become the axis of the middle segment (green line). To find the metaphyseal deformity, a new distal axis must be drawn. Draw the distal joint line and create a normal PDFA (83°) starting at a point one-third the length of the joint line from the anterior cortex. This is the new distal axis (blue line).

**Step 4:** Mark Apex[1] at the intersection of the proximal and middle axis lines. Mark Apex[2] at the intersection of the middle and distal axis lines.

**Step 5:** Measure the magnitude of the proximal (14°) and distal (15°) deformity.

**Step 6:** Bone Cuts: Place the osteotomies as close to each apex as possible. An osteotomy is performed at the level of Apex[1] and proximal to Apex[2]. Since the osteotomy is not performed at the level of Apex[2], obligatory bony translation will occur during the correction. The amount of translation is the distance between the proximal and distal axis lines at the level of the osteotomy site.

**Step 7:** Correction (part 1): Draw the C-levels. The proximal thumbtack is placed along the C-level on the convex side of the proximal deformity, and the distal thumbtack is placed along the C-level on the convex side of the distal deformity.

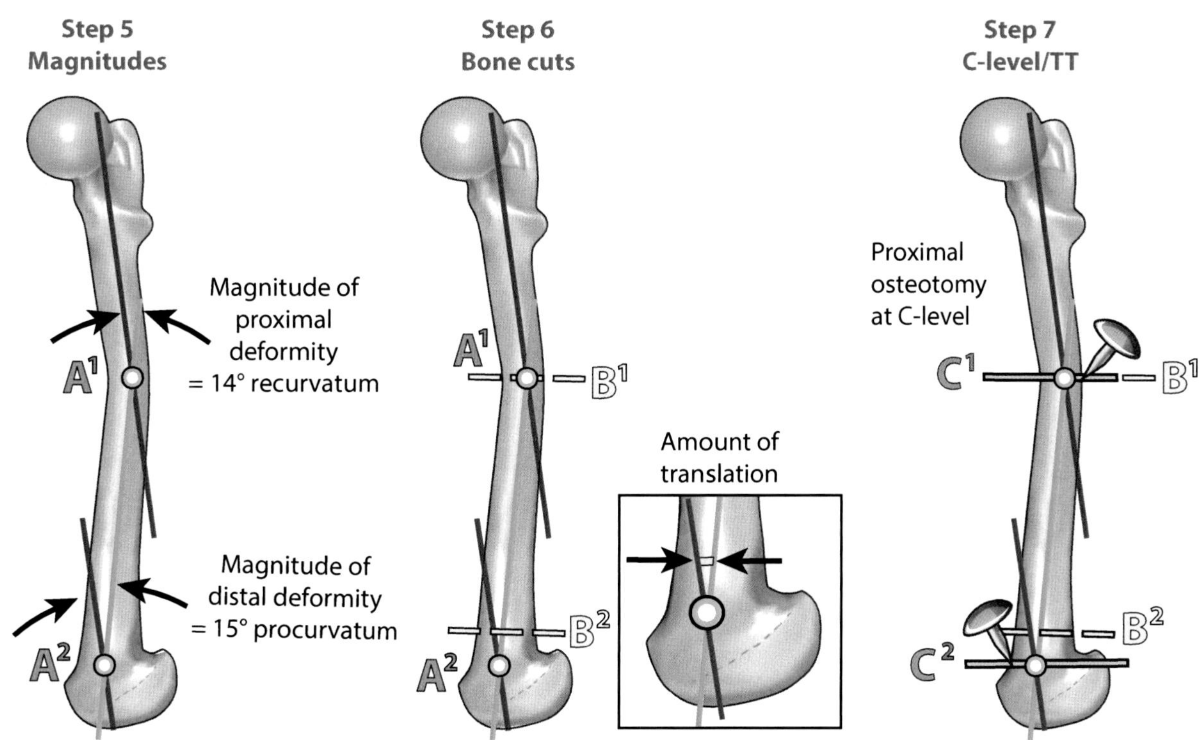


**Fig. 20 (continued):** The proximal bone cut is made at the level of Apex[1], and the distal bone cut is made proximal to Apex[2]. The proximal and distal thumbtacks are placed along the C-levels on the convex side of the deformities. A, apex; B, bone cut; C, C-level; TT, thumbtack.

© 2023 Sinai Hospital of Baltimore

**Step 8:** Correction (part 2): Angulating the bone segments around the thumbtacks results in two opening wedge osteotomies with complete alignment of the axes. Bony translation occurs at the distal osteotomy site since the osteotomy was proximal to the apex.

**Step 9:** Check the PDFA and the alignment to confirm that correction was achieved.

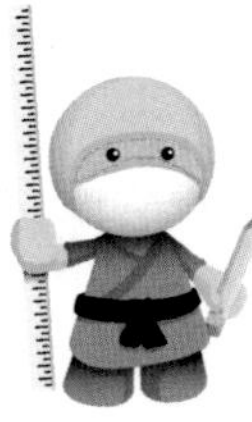

***Sensei says,***

*"Similar to the frontal plane, if the bony deformity is obvious, then the apex of the deformity should correlate with this level. If the apex is not associated with the obvious deformity, then a more complex deformity is present. The surgeon must understand this warning sign and investigate the possibility of a second, hidden angular or translational deformity in the same bone segment."*

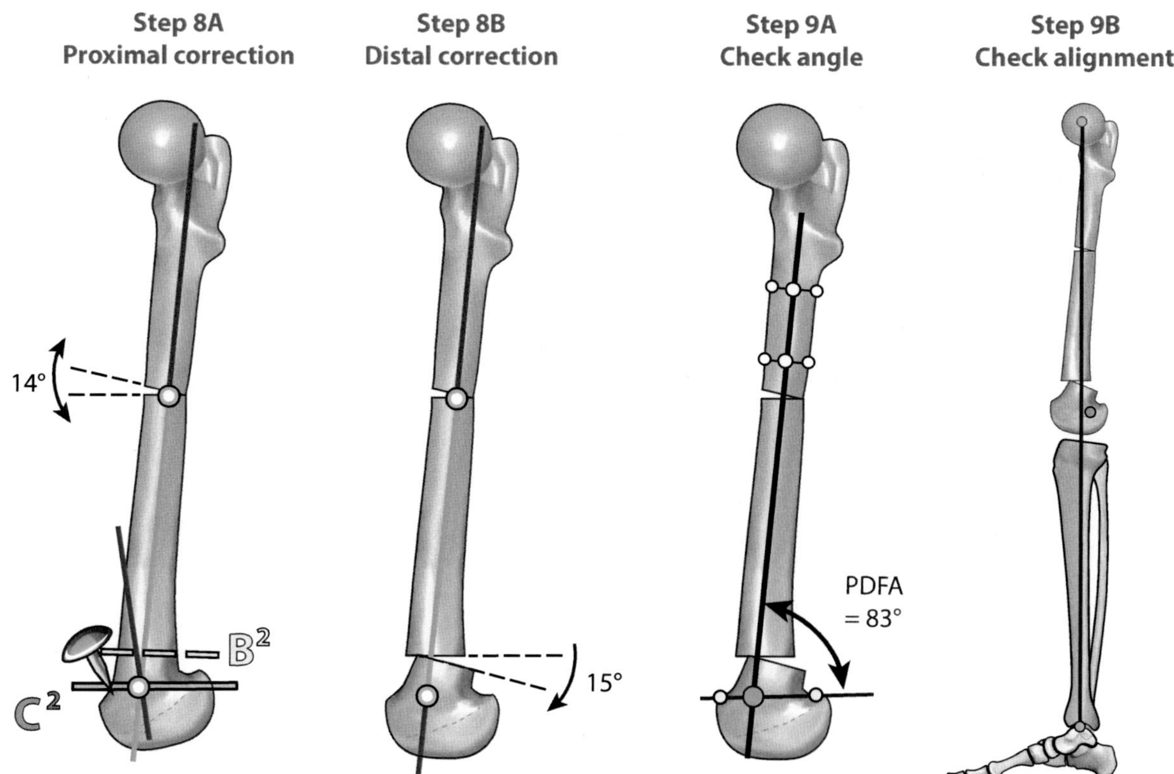


**Fig. 20 (continued):** Angulating the bone segments around the thumbtacks results in two opening wedge osteotomies. Complete alignment is achieved, but bony translation occurs at the distal osteotomy site because the osteotomy was not performed at the level of the apex. B, bone cut; C, C-level.

# Chapter 10

# Deformity Analysis in the Oblique Plane

Janet D. Conway, MD
Shawn C. Standard, MD
Philip K. McClure, MD

A limb has an oblique plane deformity if abnormalities are noted on both the AP and lateral view x-rays. Posttraumatic and congenital deformities often have deformities in both the frontal and lateral planes. For example, a tibial malunion may have both procurvatum and varus deformities. The bone does not really have two separate deformities; it has only one deformity. The deformity or bend lies in a plane that is neither frontal nor sagittal. Thus, the correct description is a deformity in the oblique plane. Standard x-rays (true AP and true lateral views) are orthogonal to each limb segment, but they are not orthogonal to the deformity. Since the standard x-rays do not delineate the true deformity or the plane of the deformity, a method must be used to analyze the oblique plane deformity.

In the classic method of Ilizarov, a deformity in the oblique plane needs to be "resolved" or analyzed to determine the exact plane of the deformity. After the plane of deformity is defined, the placement of mechanical hinges can be determined to create a hinge axis orthogonal to the plane of deformity. This will allow complete correction of the oblique plane deformity.

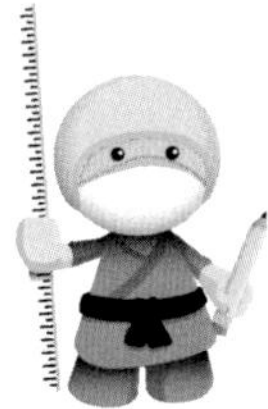

*Sensei says,*
*"Oblique plane deformities can be visualized as two separate deformities on the AP and lateral view x-rays, but the deformity is really made up of one bend in the bone."*

The easiest way to understand how to analyze an oblique plane deformity is to start with an example of how a deformity can be analyzed intraoperatively using fluoroscopy. Figure 1 shows a tibia with 17° varus (Fig. 1A) and 15° procurvatum (Fig. 1B). Start with the patient positioned supine on a radiolucent table and the limb positioned patella facing up (perpendicular to the table) (Fig. 2A). The

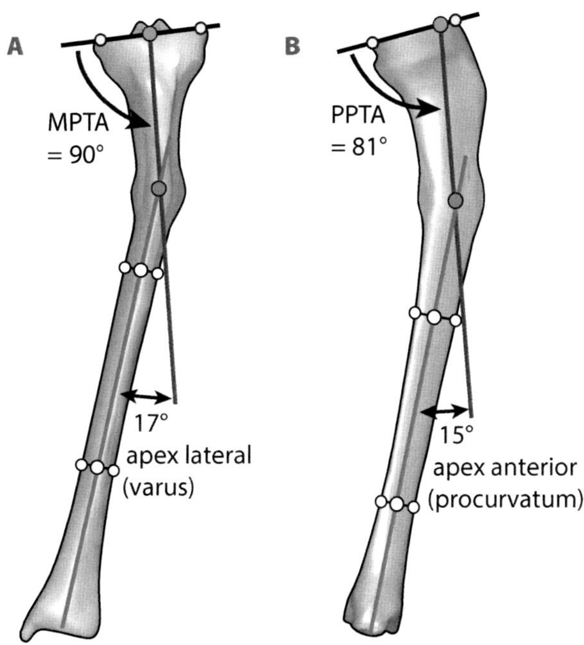


**Fig. 1:** Oblique plane deformity in the tibia. This tibia has 17° of varus (**A**) and 15° of procurvatum (**B**).

© 2023 Sinai Hospital of Baltimore

x-ray tube is positioned directly above the limb (x-ray tube in an AP position) (Figs. 2A and 2B). To analyze an oblique plane deformity, first we need to find the zero deformity plane. The zero deformity plane image is the x-ray where no deformity is seen. To obtain the zero deformity plane image, the limb should be rotated while being observed under fluoroscopy (Fig. 2C) until the bone segment appears perfectly straight and no deformity can be seen in the fluoroscopic view (Fig. 2D). In this example, when we have the x-ray tube in a AP view position and internally rotate the tibia, we are able to obtain the zero deformity plane image. The next goal is to determine the maximum deformity plane in which the maximum angulation of the deformity (i.e., magnitude of the deformity) can be seen. To obtain the maximum deformity plane image, the bone is held in the same position that was used for the zero deformity plane image (Fig. 2E). Then the x-ray tube is moved so that it is positioned 90° from

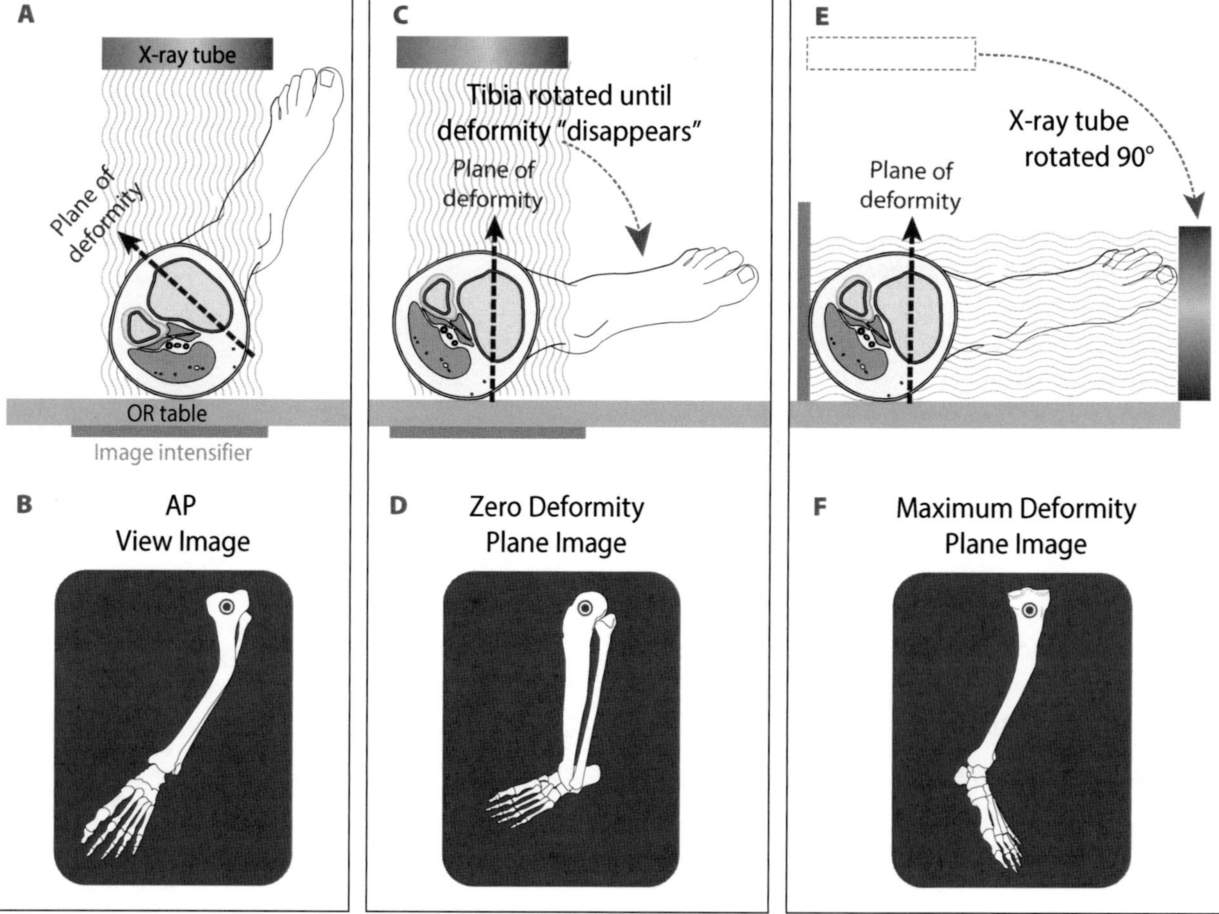


**Fig. 2:** Approach to analyze an oblique plane deformity intraoperatively using fluoroscopy with the x-ray tube positioned directly above the limb (x-ray tube in an AP position). **A**, The limb is positioned patella facing up on a radiolucent table. The x-ray tube is positioned directly above the limb (x-ray tube in an AP position). **B**, AP view image that is obtained when the limb and x-ray tube are positioned as shown in panel A. **C**, To obtain the zero deformity plane image, the limb is rotated while being observed under fluoroscopy until no deformity can be seen in the fluoroscopic view. In this example, the limb is rotated internally. **D**, Zero deformity plane image that is obtained when the bone is rotated until no deformity can be observed. **E**, To obtain the maximum deformity plane image, the bone is held in the same position that was used for the zero deformity plane image and the x-ray tube is moved so that it is positioned 90° from the zero deformity plane (orthogonal to the plane of deformity). In this case, the x-ray tube moves from an AP position to a lateral position. **F**, Maximum deformity image shows magnitude of the oblique plane deformity.

the zero deformity plane (orthogonal to the plane of deformity). To obtain the maximum deformity plane image in this example, hold the limb stable and swing the x-ray tube 90° to a lateral position (Fig. 2E). The image obtained is the maximum deformity plane image and allows the apex of the deformity to be visualized (Fig. 2F).

In Figure 2, we started with the x-ray tube positioned directly above the limb (x-ray tube in an AP position). Alternatively, we could have started with the x-ray tube positioned medial to the limb (x-ray tube in a lateral position) (Fig. 3A) so that a lateral view image is obtained first (Fig. 3B). To obtain the zero deformity plane image in this example, we externally rotate the tibia (Fig. 3C) until the tibia does not appear to have any deformity (Fig. 3D). Next, the maximum deformity plane image should be obtained by moving the x-ray tube so that it is positioned 90° from the zero deformity

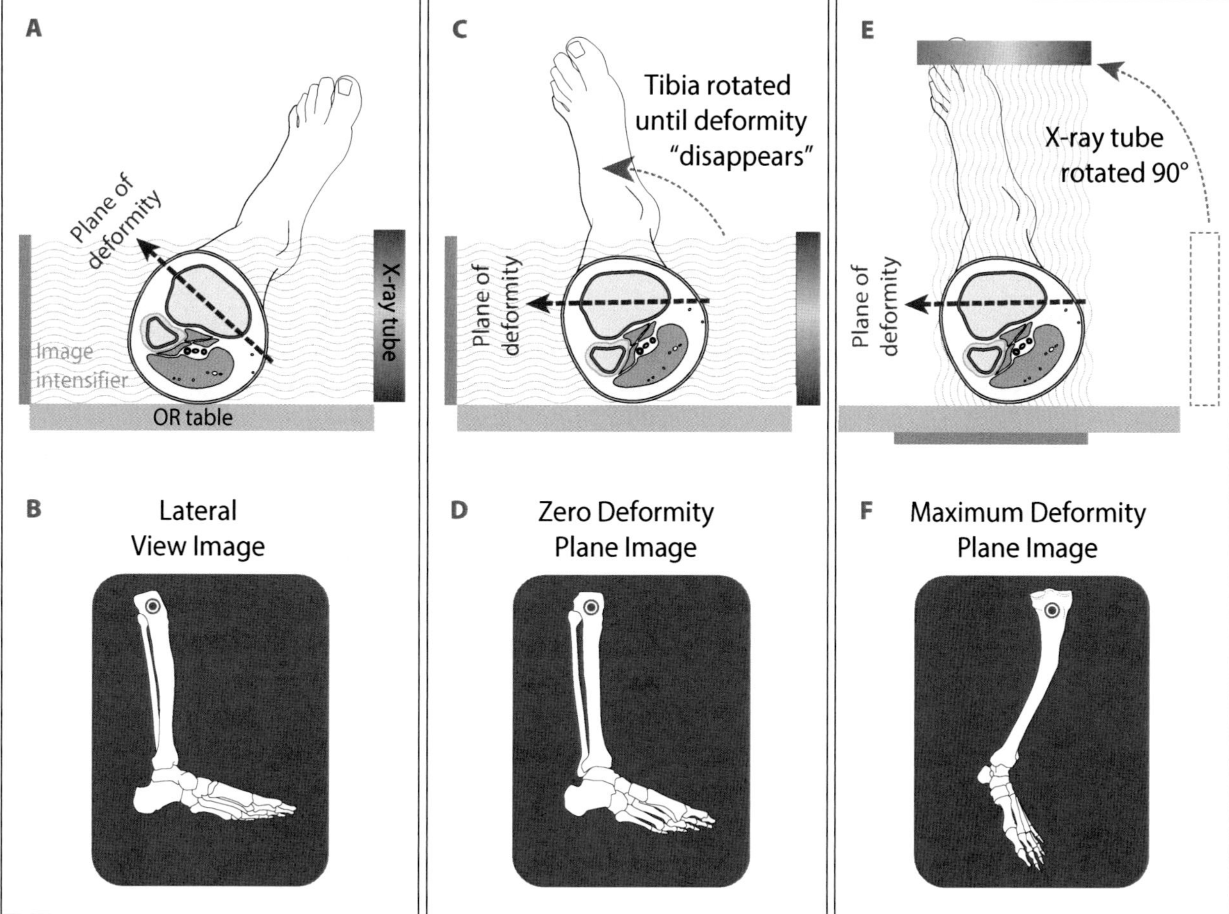


**Fig. 3:** Approach to analyze an oblique plane deformity intraoperatively using fluoroscopy with the x-ray tube positioned medial to the limb (x-ray tube in a lateral position). **A**, The limb is positioned patella facing up on a radiolucent table. The x-ray tube is positioned medial to the limb (x-ray tube in a lateral position). **B**, Lateral view image that is obtained when the limb and x-ray tube are positioned as shown in panel A. **C**, To obtain the zero deformity plane image, the limb is rotated while being observed under fluoroscopy until no deformity can be seen in the fluoroscopic view. In this example, the limb is rotated externally. **D**, Zero deformity plane image that is obtained when the bone is rotated until no deformity can be observed. **E**, To obtain the maximum deformity plane image, the bone is held in the same position that was used for the zero deformity plane image and the x-ray tube is moved so that it is positioned 90° from the zero deformity plane (orthogonal to the plane of deformity). In this case, the x-ray tube moves from a lateral position to an AP position. **F**, Maximum deformity image shows magnitude of the oblique plane deformity.

© 2023 Sinai Hospital of Baltimore

plane (orthogonal to the plane of deformity) but the limb remains in the same position that was used to obtain the zero deformity plane image. In Figure 3C, the x-ray tube is in a lateral view position to obtain the zero deformity plane image. To obtain the maximum deformity plane image, the x-ray tube is moved 90° so that it is in the AP view position (Fig. 3E). Note that the maximum deformity plane image obtained in Figure 3F matches the one obtained in Figure 2F, even though the initial position of the x-ray tube was different (Fig. 2A vs. 3A) and the limb was rotated differently (internal versus external) (Fig. 2C vs. 3C) to obtain the zero deformity plane image.

After the zero deformity plane image and maximum deformity plane image have been obtained, the magnitude of the deformity (22°) is measured on the maximum deformity image (Fig. 4) and the level of the apex is marked on the skin (Fig. 5A). A circular external fixator can now be applied by placing the hinge axis 90° (orthogonal) to the zero deformity plane at the level of the apex. In the lateral view (90° to the zero deformity plane), the hinges are positioned at the level of the cortex on the convex side of the deformity to achieve an opening wedge osteotomy with lengthening (Fig. 5B). When placed correctly, the hinges should be overlapped in the maximum deformity image (Fig. 5C). Alternatively, the hinges can be placed to achieve a neutral wedge (Fig. 5D) or closing wedge osteotomy (Fig. 5E).

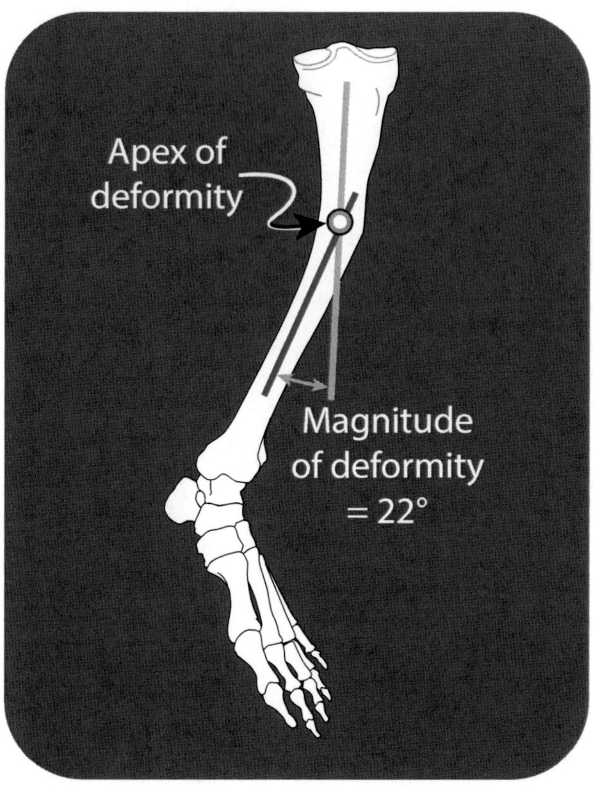


**Fig. 4:** The magnitude of the oblique plane deformity is measured on the maximum deformity image.

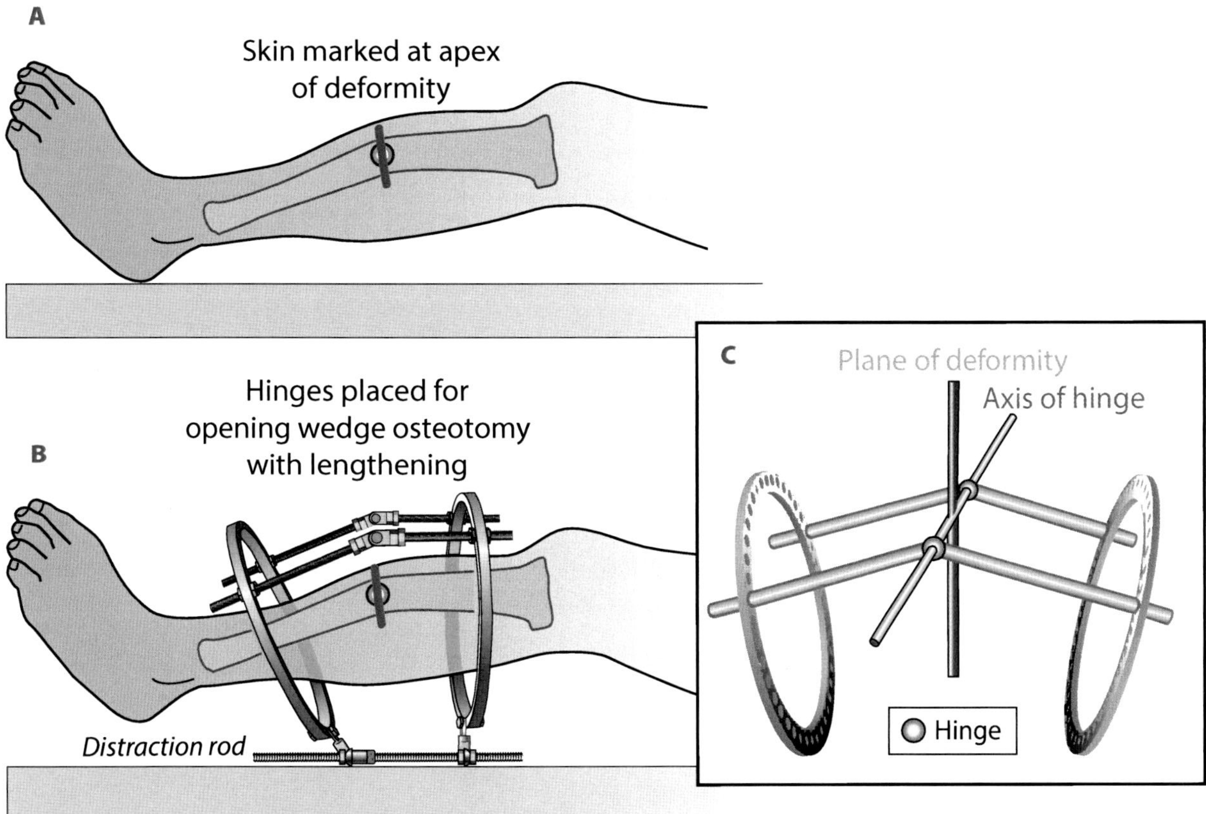


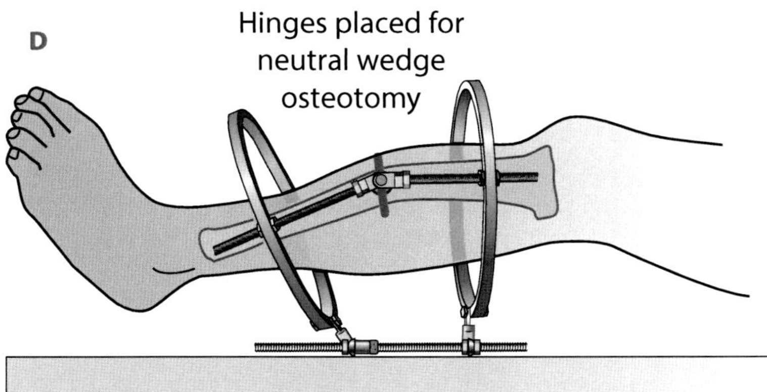


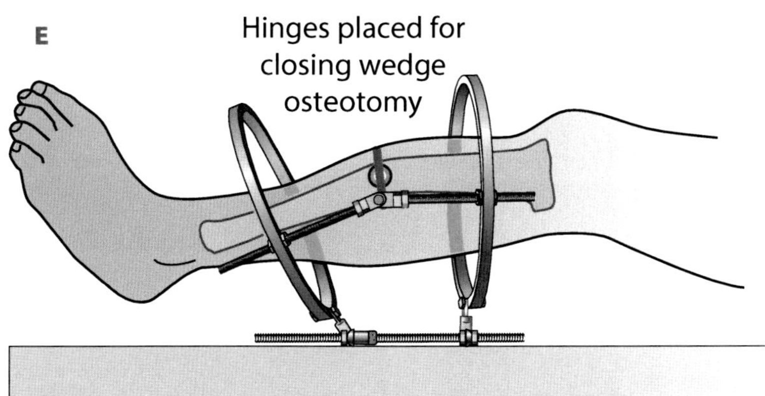


**Fig. 5: A**, Level of the apex is marked on the skin (*purple line*). **B**, Placement of hinges for opening wedge osteotomy with lengthening. **C**, Detailed view of the placement of hinges for an opening wedge osteotomy. **D**, Placement of hinges for neutral wedge osteotomy. **E**, Placement of hinges for closing wedge osteotomy.

© 2023 Sinai Hospital of Baltimore

Although a surgeon could choose to use only the fluoroscopic method/intra-operative frame assembly method that is described above to analyze an oblique plane deformity, we recommend that most surgeons also analyze the deformity using the graphic method prior to performing surgery. The graphic method allows the surgeon to simplify the three-dimensional oblique plane deformity by converting it into a schematic. The graphic method is based on the premise that any value with magnitude and direction can be considered a vector and can be represented with a simple graph. It is accurate to within 4° with clinical deformities that are less than 45°. To perform the graphic method, you will need to know the magnitude of deformity on the AP and lateral view x-rays. To demonstrate the method, the deformity shown in Figures 1 through 5 will be analyzed.

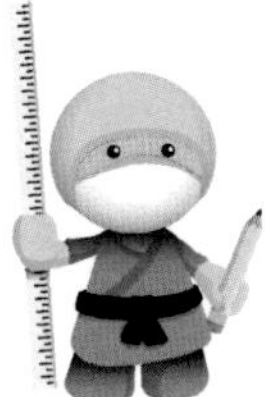

*Sensei says,*

*"For oblique plane deformities, look at your own foot and use the graphic method to determine the plane of the one bend in the bone."*

**Step 1:** Draw a schematic foot (left or right) of the limb that has the deformity. The foot should be drawn as it would appear if you were looking down at your own foot (bird's eye view) (Fig. 6, Step 1).

**Step 2:** Draw x- and y-axes centered on the foot. Designate the anterior, posterior, medial, and lateral sides of the x- and y-axes (Fig. 6, Step 2).

**Step 3:** Draw a vector along the x-axis that represents the tibial deformity in the AP view. Figure 1A showed a 17° varus deformity with the apex of the deformity pointing lateral. Draw a 17-mm line (1° = 1 mm) along the x-axis that points lateral (Fig. 6, Step 3).

**Step 4:** Draw a vector along the y-axis that represents the tibial deformity in the lateral view. Figure 1B shows a 15° procurvatum deformity with the apex pointing anterior. Draw a 15-mm line along the y-axis that points anterior (Fig. 6, Step 4).

**Step 5:** Summate the two vectors to determine the direction of the oblique plane deformity (Fig. 6, Step 5). This new vector is the plane of the deformity. In this case, the oblique plane deformity has an apex that is directed in an anterolateral direction. The direction of the deformity is the summated vector that extends from the apex.

**Step 6:** Measure the length of the summated vector to determine the magnitude of the oblique plane deformity (1 mm = 1°). The summated vector measures 23 mm, which equals a 23° deformity (Fig. 6, Step 6).

**Step 7:** Determine the exact position of the oblique plane deformity by measuring the angle between the summated vector and the x- or y-axis (Fig. 6, Step 7A). This measurement shows that the oblique plane deformity points in an anterolateral direction 41° from the coronal plane (x-axis) or 49° from the sagittal plane (y-axis) (Fig. 6, Step 7B). With a patient supine on the operating room table, the deformity lies 41° from the horizon or horizontal plane or 49° from the vertical plane.

The direction of the hinge axis and the Ilizarov hinge placement can now be determined. The hinge axis is placed perpendicular to the plane of deformity (Fig. 7A). An Ilizarov ring is superimposed on the graph to determine the hole placement for the hinges to create an oblique plane correction (Fig. 7B and 7C). The hinges can be placed to create an opening, closing, or neutral wedge osteotomy. (Fig. 7D).

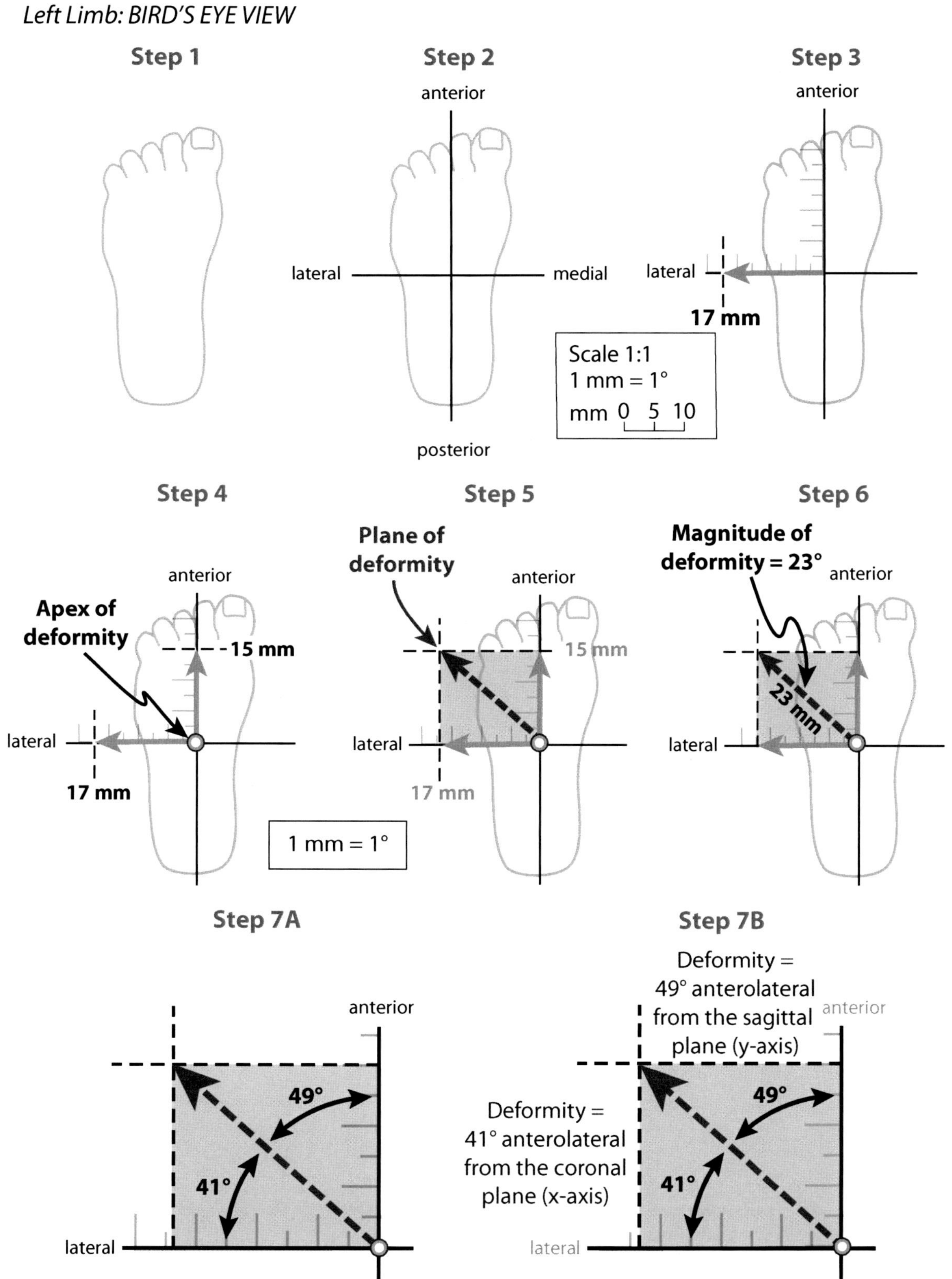


**Fig. 6:** Graphic method is used to analyze the same oblique plane deformity that is shown in Figures 1 through 5. Typically, when you use the graphic method, 1 mm is equal to 1 degree.

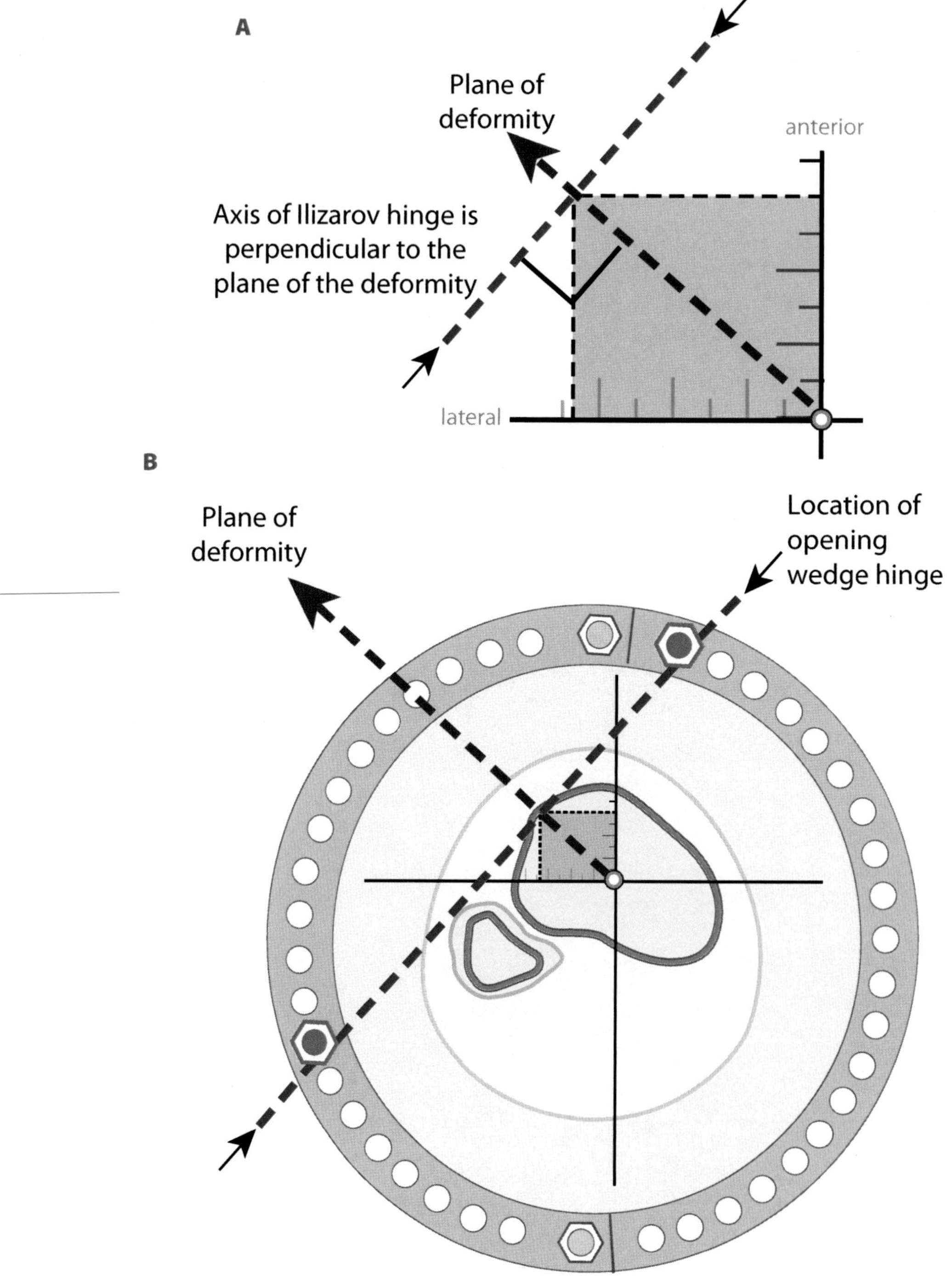


**Fig. 7:** The graphic method can be used to determine hinge placement. **A**, On the graph, the axis of the Ilizarov hinge should be perpendicular to the plane of deformity. **B**, Location of hinge in relation to the ring for an opening wedge osteotomy.

C

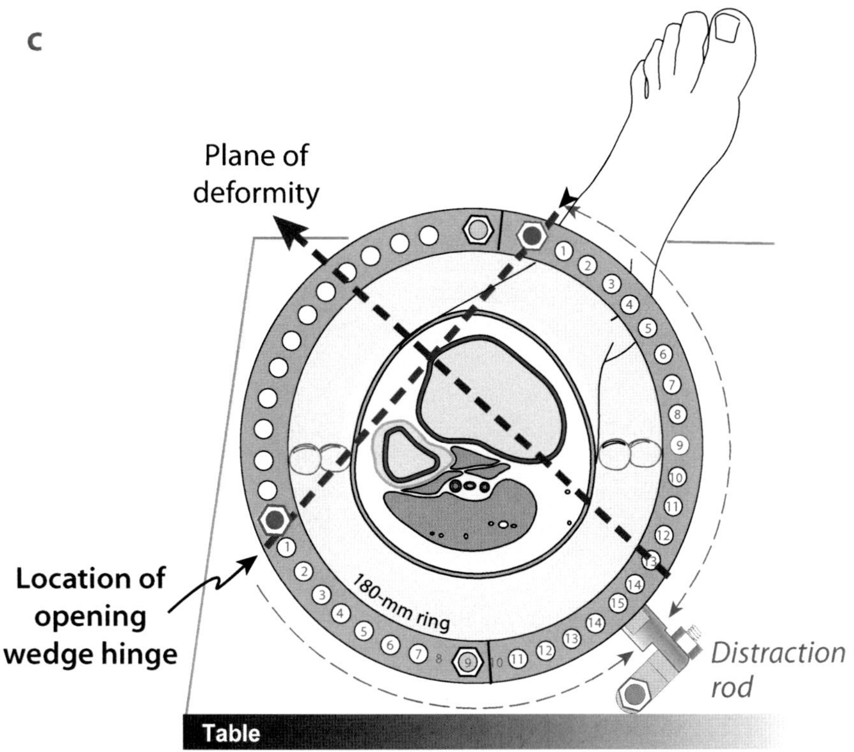


D

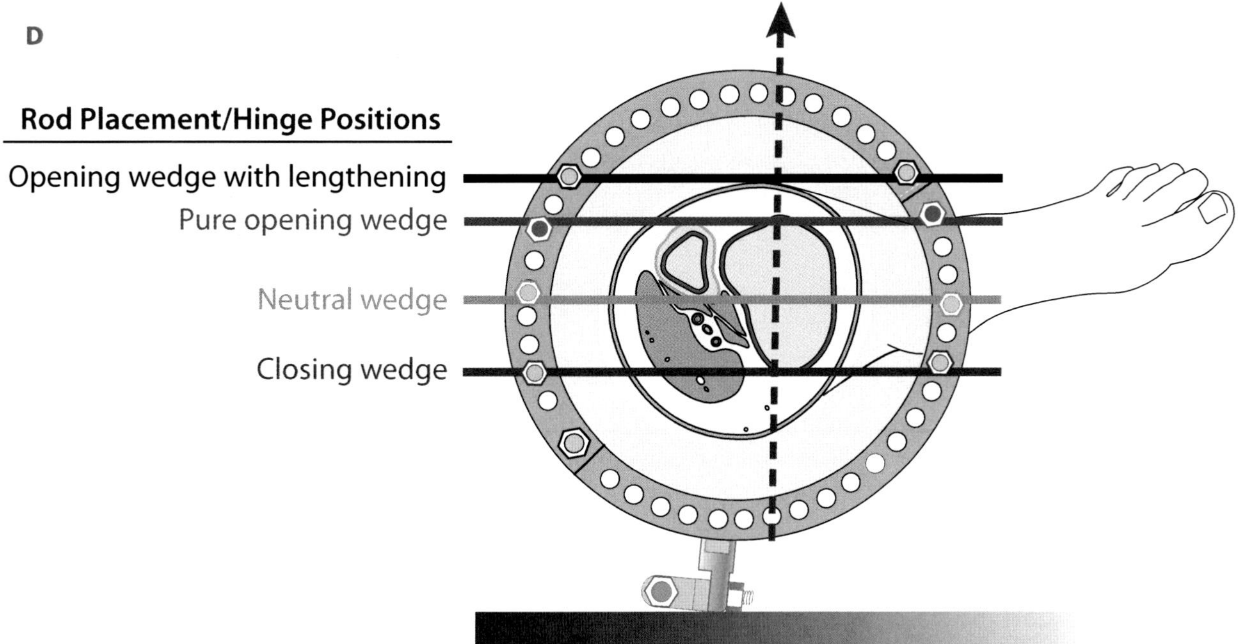


**Fig. 7 (continued): C**, Placement of ring, distraction rod, and hinge for pure opening wedge osteotomy. **D**, Rod and hinge placement for opening wedge with lengthening, pure opening wedge, neutral wedge, and closing wedge osteotomies.

© 2023 Sinai Hospital of Baltimore

To better understand the oblique plane, let's examine two x-ray examples. Figure 8 shows a patient who has proximal tibial procurvatum and a valgus deformity. For the MAP analysis, the first step is to perform the "M" step, which consists of measuring the MAD (4.8 cm lateral) (Fig. 8A). The next step is the "A" of the MAP analysis, which is to analyze the frontal and sagittal plane joint angles (Figs. 8B and 8C). The tibia is in valgus with an MPTA of 105° and procurvatum with a PPTA of 64°. The 24° SJLA is used to determine the 8° hyperextension soft-tissue contribution (Fig. 8D). For "P" (pick the bone), the tibia is selected for correction.

Next, the ABC analysis is performed. To perform the "A" step (finding the apex), the proximal and distal axis lines are drawn on the AP and lateral view x-rays (Figs. 8E and 8F). The apex is located at the intersection of the proximal and distal axis lines. The apex is close to the level of the joint on the lateral view but is slightly more distal on the AP view. This denotes the presence of the mild residual translational deformity, commonly seen in malunited fractures. For "B", the bone cut was planned in the metaphyseal bone with enough bone in the proximal fragment to allow for adequate fixation (Figs. 8G and 8H). For the "C" step, the correction is planned by drawing the C-levels and placing a thumbtack along each C-level on the convex side of the deformity on both the AP and lateral view x-rays (Figs. 8G and 8H). The C-level on the AP and lateral views works when using a device such as a Taylor Spatial Frame (Smith & Nephew, Memphis, TN), a Multi-Axial Correction (MAC) Fixation System (Biomet, Warsaw, IN), or a TL-HEX (Orthofix, Lewisville, TX). However, the hinge placement on the C-level should be determined with the graphic method when using a hinged external fixator such as an Ilizarov or TrueLok (Orthofix, Inc., Lewisville, TX). When the graphic method is used to analyze this deformity using the values obtained in Figures 8E and 8F, the magnitude of the deformity is determined to be 22° with the deformity 44° anteromedial from the frontal plane (Fig. 8I).

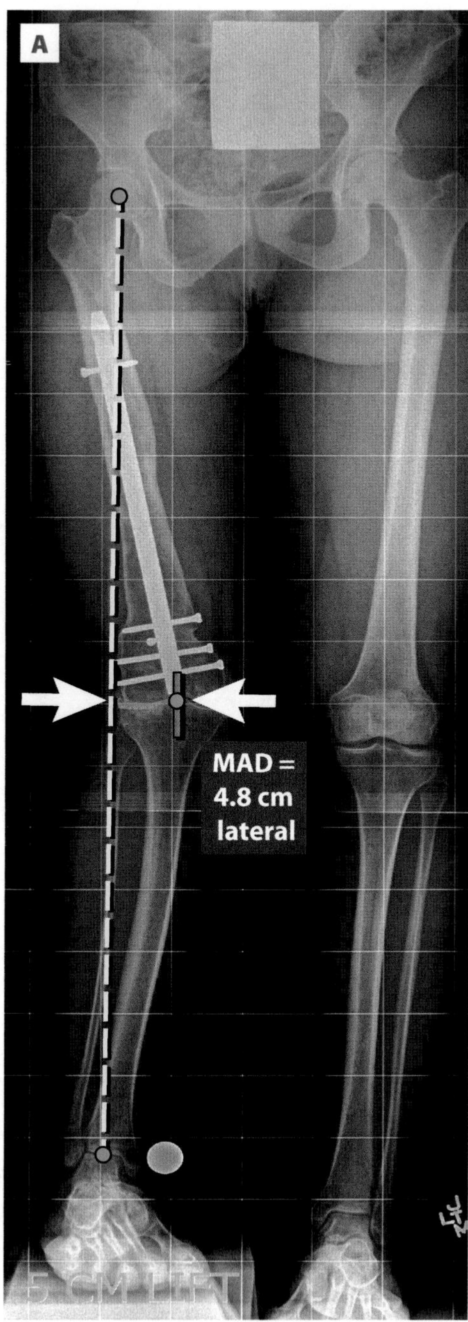


**Fig. 8:** Patient with congenital femoral deficiency status post femoral deformity correction and lengthening. **A**, Full length standing AP view x-ray shows the limb has 4.8 cm of lateral MAD.

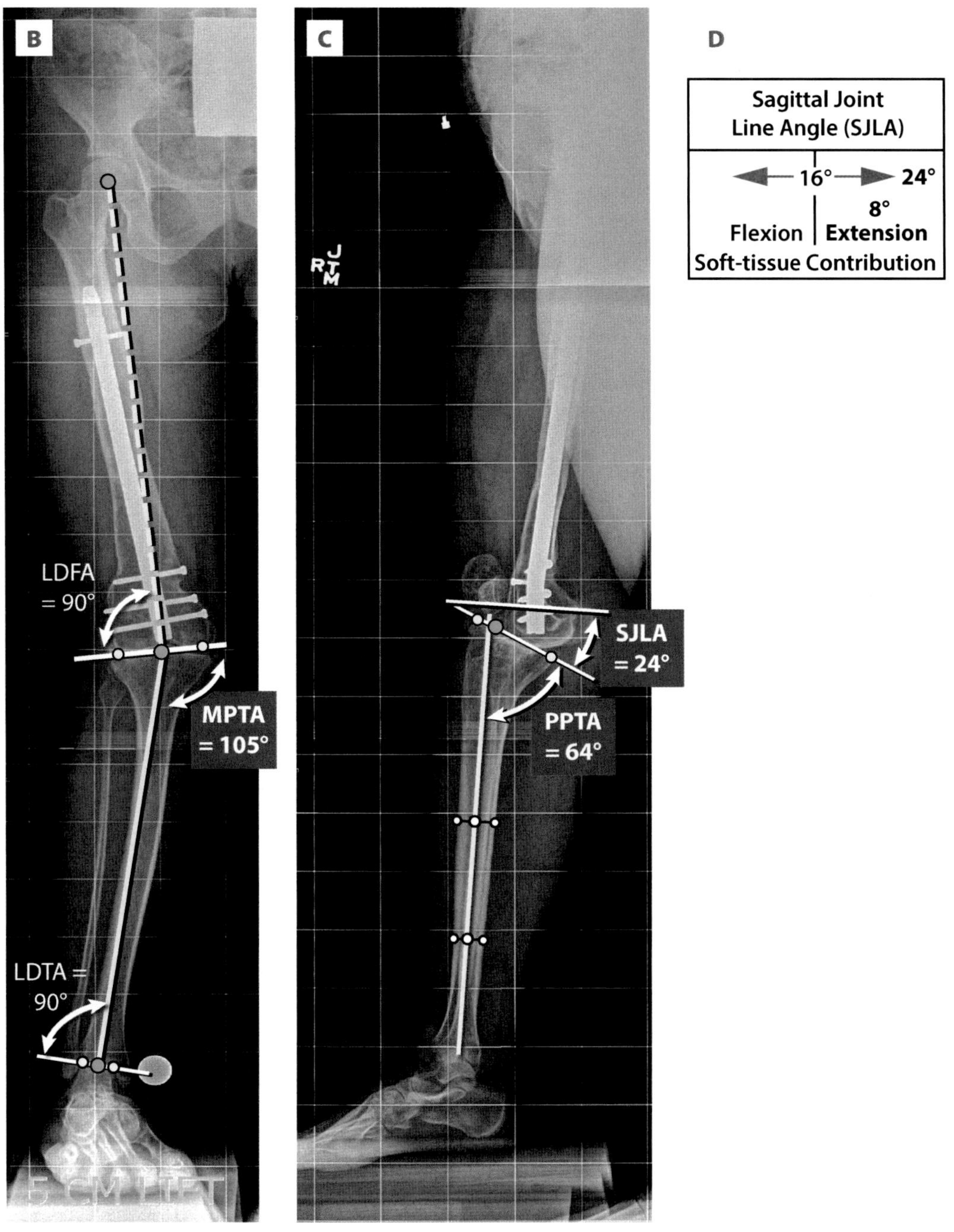


**Fig. 8 (continued): B**, Initial AP view x-ray shows the MPTA is 105° (normal range, 85–90°). **C**, Initial lateral view x-ray shows the PPTA is 64° (normal range, 77–84°) and the sagittal joint line angle (SJLA) is 24° (normal 16°). **D**, SJLA is used to determine that the soft-tissue contribution is 8° of hyperextension.

© 2023 Sinai Hospital of Baltimore

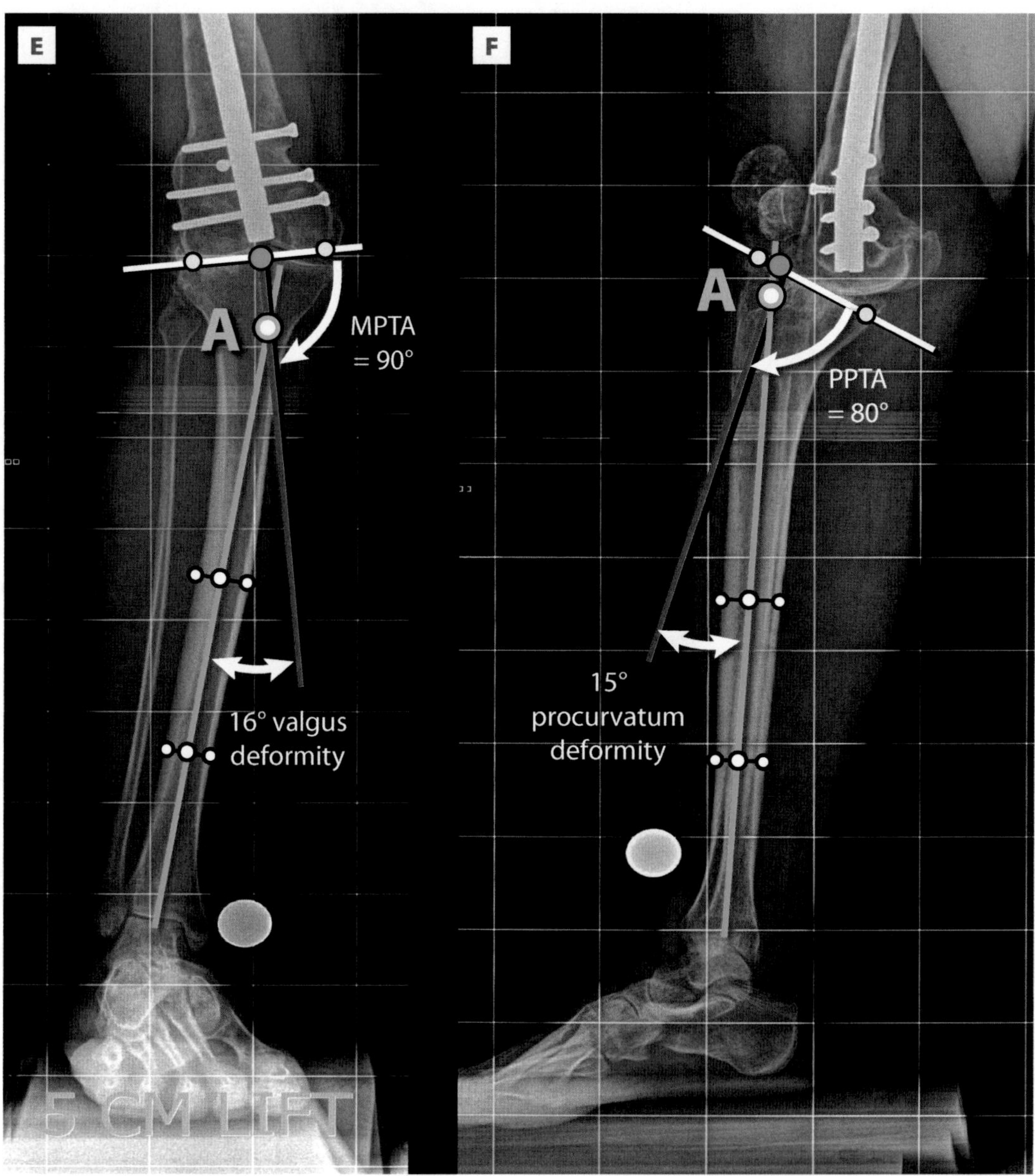


**Fig. 8 (continued): E** and **F**, To find the apex, the proximal and distal axis lines are drawn on the AP and lateral view x-rays. Note the apexes on the AP and lateral view x-ray are at two different locations. The apex is close to the level of the joint on the lateral view but is slightly more distal on the AP view. A, apex.

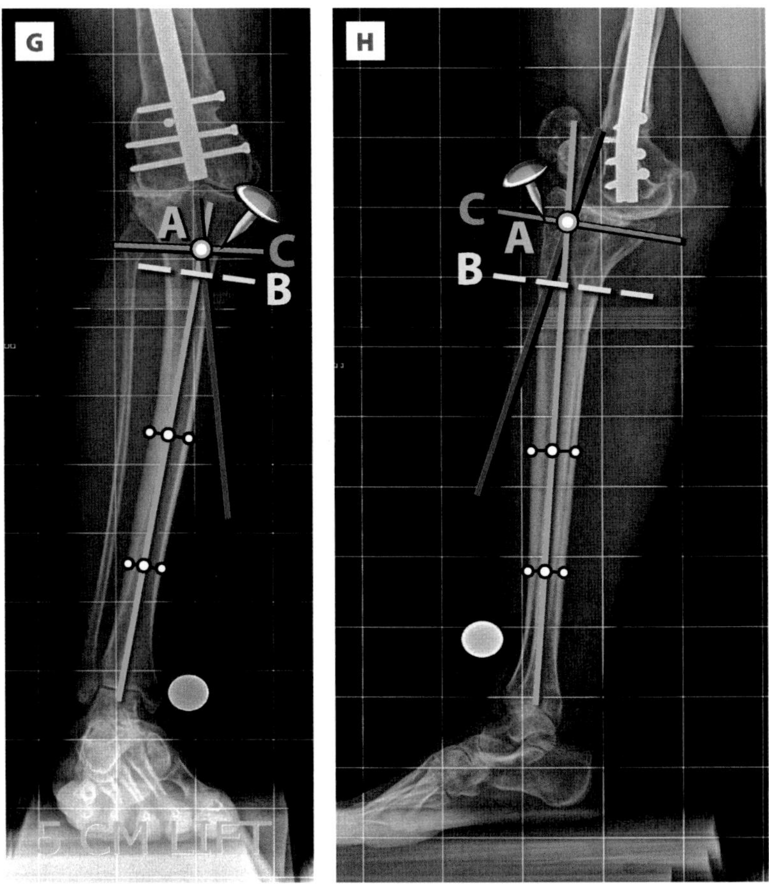


**Fig. 8 (continued): G** and **H**, The location of the bone cut is planned. Note that the bone cut is below the apexes on both the AP and lateral views. The C-levels are drawn, and the thumbtacks are placed along each C-level on the convex side of the deformity. A, apex; B, bone cut; C, C-level.

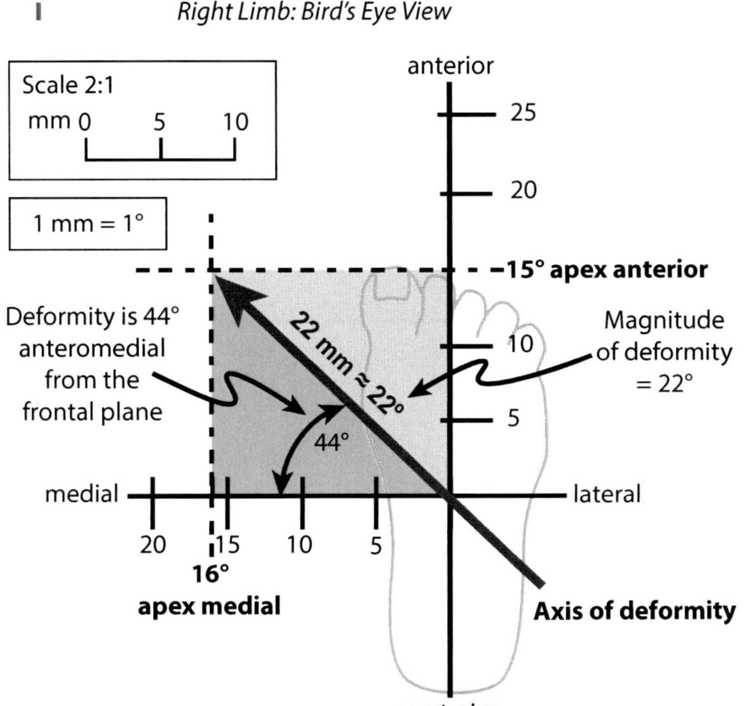


**Fig. 8 (continued): I**, When the graphic method is used to analyze this deformity using the values obtained in panels 8E and 8F, the magnitude of the deformity is determined to be 22° with the deformity 44° anteromedial from the frontal plane. When the trigonometric method (discussed at the end of this chapter) is used, the magnitude of deformity is 21.4° with the deformity 43.1° anteromedial from the frontal plane.

© 2023 Sinai Hospital of Baltimore

The bone was cut (Figs. 8J and 8K), and the bone segment was rotated around the thumbtack, which resulted in an opening wedge osteotomy with complete alignment of the bone and the axes.

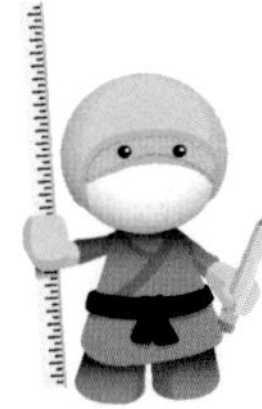

***Sensei says,***
*"Select the level of your bone cut with your fixation in mind. Also account for the translation that will occur at the osteotomy level as you correct through the apex in both planes."*

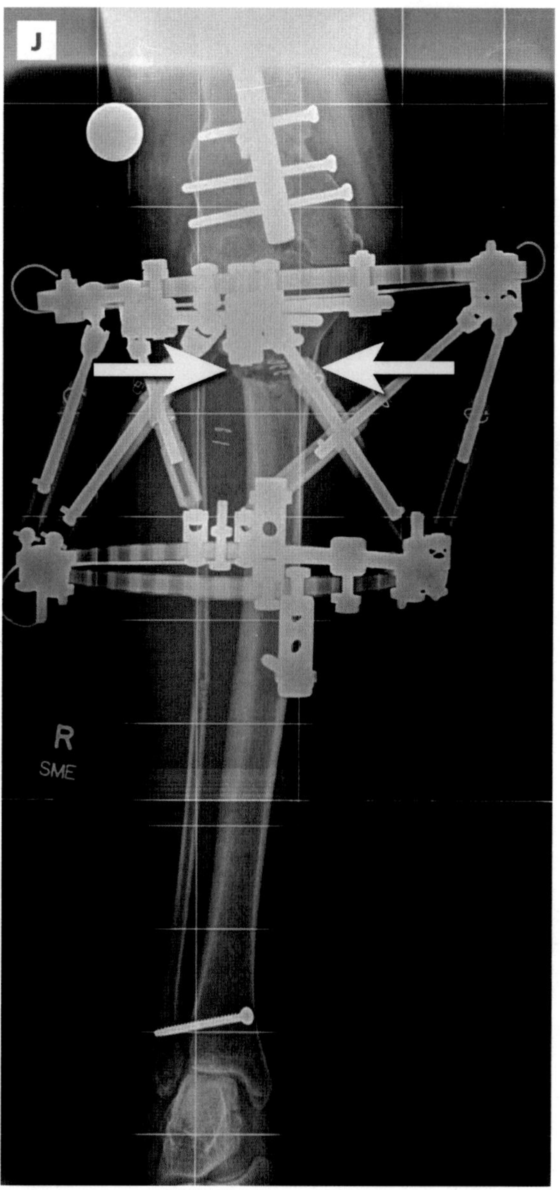


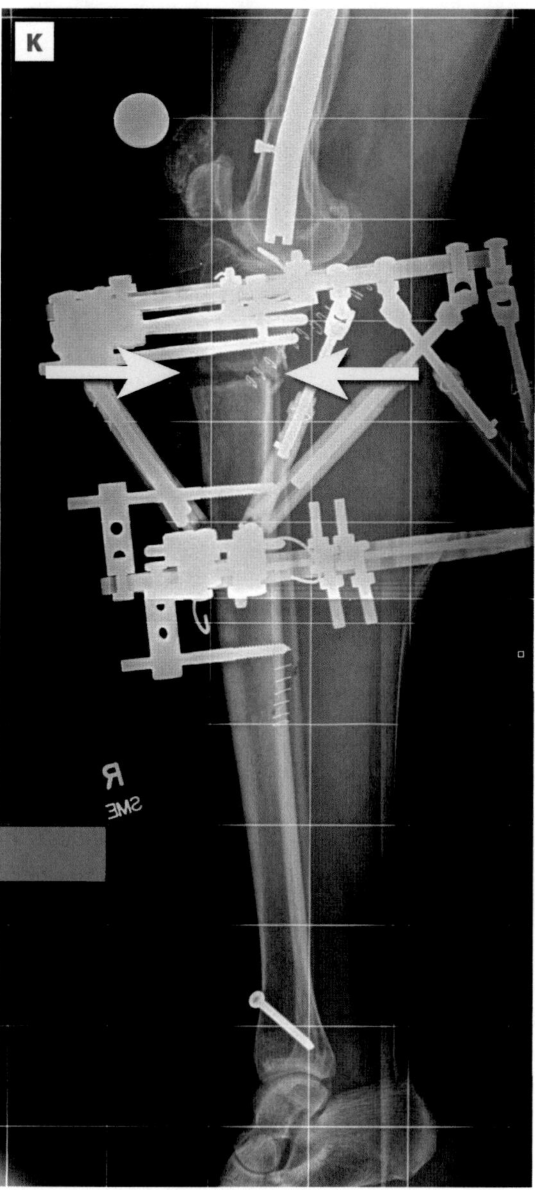


**Fig. 8 (continued):** **J** and **K**, The osteotomy is shown on the AP and lateral view x-rays (*yellow arrows*).

In the final postoperative x-rays (Figs. 8L and 8M), more translation is observed on the lateral view than on the AP view. This increased amount of translation on the lateral view x-ray occurred because the correction of the underlying translational deformity and the osteotomy were farther away from the apex on the lateral view as opposed to the AP view. When the alignment and angles are checked in Figures 8L and 8M, the MPTA of 90° matches the preoperative LDFA of 90°. Also, the MAD and PPTA are now normal.

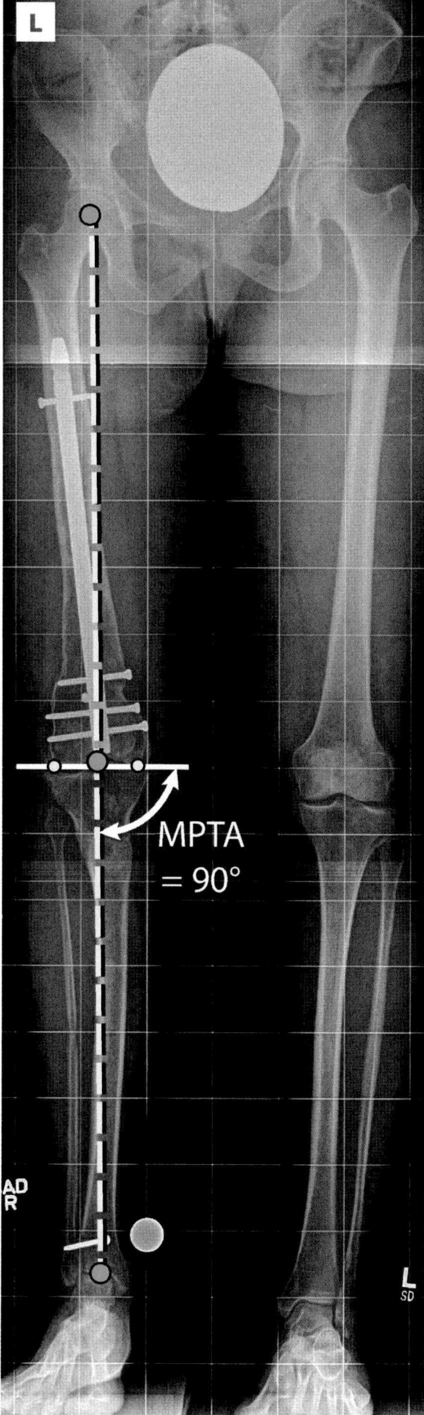


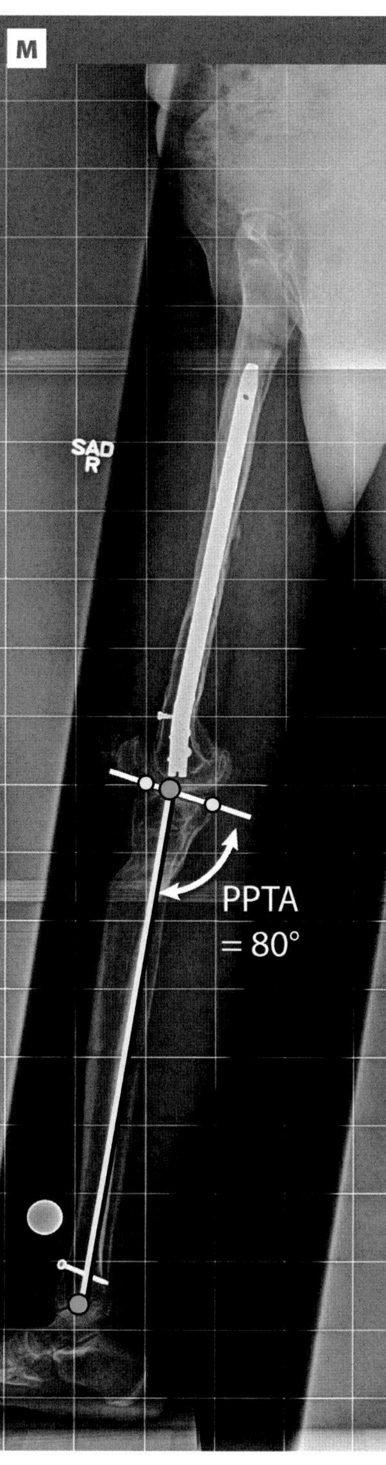


**Fig. 8 (continued): L**, AP view x-ray obtained after correction shows the corrected mechanical axis of the limb and a normal MPTA. Note the addition of length in the tibia which makes the translation difficult to appreciate since the bone cut was away from the apex but corrected with the hinge point on the correction level. **M**, Lateral view x-ray obtained after correction shows a normal PPTA. More translation is observed on the lateral view than on the AP view. This increased amount of translation on the lateral view x-ray occurred because the osteotomy was farther away from the apex on the lateral view as opposed to the AP view.

© 2023 Sinai Hospital of Baltimore

In this next example, the patient has a distal femoral deformity. For the MAP analysis, the first step is to perform the "M" step, which consists of measuring the MAD (5 cm lateral) (Fig. 9A). The MAD on the sagittal view is 19 mm posterior (Fig. 9B). The next step is the "A" of the MAP analysis, which is to analyze the frontal and sagittal plane joint angles (Figs. 9C and 9D). The LDFA is 76° (abnormal), the PDFA is 75° (abnormal), the SMAA is -13° (abnormal), and the SJLA is 13° (abnormal).

The soft-tissue contribution can be calculated using the formula method:

Soft-tissue Contribution About the Knee = SMAA – (Femoral Bony Deformity + Tibial Bony Deformity)

Soft-tissue Contribution About the Knee = -13° - (-8° + -2°)

Soft-tissue Contribution About the Knee = -3° (flexion)

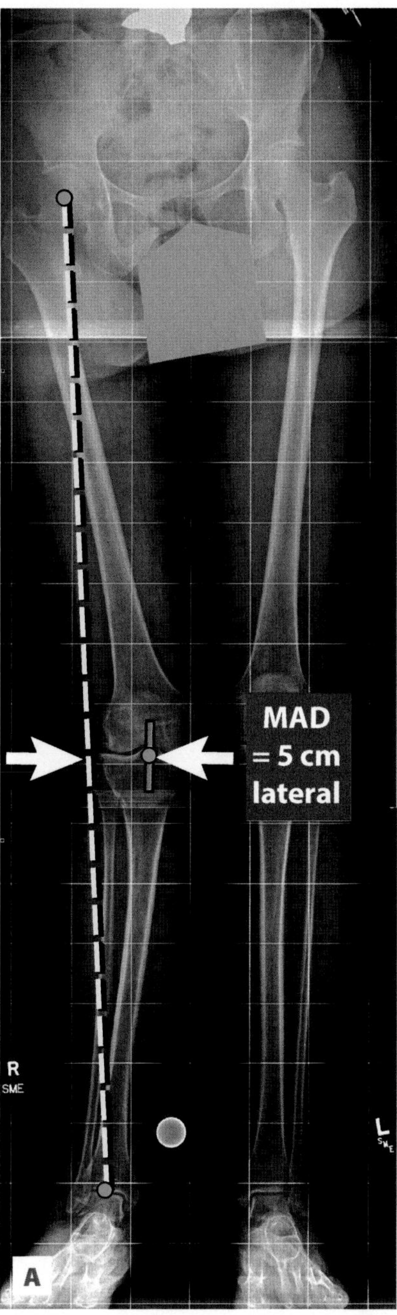


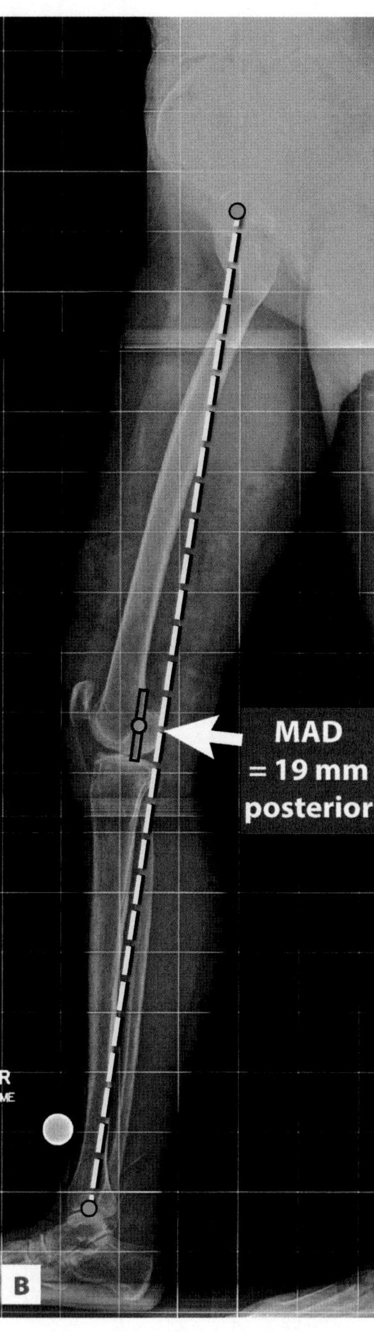


**Fig. 9:** Woman with a right distal femoral deformity and knee flexion contracture. **A**, Full length standing AP view x-ray shows the limb has a lateral MAD (5 cm lateral). **B**, Full length standing lateral view x-ray with a sagittal plane MAD of 19 mm posterior.

A limb has an oblique plane deformity if abnormalities are noted on both the AP and lateral view x-rays. For "P" (pick the bone), the femur is selected for correction. Next, the ABC analysis is performed.

To perform the "A" step (finding the apex) on the AP view x-ray, the proximal and distal axis lines need to be drawn. To determine the proximal axis, the three-line method is used (described in the chapter entitled "Femoral Axis Planning: Frontal and Sagittal Planes") (Figs. 9E and 9F). To draw the distal axis, the normal tibial mechanical axis is extended into the distal femur (Fig. 9G). This is possible because the JLCA and MPTA are normal. The apex is located at the intersection of the proximal and distal axis lines (Fig. 9H). Figure 9H shows a 14° valgus deformity of the femur on the AP view x-ray. For "B", the bone cut is planned proximal to the apex (Fig. 9I). Note how close the apex is to the joint line. The bone cut must be moved more proximal in order to allow the chosen fixation device to gain purchase in the distal fragment (Fig. 9I). The

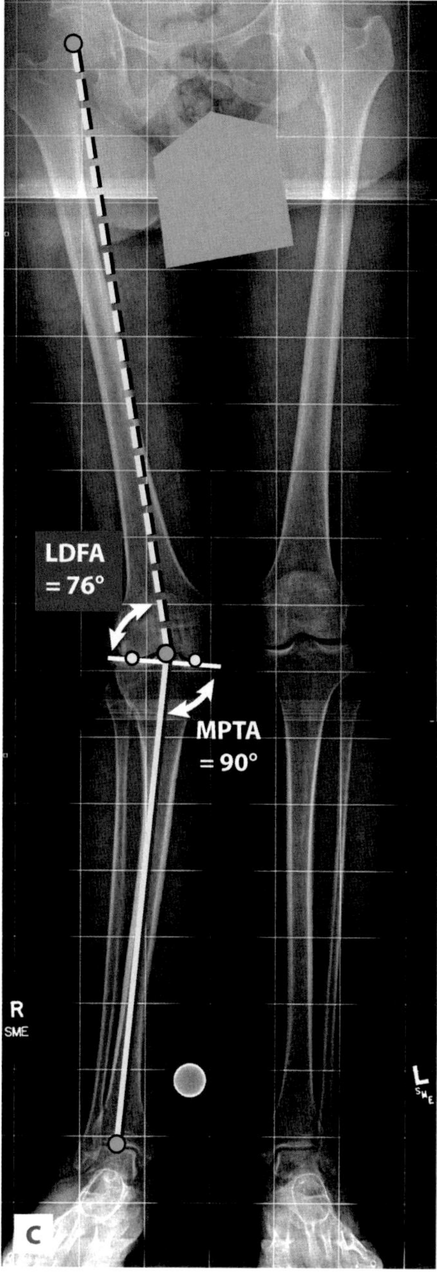


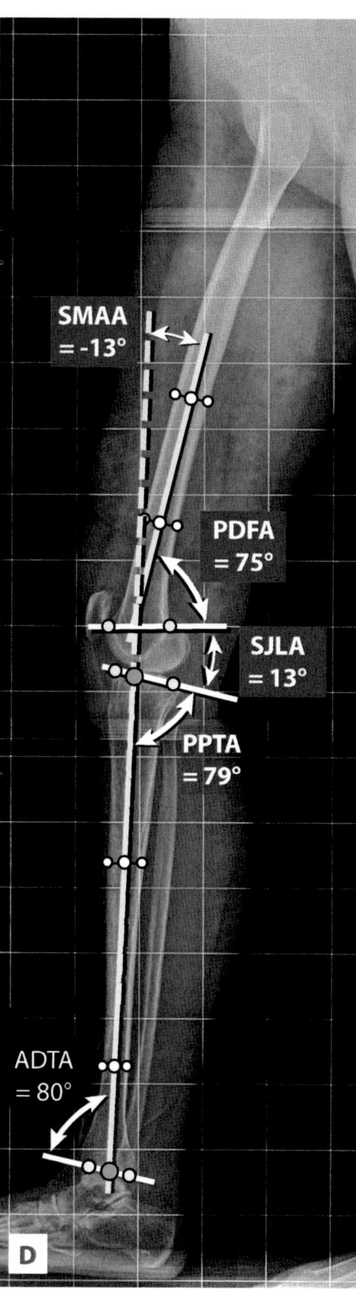


**Fig. 9 (continued): C**, Initial AP view x-ray shows that the LDFA is abnormal (76°) (normal range, 85–90°) and MPTA is normal. **D**, Initial lateral view x-ray shows the PDFA is abnormal (75°) (normal range, 79–87°), the SMAA is abnormal (-13°) (normal 0°), the SJLA is abnormal (13°) (normal 16°), the PPTA is normal, and the ADTA is normal.

© 2023 Sinai Hospital of Baltimore

type of fixation and the bone cut must be considered together. For the "C" step, the correction is planned on the AP view x-ray by drawing the C-level and placing a thumbtack along the C-level on the convex side of the deformity (Fig. 9I).

To perform the "A" step (finding the apex) on the lateral view x-ray, the proximal axis is drawn as the mid-diaphyseal line of the distal femur (Fig. 9J). The distal axis is determined by drawing the distal joint line and creating a normal PDFA starting at a point one-third of the length of the joint line from the anterior cortex (Fig. 9J). The apex is located at the intersection of the proximal and distal axis lines (Fig. 9K). Figure 9K shows 7° of procurvatum of the distal femur on the lateral view x-ray. Therefore, the patient has a distal femoral deformity. For "B", the bone cut is planned proximal to the apex (Fig. 9L). When performing the ABCs on both the AP and lateral view x-rays, the bone cut chosen on one view must be reproduced on the other view. For the "C" step, the correction is planned by drawing the C-level and placing a thumbtack along the C-level on the convex side of the deformity (Fig. 9L). Both components of the deformity (valgus and procurvatum) must be addressed. Notice that the location of the apex on the AP (Fig. 9H) and lateral view (Fig. 9K) x-rays is different, which often happens with oblique plane deformities and denotes a translational component to the deformity.

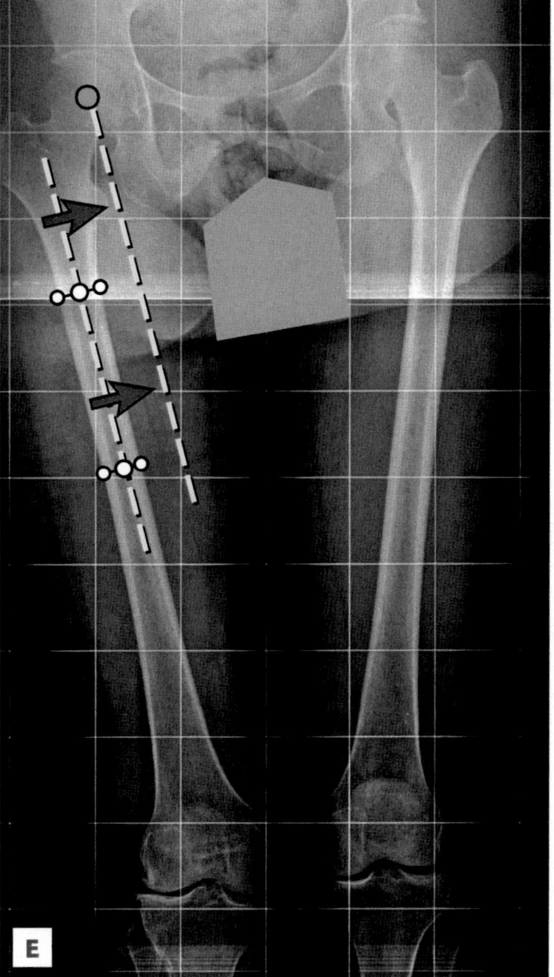


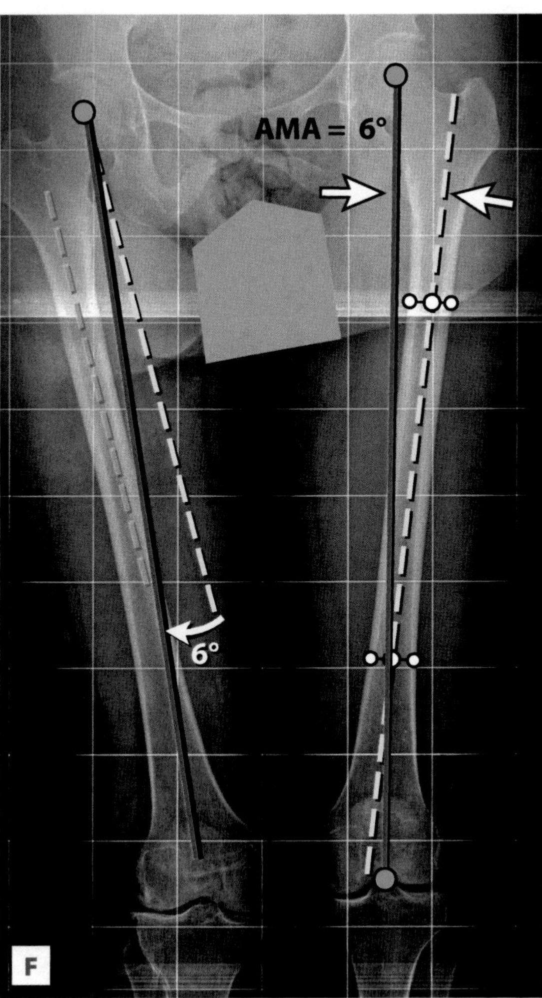


**Fig. 9 (continued): E** and **F**, The proximal axis line needs to be drawn by using the three-line method (described in the chapter entitled "Femoral Axis Planning: Frontal and Sagittal Planes"). The AMA is 6° on the normal left femur. Therefore, 6° is used for the three-line method of the right femur.

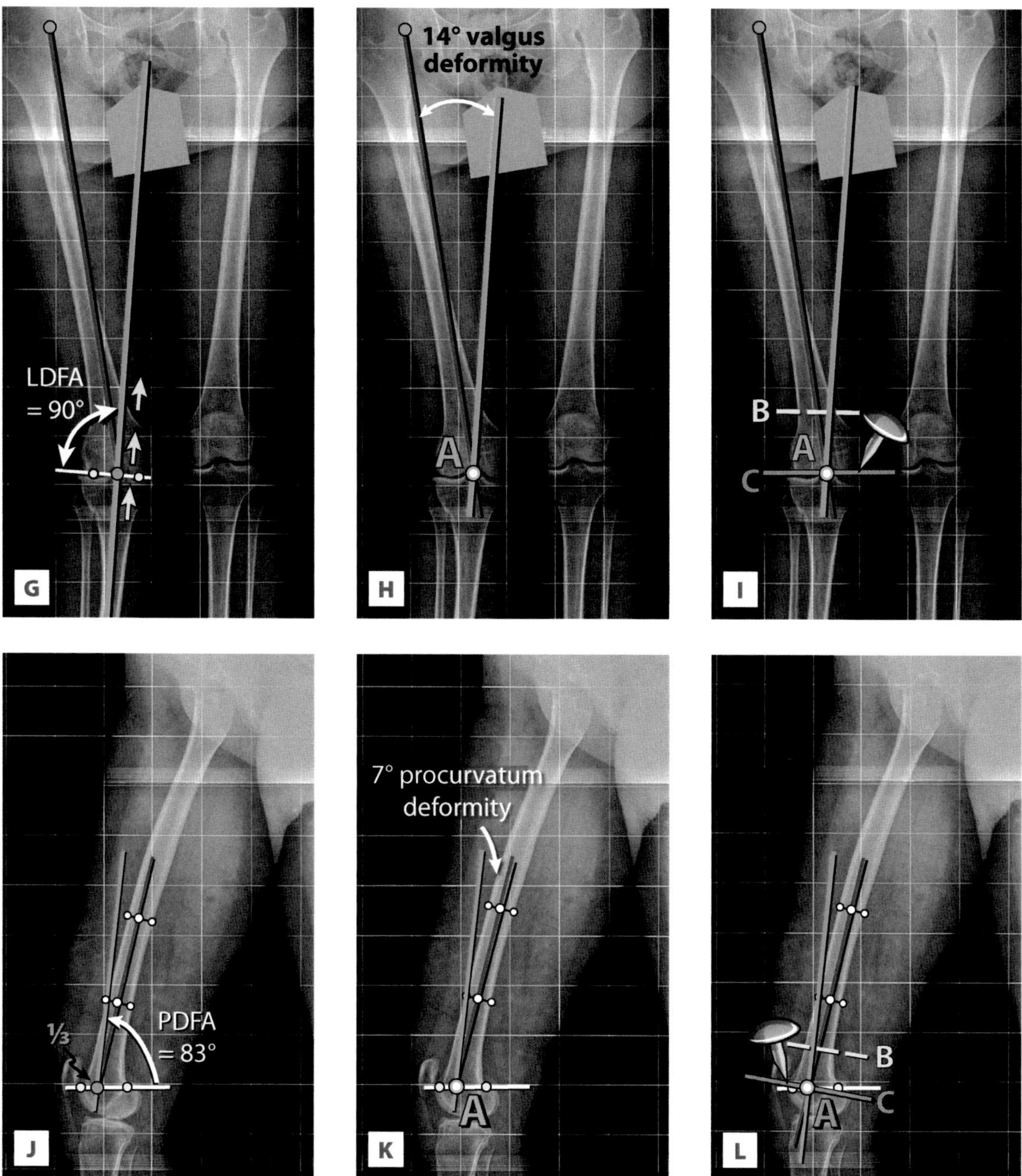


**Fig. 9 (continued): G**, To draw the distal axis, the normal tibial mechanical axis is extended into the distal femur. This is possible because the JLCA and MPTA are normal. **H**, The apex is located at the intersection of the proximal and distal axis lines. The magnitude of the deformity is 14° valgus on the AP view x-ray. **I**, The bone cut is planned proximal to the apex in order to allow the chosen fixation device to gain purchase in the distal fragment. The correction is planned by drawing the C-level and placing a thumbtack along the C-level on the convex side of the deformity. **J**, To find the apex on the lateral view x-ray, the proximal and distal axis lines need to be drawn. The proximal axis is the mid-diaphyseal line of the distal femur. The distal axis is determined by drawing the distal joint line and creating a normal PDFA starting at a point one-third of the length of the joint line from the anterior cortex. **K**, The apex is located at the intersection of the proximal and distal axis lines. The patient has 7° of procurvatum of the distal femur on the lateral view x-ray. **L**, The bone cut is planned proximal to the apex. The correction is planned by drawing the C-level and placing a thumbtack along the C-level on the convex side of the deformity. A, apex; B, bone cut; C, C-level.

*© 2023 Sinai Hospital of Baltimore*

When the graphic method is used to analyze this deformity using the values obtained in Figures 9H and 9K, the magnitude of the deformity is determined to be 15.5° with the deformity 27° anteromedial from the frontal plane (Fig. 9M).

For the correction, the bone segment was rotated around the thumbtack, which resulted in an opening wedge osteotomy with complete alignment of the bone and the axes. By observing each individual thumbtack's placement on the AP and lateral view x-rays (Figs. 9I and 9L), one can see that the oblique hinge is in an anterior medial position. In the final postoperative x-rays (Figs. 9N and 9O), the MAD, LDFA, and PDFA are normal. Plate fixation was chosen. A fixator was used in the operating room to accurately hold the correction for plate placement. Moving the bone cut more proximally allowed the plate to capture the distal fragment with six screws to provide good fixation. Note the mandatory translation that had to occur to completely and accurately correct the deformity (Figs. 9N and 9O). The locking plate was placed off the bone proximally to accommodate this mandatory translation.

Note that if the bone cut is made at the apex on the AP view but not at the apex on the lateral view, some sagittal plane translation will need to occur. With acute translation correction, the anteroposterior and lateral apexes are brought to the same level. This consideration is important with oblique plane deformity analysis because knowing the amount of translation will help you choose the best method for fixation. For example, too much translation in the sagittal plane will not allow a rod to be used for fixation.

*Sensei says,*

*"Oblique plane deformities have one apex that can be analyzed as two apexes: one on the AP view x-ray and one on the lateral view x-ray. Often these apexes are not at the same level in the bone. This is particularly true if there is angulation and translation in different planes."*

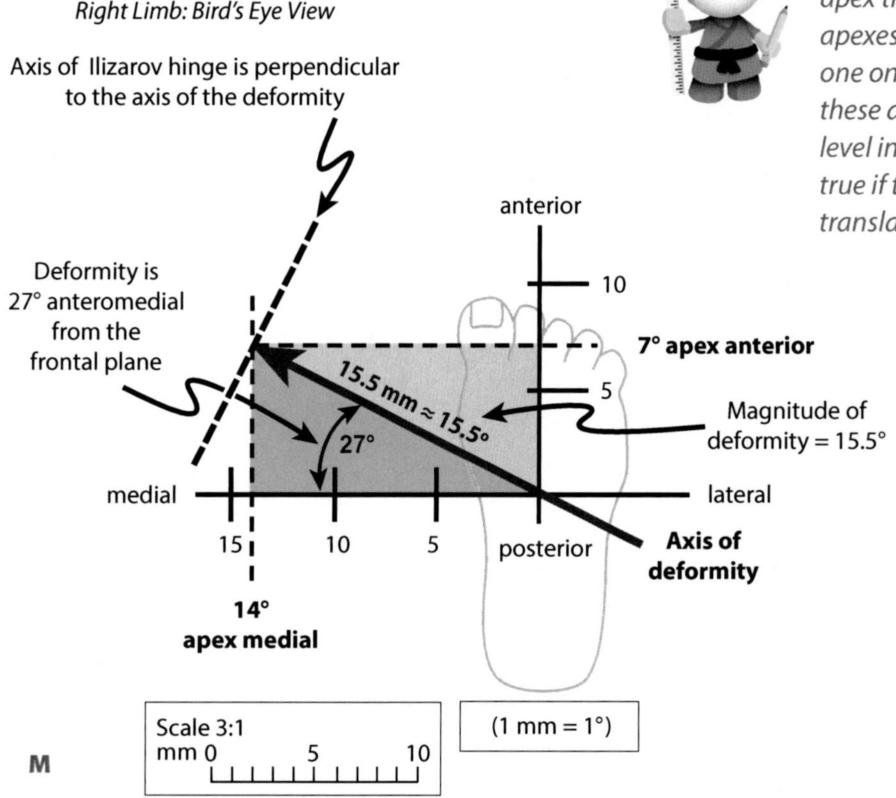


**Fig. 9 (continued): M,** When the graphic method is used to analyze this deformity using the values obtained in Figures 9H and 9K, the magnitude of the deformity is determined to be 15.5° with the deformity 27° anteromedial from the frontal plane. When the trigonometric method (discussed at the end of this chapter) is used, the magnitude of deformity is 15.5° with the deformity 26.2° anteromedial from the frontal plane.

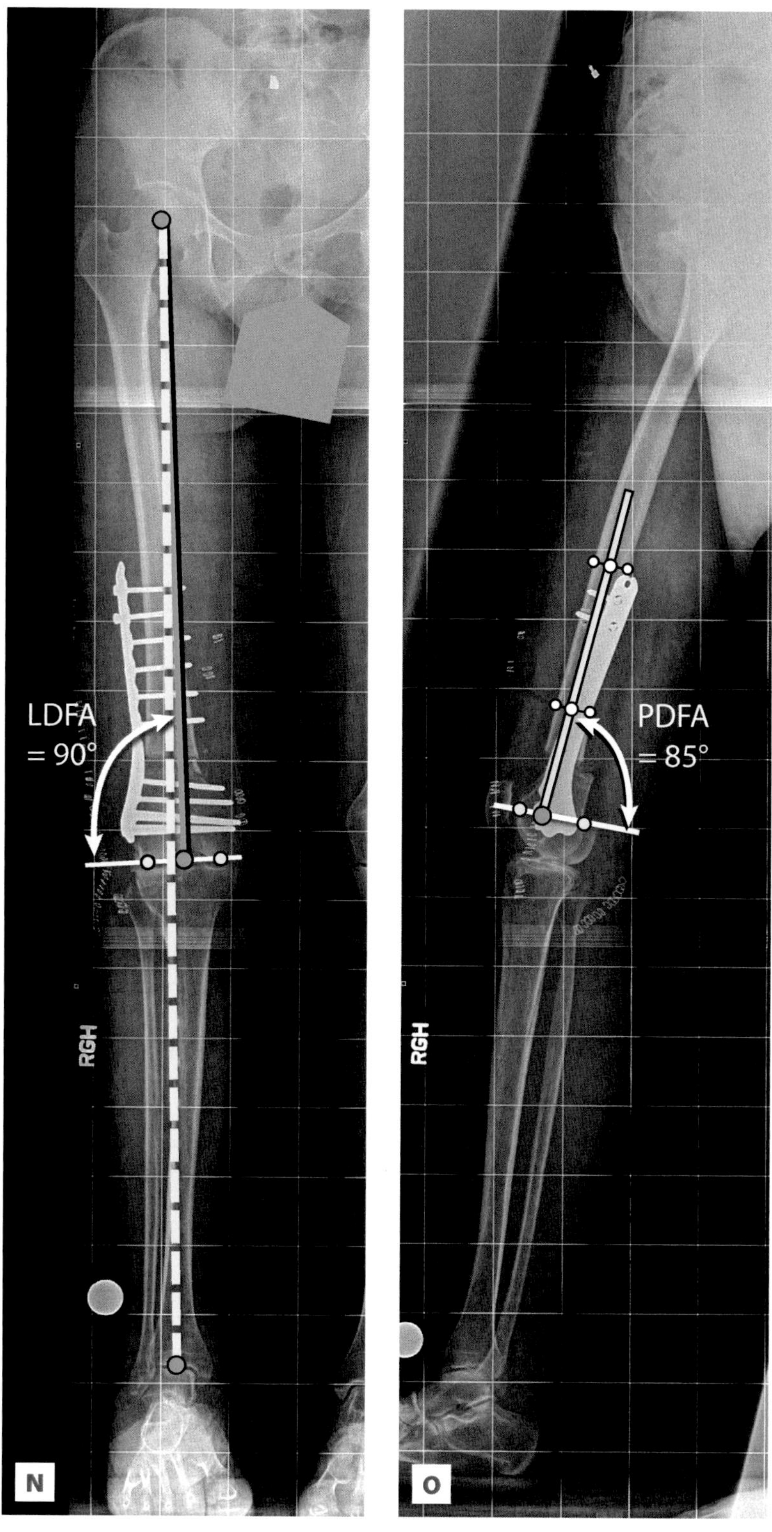


**Fig. 9 (continued): N**, AP view x-ray obtained after correction shows corrected mechanical axis of limb and LDFA of 90° (normal). Note the translation of the distal femoral segment with the plate appropriately fixed off the bone proximally. **O**, Lateral view x-ray obtained after correction shows the bone cut at the metadiaphyseal femur. PDFA is 85° (overcorrected). Note the posterior translation of the distal fragment.

*© 2023 Sinai Hospital of Baltimore*

As an alternative to the graphic method, you can input the AP and lateral view deformity magnitudes and the directions of the apexes into a trigonometric formula to give you the true magnitude and direction of the oblique plane deformity and the orientation of the oblique plane from the frontal plane. The Multiplier App (available through iTunes and Google Play) includes this formula to spare you the difficulty of trigonometric calculations. For most common deformities with smaller magnitudes (<45°), the graphic method is satisfactory. For oblique plane deformities with larger magnitudes, the accuracy of the graphic method starts to deteriorate somewhat.

Modern day deformity correction thankfully does not need to be this complicated. Using a six-axis frame, for example, eliminates the complexity of calculating the exact location of the deformity in the oblique plane. Accurate and reproducible x-rays, however, are essential when correcting oblique plane deformities. X-rays should be obtained orthogonal to the primary deformity segment. In the case of proximal deformities, both the AP and lateral view x-rays should be obtained orthogonal to the proximal joint segment. In the case of distal deformities, both the AP and lateral view x-rays should be obtained orthogonal to the distal joint segment.

# Chapter 11

# Determining Limb Length Discrepancy: MAP the LLD

Shawn C. Standard, MD

Untreated limb length discrepancy (LLD) can lead to long-term detrimental effects on the spine, hips, knees, and ankles. The ultimate goal of limb lengthening is to produce a pelvic line that is parallel to the ground (horizontal) during a double-leg stance. An uneven pelvic line produces pelvic obliquity that results in compensatory spinal curves and decreasing hip coverage of the long leg. Conversely, compensation for LLD can occur and the pelvic line can be made level by either the short leg having the foot and ankle in an equinus position or the long leg having a flexed knee. Determining the amount and location of LLD enables the surgeon to formulate a correct surgical strategy to address the LLD and any concurrent limb deformities in the appropriate limb segments.

Several studies have shown that LLD can have a normal variation of ≤ 2 cm without apparent harm. Other research has reported detriment to the hip when an LLD results in significantly decreasing hip coverage, regardless of the exact amount of LLD.[1] The goal while ambulating is energy conservation, which is accomplished by minimizing the vertical excursion of the body's center of gravity. This vertical excursion of the center of gravity can double in the presence of a non-compensated LLD, thereby increasing energy consumption.[2] In our clinical experience, LLD that is < 1.5 cm does not require treatment unless clinical symptoms dictate otherwise.

Once the total LLD has been calculated, the shoe lift prescription can be determined by subtracting 1 cm from the calculated LLD. The rationale for the 1 cm subtraction is to improve clearance of the foot during the swing phase and prevent the lifted shoe from "stubbing" the ground.

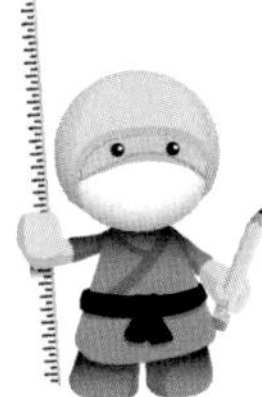

***Sensei says,***
*"He who has a pelvic line that is parallel to the horizon and is not standing on blocks has equal limb lengths and balance."*

## X-ray Assessment of LLD

An accurate assessment of LLD begins with an adequate full-length standing AP x-ray of both lower limbs with the patellae facing forward. If significant LLD is present, blocks should be placed under the short limb to "lift" the pelvis on incrementally increasing 1 cm blocks until the iliac crests are leveled. The height of the blocks required to level the pelvis should be noted on the x-ray. It also should be noted if no blocks were used. The height of the blocks represents the x-ray assessment of the LLD and can be quite accurate if performed by an experienced technician.

© 2023 Sinai Hospital of Baltimore

Calculating the LLD may be confusing if blocks were inadvertently used under the long leg or if the short leg was overlifted. In these situations, you have two options:

1. The patient can be repositioned and a second x-ray can be obtained. This option is not optimal as it will expose the patient to additional radiation from repeat radiographs.

2. You can use the formula/method described in this chapter to prevent the need for a new x-ray.

You will not be able to determine total LLD if you only have a bilateral ankle AP x-ray instead of a full-length standing AP x-ray of both limbs. However, you can still determine the foot segment contribution to LLD by using a method described near the end of this chapter.

## MAP the LLD

The lower extremity length is the result of the additive effect of four individual segments of the lower limb: the pelvis, femur, tibia, and foot. An increase or decrease in length can occur in any of these segments. Each segment must be analyzed, and its additive effects calculated. This calculation then must be compared to the contralateral lower extremity. Suddenly, the simple task of determining LLD has become a daunting task with multiple variables. However, the same strategy that has been introduced for deformity analyses—the mnemonic MAP—will be used to assist in evaluating a patient's LLD. This mnemonic (shown in Table 1) will allow for a simple, consistent, and accurate approach to determining LLD.

## Measure the Limb Length Discrepancy Using the Total LLD Method

The Total LLD Method accounts for all segments of the lower limb and calculates the absolute LLD. This method uses the pelvic line as the reference for measurement. A disadvantage of this method is the potential difficulty one may have when trying to visualize the inferior aspects of the sacroiliac (SI) joints with different radiographic qualities. Other bony landmarks can also be used to draw the pelvic line, such as the first sacral foramen, the upper end plate of the S1, or the inferior end plate of L5.

**Table 1**

**MAP the LLD**

**M**easure the limb length discrepancy using the Total LLD Method

**A**nalyze the lengths of the four individual bone segments

- Pelvis
- Femur
- Tibia
- Foot (foot contribution can be measured directly or indirectly)

**P**ick the bone segment that has the greatest discrepancy

- Goal of lengthening is to level the pelvis
- Discrepancies in the feet and tibiae are addressed with tibial lengthening.
- Discrepancies in the pelvis and femora are addressed with femoral lengthening.

### Introduction to the Total LLD Method (Fig. 1)

**Step 1:** Place two points on the inferior aspect of each SI joint. Draw a pelvic line by connecting these two points.

**Step 2:** Determine which limb **appears** to be the short limb in the x-ray. You can determine the short limb by imagining a ball being placed on the pelvic line. The ball will roll toward the limb that appears shorter in this x-ray. If the blocks/lifts were placed incorrectly, the ball may roll towards the limb that you know is actually longer (based on your clinical evaluation). However, the goal of this step is to determine which limb **appears** shorter in this x-ray.

**Step 3:** Locate the center of each femoral head (blue points). Draw two points (orange points) that are on the pelvic line and are placed directly over the center of each femoral head.

**Step 4:** Draw a line (Line A) that starts on the pelvic line at a point directly over the

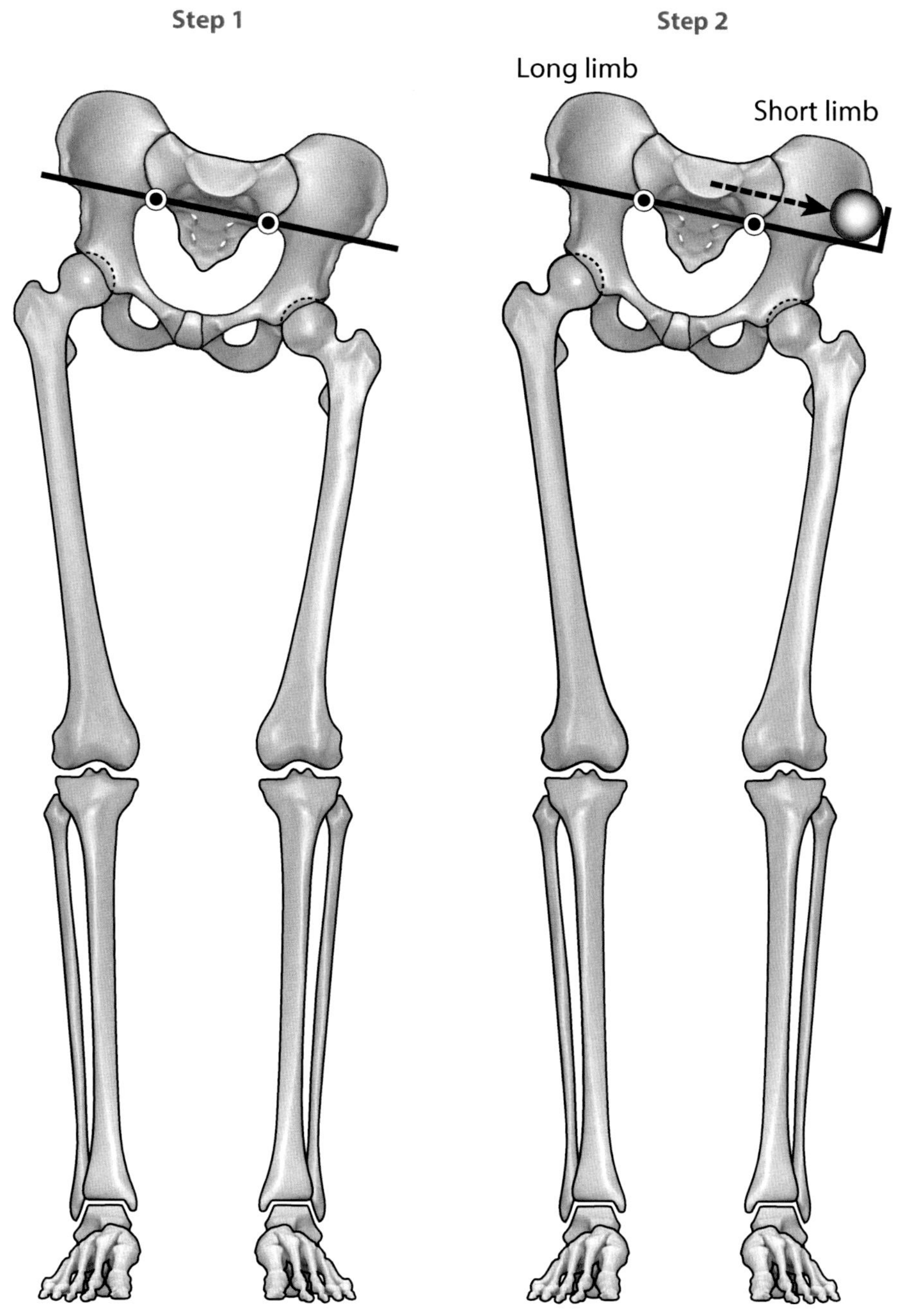


**Fig. 1:** Steps 1 and 2 to calculate the total LLD.

© 2023 Sinai Hospital of Baltimore

center of the right femoral head. Direct the line proximally and end it at a grid line on the x-ray or the top of the x-ray. Create a second line (Line B) that starts at a point on the pelvic line directly over the left femoral head and is directed proximally. Line B should end at the same common grid line where Line A ends.

**Step 5:** Measure the lengths of Line A and Line B. Remember that the goal of this step is to determine which limb **appears** shorter in this x-ray, even if it does not match your clinical observations.

- The longer line is above the shorter leg. The length of that line is designated $T_{Short}$. In our calculations, all values (length of line A or B, height of the blocks/lifts) for the short limb will be assigned **positive values.**
    - Line B = left limb = $T_{Short}$ = +20 cm
- The shorter line is above the longer leg. The length of that line is designated $T_{Long}$. In our calculations, all values (length of line A or B, height of the blocks/lifts) for the longer limb will be assigned **negative values.**
    - Line A = right limb = $T_{Long}$ = -16 cm

**Step 6:** Check for the presence of a lift or blocks in the x-ray. The height of the blocks will be assigned a positive or negative value depending on whether the blocks were placed under the limb designated as the short limb or the long limb (if an unintended mistake caused selection of the incorrect short limb).

- If blocks were placed under the short limb ($T_{Short}$), then the height of the blocks ($B_{Height\ of\ Blocks}$) should be included in the formula below as a **positive value.**
- If blocks were placed under the long limb ($T_{Long}$), then the height of the blocks should be a **negative value.**

In this example, no blocks were used.

$B_{Height\ of\ Blocks}$ = 0 cm

**Step 7:** Calculate the total LLD:

Total LLD = $T_{Short} + T_{Long} + B_{Height\ of\ Blocks}$

= (+20 cm) + (-16 cm) + 0 cm

Total LLD = +4 cm

- If the total LLD value is positive, then the limb labeled $T_{Short}$ is short by this amount.
- If the total LLD value is negative, then the limb labeled $T_{Long}$ is short by this amount. This situation can happen if a short limb was overlifted, which causes us to label it as $T_{Long}$ when evaluating the x-ray.

**Conclusion:**

The left limb ($T_{Short}$) is 4 cm shorter than the right limb ($T_{Long}$).

## Four Examples of Calculating Total LLD With the Three Line Method

The same deformity is assessed for total LLD using the Three Line Method in the following four examples. The Three Line Method eliminates the need to measure to a common grid line or the top of the x-ray. Each example shows a different scenario for the placement of the blocks: no lift is used, the lift is used correctly on the short side to make the pelvis level, the short limb is overlifted, and the long limb is lifted. The same deformity is handled in four different ways when positioning the patient for the x-ray, but you can still use the formula to correctly calculate total LLD.

**Step 3**

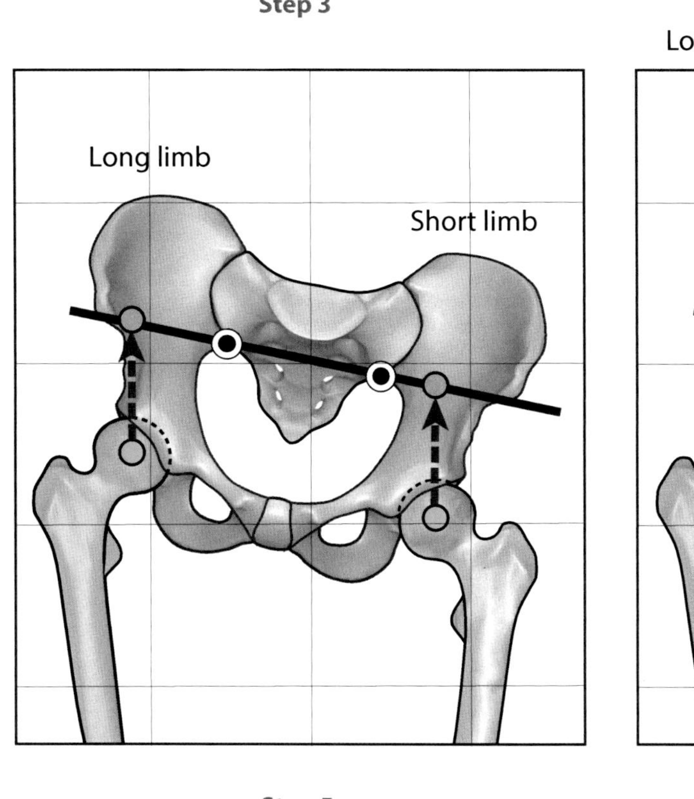


**Step 4**

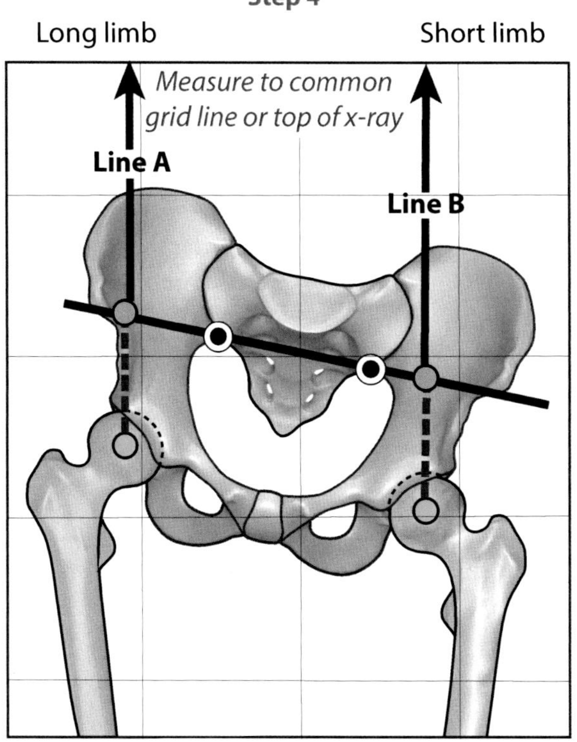


**Step 5**

Long limb

Short limb

**Negative values**

$T_{Long}$ = -16 cm

Positive values

$T_{Short}$ = +20 cm

**Steps 6 and 7**

Total LLD = $T_{Short} + T_{Long} + B_{Height\ of\ Blocks}$
= (+20 cm) + (-16 cm) + (0 cm)
= +4 cm (positive value)

**Left limb ($T_{Short}$) is shorter than the right limb by 4 cm**

**Fig. 1 (continued):** Steps 3 through 6 to calculate the total LLD.

*© 2023 Sinai Hospital of Baltimore*

### No Blocks Were Used to Lift the Short Limb (Fig. 2)

**Step 1:** Place two points on the inferior aspect of each SI joint. Draw a pelvic line (Line 1) by connecting these two points. Determine which limb **appears** short in the x-ray.

**Step 2:** Move Line 1 so it passes through the center of the femoral head of the long leg. This is our current pelvic line.

**Step 3:** Create a horizontal line (Line 2) that passes through the center of the femoral head of the long leg. This is our desired pelvic line.

**Step 4:** Create Line 3 by drawing a vertical line that passes through the femoral head of the short leg as well as both Lines 1 and 2. Measure the amount of Line 3 that exists between Lines 1 and 2.

**Step 5:** In this example, blocks were not used to lift either leg ($B_{\text{Height of Blocks}}$ = 0 cm).

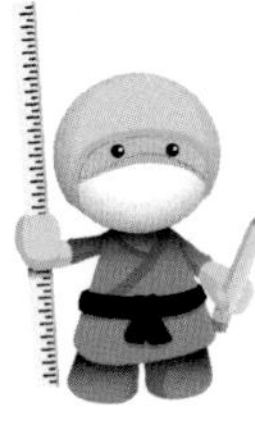

*Sensei says,*

*"When calculating total LLD, values for the height of the blocks/lifts of the limb that appears short will be assigned **positive values.** All values for the limb that appears longer will be assigned **negative values.**"*

**Step 6:** Calculate the total LLD:

Total LLD = Line 3 + $B_{\text{Height of Blocks}}$

= 3 cm + 0 cm

Total LLD = +3 cm

If the total LLD value is positive, then the limb labeled $T_{\text{Short}}$ is short by this amount.

**Conclusion:**

The right limb ($T_{\text{Short}}$) is 3 cm shorter than the left limb ($T_{\text{Long}}$).

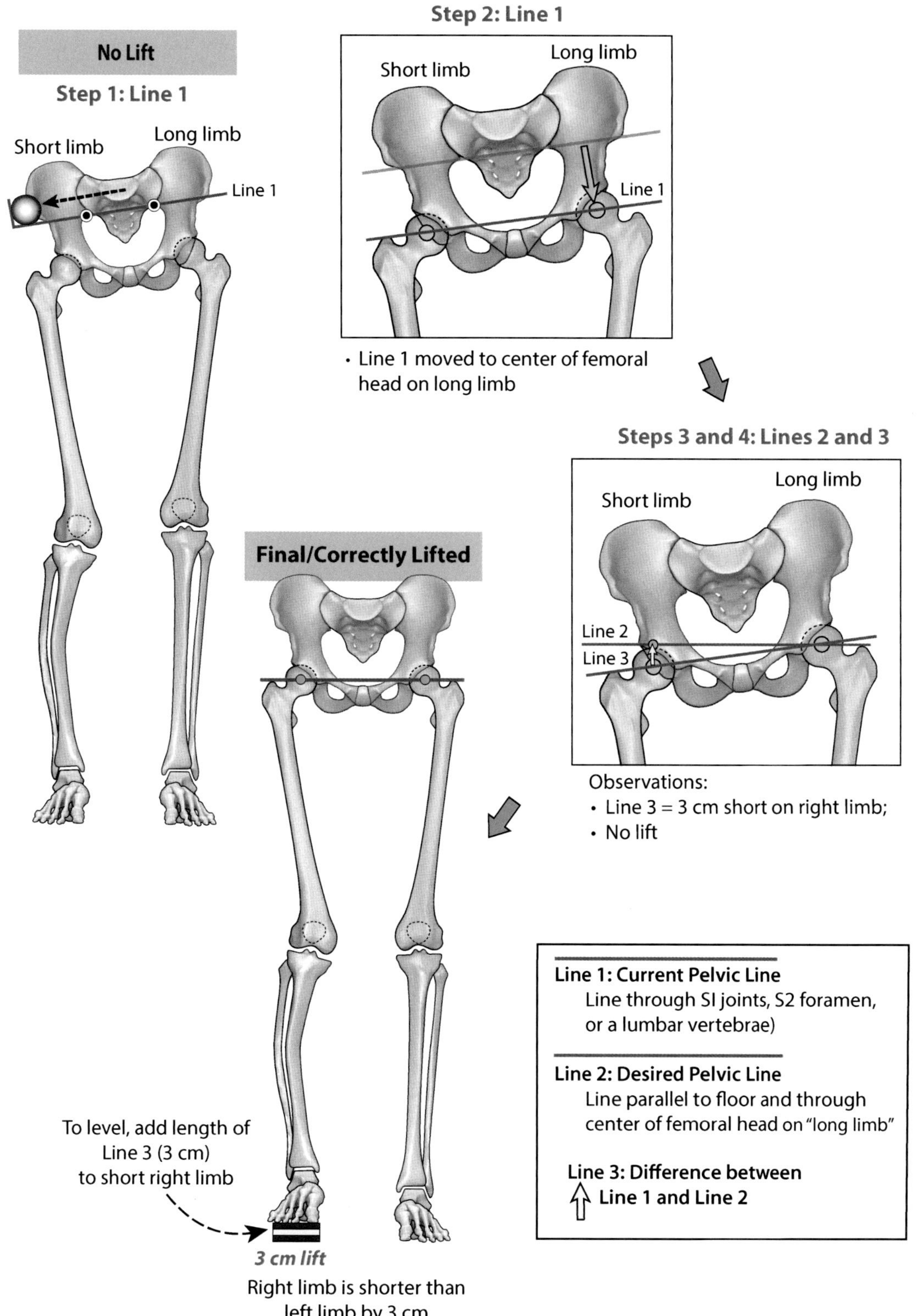


**Fig. 2:** Example of calculating total LLD when no blocks are used to position the limbs in the x-ray.

© 2023 Sinai Hospital of Baltimore

## Short Limb Correctly Positioned on Blocks (Fig. 3)

**Step 1:** Draw a pelvic line (Line 1). Determine which limb **appears** short in the x-ray. In this example, the short limb is placed correctly on blocks, which makes the pelvic line level.

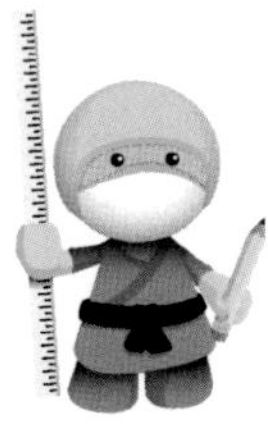

***Sensei says,***
*"If the pelvic line is horizontal, then either the limb lengths are equal or the limb that is lifted is short by exactly the height of the blocks that are placed under that limb."*

Note: Because the pelvic line is horizontal, the LLD is equal to the amount of lift used. We can skip steps 2–4 from the previous example and go directly to step 5.

**Step 5:** Calculate the total LLD:

$$\text{Total LLD} = \text{Line 3} + B_{\text{Height of Blocks}}$$

$$= 0 \text{ cm} + 3 \text{ cm}$$

$$\text{Total LLD} = +3 \text{ cm}$$

**Conclusion:**

The right limb ($T_{Short}$) is 3 cm shorter than the left limb ($T_{Long}$).

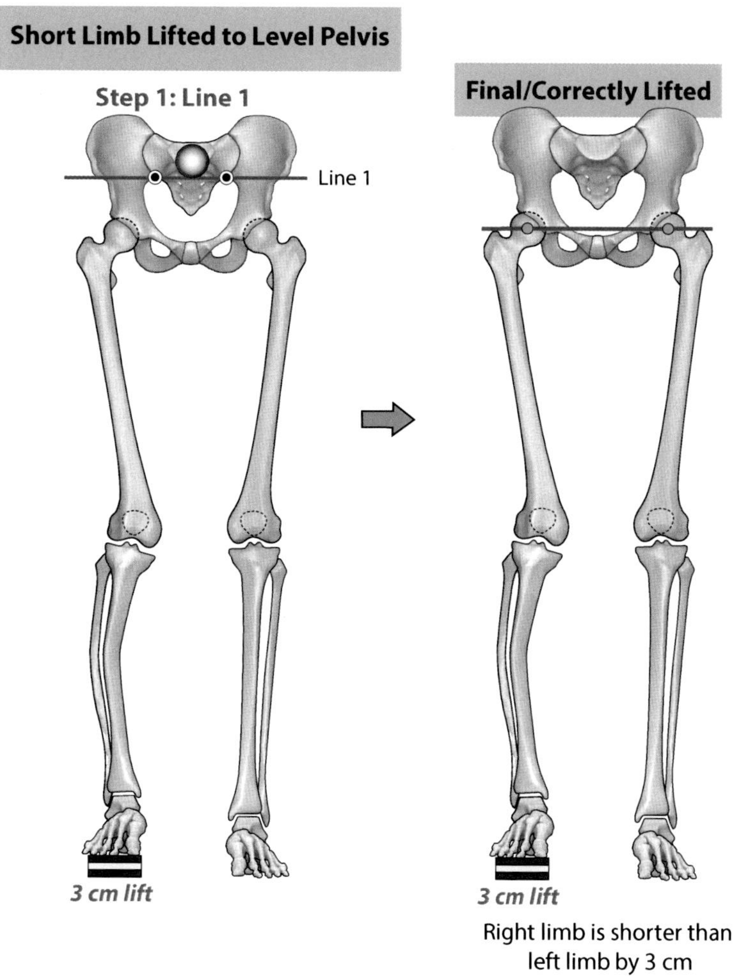


**Fig. 3:** Example of calculating total LLD when blocks are used correctly under the short limb to level the pelvis. Note this is the same deformity shown in Figure 2.

© 2023 Sinai Hospital of Baltimore

## Short Limb Overlifted on Blocks (Fig. 4)

**Step 1:** Draw the pelvic line (Line 1). Determine which limb **appears** short in the x-ray. In this example, we know that the short limb is overlifted. However, the goal of this step is to determine which limb **appears** shorter in this particular x-ray, even if it does not match the clinical assessment. If a ball were to be placed on the pelvic line, it would roll toward the left side. Therefore, the left limb is designated the "short" side in this x-ray. This is very important because it means that the line length and lift height values for the left limb will be assigned positive values.

**Step 2:** Move Line 1 so it passes through the center of the femoral head of the long leg. This is our current pelvic line.

**Step 3:** Create a horizontal line (Line 2) that passes through the center of the femoral head of the long leg. This is our desired pelvic line.

**Step 4:** Create Line 3 by drawing a vertical line that passes through the femoral head of the short leg as well as both Lines 1 and 2. Measure the amount of Line 3 that exists between Lines 1 and 2.

**Step 5:** Determine the height of the blocks. In this case, blocks were placed under $T_{Long}$, which means their height is assigned a negative value.

$B_{Height\ of\ Blocks}$ = -5 cm

**Step 6:** Calculate the total LLD:

Total LLD = Line 3 + $B_{Height\ of\ Blocks}$

= (+2 cm) + (-5 cm)

Total LLD = -3 cm

The total LLD value is negative, which means the limb labeled $T_{Long}$ is actually short by this amount. This situation happens when a short limb was overlifted, which caused the short limb to appear to be the long limb in this x-ray.

**Conclusion:**

The right limb ($T_{Long}$) appears longer in this x-ray because of overlifting. The right limb is actually shorter than the left limb by 3 cm. Therefore the total LLD value is negative.

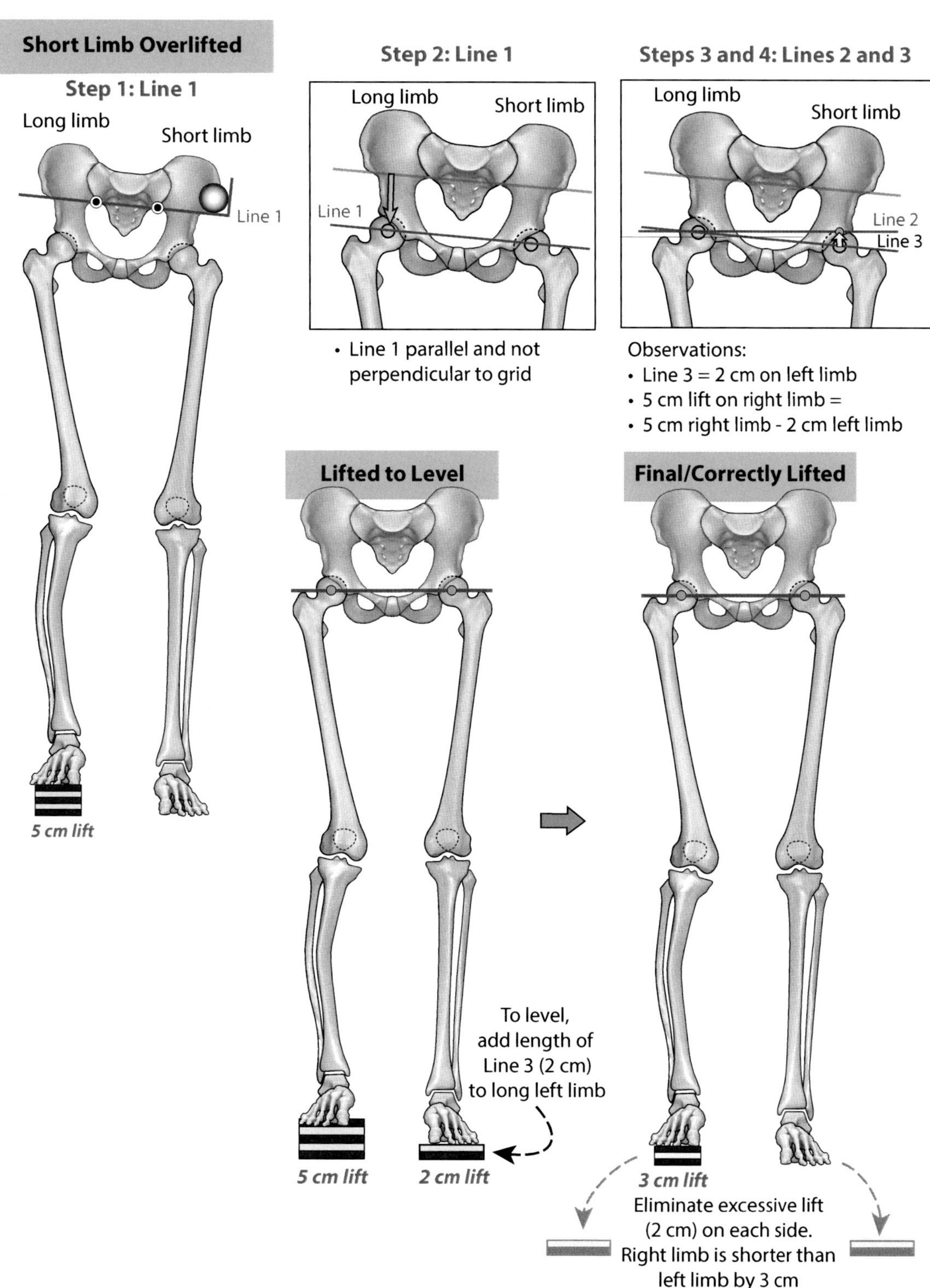


**Fig. 4:** Example of calculating total LLD when the blocks placed under the short limb have caused it to be overlifted (pelvic line is not level). Note this is the same deformity shown in Figures 2 and 3.

### Long Limb Lifted on Blocks (Fig. 5)

**Step 1:** Draw the pelvic line (Line 1). Determine which limb **appears** short in the x-ray.

**Step 2:** Create a horizontal line (Line 2) that passes through the center of the femoral head of the long leg. This is our current pelvic line.

**Step 3:** Create a horizontal line (Line 2) that passes through the center of the femoral head of the long leg. This is our desired pelvic line.

**Step 4:** Create Line 3 by drawing a vertical line that passes through the femoral head of the short leg as well as both Lines 1 and 2. Measure the amount of Line 3 that exists between Lines 1 and 2.

**Step 5:** Determine the height of the blocks. In this case, blocks were placed under $T_{Long}$, which means that the height of the blocks is assigned a negative value.

$B_{\text{Height of Blocks}}$ = -3 cm

**Step 6:** Calculate the total LLD:

Total LLD = Line 3 + $B_{\text{Height of Blocks}}$

= (+6 cm) + (-3 cm)

Total LLD = +3 cm

The total LLD value is positive, which means that the limb labeled $T_{Short}$ is short by this amount.

**Conclusion:**

The right limb ($T_{Short}$) is 3 cm shorter than the left limb ($T_{Long}$).

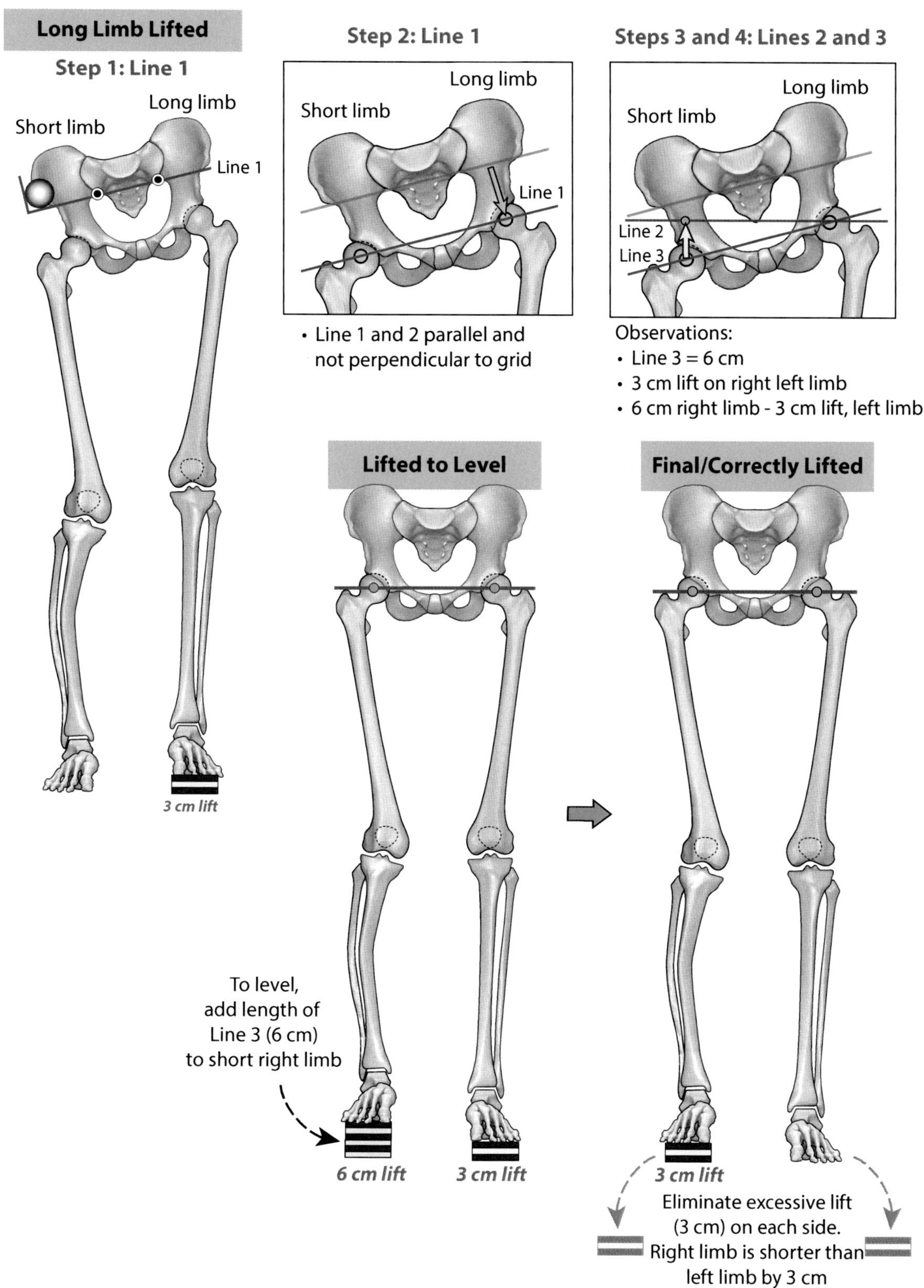


**Fig. 5:** Example of calculating total LLD when blocks were placed under the long limb instead of the short limb. Note this is the same deformity shown in Figures 2–4.

© 2023 Sinai Hospital of Baltimore

## Measure the Total LLD Using the Desired Horizontal Pelvic Line Method (Nelson Line Method)

Another strategy to calculate the total LLD utilizes a simple horizontal line. This method is called the Desired Horizontal Pelvic Line Method, or the Nelson Line Method (named after Dr. Scott Nelson at Loma Linda University). This method is helpful when radiopaque grids are not utilized in full-length standing AP x-rays.

When an x-ray grid is not present and a reproducible landmark, such as the edge of the x-ray, is not in proximity to the pelvic line, then a simple horizontal line can be drawn. This horizontal line is easily created on most digital radiographic viewing programs. When this horizontal line is placed in the proper position, it becomes the desired horizontal pelvic line. The distance between the current pelvic line and the desired horizontal pelvic line equals the limb length discrepancy. This technique eliminates any math, but the x-ray magnification needs to be taken into consideration. If blocks are used during the radiographic examination, a simple final calculation is needed.

### Introduction to the Desired Horizontal Pelvic Line Method (Nelson Line Method) (Fig. 6)

**Step 1:** Place a point on the inferior aspect of each SI joint or at the apex of each sciatic notch. Draw the current pelvic line by connecting these two points.

**Step 2:** Determine which limb appears long and which **appears** short (based on this x-ray, not the clinical exam). Remember that the imaginary ball rolls down the pelvic line towards the side that should be labeled "short." Note the presence of any blocks under the limbs.

**Step 3:** Simply move the current pelvic line to the center of the femoral head of the long leg. Note that in this method, the long limb will be assigned negative values and the short limb will be assigned positive values.

**Step 4:** Draw a simple horizontal line that starts at the center of the femoral head of the long leg. This line should be level (slope is 0°). This now represents the desired horizontal pelvic line. In other words, if this desired horizontal pelvic line was the true pelvic line, then the limb lengths would be equal.

**Step 5:** Measure the distance between the current pelvic line and the desired horizontal pelvic line at the position of the center of the femoral head of the short leg.

Distance = $T_{Short}$ = +3 cm

Check for the presence of a lift or blocks in the x-ray.

- If blocks were placed under the short limb, the height of the blocks should be added to the measured distance. The height of the blocks used is a positive value (values associated with the short limb are assigned positive values).

**Conclusion:**

The left limb (labeled the short limb) is 3 cm shorter than the right limb (labeled the long limb).

## Analyze the Lengths of Individual Bone Segments

If the total LLD has been determined, why do the individual limb segments need to be analyzed and measured? The total LLD represents the overall discrepancy in the entire limb, but it does not tell us where those discrepancies are located. The analysis of the individual bone segments will help determine which segment is contributing to the LLD. This information is essential to create a surgical strategy that achieves limb equalization and a horizontal pelvic line.

The lower limb has four segments that contribute to limb length: the pelvis, femur, tibia, and foot.

Pelvic segment = distance from the sacroiliac joint to the roof of the acetabulum (the iliac crests do not contribute to limb length)

Femoral segment = distance from the superior portion of the femoral head to the distal femoral joint line

Tibial segment = distance from the distal femoral joint line to the distal tibial joint line

Foot segment = distance from the distal tibial joint line to the floor

The height of the pelvis, femur, and tibia can each be measured directly from a full-length standing AP x-ray by using the Total LLD Method. The foot height cannot be measured directly on a full-length standing AP x-ray because it is difficult to discern where the bottom of the foot or the floor is located on the x-ray. However, the foot height contribution can be calculated.

In the following example, the total LLD will be calculated first. Then the lengths of the individual segments will be determined, and a surgical strategy will be formulated.

© 2023 Sinai Hospital of Baltimore

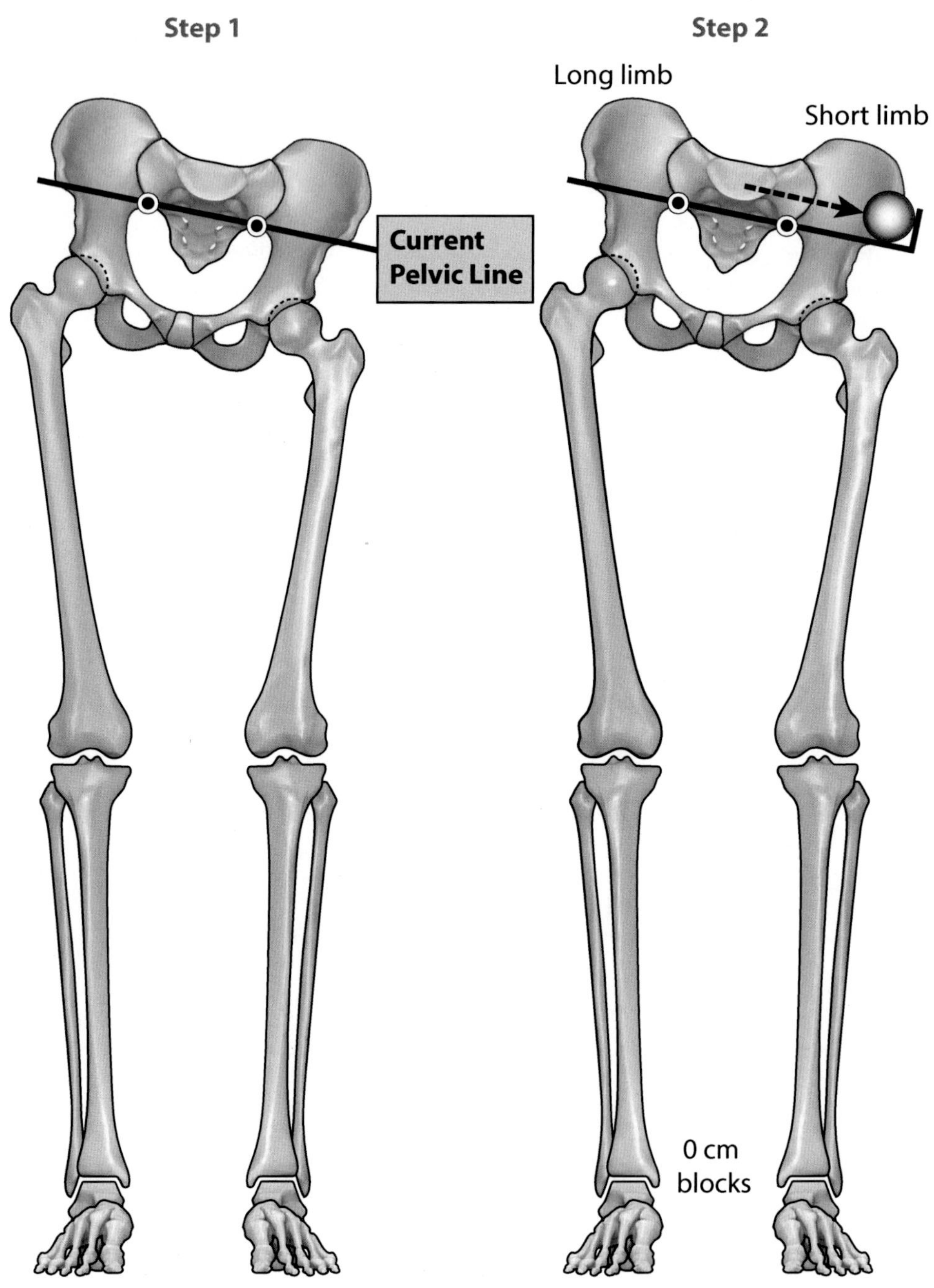


**Fig. 6:** Steps 1 and 2 to calculate the total LLD using the Desired Horizontal Pelvic Line Method.

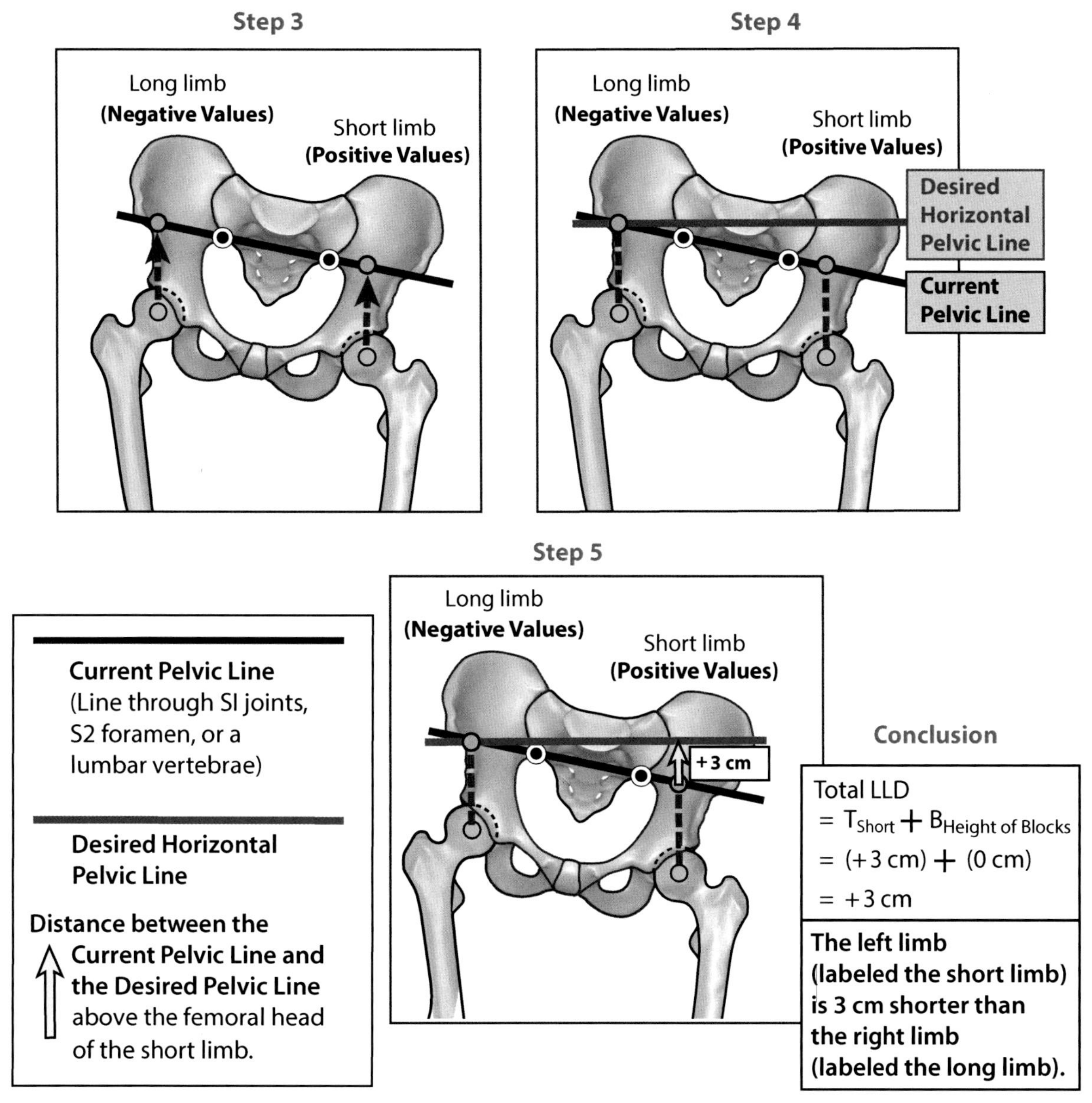


**Fig. 6 (continued):** Steps 3 through 5 using the Desired Horizontal Pelvic Line Method.

© 2023 Sinai Hospital of Baltimore

Steps 1–4

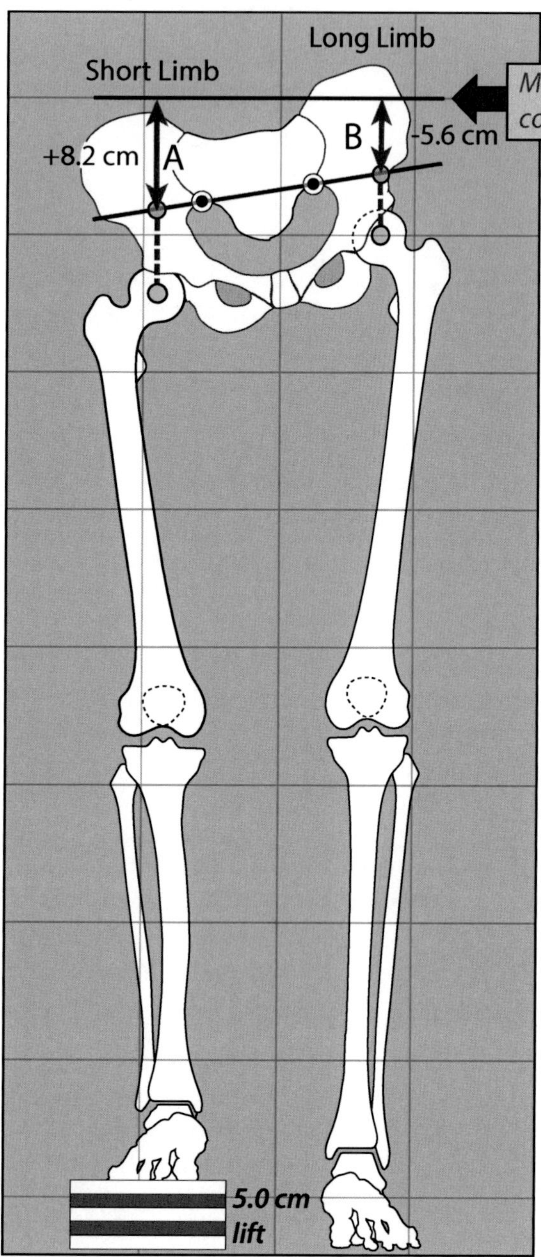


**Fig. 7:** Steps 1 through 4 to calculate the total LLD.

## Determine Total LLD (Fig. 7)

**Step 1:** Draw the pelvic line. Note that the right limb **appears** short in the x-ray.

**Step 2:** Draw two points (orange points) that are on the pelvic line and are placed directly over the center of each femoral head (blue points).

**Step 3:** Draw Line A and Line B (red lines) and measure their lengths.

- The longer line is above the leg that **appears** shorter in the x-ray. The length of that line is assigned a positive value.
  - Line A = right limb = $T_{Short}$ = +8.2 cm
- The shorter line is above the leg that **appears** longer in the x-ray. The length of that line is assigned a negative value
  - Line B = left limb = $T_{Long}$ = -5.6 cm

**Step 4:** Determine the height of the blocks under the right leg. In this case, blocks were placed under $T_{Short}$, which means the block height is assigned a positive value.

$B_{Height\ of\ Blocks}$ = +5.0 cm

**Step 5:** Calculate the total LLD:

$= T_{Short} + T_{Long} + B_{Height\ of\ Blocks}$
= (+8.2 cm) + (-5.6 cm) + (+5.0 cm)
= +7.6 cm total LLD

The total LLD value is positive, which means that the limb labeled $T_{Short}$ is short by this amount.

**Conclusion:**

The right limb ($T_{Short}$) is 7.6 cm shorter than the left limb ($T_{Long}$). The overall discrepancy in the entire limb is 7.6 cm but does not tell us where those discrepancies are located. The next step, analyzing the lengths of the individual bone segments, will show us length contributions and losses in length from the pelvis, femur, tibia, and foot segments.

## Analyze the Lengths of Individual Segments (Fig. 8)

**Step 1:** Draw the pelvic line. Draw the femoral head line for each limb at the superior margins of the femoral head. Also, draw the distal femoral joint line and the distal tibial joint line for each limb.

**Step 2:** Draw two points (orange points) that are on the pelvic line and are placed directly over the center of each femoral head. Measure the distance between each femoral head line and the orange points above each femoral head.

**Step 3:** Measure the distance between each femoral head line and each distal femoral joint line.

**Step 4:** Measure the distance between each distal femoral joint line and each distal tibial joint line.

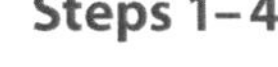


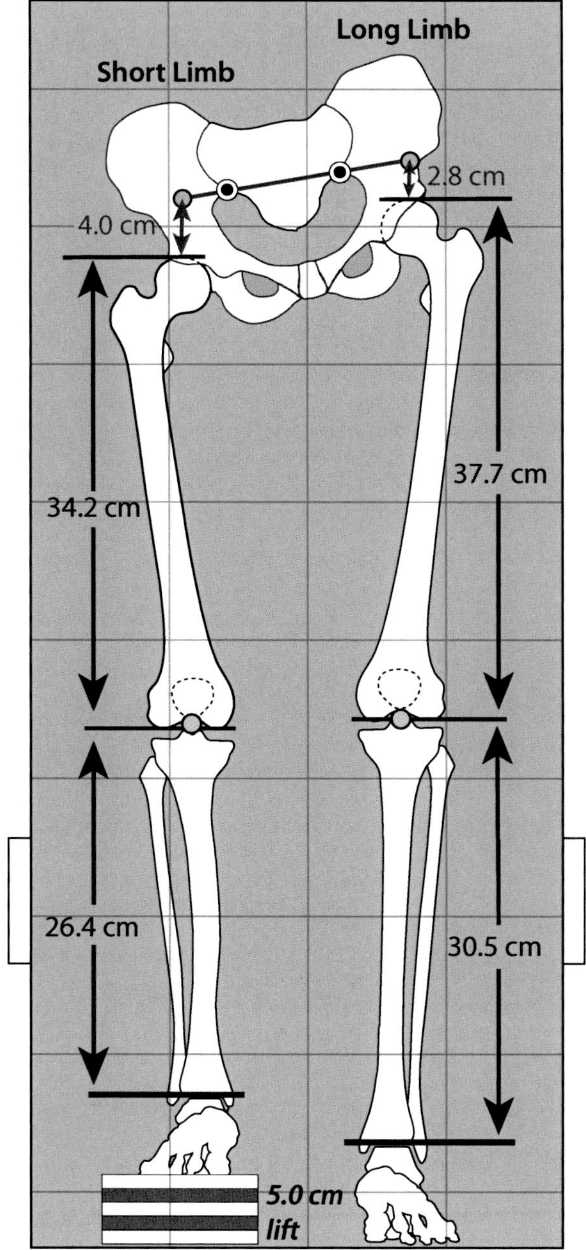


**Fig. 8:** Steps 1–4 to determine the lengths of the individual segments. Note this is the same deformity shown in Figure 7.

© 2023 Sinai Hospital of Baltimore

**Step 5:** Calculate the differences in each segment and designate them as ΔP, ΔFemur, and ΔT. The length contribution and length loss are always looked at relative to the "abnormal" limb. To ensure that the ΔP, ΔFemur, and ΔT have the correct positive/negative values, take the lengths from the "abnormal" limb and subtract the lengths from the "normal" side (see Table below). A plus sign denotes length contribution and a minus sign denotes length loss.

**Step 5**

| Calculating Pelvic, Femoral, and Tibial Length Contribution and Length Loss in the "Abnormal" Limb | | | | |
|---|---|---|---|---|
| | Length of Abnormal Side (cm) | | Length of Normal Side (cm) | Length Loss (Negative Value) or Length Contribution (Positive Value) from Each Segment (cm) |
| Pelvic Segments | 4.0 | - | 2.8 | +1.2 |
| Femoral Segments | 34.2 | - | 37.7 | -3.5 |
| Tibial Segments | 26.4 | - | 30.5 | -4.1 |

**Step 6:** The foot segment length loss/contribution can be calculated by using the formula below. Note that the height of the blocks (if any) does not need to be factored into the formula because the total LLD value (already determined to be +7.6 cm) has already accounted for the blocks.

**Step 6**

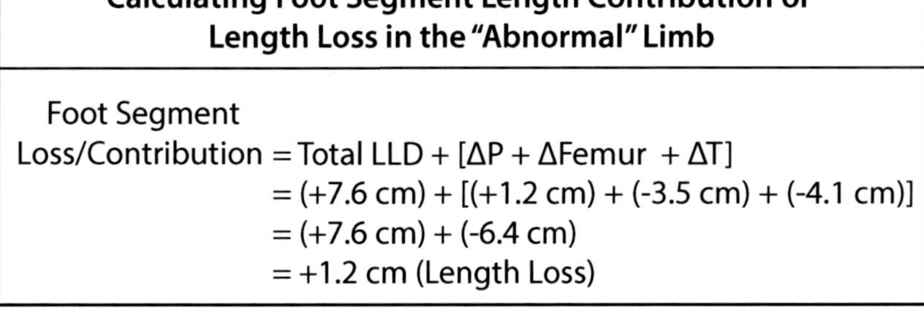

**Calculating Foot Segment Length Contribution or Length Loss in the "Abnormal" Limb**

Foot Segment Loss/Contribution = Total LLD + [ΔP + ΔFemur + ΔT]
= (+7.6 cm) + [(+1.2 cm) + (-3.5 cm) + (-4.1 cm)]
= (+7.6 cm) + (-6.4 cm)
= +1.2 cm (Length Loss)

In this example, the foot segment contributes a 1.2 cm loss of length to the "abnormal" (right) limb.

- If the foot segment contribution is positive, then the foot of the "abnormal" limb is short by that amount.
- If the foot segment contribution is negative, then the foot of the "abnormal" limb contributes that much length to the "abnormal" limb.

To determine the correct sign for ΔFoot, the length contribution or length loss is always looked at relative to the "abnormal" limb. Since the foot of the abnormal limb is shorter than the contralateral foot, this means that ΔFoot = -1.2 cm (this is a negative value because there is a loss of length in the right foot). This negative value for ΔFoot will be used in the next section to determine the surgical strategy.

## MAP the LLD: Pick the Shortened Bone Segment

Once the LLD measurement and the analysis of the individual bone segments have been completed, the LLD's contributing factors can be identified. When creating a surgical lengthening strategy, the pelvis and femur are considered one functional unit, and the tibia and foot are another functional unit. This means that any loss of length in the pelvis and femur is usually gained in the femur. Any loss of length in the foot and tibia is gained in the tibia. This is not an absolute rule. If significant deformity lies in the pelvis or foot, then corrective osteotomies could gain length from these segments simultaneously.

In the previous example, the total LLD was calculated to be a 7.6 cm discrepancy in the right leg. The right hemipelvis contributed 1.2 cm of length, and the femur contributed 3.5 cm loss of length:

ΔP = +1.2 cm (right pelvis contributing length)

ΔFemur = -3.5 cm (right femoral discrepancy)

ΔP + ΔFemur = pelvic and femoral contribution to total LLD

(+1.2 cm) + (-3.5 cm) = -2.3 cm pelvic and femoral contribution to total LLD

The tibia contributed a loss of length of 4.1 cm, and the foot contributed a 1.2 cm loss of length.

ΔT = -4.1 cm (right tibial discrepancy)

ΔFoot = -1.2 cm (right foot discrepancy)

ΔT + ΔFoot = tibial and foot contribution to total LLD

(-4.1 cm) + (-1.2 cm) = -5.3 cm tibial and foot contribution to total LLD

The pelvis and femur contribute 2.3 cm to the 7.6 cm discrepancy. The tibia and foot contribute 5.3 cm to the 7.6 cm discrepancy. The most problematic segment in this example is the tibia/foot segment. The surgical strategy would be a 5.3 cm tibial lengthening. This would address the significant limb length difference. The femoral difference can be addressed in the future with either a contralateral femoral epiphysiodesis or ipsilateral femoral lengthening at skeletal maturity.

## Correcting Significant Deformities Can Result in a Gain in Length

The presence of a significant deformity in the limb of interest should be taken into consideration when developing a surgical strategy. Significant deformities require realignment for functional improvement but are also a source of hidden length that must be identified and calculated. The amount of limb length that will be gained from a deformity correction can be calculated by using segmental measurements and a simple formula.

$M_2 - M_1$ = amount of length gained from deformity correction

Where:

$M_1$ = length of the limb's mechanical axis

$M_2$ = femoral and tibial axis lengths on the convex side of the limb. The measurements on the convex side of the limb may consist of multiple segments. The segments are simply added.

© 2023 Sinai Hospital of Baltimore

## Example of Calculating Length Gain After Correction of a Significant Deformity (Fig. 9)

The segmental lengths of the femur and tibia on the convexity of the deformity are added together ($M_2$).

$M_2$ = 35.4 cm + 7.0 cm + 30.5 cm = 72.9 cm

The length of the lower limb's overall mechanical axis ($M_1$) is measured.

$M_1$ = 70.3 cm

The formula for estimating length gain from deformity correction:

$M_2 - M_1$ = amount of length gained from deformity correction

72.9 cm – 70.3 cm = 2.6 cm gained from deformity correction

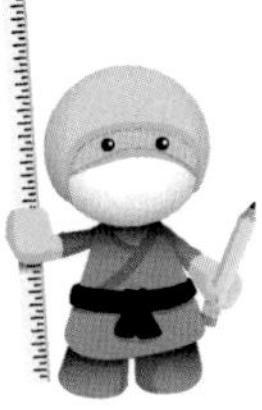

*Sensei says,*
*"He who has limb deformity has hidden length."*

## Alternate Strategy to Determine Foot Segment Length Loss/Contribution With Bilateral Ankle AP X-ray

If you do not have a full-length standing AP x-ray of both limbs, you can still determine the foot segment length loss/contribution by examining a bilateral ankle AP x-ray. The same deformity is assessed in the following three examples. Each example shows a different scenario for the placement of the blocks: no lift is used, the short foot is overlifted, and the long foot is lifted. The same deformity is handled in three different ways when positioning the patient for the x-ray, but you can still use the same formula.

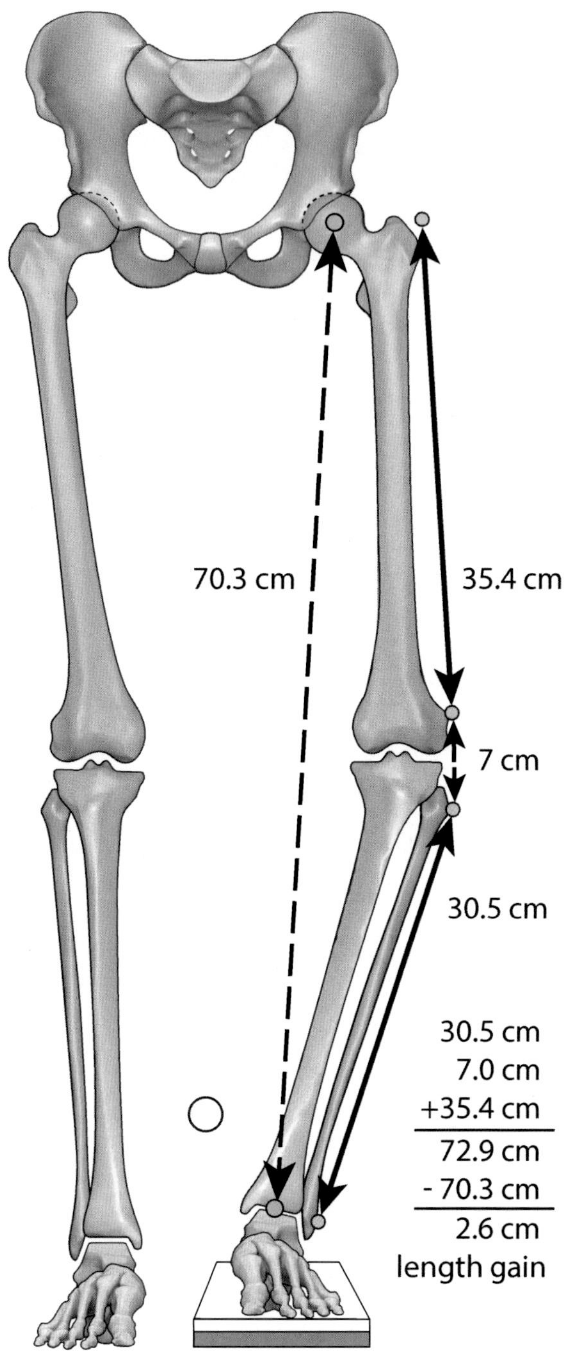


**Fig. 9:** Length can be gained when a significant deformity is corrected. To calculate the amount of length that will be gained, measure the length of the limb's mechanical axis, measure the lengths of the femur/knee/tibia on the convex side of the limb, and then use the formula.

## Direct Method of Determining Foot Segment Contribution When Lift Is Not Used in the X-ray (Fig. 10)

**Step 1:** Draw the distal tibial joint line for each limb.

**Step 2:** Draw a line (Line A) that starts at the right distal tibial joint line. Direct the line proximally and end it at a grid line on the x-ray. Create a second line (Line B) that starts at the left distal tibial joint line and is directed proximally. Line B should end at the same common grid line on the x-ray that Line A ends on.

**Step 3:** Measure the lengths of Line A and Line B. This step aims to determine which foot segment **appears** shorter and which **appears** longer in this x-ray. The short/long labels on the foot segments may not match which limb was determined to be short after the clinical assessment, or which limb was determined to be short when calculating total LLD using a full-length standing x-ray.

- The longer line is above the foot segment that appears shorter (right foot) and is given a positive value
    - Line A = right foot = $F_{Short}$ = +7.4 cm
- The shorter line is above the foot segment that appears longer (left foot) and is given a negative value.
    - Line B = left foot = $F_{Long}$ = -6.2 cm

**Step 4:** Note that no blocks were used to lift either foot ($B_{Height\ of\ Blocks}$ = 0 cm). Calculate the foot segment contribution:

$F_{Short} + F_{Long} + B_{Height\ of\ Blocks}$ = foot segment contribution

(+7.4 cm) + (-6.2 cm) + 0 cm = +1.2 cm

The foot segment contribution has a positive value, which means that the right foot segment labeled $F_{Short}$ is shorter than the left foot segment.

**Conclusion:**

The right foot ($F_{Short}$) is 1.2 cm shorter than the left foot ($F_{Long}$).

© 2023 Sinai Hospital of Baltimore

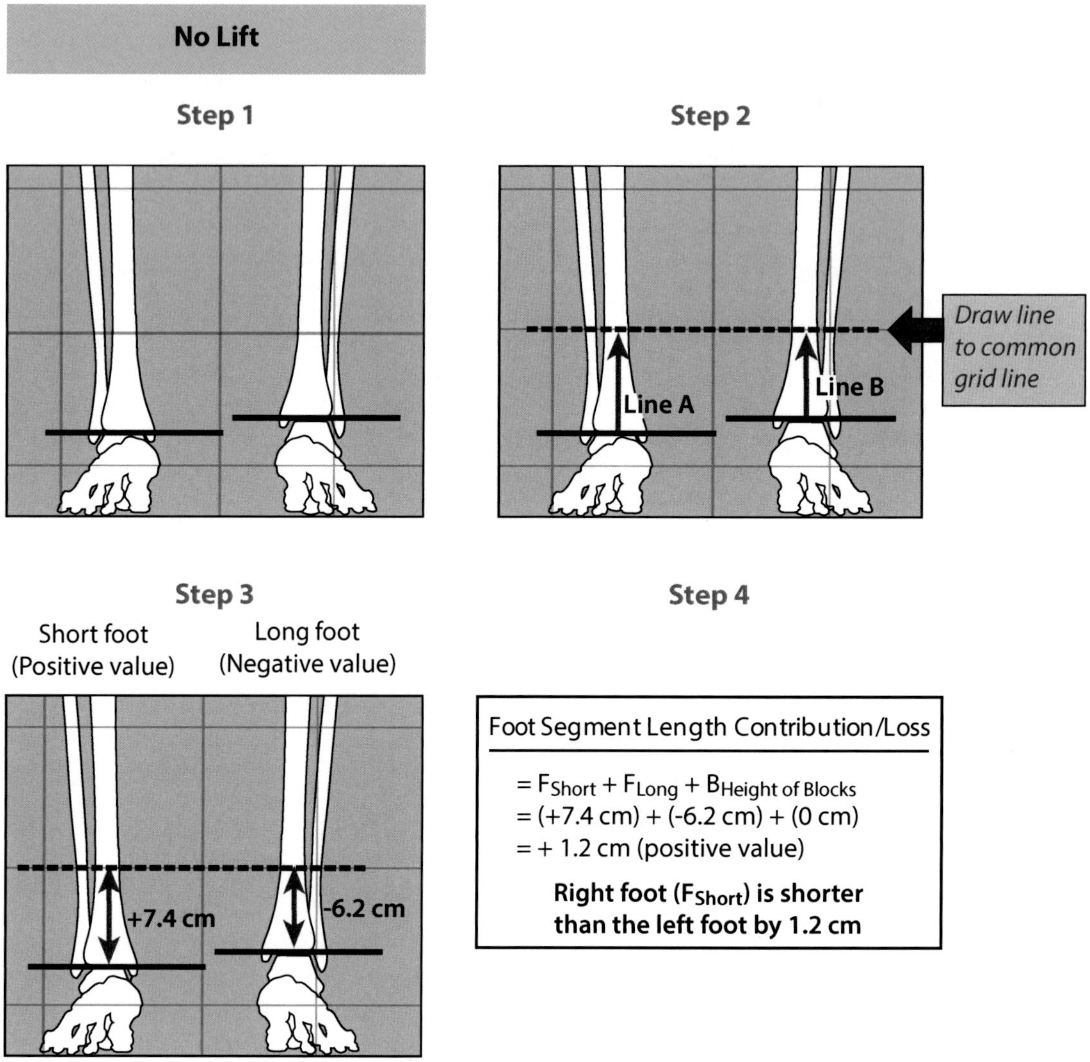

No Lift

Step 1

Step 2

Draw line to common grid line

Line A

Line B

Step 3

Short foot (Positive value)

Long foot (Negative value)

+7.4 cm

-6.2 cm

Step 4

Foot Segment Length Contribution/Loss

$= F_{Short} + F_{Long} + B_{Height\ of\ Blocks}$
$= (+7.4\ cm) + (-6.2\ cm) + (0\ cm)$
$= +\ 1.2\ cm$ (positive value)

**Right foot ($F_{Short}$) is shorter than the left foot by 1.2 cm**

**Fig. 10:** Example of calculating foot segment contribution/loss when no blocks are used to position the feet in the x-ray.

## Direct Method: Short Foot Overlifted (Fig. 11)

**Step 1:** Draw the distal tibial joint line for each limb. Draw Line A and Line B so that they both end at the same common grid line on the x-ray.

**Step 2:** Measure the lengths of Line A and Line B. This step's goal is to determine which foot segment **appears** shorter and which **appears** longer in this x-ray.

- The shorter line is above the longer foot segment and is given a negative value.
   - Line A = right side = $F_{Long}$ = -2.4 cm
- The longer line is above the shorter foot segment and is given a positive value.
   - Line B = left side = $F_{Short}$ = +6.2 cm

**Step 3:** In this example, the blocks were placed under the long foot segment ($F_{Long}$). This means the height of the blocks (5.0 cm) should be assigned a negative value.

- If blocks were placed under the foot segment that we labeled short ($F_{Short}$), then the height of the blocks ($B_{Height\ of\ Blocks}$) should be included in the formula as a **positive value**.

## Short Foot Over Lifted

**Step 1**

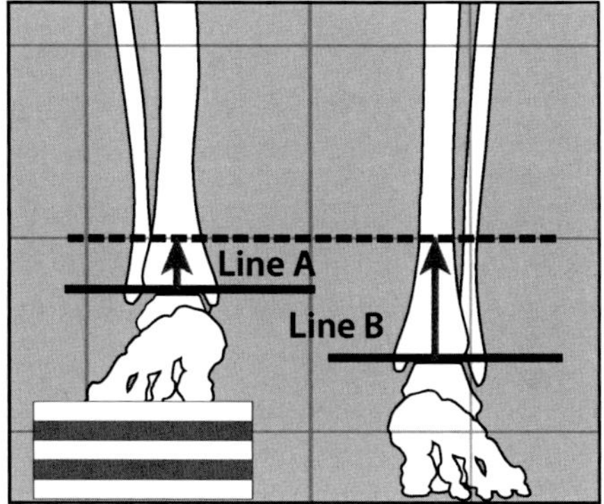


**Steps 2 and 3**

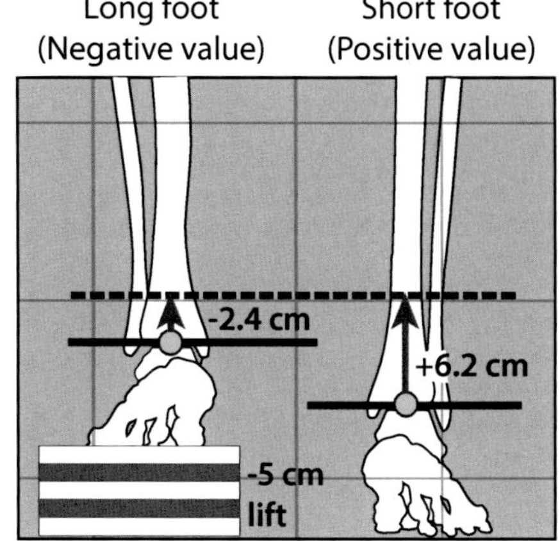


**Step 4**

Foot Segment Length Contribution/Loss

$= F_{Short} + F_{Long} + B_{Height\ of\ Blocks}$
$= (+6.2\ cm) + (-2.4\ cm) + (-5\ cm)$
$= -1.2$ cm (negative value)

**Right foot ($F_{Long}$) is shorter than the left foot by 1.2 cm**

**Fig. 11:** Example of calculating foot segment contribution/loss when the blocks that are placed under the short foot have caused it to be overlifted. Note this is the same deformity shown in Figure 10.

- If blocks were placed under the foot segment that we labeled long ($F_{Long}$), then the height of the blocks should be assigned a **negative value**.

**Step 4:** Calculate the foot segment contribution:

$$F_{Short} + F_{Long} + B_{Height\ of\ Blocks} = \text{Foot segment contribution}$$

(+6.2 cm) + (-2.4 cm) + (-5.0 cm) = -1.2 cm

The foot segment contribution has a negative value, which means that the right foot segment labeled $F_{Long}$ is shorter than the left foot segment ($F_{Short}$).

**Conclusion:**

The right foot ($F_{Long}$) is 1.2 cm shorter than the left foot ($F_{Short}$).

**Long Foot Lifted**

**Step 1**

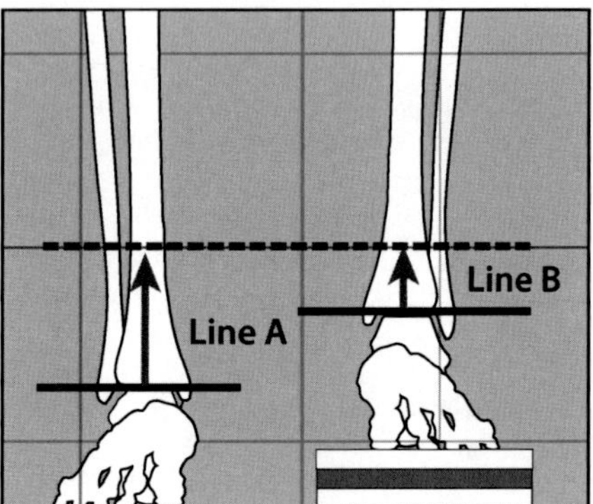


**Steps 2 and 3**

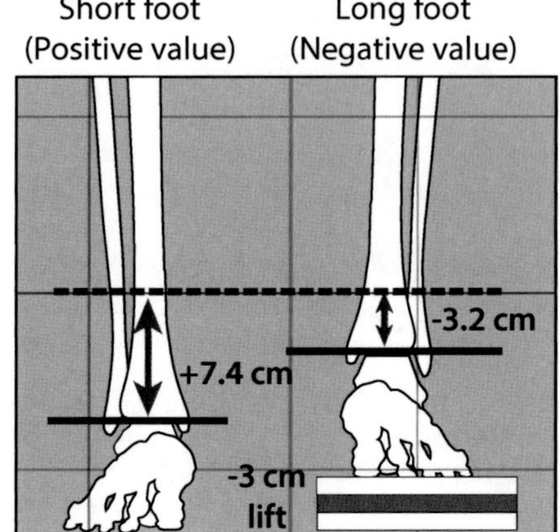


**Step 4**

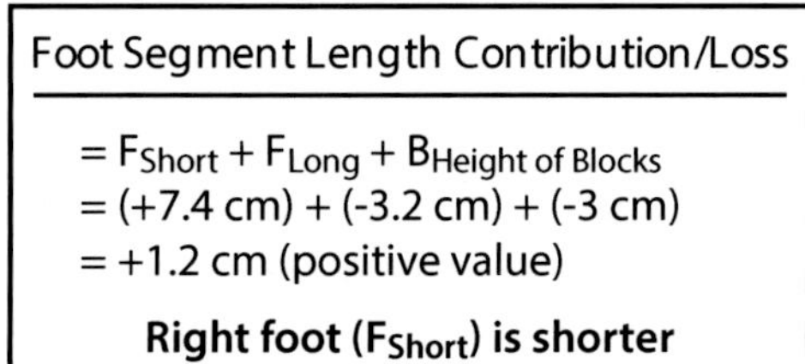


**Fig. 12:** Example of calculating foot segment contribution/loss when blocks are placed under the long foot. Note this is the same deformity shown in Figures 10 and 11.

## Direct Method: Long Foot Lifted (Fig. 12)

**Step 1:** Draw the distal tibial joint line for each limb. Draw Line A and Line B so that they both end at the same common grid line on the x-ray.

**Step 2:** Measure the lengths of Line A and Line B.

- The shorter line is above the longer foot segment and is given a negative value.
  - Line B = left side = $F_{Long}$ = -3.2 cm
- The longer line is above the shorter foot segment and is given a positive value.
  - Line A = right side = $F_{Short}$ = +7.4 cm

**Step 3:** In this example, the blocks were placed under the long foot segment ($F_{Long}$). This means that the height of the blocks (3.0 cm) should be assigned a negative value.

**Step 4:** Calculate the foot segment contribution:

$F_{Short} + F_{Long} + B_{Height\ of\ Blocks}$ = foot segment contribution

(+7.4 cm) + (-3.2 cm) + (-3.0 cm) = +1.2 cm

The foot segment length contribution/loss has a positive value, which means that the right foot segment labeled $F_{Short}$ is shorter than the left foot segment.

**Conclusion:**

The right foot ($F_{Long}$) is 1.2 cm shorter than the left foot ($F_{Long}$).

## Pitfalls in Determining Limb Length Discrepancy: MAP the LLD

Inferior assessment techniques are common pitfalls in the determination of LLD. These include inferior x-ray quality, improper positioning of a patient when an x-ray is obtained, incorrect x-ray technique, and incorrect use of blocks. Other confounding factors include soft-tissue contractures and significant deformities in the lower extremities. However, the most common pitfall is not understanding the process for assessing LLDs. By following the mnemonic MAP the LLD, the determination of limb length discrepancies will become consistent, straightforward, and accurate.

## References

1. Shapiro F. Lower extremity length discrepancies. In: Shapiro F, ed. *Pediatric Orthopedic Deformities*. 1st ed. Cambridge, MA: Academic Press, 2001:606-608.

2. Paley D. *Principles of Deformity Correction*. 1st ed. Berlin, Germany: Springer, 2002.

© 2023 Sinai Hospital of Baltimore

# Chapter 12

# Reverse Planning for Femoral Deformity

Philip K. McClure, MD

"Reverse planning" entails correcting length and deformity through the creation of the final corrected alignment, and then "reversing" the lengthening to generate the operative plan. This concept may be further simplified to "beginning with the end in mind." The reverse planning method for lengthening and deformity correction was initially introduced to the literature by Rainer Baumgart in 2009.[1] It is particularly important to the femur because the anatomic and mechanical axes of normal femora deviate from each other by 5° to 7°. This discrepancy causes an obligatory mechanical axis deviation to occur if lengthening is performed along the anatomic axis (Fig. 1).[2] When lengthening with an external fixator, the skilled surgeon has the option to choose which axis the lengthening follows, inclining the pins to the mechanical axis if necessary to maintain or obtain neutral alignment at the completion of lengthening.

Options for deformity correction and lengthening include restoration of the neutral mechanical axis prior to lengthening, at the completion of lengthening, or after the initial lengthening has healed (Fig. 2). The surgeon's choice of methods may depend on multiple factors: severity and nature of the patient's presenting complaint (length or deformity), knee stability, hip stability, severity of deformity if present, apex of deformity (proximal, distal, or diaphyseal), and the functional status of the distal femoral growth plate. It is important to note that age is not necessarily a primary factor, though generally it is a surrogate for physeal function. Complete distal femoral growth arrests are common in the settings of various causes of limb length discrepancy (e.g., posttraumatic and post-septic deformity), and retrograde lengthening is an option in this setting regardless of patient age.

© 2023 Sinai Hospital of Baltimore

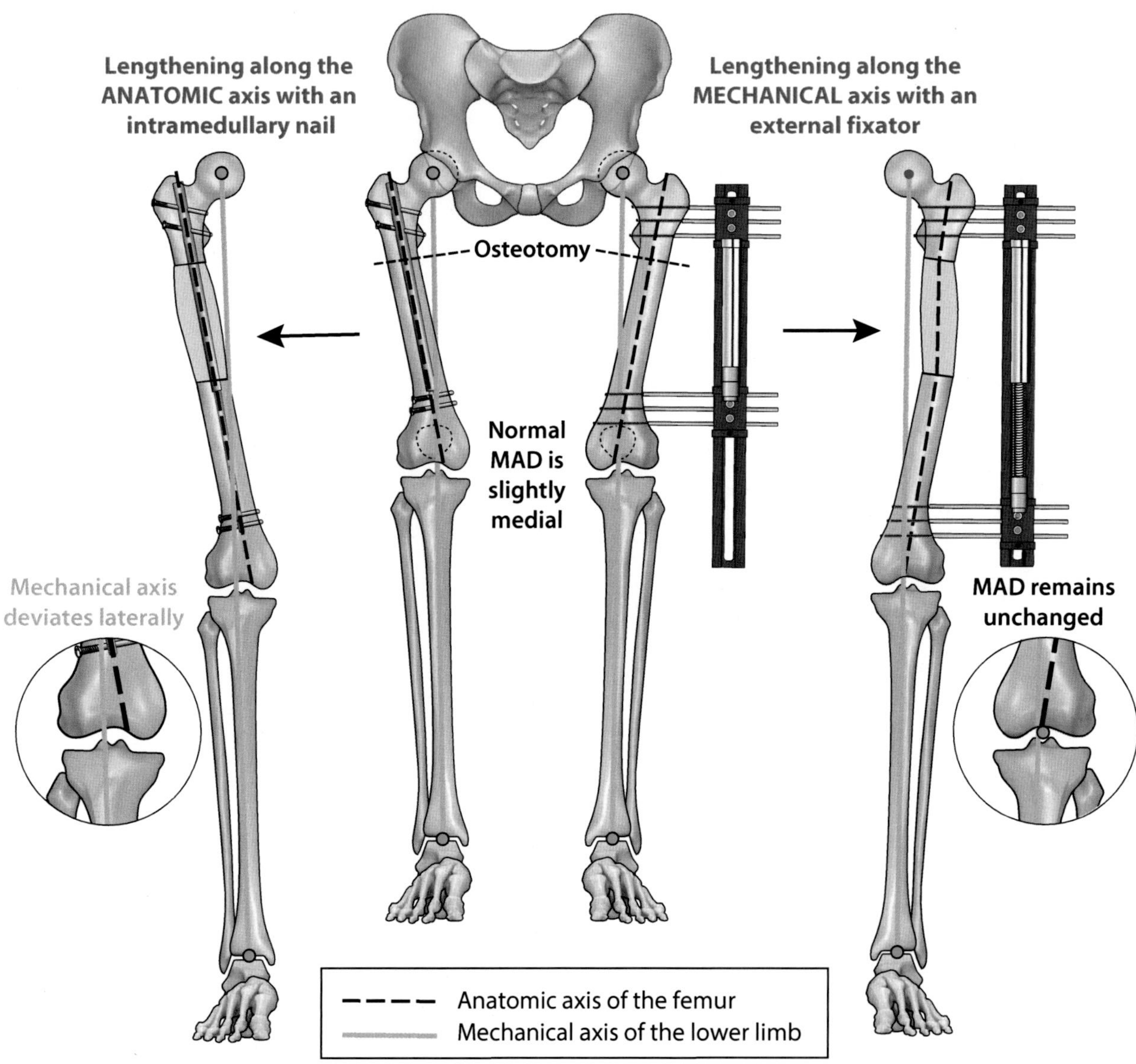


**Fig. 1:** When lengthening along the anatomic axis, the mechanical axis shifts laterally. When lengthening along the mechanical axis, the mechanical axis does not change. MAD, mechanical axis deviation.

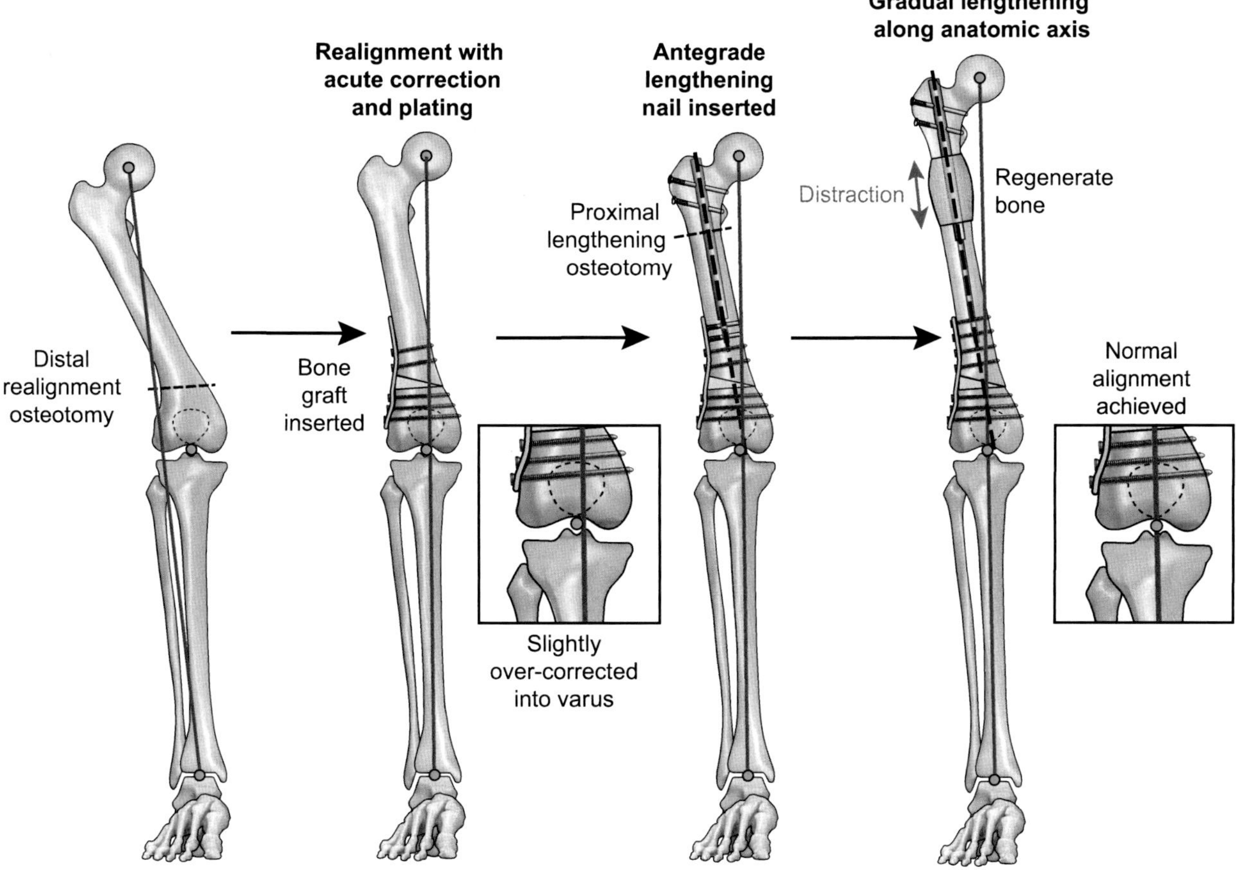


**Fig. 2: A**, Realignment with distal femoral osteotomy and then antegrade femoral lengthening.

© 2023 Sinai Hospital of Baltimore

B

Angular Correction and Femoral Lengthening with Retrograde Nail in One Stage

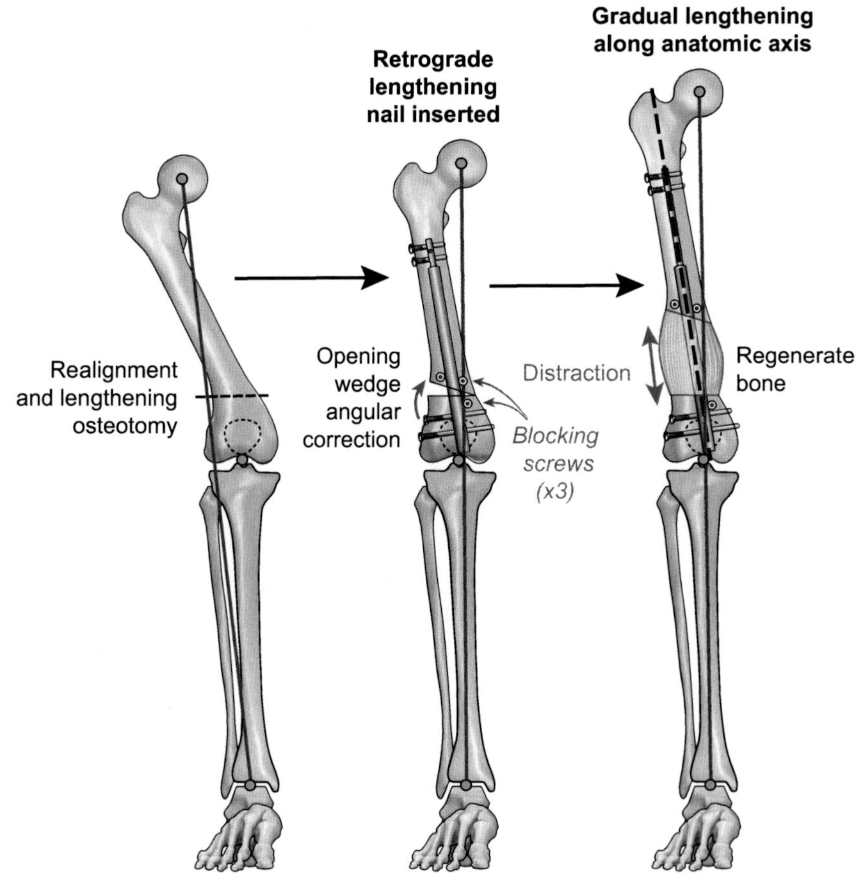


**Fig. 2 (continued): B**, Reverse planning and angular correction with one-stage lengthening.

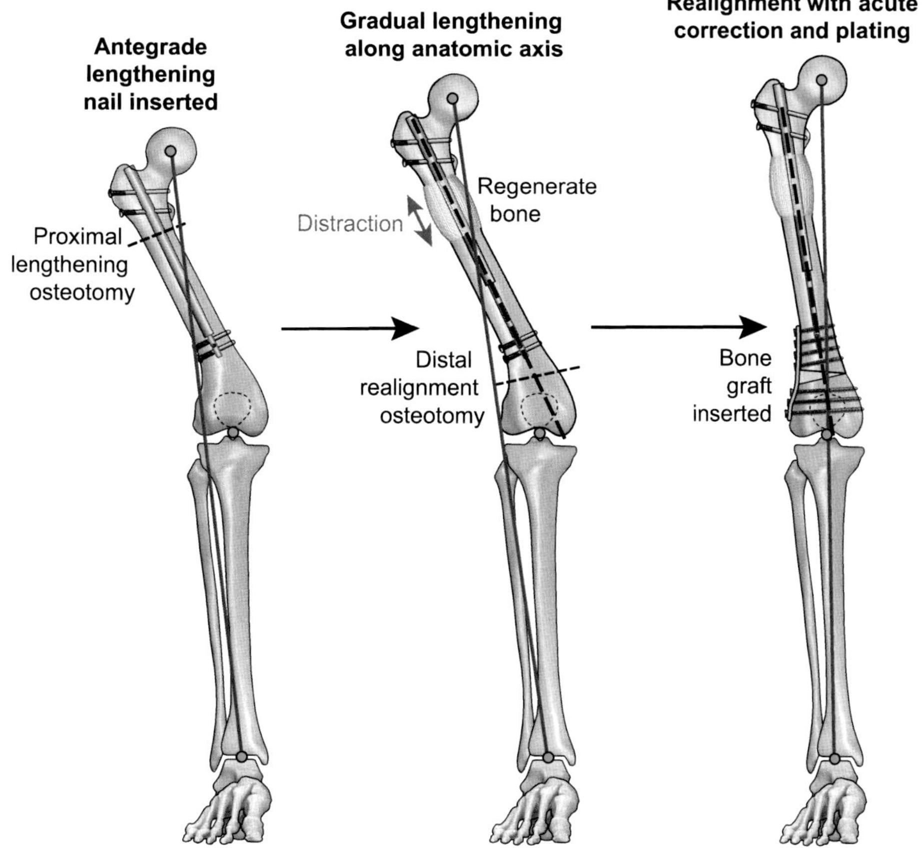


**Fig. 2 (continued): C**, Antegrade lengthening followed by distal femoral osteotomy for angular correction.

An important component when considering reverse planning is to be sure to carefully analyze your deformities as outlined throughout this book to ensure the technique is applicable to your patient's problem. In Figure 3, an isolated deformity of the distal femur on the short side is present. This is an ideal situation for the reverse planning technique.

The reverse planning method is an important concept to understand and will be outlined here using digital planning software.[3] The initial publication by Baumgart[1] can be referenced if manual planning using paper is preferred (Fig. 4), as the primary concepts are the same in both the classic and modified methods. That method for femoral lengthening requires modification to improve the accuracy of the lengthening magnitude. The requite modification is presented in this chapter (Fig. 5). In general, the take-home message is to "begin with the end in mind." While the reverse planning concept can be applied to antegrade and retrograde femoral lengthening, the mechanical constraints of lengthening nails make it most applicable to retrograde femoral lengthening.

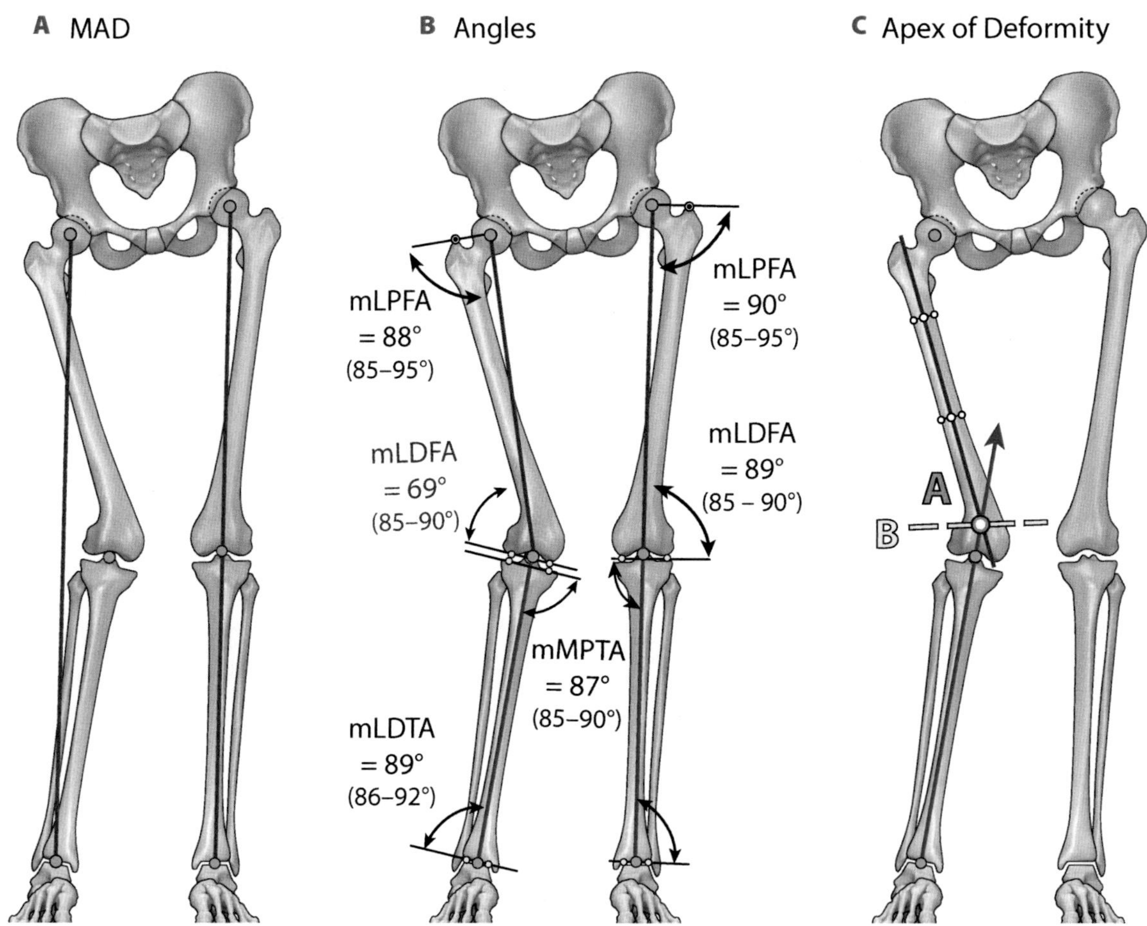


**Fig. 3: A**, The mechanical axis of the right leg falls well lateral to the knee, indicating valgus alignment of the lower limb. Leg length discrepancy also is present. **B**, Analysis of individual bone segments reveals a normal tibia bilaterally, a normal femur on the left, and a deformed femur on the right side. **C**, The apex of the femoral deformity is at the level of the distal metaphysis.

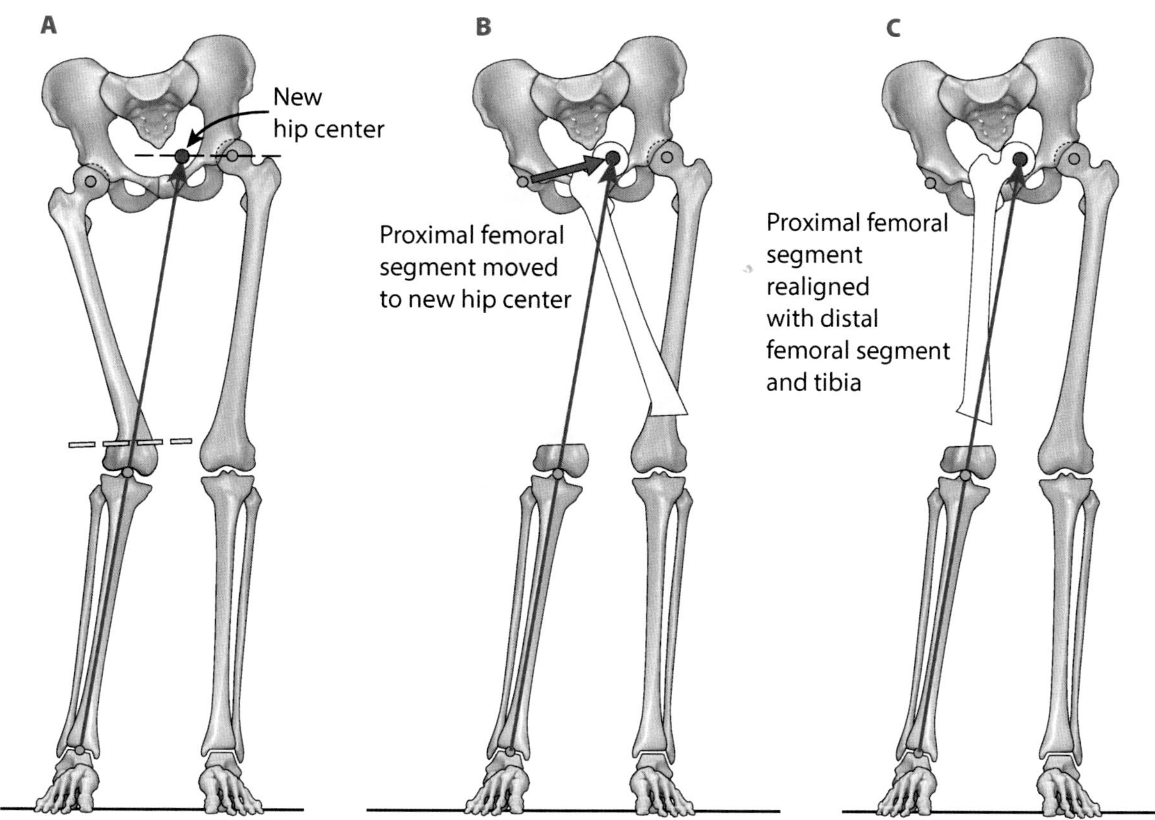


**Fig. 4:** "Classic" Baumgart reverse lengthening planning. **A**, Having determined an acceptable tibia, the new mechanical axis of the limb is extended proximally. A new hip center is drawn where this line intersects with a horizontal line at the level of the contralateral hip. **B**, The operative hip center is moved to the "new hip center." **C**, The operative femur is rotated until an appropriate position is identified for intramedullary nail placement.

© 2023 Sinai Hospital of Baltimore

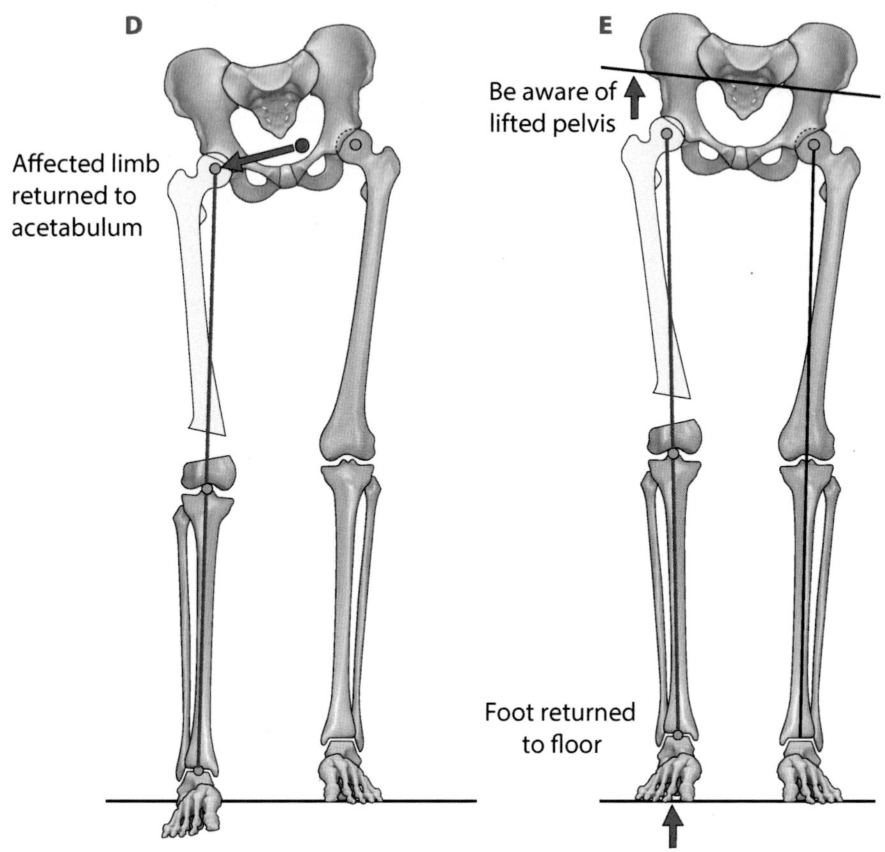


**Fig. 4 (continued): D**, For illustration purposes, the final femur alignment is moved to the old hip center, without changing its alignment or length. **E**, With the operative limb restored to the floor, overlengthening is evident. This results from the original deviation of the tibial axis from the vertical axis, and the error becomes larger as that angle increases.

Ideally, radiographs to use in planning are obtained with the tibia oriented vertically perpendicular to the floor, as this improves the accuracy of length correction. When this position cannot be captured on the film, the surgeon should plan the length along the planned mechanical axis from the ankle (Fig. 5) rather than using the Baumgart method[1] of horizontally moving the new hip center across from the contralateral side. The latter technique can be imprecise in a manner that becomes strikingly conspicuous when the tibia is not vertically oriented by greater than 5-10°, as seen in Figure 5. More significant deviations from vertical position demonstrate more striking errors.

If using digital planning software, the first step is to import the images. The preferred method is exporting jpeg images from a picture archive and communication system (PACS). Taking a photograph of the screen is not recommended, but may be adequate if the picture is taken with the line of imaging "normal" to the center of the image being captured. Deviation from this results in parallax, similar to a poorly obtained radiograph. An extreme example is shown in Figure 6, where the neutral grid is distorted significantly by an off-angle photograph. The effects of this on planning can be subtle yet significant.

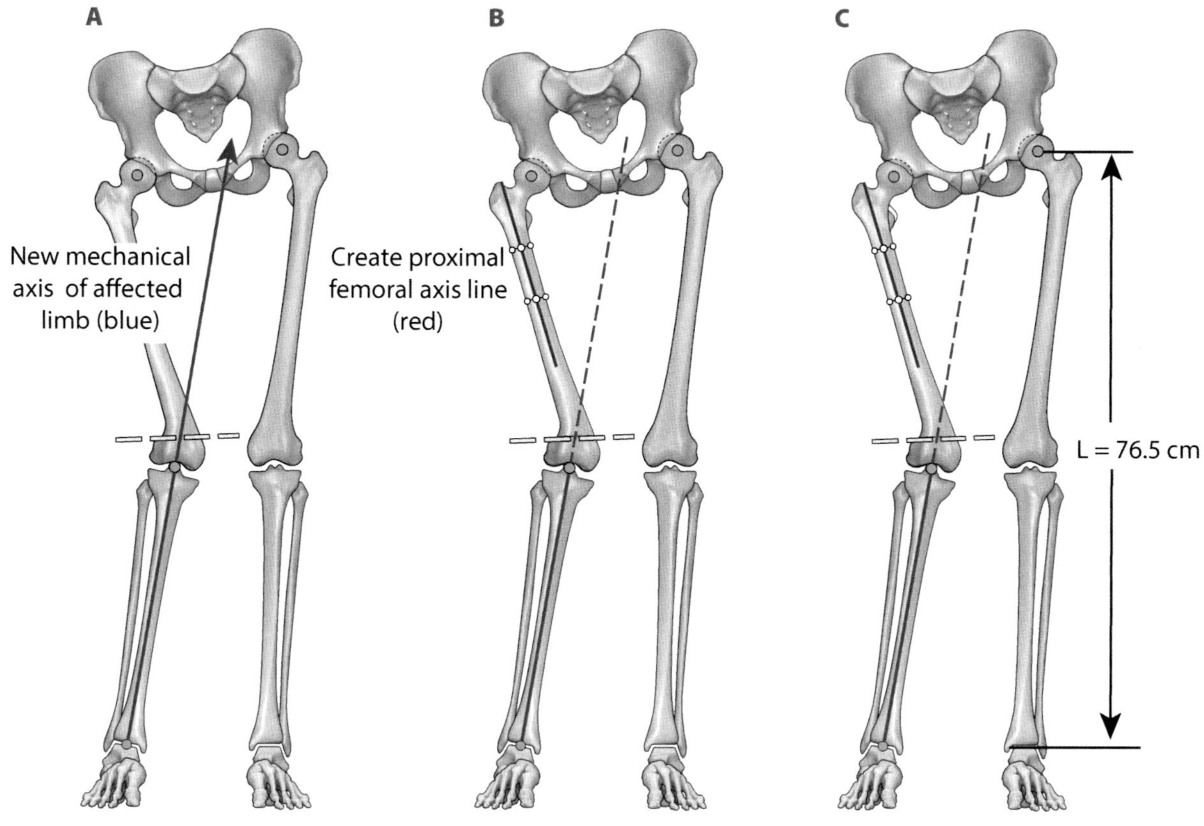


**Fig. 5:** The modified Baumgart reverse planning technique. **A**, Extend the mechanical axis of the tibia proximally to define the new mechanical axis of the limb. **B**, Create a proximal femoral axis. **C**, Measure the length of the contralateral limb (be sure to account for future growth if applicable).

© 2023 Sinai Hospital of Baltimore

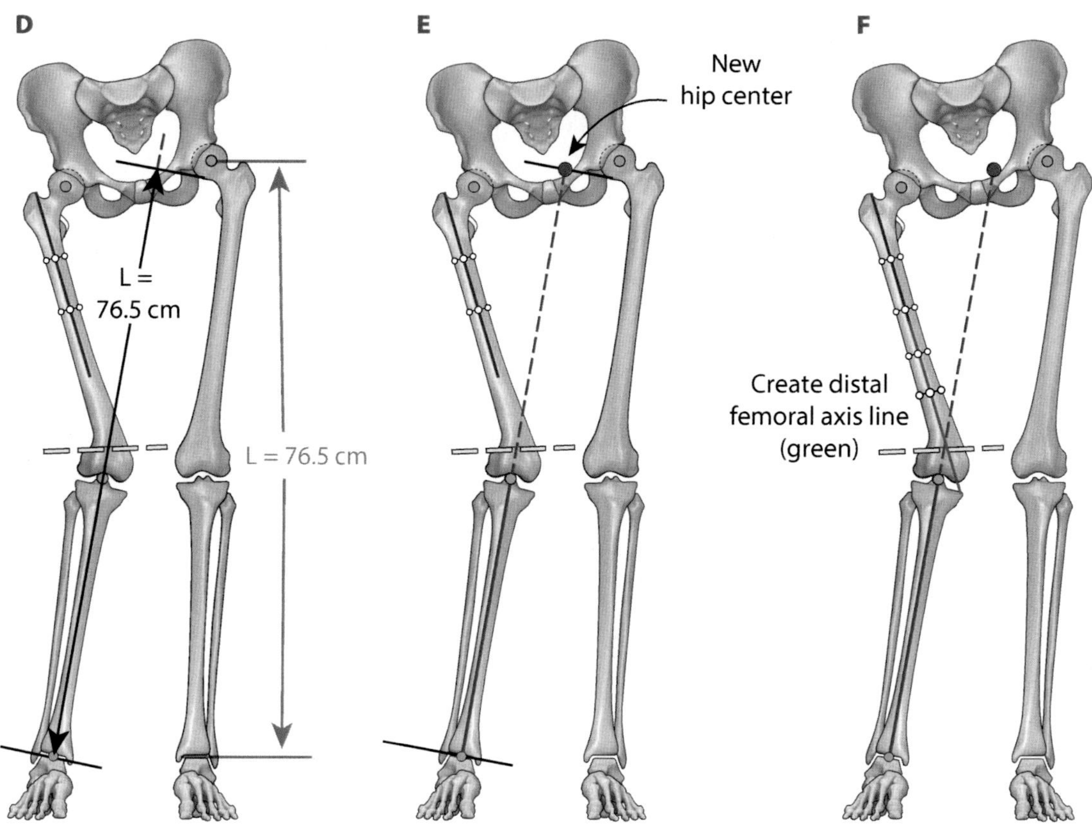


**Fig. 5 (continued): D**, Measure this length (planned lengthening) along the new mechanical axis of the short limb. **E**, Mark the new hip center accordingly. **F**, Create a new distal femoral axis line that is colinear with the proximal femoral axis line.

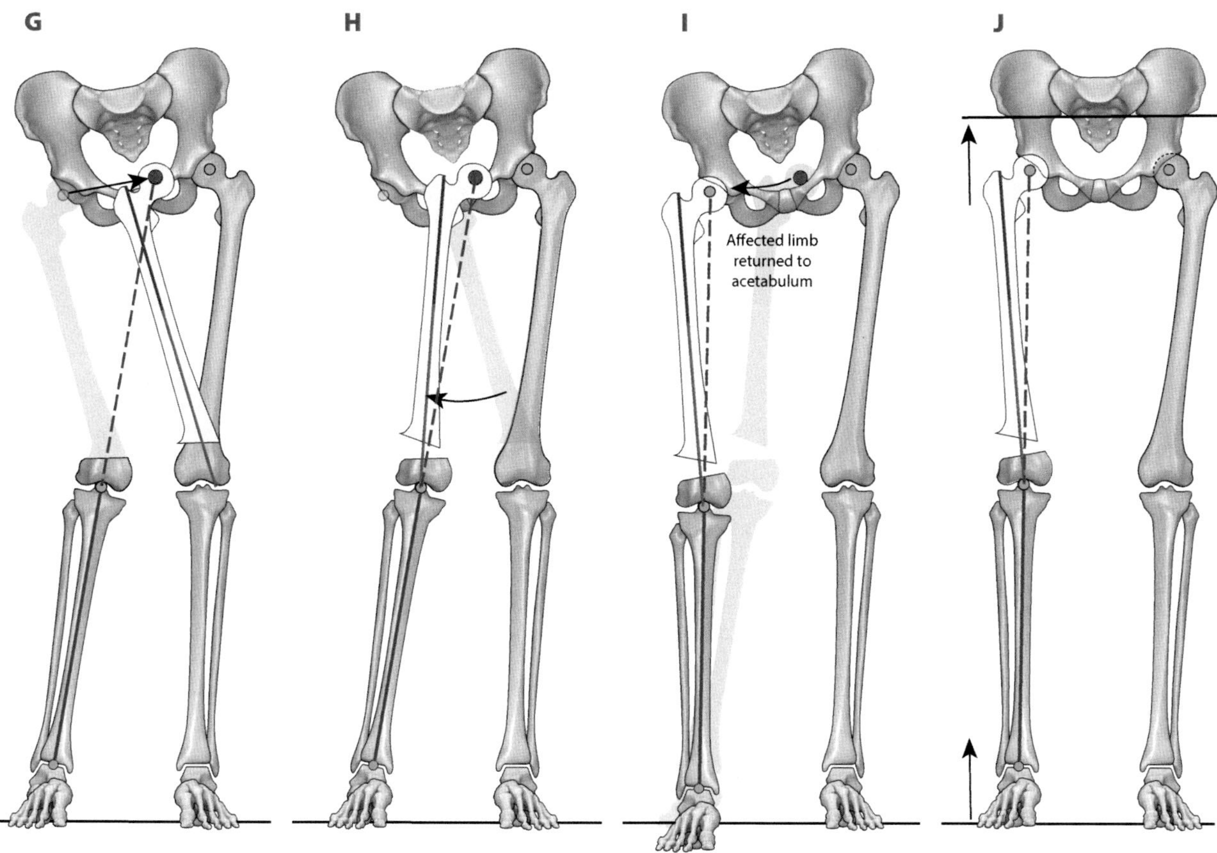


**Fig. 5 (continued): G**, Create an osteotomy line 6–8 cm up from the joint line, and move the entire proximal segment along with the femoral axis lines to the new hip center. **H**, Rotate the proximal segment until the distal femoral axis line (nail line) goes through the notch of the distal femur. This generates your final femoral alignment after lengthening. **I**, The lower limb and **J**, pelvis are returned to normal alignment to demonstrate and confirm adequate correction of deformity and length.

© 2023 Sinai Hospital of Baltimore

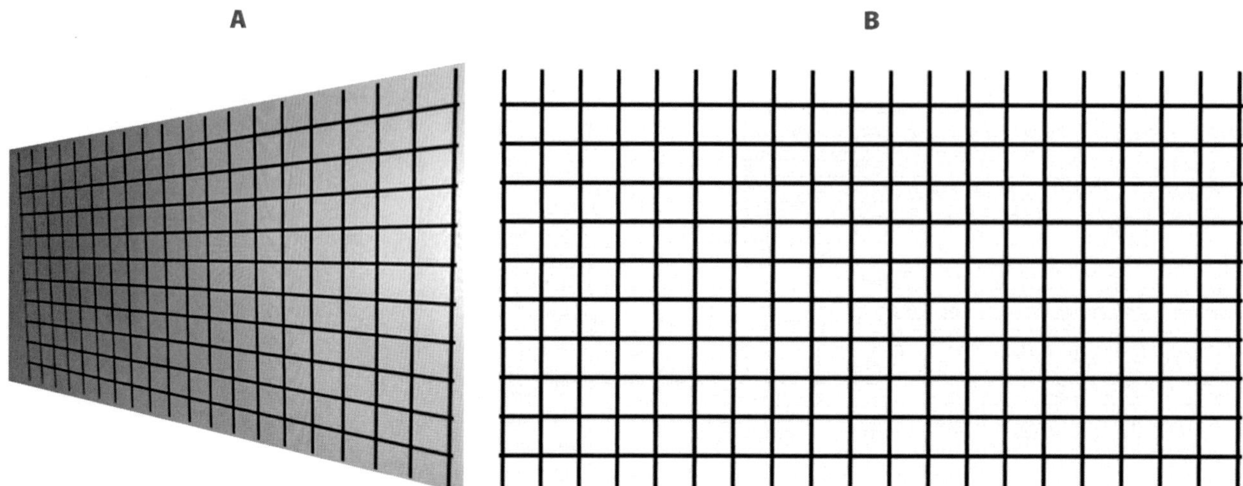


**Fig. 6: A**, A neutral grid is distorted significantly when an off-angle image is captured. **B**, A neutral grid with the line of imaging "normal" to the center of the image.

Once the images are imported into the software and opened, the first step is to calibrate the images to allow accurate measurements of length (Fig. 7). After you press the calibrate button, a circle tool will appear. Grab the blue calibration circle tool by the dotted circumferential line and drag it over the magnification marker. Resize the dashed circular line so that it is centered on the edge of the magnification marker by using the two solid blue balls on either side of the circle. Next, enter the diameter of the magnification marker in the calibrate field at the top of the screen. Alternatively, the circular marker can be used to measure a 5-cm grid line, again being careful to use the center of the dotted line as the measurement point.

Once the images are appropriately obtained and calibrated, the next critical step is deformity analysis. This process is completed following the methods that are presented in previous chapters ("Deformity Analysis in the Sagittal Plane," "Tibial Axis Planning: Frontal and Sagittal Planes," and "Femoral Axis Planning: Frontal and Sagittal Planes").

The reverse planning method typically does not plan sagittal alignment independently. Regardless, the images must be scrutinized for apex of deformity, soft-tissue contractures/compensations, and canal fit. The surgeon should be sure that the planned coronal correction correlates with the sagittal apex (if present) and plan for soft-tissue considerations accordingly. In rare cases, severe sagittal deformity results in "found length" upon its correction, and this would need to be taken into account. The amount of length to be obtained comes from a combination of radiographic measurements and clinical data. The radiographic measurements can be made in PACS or within the software after calibration. In cases with complex anatomy, the use of a preoperative shoe lift can be valuable to determine the appropriate amount of length needed. This typically requires several months and multiple adjustments of the lift to garner useful data. Though time-consuming, it is difficult to get better data regarding ideal leg lengths in the setting of complex skeletal abnormalities (e.g., congenital scoliosis, abnormal hip centers, posterior pelvic variations).

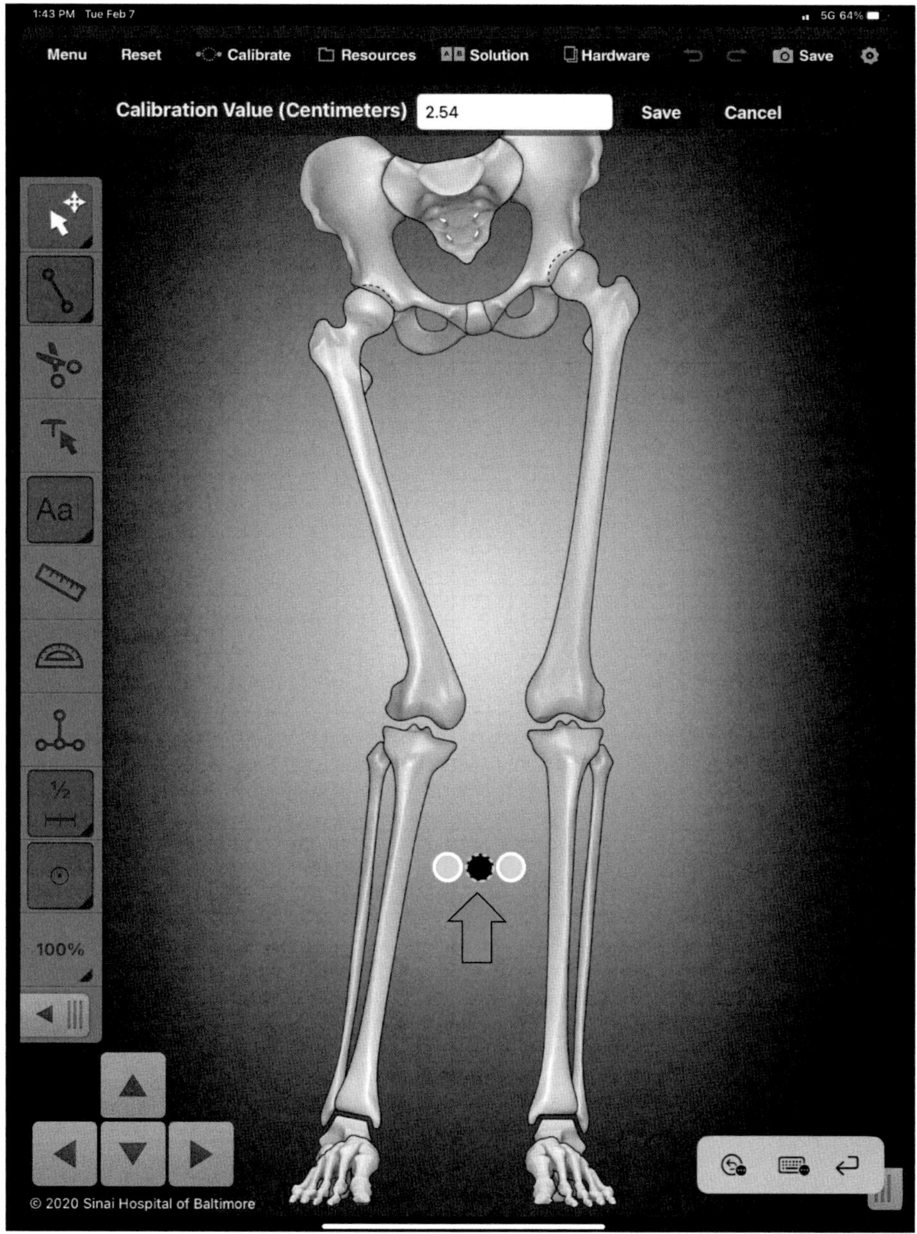


**Fig. 7:** If using the Bone Ninja app, the image needs to be calibrated *(blue arrow)* by using either the magnification marker or a grid line as a reference. This screenshot shows the circular calibration tool can be used to measure a 5-cm grid line. Be sure to resize the dashed circular line so that it is centered on the edge of each grid line.

Analysis of the femoral apex of deformity can be done either mechanically (Fig. 8A) or anatomically (Fig. 8B), depending on surgeon preference as the anatomic and mechanical apexes generally coincide. It is important to evaluate the tibia in both the coronal and sagittal planes as well, since femoral tunnel vision in the setting of limb length discrepancy can lead to regrettable consequences (Fig. 8C).

Once the tibia has been deemed "acceptable," the next step is to define the new mechanical axis of the limb (Fig. 9). Of note, if the tibia is also deformed and will undergo correction, this planning should be done before reverse planning of the femur. The corrected tibia can then be used to set the new mechanical axis of the limb. The reverse planning concept of "beginning with the end in mind" can be applied to the tibia as well, but since the

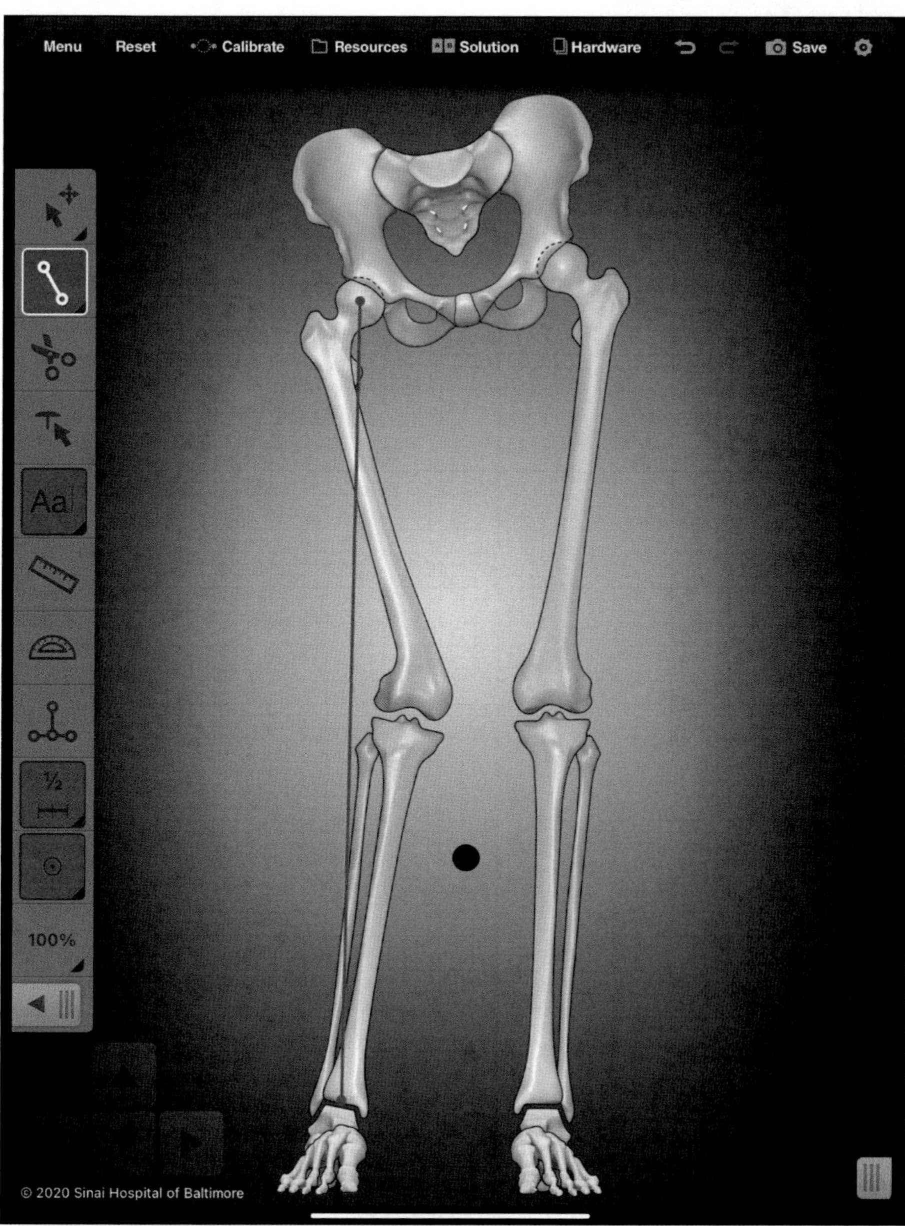


**Fig. 8: A,** Mechanical analysis of the femoral apex of deformity.

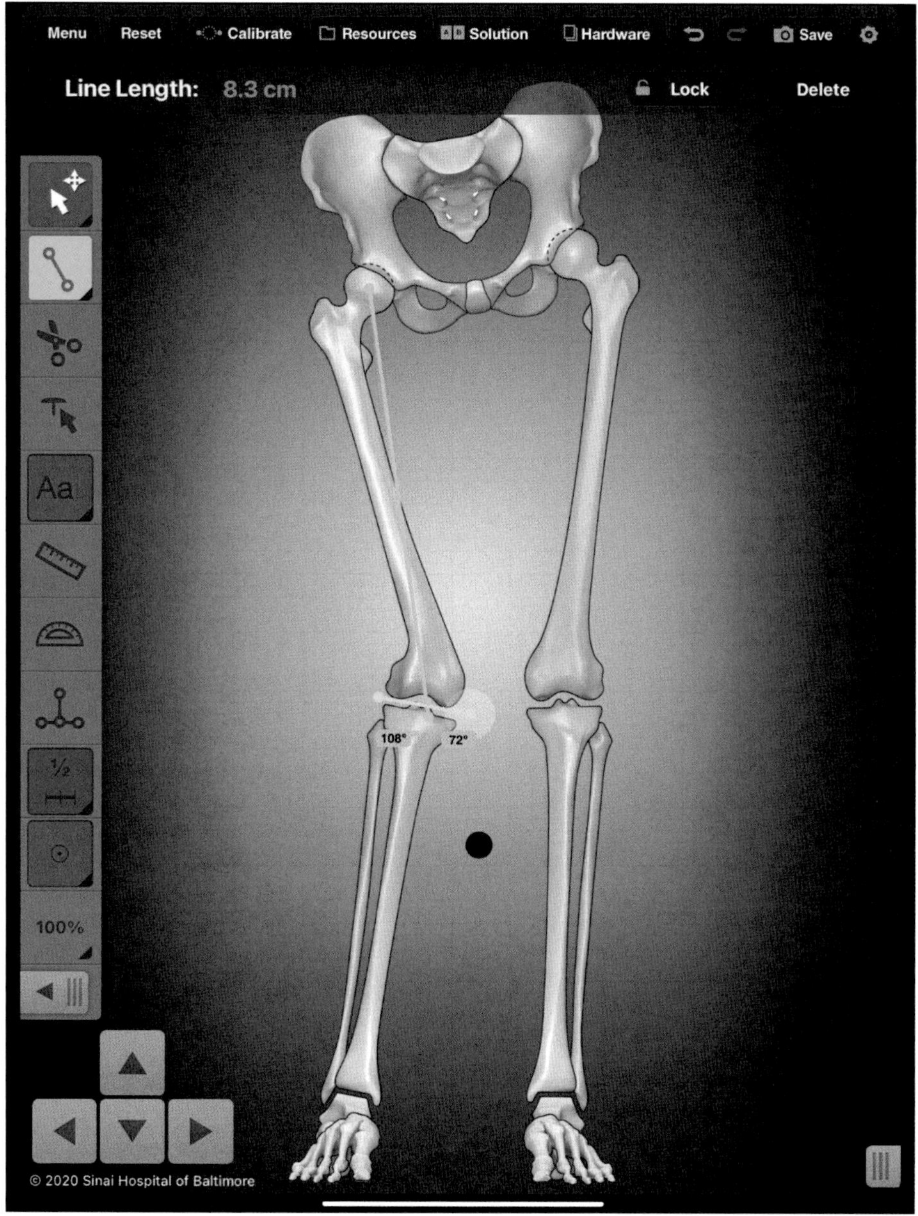


**Fig. 8: B**, Anatomic analysis of the femoral apex of deformity.

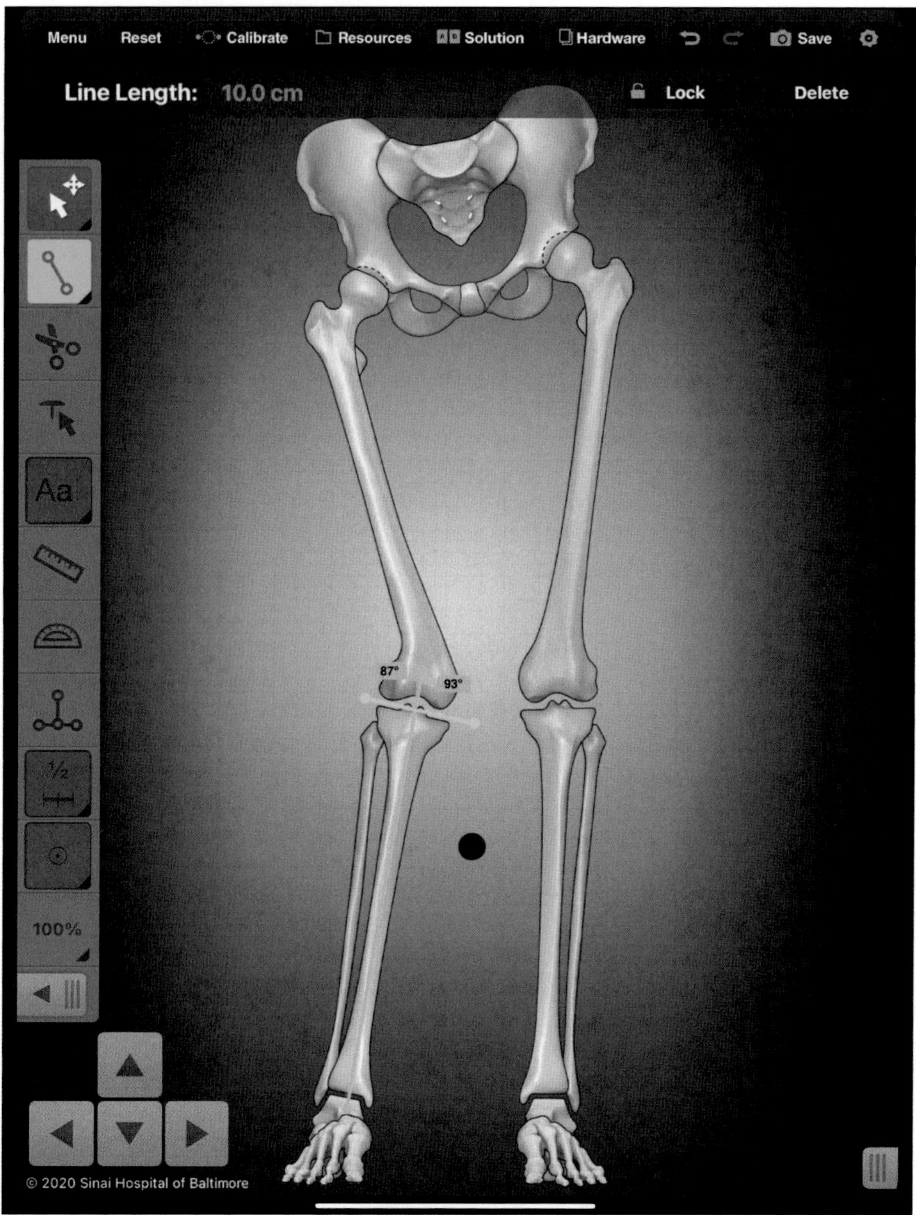


**Fig. 8:** C, Anatomic analysis of the tibia. Evaluate the tibia in both the coronal and sagittal planes; failing to analyze the tibia in limb length discrepancy cases can lead to regrettable consequences.

intramedullary lengthening axis and the mechanical axis are essentially the same, it is a more intuitive process.

The length of the contralateral limb is measured and is used as the template for the length to be gained. This prevents the inaccuracy of the classic method, as discussed above. The new hip center is marked along the new mechanical axis and is measured from the ankle to the new hip center. After defining the new mechanical axis of the limb and hip center, the next step is to define the anatomic axis of the proximal femur. This is done

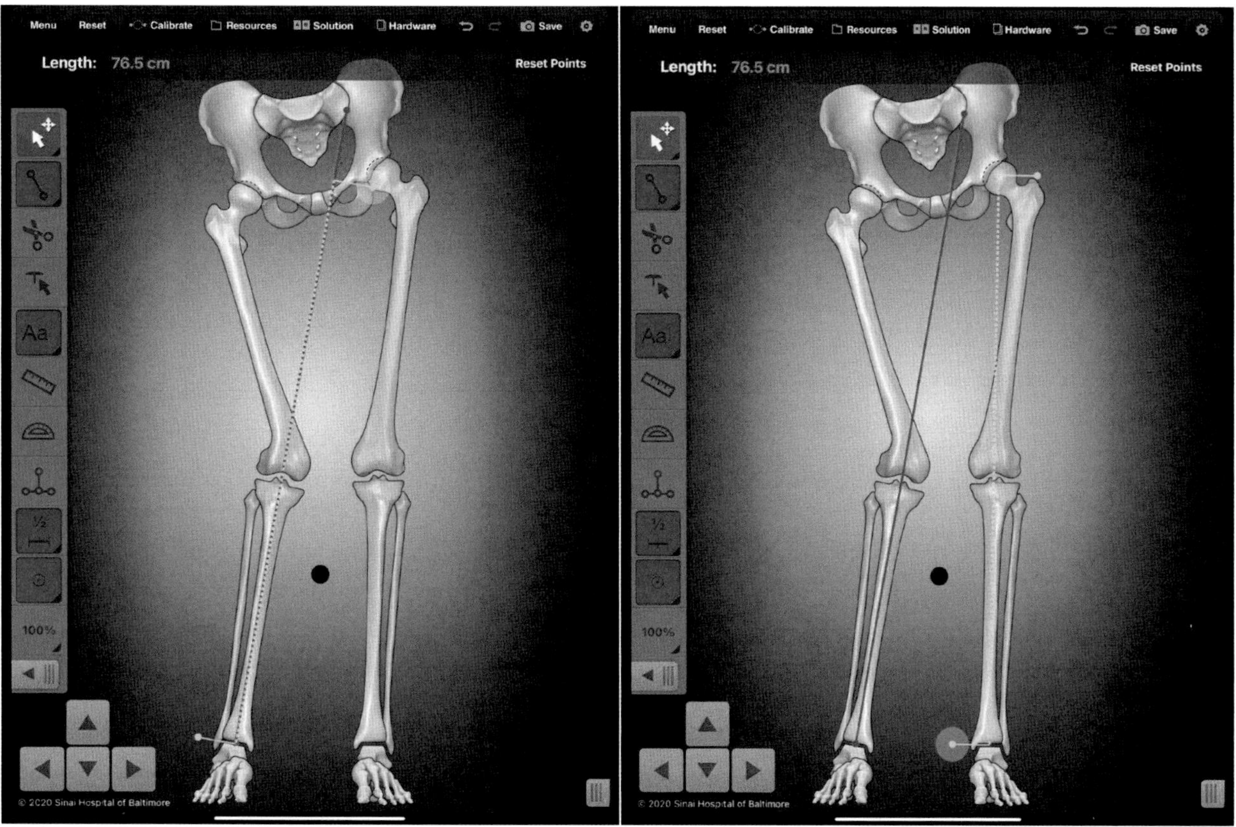


**Fig. 9:** Define the new mechanical axis of the limb.

by creating a mid-diaphyseal line of the proximal segment, which should exit out the piriformis fossa of the proximal femur. This line needs to be drawn carefully and should follow the anticipated pathway of the proximal aspect of the nail. We will call this line the proximal nail line during reverse planning. In the software, the line should be brought well proximal to the greater trochanter of the femur, allowing for easier manipulation (Fig. 10).

A distal "nail line" is then drawn as a collinear extension of this line and brought out the distal aspect of the femur. At this juncture, the exit point of the nail is not important, and care should be taken to avoid the temptation to place it in reference to the distal femur. The interplay between the proximal nail line and the distal nail line is essential to the reverse planning method.

To define the new hip center in skeletally mature patients, the length of the contralateral limb should be used. In immature patients, the calculated length of the contralateral limb will need to be used. This distance is measured up from the ankle on the operative side along the new mechanical axis. A dot is placed along the new mechanical axis at the desired length from the ankle joint and represents the new hip center. To adequately address limb length discrepancy, surgeons should be careful to include foot height and pelvic height contributions, as well as the impact of congenital scoliosis on planned lengthening (Fig. 11).

The next step is to choose the osteotomy. As a general rule, the osteotomy is in the metadiaphyseal junction 6 to 8 cm above the joint line. Considerations include a desire to remain

© 2023 Sinai Hospital of Baltimore

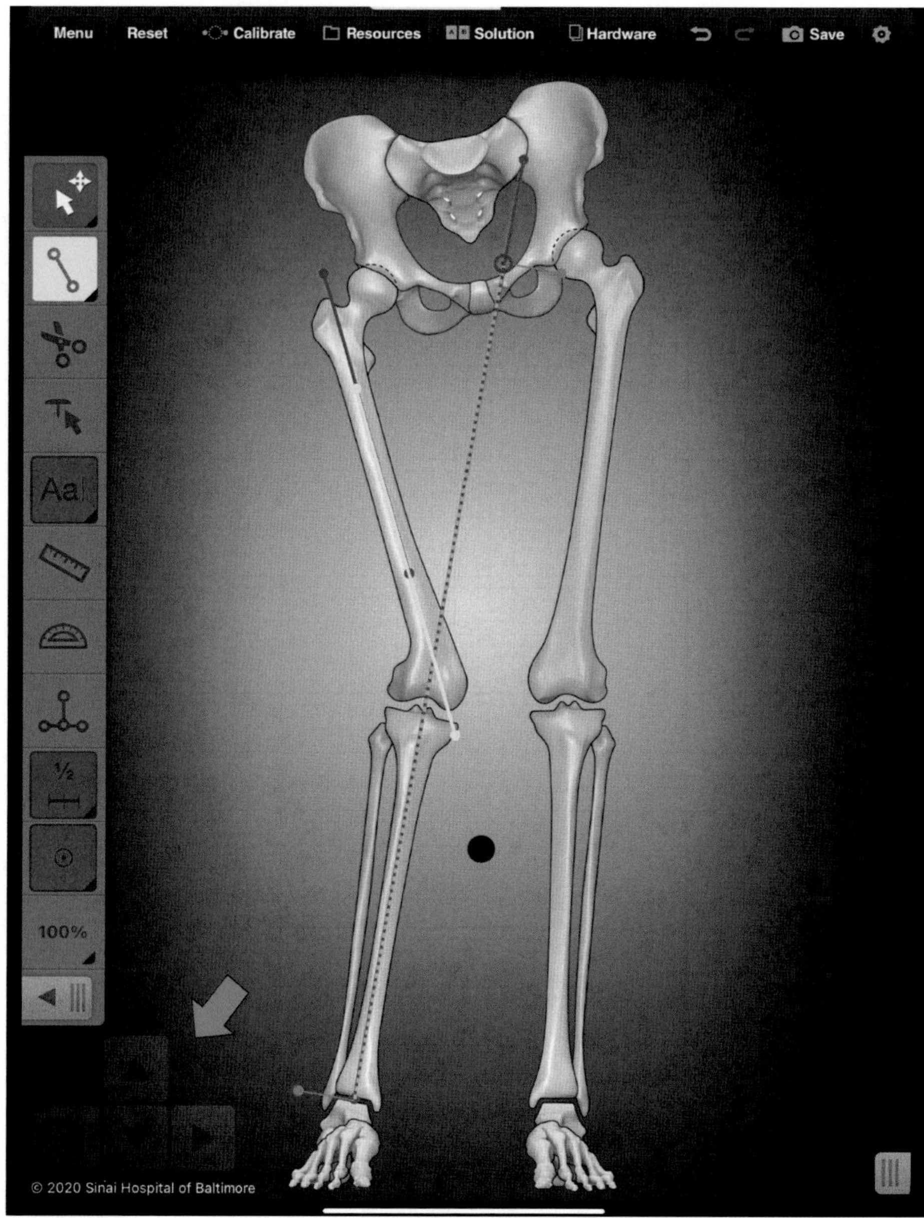


**Fig. 10:** Draw the proximal nail line, which is a mid-diaphyseal line *(purple line)* in the proximal femoral segment that exits out the piriformis fossa and follows the anticipated pathway of the nail. Draw a distal nail line *(yellow line)* that extends the proximal mid-diaphyseal line until it exits the distal femur. Note that this distal line does not have to pass through the notch. Precision is required for this step; be sure to zoom in and use the nudge tools *(blue arrow)*. The new mechanical axis of the limb *(orange line)* is also shown.

extra-articular, the severity of the deformity, soft-tissue constraints, and locking patterns of the lengthening device. An excessively high osteotomy will limit the ability to correct the deformity and risk running into weakness at the socket/plug junction of the lengthening device.

In the Bone Ninja app, as well as other digital planning programs, this step is completed by outlining the entire moving fragment (Fig. 12). It is often helpful to measure with the ruler tool and mark the osteotomy with a transverse line to avoid simple mistakes when using the cut tool.

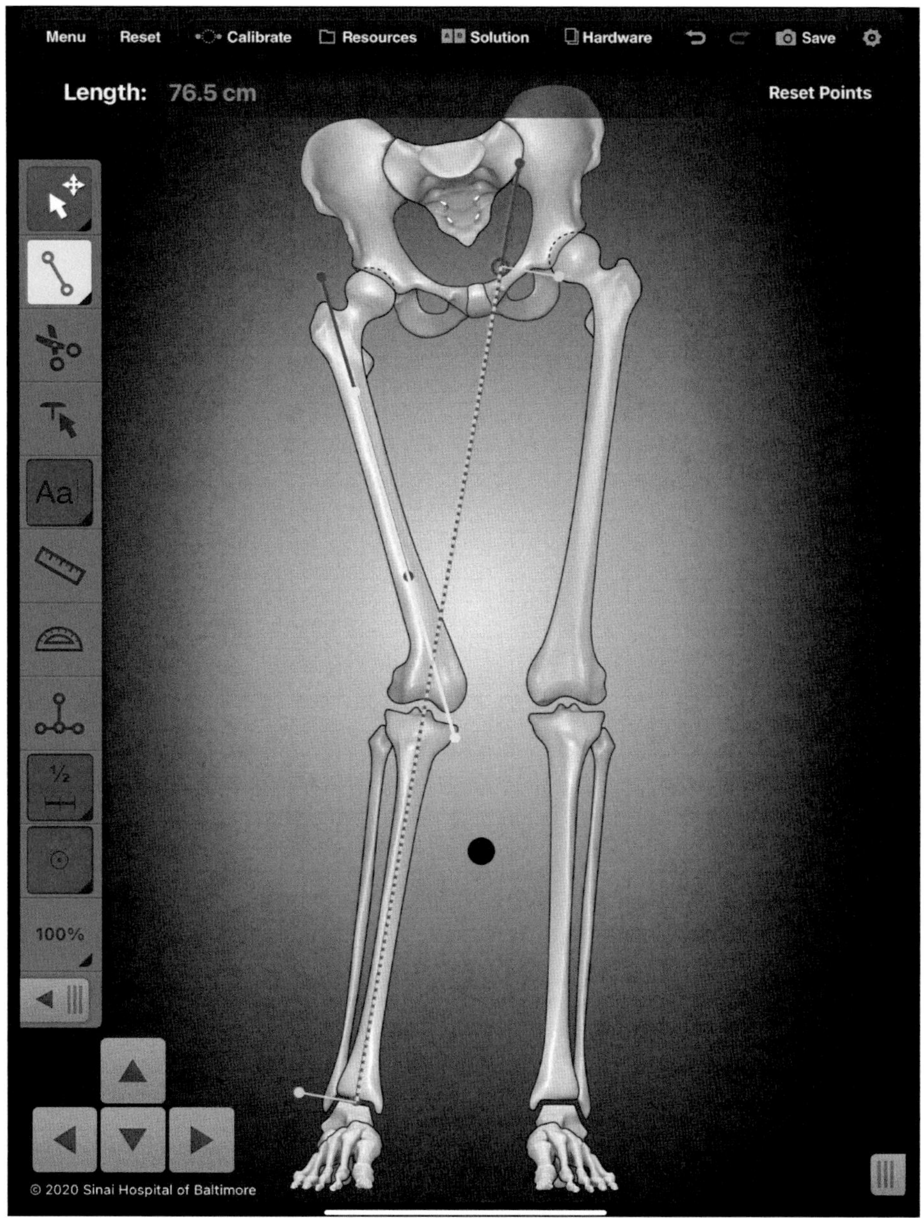


**Fig. 11:** The nail lines (proximal and distal), as well as the new hip center level along the new mechanical axis as measured from the ipsilateral plafond should be reviewed for accuracy.

Once the osteotomy is made, select the proximal femoral segment, the proximal nail line, and the distal nail line. Move the old hip center (along with the proximal femoral fragment and associated lines) to coincide with the new hip center using translation tools only. It is typically enough to click and drag, though "nudge" tools are helpful for fine control if a stylus is not being used (Fig. 13).

With the new and old hip centers currently coincident, the deformity correction is now executed by swinging the moving fragment around a rotation point at the hip center (Fig. 14). The center of the thumbtack tool should be placed carefully over the center of the hip. The proximal fragment, proximal nail line, and distal nail line are all rotated as one unit until the nail line exits the distal

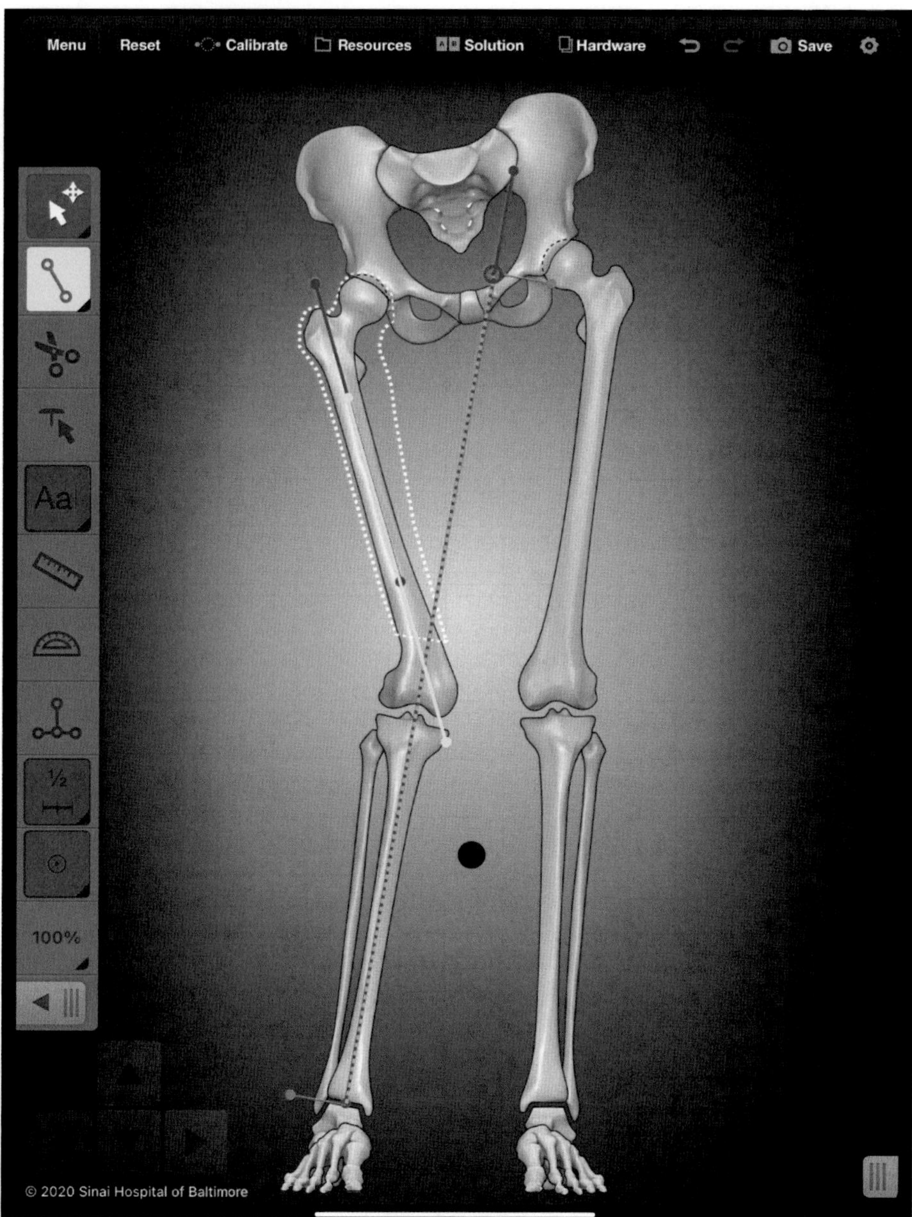


**Fig. 12:** To simulate the osteotomy and create a moving fragment, outline the proximal femoral segment using the cut tool in the Bone Ninja app. Also select the proximal nail line *(purple line)*, distal nail line *(yellow line)*, proximal femur, and current hip center. Avoid grabbing the rotation markers. If you make a mistake, there are undo and redo buttons at the top of the screen.

femur through the notch. If the nail line goes through the cortex of the distal femoral segment, the osteotomy will need to be moved more distally to allow full correction. Failure to modify the cut at this juncture will lead to under-correction of the deformity or a need to ream cortical bone to restore the planned nail pathway.

The image resulting from the rotation step is the anticipated end alignment and length gained. It can be helpful to "cut out" the entire distal femur and tibia to allow moving the femoral head back into the acetabulum to double-check the length gained (Fig. 15A). Occasionally, rotating the pelvis on the radiograph using the cut tool is also useful (Fig. 15B).

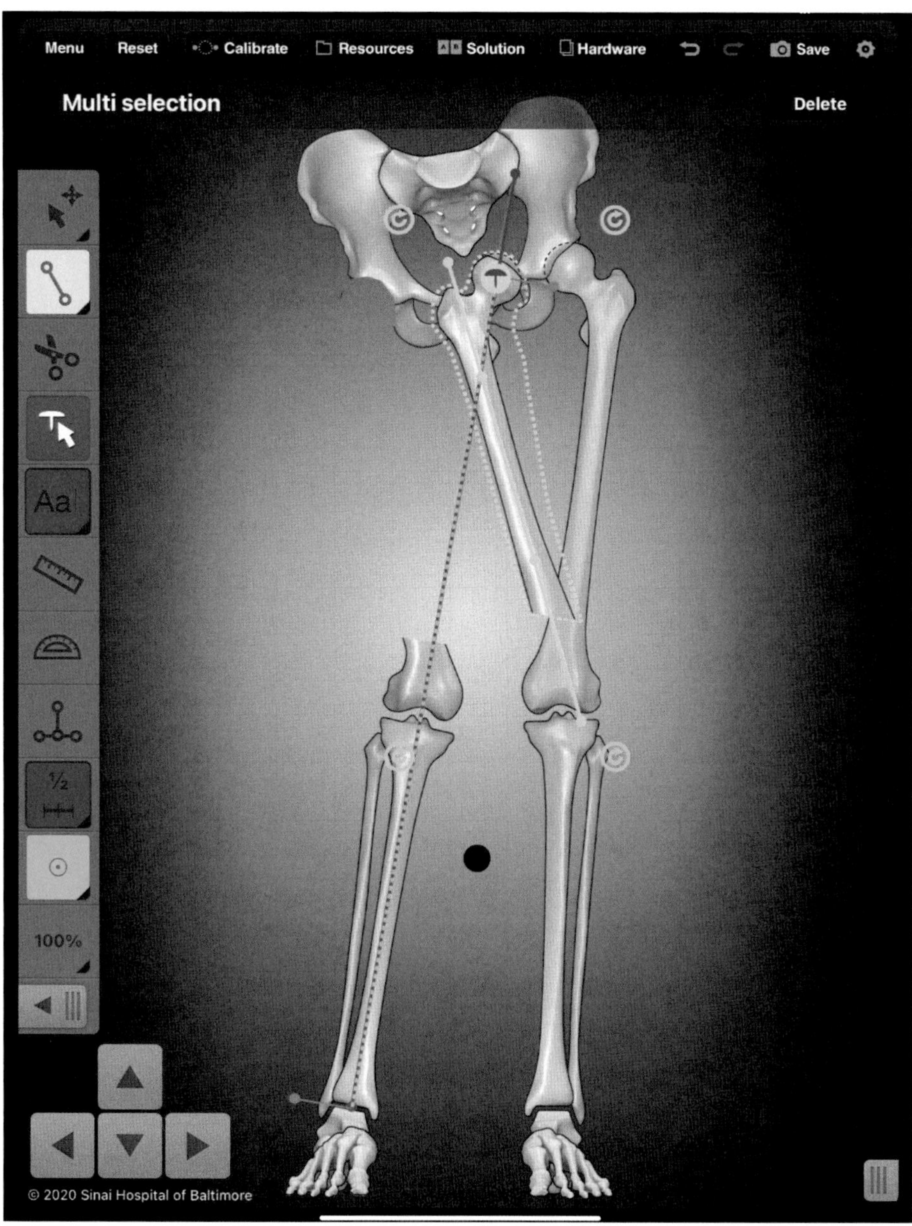


**Fig. 13:** Translate the current hip center so that it coincides with the new hip center.

The length gained is then reversed using the nudge tool (Fig. 16). The proximal nail line and the proximal femoral segment should be moved down the distal nail line, which needs to be deselected prior to undoing the lengthening process. In this representation, the proximal femur and proximal nail line "move" down the lengthening nail to dock with the distal fragment. This produces the anticipated position in the operating room after osteotomy and rod placement (Fig. 17). Note that after reversing the planned lengthening, the hip center is no longer on the "new" mechanical axis line.

This highlights the key concept of reverse planning. The surgeon should evaluate this plan for feasibility (e.g., osteotomy level, requirement for cortical reaming, need for blocking screws).

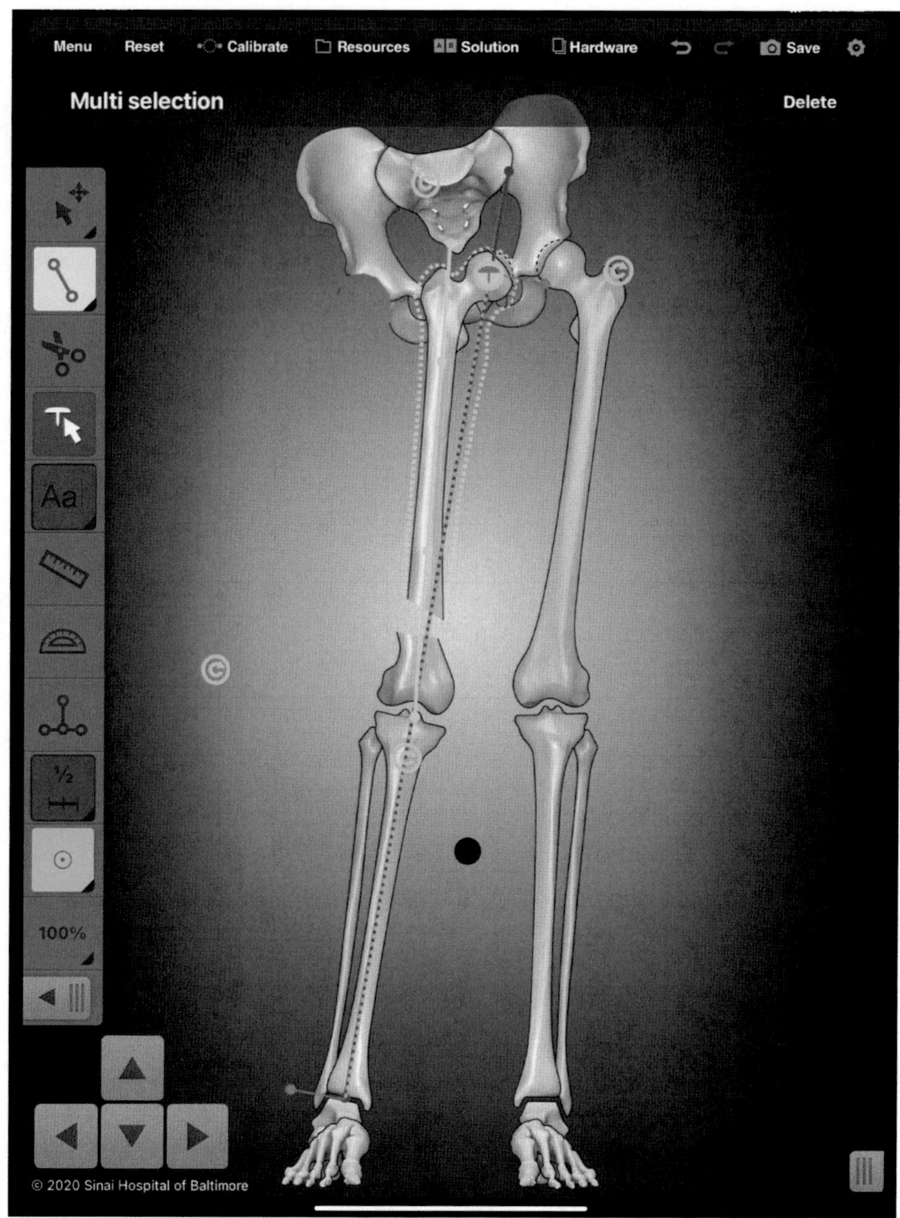


**Fig. 14:** Place the thumbtack tool (point of rotation) on the new hip center. Rotate the moving fragment until the anatomic proximal nail line and distal nail line pass through the planned nail entry point. After translating and rotating, the Bone Ninja image shows the anticipated end alignment and length gained.

This image becomes the operative plan (Fig. 17). The limitations of the lengthening device chosen (e.g., tendency to bend, locking pattern) are of critical importance to an optimal outcome. Once mastered, the reverse planning concept will allow the surgeon to be confident in the outcome while minimizing the risk of unwanted mechanical axis deviation secondary to the anatomic-mechanical axis divergence.

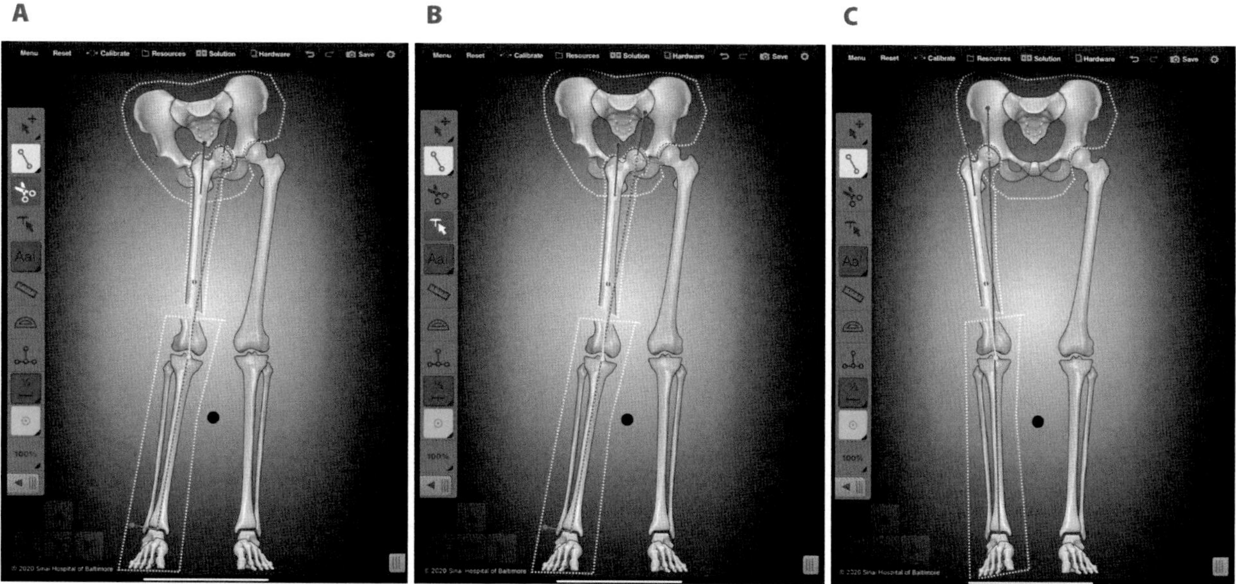


**Fig. 15:** As an extra check, the surgeon can **A**, cut out the pelvis and **B**, rotate it on the center of the left femoral head to a horizontal position. **C**, The surgeon can then cut out the distal femur and tibia and move them along with the proximal segment into an anatomic position. This is a useful tool for education patients about the planned result.

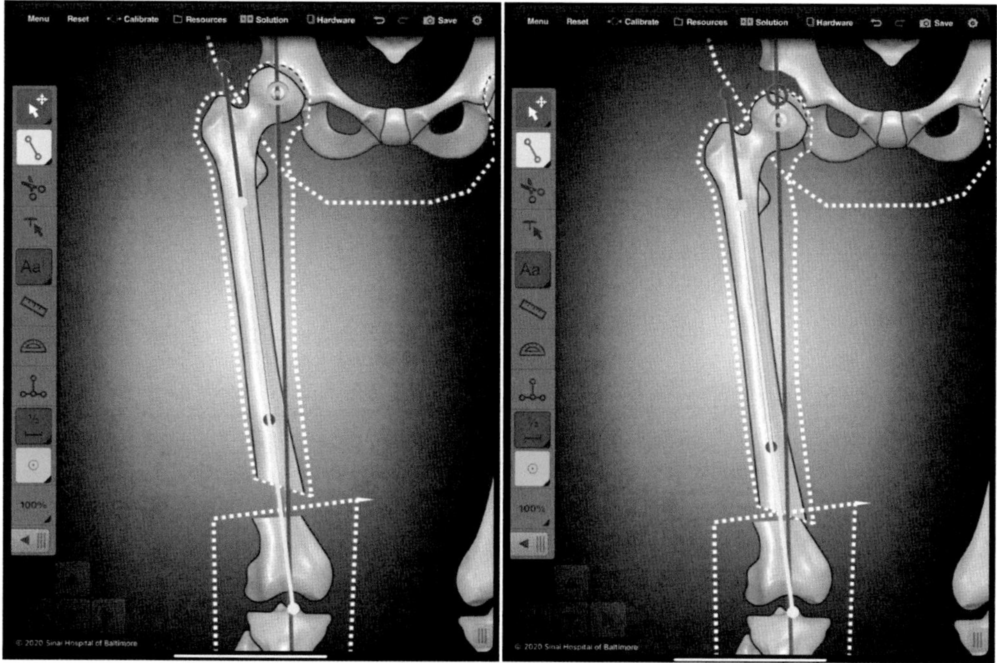


**Fig. 16:** To show the anticipated position after osteotomy and rod placement in the operating room, use the nudge tool to realign the proximal and distal nail lines. Typically, translation will be necessary to align the axes.

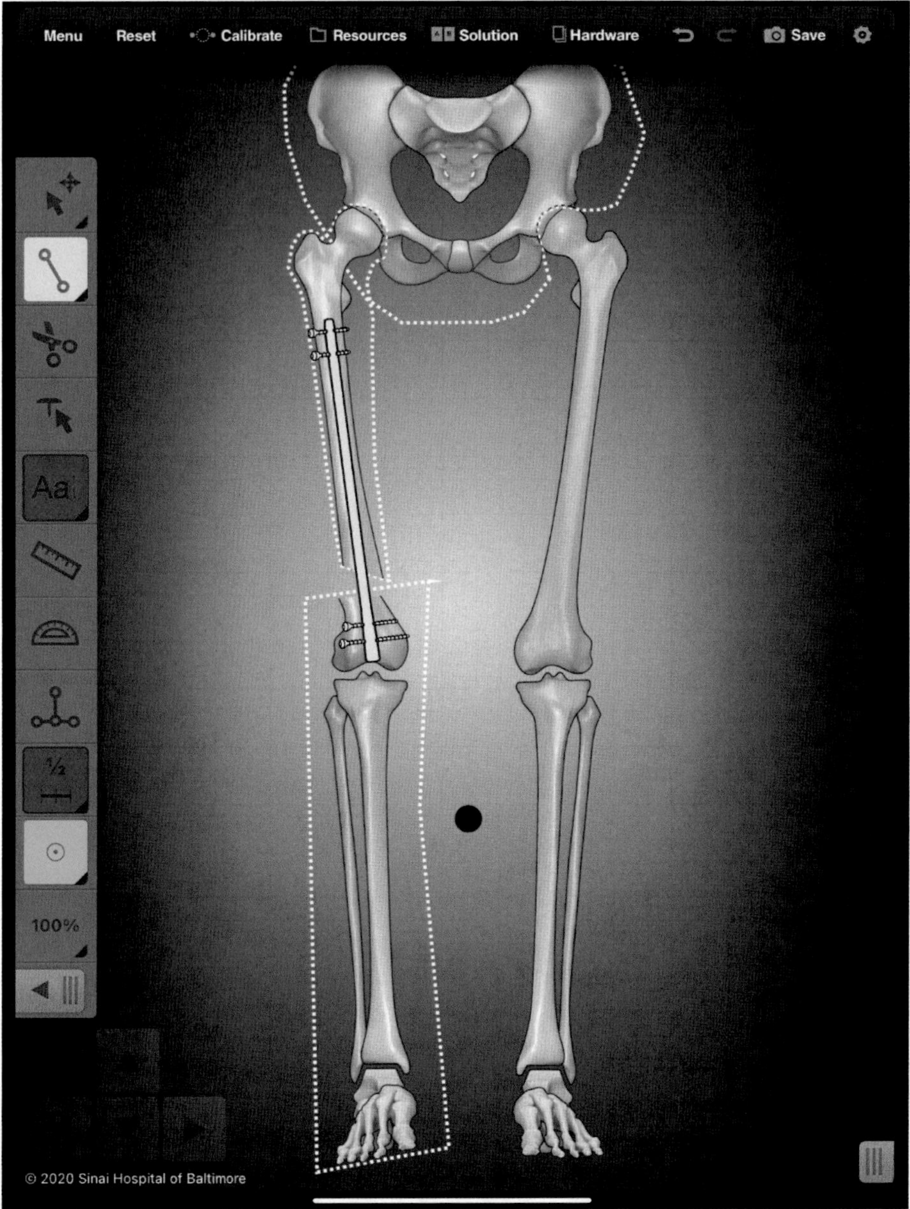


**Fig. 17:** The anticipated position at the end of lengthening is shown after the osteotomy and rod placement. The operative plan should be evaluated for feasibility.

## References

1. Baumgart R. The reverse planning method for lengthening of the lower limb using a straight intramedullary nail with or without deformity correction. A new method. Oper Orthop Traumatol. 2009;21(2):221-33.

2. Burghardt RD, Paley D, Specht SC, Herzenberg JE. The effect on mechanical axis deviation of femoral lengthening with an intramedullary telescopic nail. J Bone Joint Surg Br. 2012;94(9):1241-5.

3. Hung AL, McClure PK, Franzone JM, Hammouda AI, Standard SC, Chau WW, Herzenberg JE. Bone Ninja mobile app for reverse planning method in internal limb deformity and lengthening surgery. Strategies Trauma Limb Reconstr. 2019;14(2):72-76.

# Chapter 13

# Foot and Ankle: Normal Alignment

Bradley M. Lamm, DPM
Noman A. Siddiqui, DPM

## Normal Angles and Relationships

Deformity planning for the foot and ankle originates from a standard set of radiographic lines, angles, and reference points. Obtaining proper weightbearing lower extremity and foot and ankle x-rays (discussed in previous chapters "Obtaining X-rays of the Lower Limbs" and "Obtaining X-rays of the Ankle and Foot for Deformity Analysis") is essential.

Frontal plane x-rays (hindfoot alignment view and long leg calcaneal axial view) provide essential information regarding the tibial-calcaneal relationship and should be routinely ordered. Preoperative frontal plane relationships are helpful to distinguish malalignment of the ankle joint, subtalar joint, tibia, talus, and calcaneus. On the long leg calcaneal axial view, a subtalar joint deformity and an osseous calcaneal tuber deformity can be identified. On the hindfoot alignment view (Saltzman view), the ankle joint deformity and calcaneal translation can be determined. Ankle and axial view x-rays should include the entire tibia for accurate planning. Understanding radiographic angular relationships is critical for appropriate evaluation and identification of the level and extent of the foot and ankle deformity.

### Lateral View Weightbearing X-ray of the Ankle to Include the Tibia

- The posterior proximal tibial angle (PPTA) is the angle formed by the modified mechanical axis of the tibia and the joint line of the proximal tibia (normal, 81° [77–84°]) (Fig. 1).
- The anterior distal tibial angle (ADTA) is the angle formed by the modified mechanical axis of the tibia and the joint line of the distal tibia (normal, 80° [78–82°]) (Fig. 1).

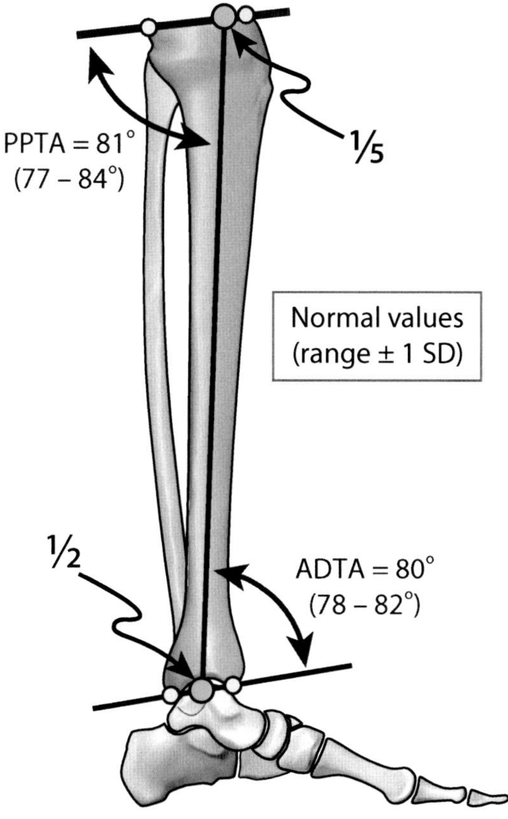


**Fig. 1:** Normal sagittal plane measurements of the tibia. PPTA, posterior proximal tibial angle; ADTA, anterior distal tibial angle; SD, standard deviation.

© 2023 Sinai Hospital of Baltimore

## Lateral View Weightbearing X-ray of the Foot (Table 1)

- The tibio-talar angle is the angle formed by the mid-diaphyseal line of the tibia and the line that bisects the talar neck (normal, 68° [64–72°]) (Fig. 2).
- The lateral process of the talus should be located along the tibial mid-diaphyseal line (normal, 3 mm anterior [±3 mm from tibial mid-diaphyseal line]) (Fig. 2).

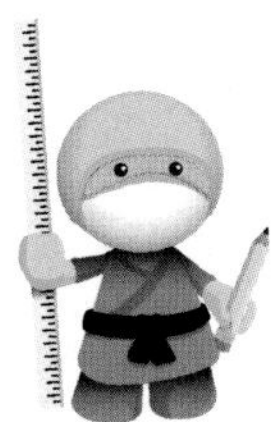

***Sensei says,***
*"The lateral process of the talus, which also serves as the center of ankle joint range of motion, should fall 3 mm anterior to the tibial mid-diaphyseal line."*

- The calcaneal inclination angle (CIA) is the angle formed by the plantar surface of the calcaneus and the weightbearing surface of the foot (normal, 18° [13–23°]) (Fig. 2).
- Navicular height is the perpendicular distance from the floor to the plantar-most portion of the navicular (normal, 4 cm [3–5 cm]) (Fig. 2).
- The metatarsal declination angle is the angle formed by the weightbearing surface of the foot and mid-diaphyseal line of the first metatarsal shaft (normal, 23° [20–26°]) (Fig. 2).
- The lateral Meary's angle is formed by the talar neck bisector line and the mid-diaphyseal line of the first metatarsal (normal, 6° [2–10°]) (Fig. 2).
- The plantigrade angle is formed by the mid-diaphyseal line of the tibia and the sole of the foot. It is normally 88° (85–91°) when standing in static stance (Fig. 3).
- The plantar distal metatarsal angle (PDMA) is the relationship between the mid-diaphyseal line of the first metatarsal and the line along the first metatarsal neck (normal, 81° [76–86°]) (Fig. 3).
- The plantar distal hallux angle (PDHA) is formed by the mid-diaphyseal line of the hallux and a line along the neck of the hallux (normal, 80° [75–85°]) (Fig. 3).
- The dorsal proximal phalangeal angle (DPPA) is formed by the mid-diaphyseal line of the distal phalanx and the proximal joint line at the base of the distal phalanx (normal, 78° [73–83°]) (Fig. 3).
- The dorsal proximal hallux angle (DPHA) is formed by the mid-diaphyseal line of the hallux and the proximal joint line at the base of the hallux (normal, 83° [77–89°]) (Fig. 3).
- The dorsal proximal metatarsal angle (DPMA) is formed by the mid-diaphyseal line of the first

**Table 1. Lateral View Measurements and Landmarks of the Foot**

| Acronym of Joint Angle | Complete Name of Joint Angle | Average Normal Value (Range ± 1 SD) |
|---|---|---|
| CIA | calcaneal inclination angle | 18° (13–23°) |
| DPHA | dorsal proximal hallux angle | 83° (77–89°) |
| DPMA | dorsal proximal metatarsal angle | 86° (81–91°) |
| DPPA | dorsal proximal phalangeal angle | 78° (73–83°) |
| - | lateral Meary's angle | 6° (2–10°) |
| - | lateral process of talus | 3 mm anterior (± 3 mm) |
| - | metatarsal declination angle | 23° (20–26°) |
| - | navicular height | 4 cm (3–5 cm) |
| PDHA | plantar distal hallux angle | 80° (75–85°) |
| PDMA | plantar distal metatarsal angle | 81° (76–86°) |
| - | plantigrade angle | 88° (85–91°) |
| - | tibio-talar angle | 68° (64–72°) |

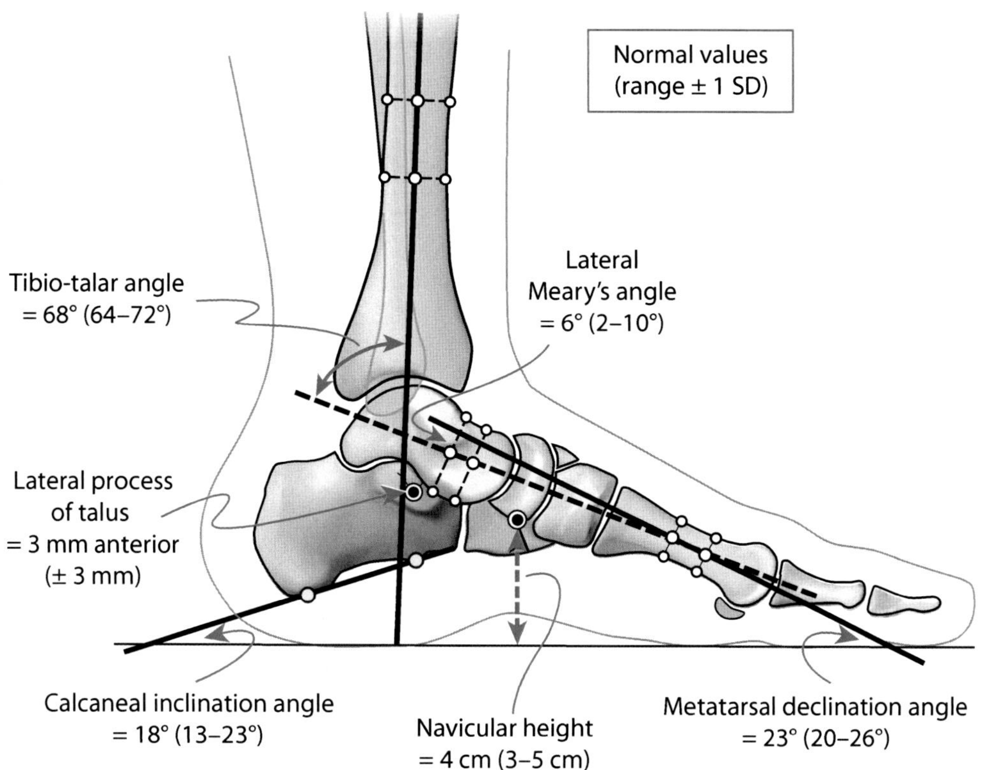


**Fig. 2:** Normal sagittal plane measurements and reference points of the foot. SD, standard deviation.

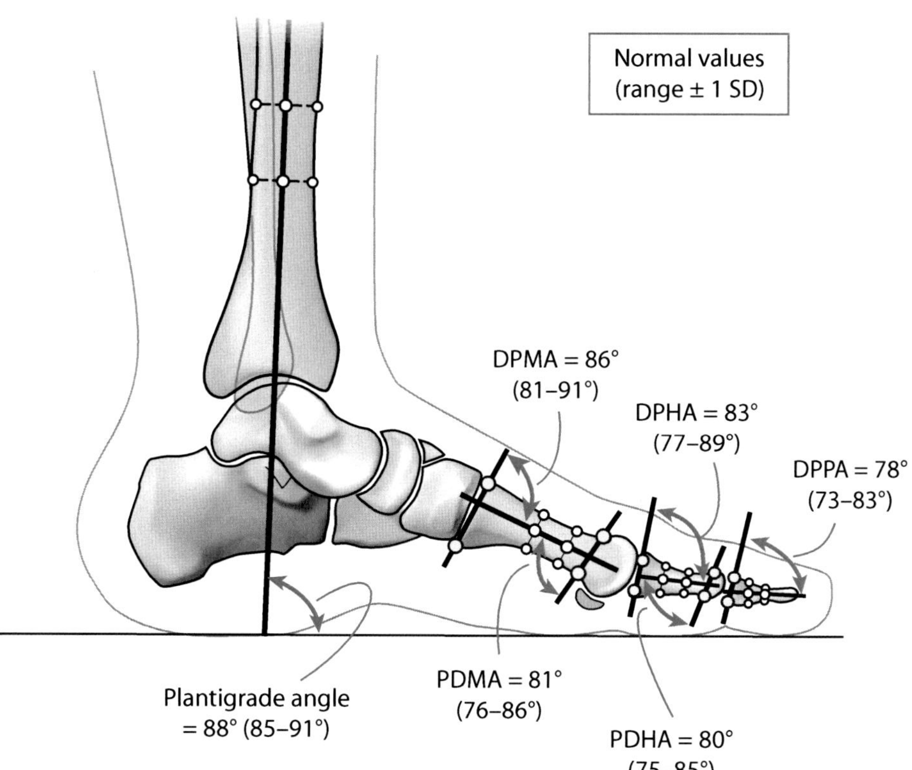


**Fig. 3:** Normal sagittal plane measurements of the foot. DPMA, dorsal proximal metatarsal angle; DPHA, dorsal proximal hallux angle; DPPA, dorsal proximal phalangeal angle; PDHA, plantar distal hallux angle; PDMA, plantar distal metatarsal angle; SD, standard deviation.

© 2023 Sinai Hospital of Baltimore

metatarsal and the joint line of the first metatarsal base (normal, 86° [81–91°]) (Fig. 3).

### Anteroposterior View Weightbearing X-ray of the Ankle to Include the Tibia

- The medial proximal tibial angle (MPTA) is formed by the tibial mid-diaphyseal line and the joint line of the proximal tibia (normal, 87° [85–90°]) (Fig. 4).
- The lateral distal tibial angle (LDTA) is formed by the tibial mid-diaphyseal line and the joint line of the distal tibia (normal, 89° [86–92°]) (Fig. 4).
- The center of the talar dome is a bisector line drawn halfway between the medial and lateral aspects of the trochlea of the talus. The center of the talar dome is slightly lateral to the tibial mid-diaphyseal line (Fig. 5A).
- The plafond malleolar angle (PMA) is the relationship between the tibial plafond and the transmalleolar axis (tip of the medial malleolus to the tip of the lateral malleolus) (normal, 15° [13–17°]) (Fig. 5B) (Table 2).

### Anteroposterior View X-ray of the Foot (Table 3)

- The talo-calcaneal angle (TCA or Kite angle) is formed by the talar bisector line and a line drawn along the lateral wall of the calcaneus (normal, 21° [15–27°]) (Fig. 6A).
- The fourth intermetatarsal angle (IMA) is the angle formed by the mid-diaphyseal line of the fourth

**Table 2. Axial View Measurements and Landmarks of the Foot**

| Acronym of Joint Angle | Complete Name of Joint Angle | Average Normal Value (Range ± 1 SD) |
|---|---|---|
| JLCA of tibia and talus | joint line convergence angle of tibia and talus | 0° ± 1° |
| PMA | plafond malleolar angle | 15° (13–17°) |
| - | tibial-calcaneal angle | 2° valgus (± 3°) |
| - | tibial-calcaneal distance | 10 mm lateral (6–14 mm lateral) |

**Table 3. AP View Measurements and Landmarks of the Foot**

| Acronym of Joint Angle | Complete Name of Joint Angle | Average Normal Value (Range ± 1 SD) |
|---|---|---|
| 1st mIMA | 1st mechanical intermetatarsal angle | 9° (6–12°) |
| 4th IMA | 4th intermetatarsal angle | 9° (6–12°) |
| - | AP Meary's angle | 7° (3–11°) |
| HAA | hallux abductus angle | 8° (4–12°) |
| HIA | hallux interphalangeal angle | 11° (7–15°) |
| LDHA | lateral distal hallux angle | 88° (84–92°) |
| LDMA | lateral distal metatarsal angle | 90° (87–93°) |
| MAD | mechanical axis deviation | 4 mm lateral (2–6 mm lateral) |
| MPHA | medial proximal hallux angle | 95° (92–98°) |
| MPMA | medial proximal metatarsal angle | 92° (88–96°) |
| MPPA | medial proximal phalangeal angle | 95° (91–99°) |
| - | metatarsal parabola angle | 140° (135–145°) |
| MAA | metatarsus adductus angle | 11° (6–16°) |
| TCA | talo-calcaneal angle | 21° (15–27°) |

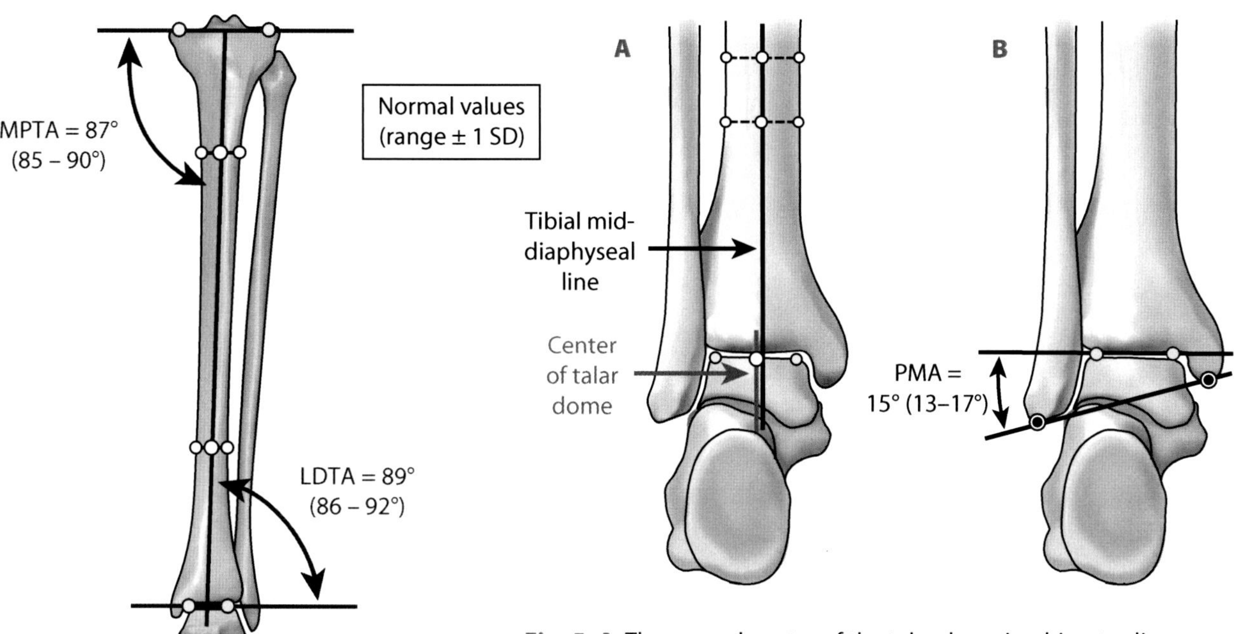


**Fig. 4:** Normal frontal plane measurements of the tibia. MPTA, medial proximal tibial angle; LDTA, lateral distal tibial angle; SD, standard deviation.

**Fig. 5: A**, The normal center of the talar dome is a bisector line drawn halfway between the medial and lateral aspects of the trochlea of the talus. **B**, Plafond malleolar angle (PMA) is the relationship between the tibial plafond and the transmalleolar axis (tip of the medial malleolus to the tip of the lateral malleolus).

**Table 4. AP View Joint Line Convergence Angle Measurements of the First Metatarsal**

| Acronym of Joint Angle | Complete Name of Joint Angle | Average Normal Value (Range ± 1 SD) |
|---|---|---|
| JLCA 1st metatarsal cuneiform joint | joint line convergence angle 1st metatarsal cuneiform joint | 1° (0–2°) open medially |
| JLCA 1st metatarsal phalangeal joint | joint line convergence angle 1st metatarsal phalangeal joint | 3° (1–5°) open medially |
| JLCA hallux interphalangeal joint | joint line convergence angle hallux interphalangeal joint | 1° (0–2°) open medially |

metatarsal and the mid-diaphyseal line of the fifth metatarsal (normal, 9° [6–12°]) (Fig. 6A).

- The first mechanical IMA is the angle formed by the mechanical axis of the first metatarsal and the mechanical axis of the second metatarsal (normal, 9° [6–12°]) (Fig. 6A).
- The lateral distal metatarsal angle (LDMA) is the angle between the mid-diaphyseal line of the first metatarsal and the distal joint line of the first metatarsal (normal, 90° [87–93°]) (Fig. 6B).
- The lateral distal hallux angle (LDHA) is formed by the hallux mid-diaphyseal line and the distal joint line of the hallux (normal, 88° [84–92°]) (Fig. 6B).
- The medial proximal phalangeal angle (MPPA) is the angle between the hallux distal phalanx mid-diaphyseal line and the proximal joint line of the distal phalanx (normal, 95° [91–99°]) (Fig. 6B).
- The joint line convergence angle (JLCA) is an angle formed by two adjacent joint surfaces

© 2023 Sinai Hospital of Baltimore

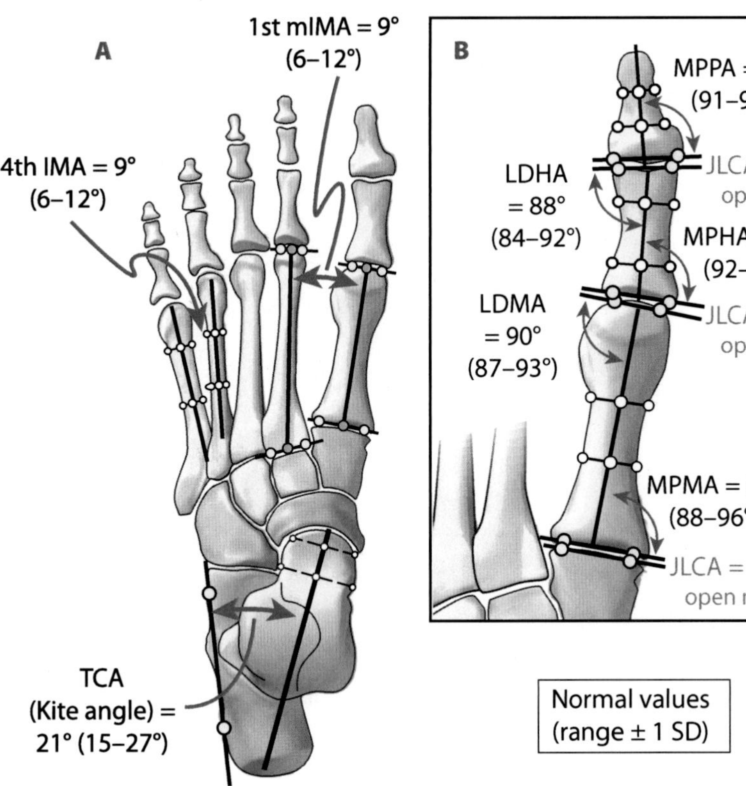


**Fig. 6:** Normal AP view measurements of the foot. TCA, talo-calcaneal angle; IMA, intermetatarsal angle; mIMA, mechanical intermetatarsal angle; LDMA, lateral distal metatarsal angle; LDHA, lateral distal hallux angle; MPPA, medial proximal phalangeal angle; JLCA, joint line convergence angle; MPHA, medial proximal hallux angle; MPMA, medial proximal metatarsal angle; SD, standard deviation.

(Fig. 6B) (Table 4). The normal value of each JLCA varies depending on the joint that it is describing.

- The medial proximal hallux angle (MPHA) is the angle between the mid-diaphyseal line of the hallux and the proximal joint line of the hallux (normal, 95° [92–98°]) (Fig. 6B).
- The medial proximal metatarsal angle (MPMA) is the angle between the mid-diaphyseal line of the first metatarsal and the proximal joint line of the first metatarsal (normal, 92° [88–96°]) (Fig. 6B).
- The metatarsus adductus angle (MAA) (normal, 11° [6–16°]) provides the angular relationship of the midfoot with respect to the second metatarsal mid-diaphyseal line (Fig. 7). This relationship is useful to determine the angulation of the forefoot with respect to the midfoot. To measure this angle, draw the mid-diaphyseal line of the second metatarsal. Then draw a line that connects the most medial aspect of the first metatarsal base and the most medial aspect of the talo-navicular joint. Next, draw a line that connects the most lateral aspect of the calcaneal-cuboid joint and the fourth metatarsal-cuboid joint. Draw a third line that connects the halfway point of the medial

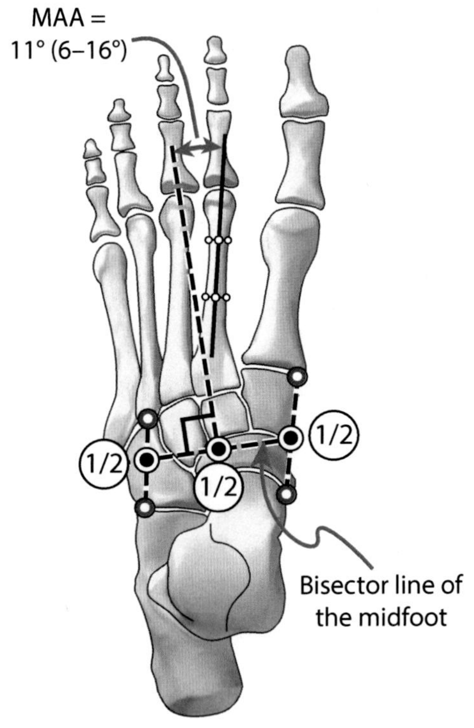


**Fig. 7:** The normal metatarsus adductus angle (MAA) is the angular relationship of the midfoot with respect to the second metatarsal mid-diaphyseal line. SD, standard deviation.

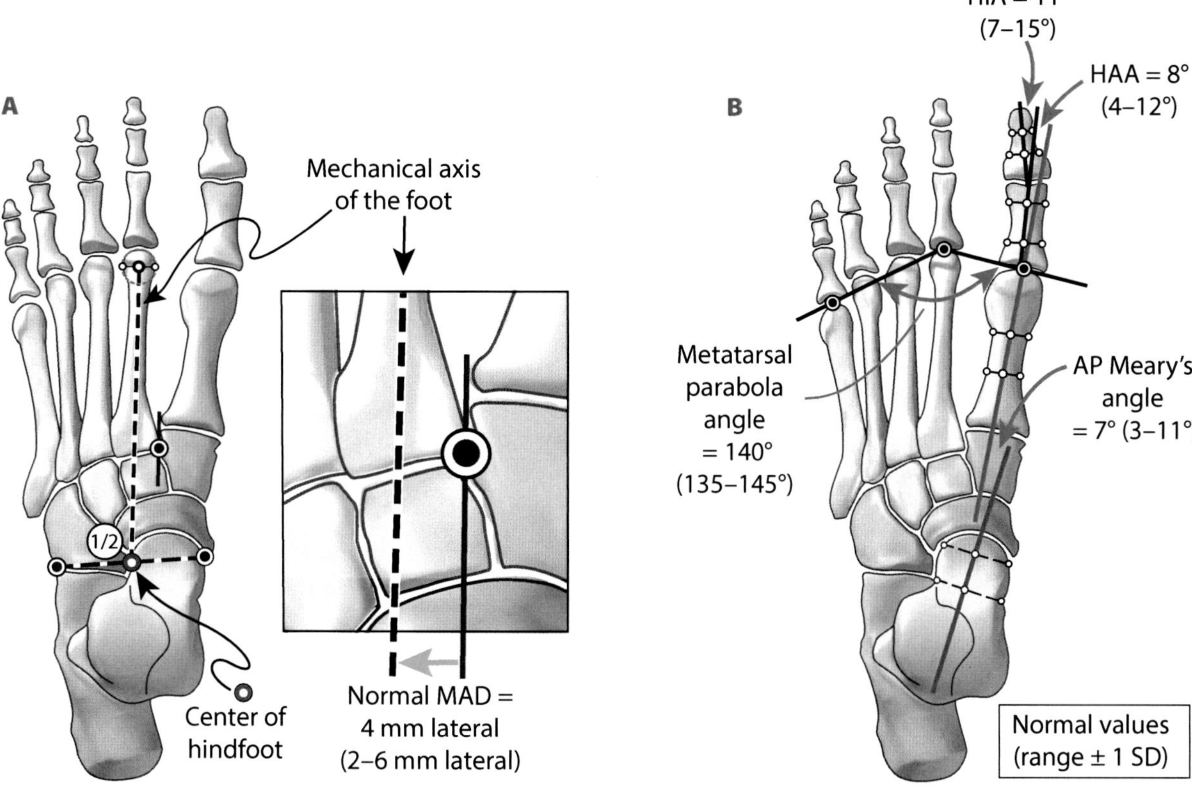


**Fig. 8: A**, Normal mechanical axis deviation (MAD) is 4 mm lateral (range, 2–6 mm lateral). **B**, AP view measurements of the foot. HIA, hallux interphalangeal angle; HAA, hallux abductus angle; SD, standard deviation.

line and the halfway point of the lateral line. This is the bisector line of the midfoot. Mark the center of this bisector line, and draw a line that extends distally from this point and is perpendicular to the bisector line. The angle created by this line and the mid-diaphyseal line of the second metatarsal is the MAA (Fig. 7).

- The mechanical axis of the foot is a line that extends from the center of the second metatarsal head to the center of the hindfoot (Fig. 8A). The center of the hindfoot is a point halfway between a point at the lateral aspect of the calcaneal-cuboid joint and the medial aspect of the talo-navicular joint (Fig. 8A, *red point*).
- The normal mechanical axis of the foot is 4 mm lateral (normal range, 2–6 mm lateral) from the most medial aspect of the second metatarsal intermediate cuneiform joint (Fig. 8A). Values outside of this range are considered abnormal mechanical axis deviation.
- The hallux interphalangeal angle (HIA) is the angle between the mid-diaphyseal line of the hallux and the mid-diaphyseal line of the distal hallux phalanx (normal, 11° [7–15°]) (Fig. 8B).
- The hallux abductus angle (HAA) is formed by the mid-diaphyseal line of the hallux and the mid-diaphyseal line of the first metatarsal (normal, 8° [4–12°]) (Fig. 8B).
- The metatarsal parabola angle is the angle formed by one line connecting the most distal aspect of the first metatarsal and the most distal aspect of the second metatarsal and another line connecting the most distal aspect of the fifth and second metatarsal (normal, 140° [135–145°]) (Fig. 8B).
- The relationship between the talar bisector line and the mid-diaphyseal line of the first metatarsal is known as the anteroposterior view Meary's angle (normal, 7° [3–11°]) (Fig. 8B).

© 2023 Sinai Hospital of Baltimore

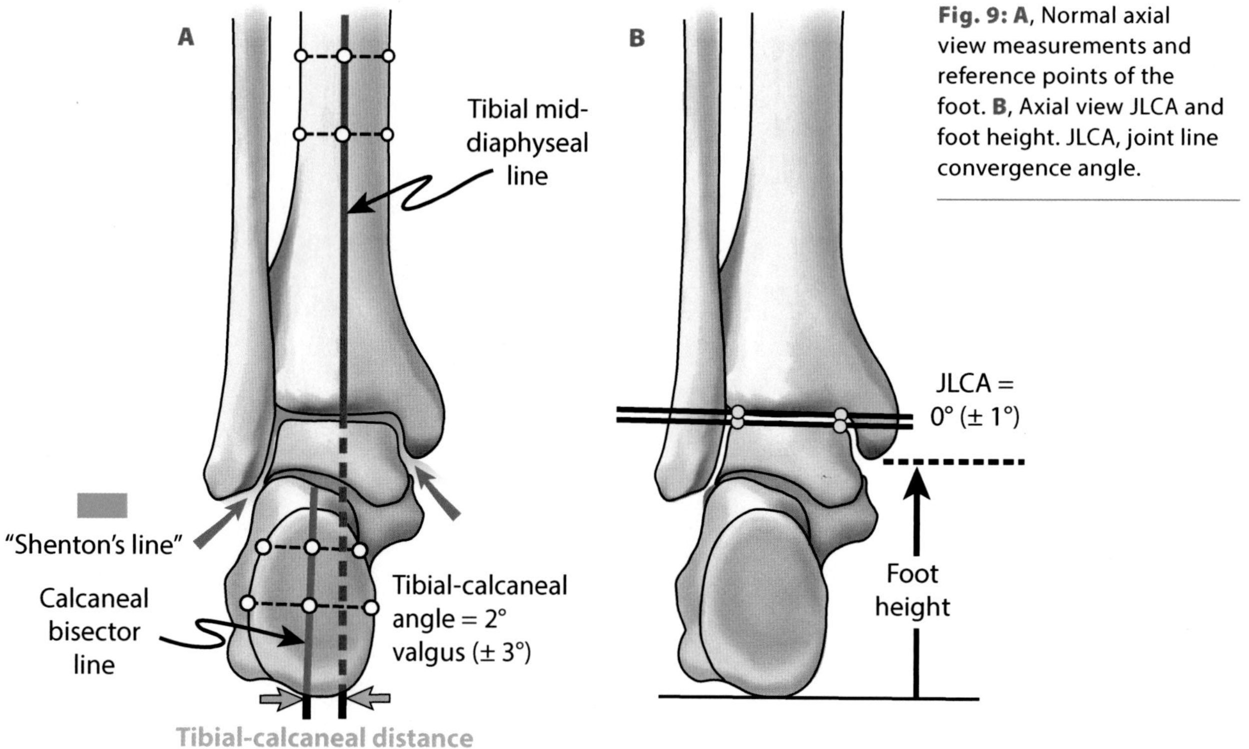


**Fig. 9: A**, Normal axial view measurements and reference points of the foot. **B**, Axial view JLCA and foot height. JLCA, joint line convergence angle.

## Long Leg Calcaneal Axial View and Hindfoot Alignment View X-rays (Table 2)

- On the hindfoot alignment view (Saltzman view), the calcaneal bisector is 10 mm lateral (6–14 mm lateral) to the tibial mid-diaphyseal line (Fig. 9A). This is called the tibial-calcaneal distance (Table 2).
- Shenton's line of the ankle is a congruent space that exists between the medial talus, medial malleolus, and extends across the tibiotalar joint space to the fibular-talar space (Fig. 9A).
- The tibial-calcaneal angle is the angle formed by the calcaneal bisector line and the tibial mid-diaphyseal line (normal, 2° valgus [± 3°]) (Fig. 9A) (Table 2).
- The joint line convergence angle (JLCA) of the ankle has a normal value of 0° (±1°) (Fig. 9B) (Table 2).
- Foot height is a clinical measure from the floor to the tip of the medial malleolus (Fig. 9B).

# Chapter 14

# Foot and Ankle Axis Planning: Frontal, Sagittal, and Transverse Planes

Bradley M. Lamm, DPM
Noman A. Siddiqui, DPM

## Frontal Plane Axis Planning

Axis planning identifies the proximal and distal axes of the deformed bone or bone segment. The intersection of the proximal and distal axes shows the location of the deformity, which is called the apex of the deformity.

A frontal plane deformity is characterized by varus or valgus malalignment of the distal tibia, ankle, talus, and calcaneus in isolation or in combination. Malalignment in the frontal plane of the ankle joint is evaluated on a weightbearing AP view ankle x-ray and an axial view x-ray (hindfoot alignment view and long leg calcaneal axial view).

LDTA measurements greater than 92° signify a varus position, while those in valgus have LDTA measurements of less than 86° (refer to the chapter entitled "Foot and Ankle: Normal Alignment," Fig. 4).

Frontal plane deformity of the hindfoot on the hindfoot alignment view or long leg calcaneal axial view is noted to be varus/valgus as measured by the relationship of the calcaneal bisector line and the mid-diaphyseal line of the tibia (Fig. 1). On the hindfoot alignment view, it is also important to note the center (solid black point in Fig. 1) of the calcaneus with respect to the tibial mid-diaphyseal line. Medial or lateral translation of the calcaneus when compared to the tibial mid-diaphyseal line is a major factor for the evaluation of axial alignment.

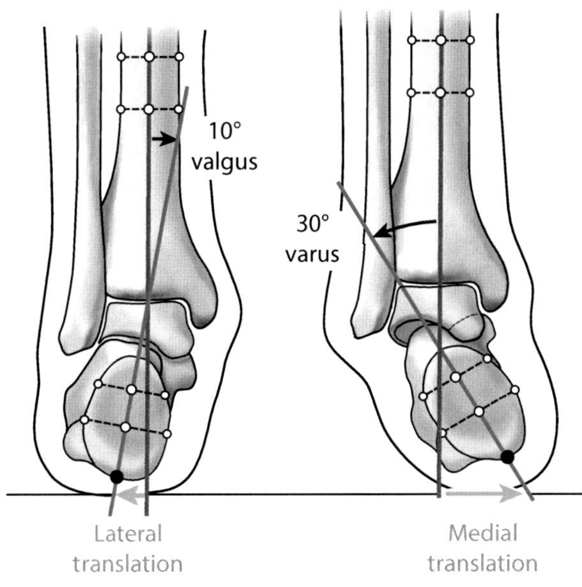


**Fig. 1:** The relationship between the calcaneal bisector line and the mid-diaphyseal line of the tibia reveals whether a hindfoot varus or valgus deformity is present. The solid black dot represents the center of the calcaneus with respect to the tibial mid-diaphyseal line.

© 2023 Sinai Hospital of Baltimore

## Identifying the Apex on an AP View Ankle X-ray

**Step 1:** Draw the mechanical axis of the tibia (Fig. 2A).

**Step 2:** Draw the joint line of the ankle and measure the LDTA. The LDTA is 84° (abnormal) (Fig. 2A).

**Step 3:** Measure the plafond malleolar angle (13°) (Fig. 2B). Note that this patient has normal medial and lateral malleolar height.

**Step 4:** Create a normal LDTA of 89° from the center of the ankle joint (Fig. 2C).

**Step 5:** Locate the apex of the deformity at the intersection of the two axes (Fig. 2D). Measure the magnitude of the deformity (5°). Note that the apex is at the level of the ankle joint.

## Identifying the Apex on a Hindfoot Alignment View X-ray

**Step 1:** Draw a mid-diaphyseal line of the distal tibia (red line) (Fig. 3A).

**Step 2:** Draw a calcaneal bisector line (blue line) (Fig. 3A). First draw the lateral and medial borders of the calcaneus. Then use these borders to draw the calcaneal bisector line.

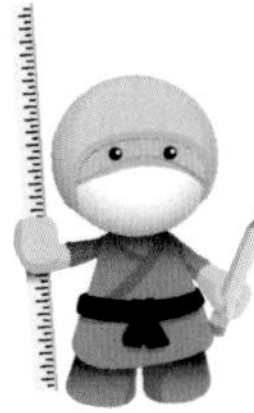

***Sensei says,***

*"When the Apex of the deformity is located at the level of the joint, an osteotomy will need to be made in a region remote from the Apex. Thus, translation will occur at the osteotomy site."*

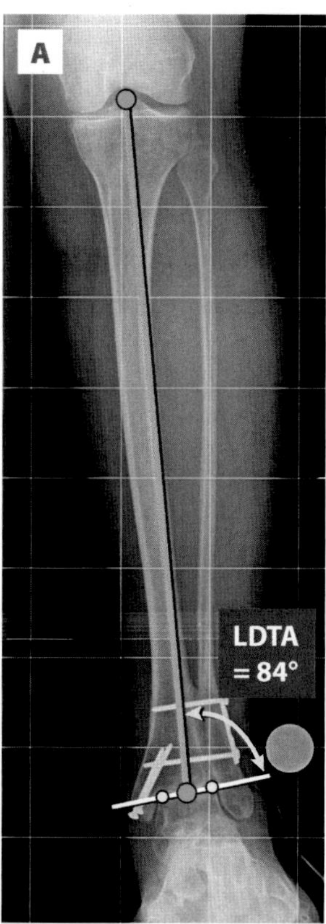


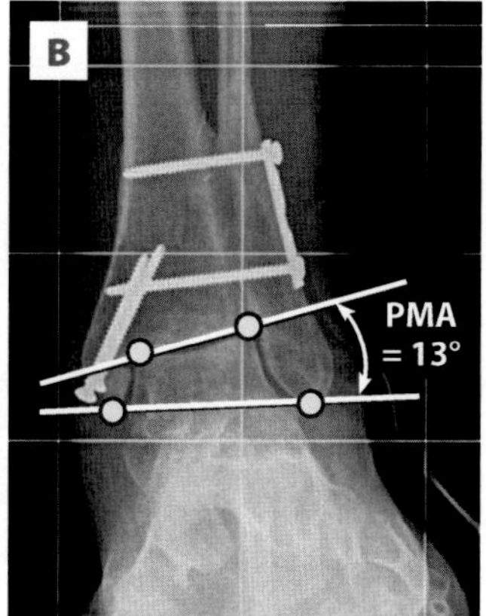


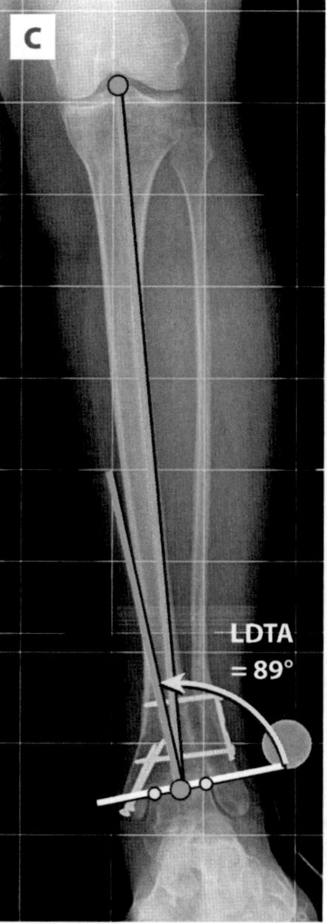


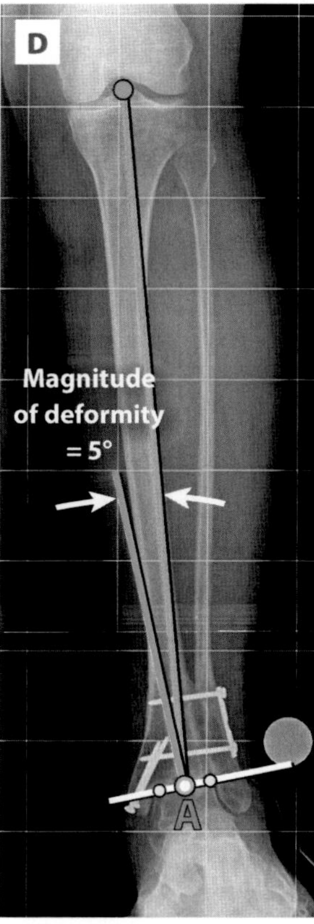


**Fig. 2:** The apex of the deformity is identified on an AP view ankle x-ray. A, apex.

**Step 3:** Measure the magnitude of the deformity (Fig. 3A). Note that this apex (intersection of red and blue lines) does not account for the normal lateral translational relationship of the calcaneus to the tibia. The normal tibial-calcaneal distance is 1.0 cm lateral.

**Step 4:** Measure the distance between the tibial mid-diaphyseal line and the calcaneal bisector line at the plantar-most level of the calcaneus (Fig. 3A). The anatomic relationship between the calcaneal bisector line and tibial mid-diaphyseal line should be maintained (10 mm lateral [6–14 mm lateral]) and accounted for during deformity correction.

**Step 5:** To locate the apex of the deformity, draw a third line (blue dashed line) that is parallel and 1 cm medial to the calcaneal bisector line (solid blue line) (Fig. 3B). The apex (A) is located at the intersection of the tibial mid-diaphyseal line and the blue dashed line.

**Step 6:** Perform the correction (Figs. 3C–E). When the deformity is corrected, the calcaneal bisector line is 1 cm lateral to the mid-diaphyseal line of the tibia (Fig. 3E).

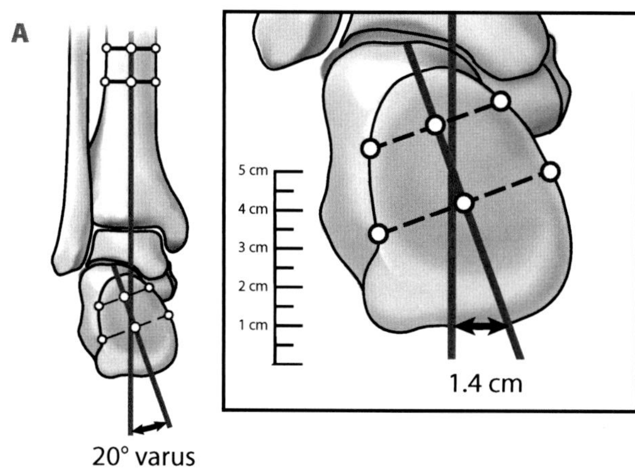


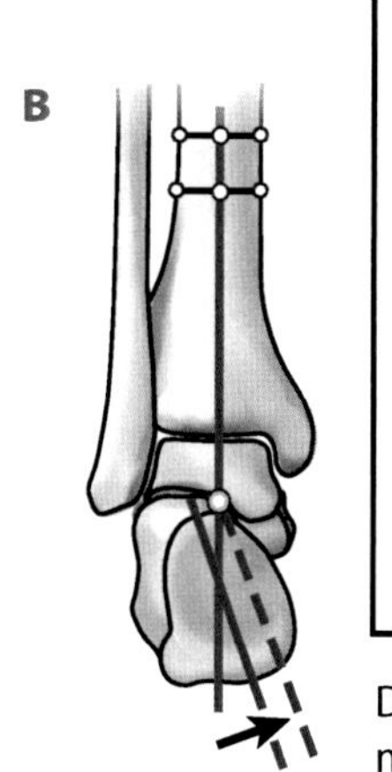


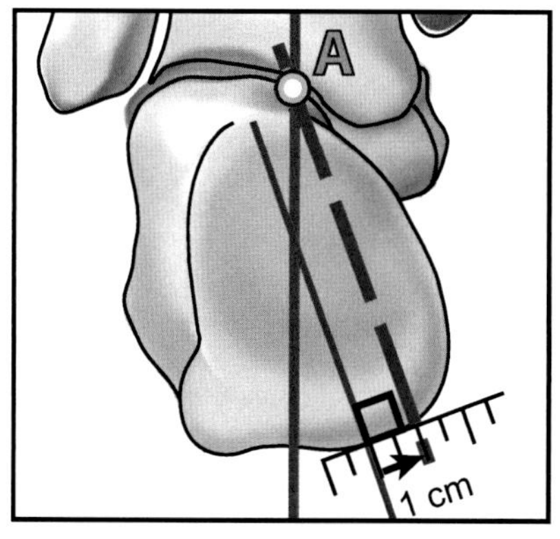


Draw a third line parallel and 1 cm medial to the calcaneal bisector line

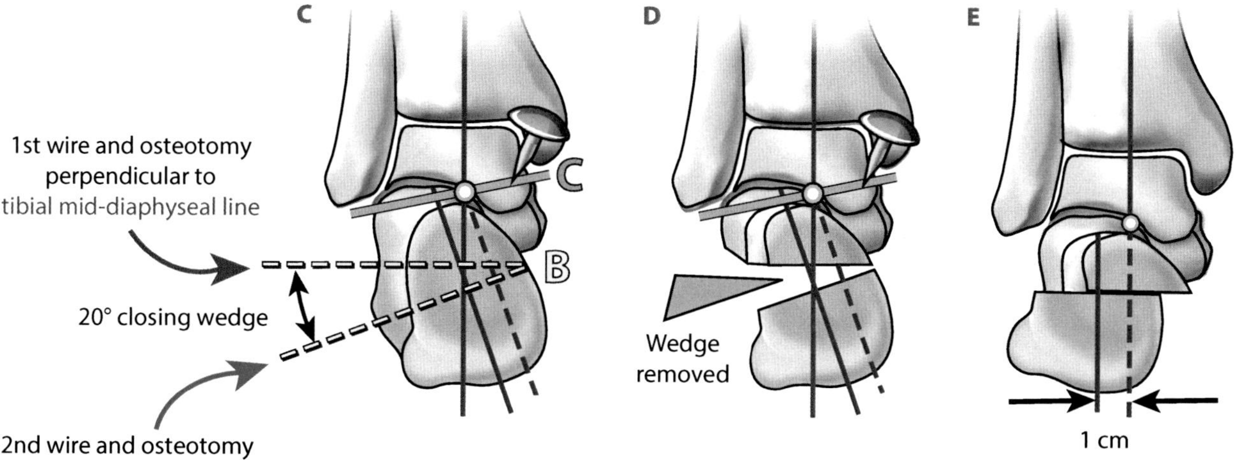


**Fig. 3:** The illustration shows how the apex of the calcaneal varus deformity is identified and corrected via a Dwyer calcaneal osteotomy on a hindfoot alignment view x-ray. A, apex; B, bone cut; C, C-level.

© 2023 Sinai Hospital of Baltimore

## Compensation for Frontal Plane Deformity

Frontal plane deformity of the distal tibia and ankle is commonly compensated by motion in the subtalar joint. The subtalar joint normally allows for 30° of inversion and 10° of eversion. In the frontal plane, valgus deformity of the distal tibia is tolerated better than varus deformity because a greater amount of subtalar joint motion is available (Fig. 4).

The subtalar joint compensates for a valgus ankle deformity by inversion and for a varus ankle deformity by eversion (Fig. 5). Distal tibial varus or valgus deformities that exceed the amount of compensation that is available at the subtalar joint result in compensatory forefoot pronation and supination, respectively.

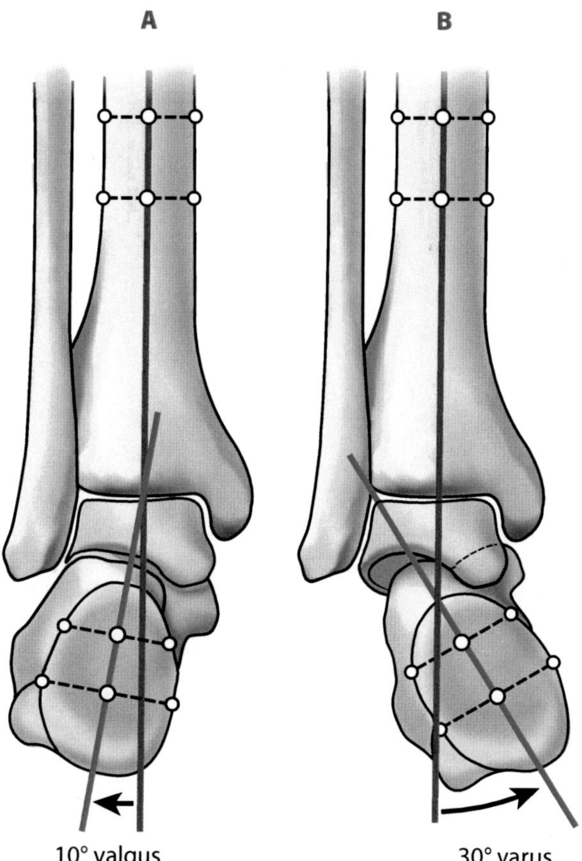


**Fig. 4:** Frontal plane deformity of the distal tibia and ankle is commonly compensated by motion in the subtalar joint. The subtalar joint normally allows for 10° of eversion (**A**) and 30° of inversion (**B**).

- In cases of distal tibial varus that do not have adequate subtalar joint eversion compensation, the first ray must compensate to bring the forefoot to the ground. The increased plantarflexion of the first ray increases the arch height, thus decreasing the weightbearing surface of the foot. This results in a cavus deformity.
- In cases of distal tibial valgus with inadequate subtalar joint inversion compensation, the forefoot supinates and the first ray dorsiflexes, which flattens the arch and increases the weightbearing surface of the foot.

## Varus and Valgus Deformities of the Distal Tibia/Ankle

In normal gait, the ground reaction force vector (GRFV) passes lateral to the ankle joint and imparts a valgus moment arm on the ankle joint, as this creates subtalar joint eversion (Figs. 5A and 5B). A valgus deformity moves the GRFV more laterally, which further increases the load on the lateral aspect of the ankle joint and laterally shifts the talus into the fibula, thereby distracting the syndesmosis (Fig. 5D). Distracting the syndesmosis results in articular destruction. This deformity is a common sequela of an ankle fracture that resulted in a shortened fibula or a valgus tilt to the tibial plafond because of incomplete reduction.

Varus deformity of the distal tibia or ankle moves the GRFV medially; however, this is not likely to result in degenerative changes (Fig. 5C). The broader medial malleolus articular surface offloads the increase in pressure and spares the ankle from degenerative changes. However, it is more symptomatic because the subtalar joint cannot compensate as much in eversion as it can in inversion. Thus, there is an increased likelihood of subtalar arthritis and early painful forefoot symptoms.

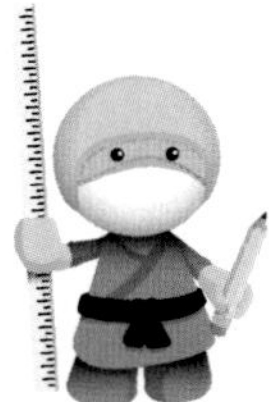

*Sensei says,*

*"The amount of compensation for a deformity at an adjacent joint is dependent on the mobility of that adjacent joint."*

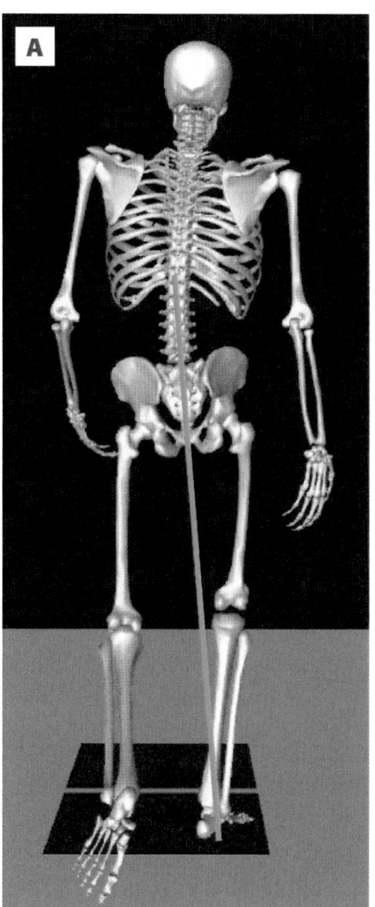


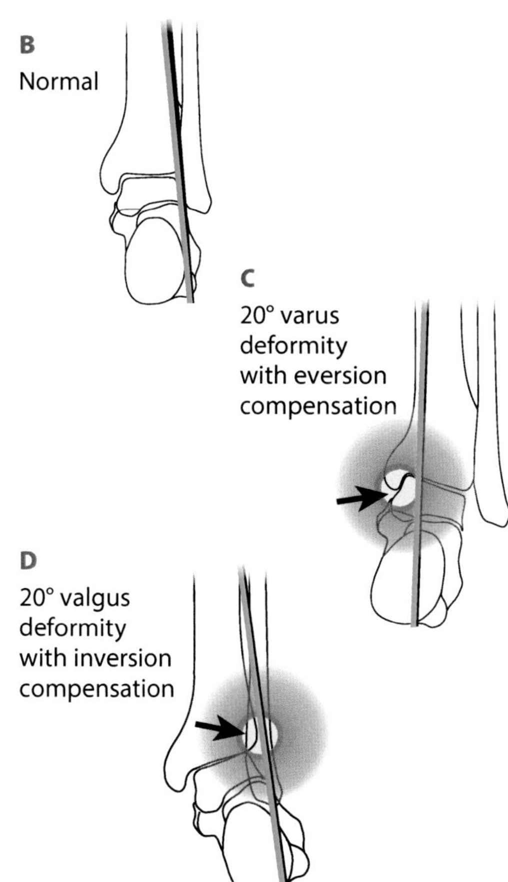


Fig. 5: A and B, In normal gait, the ground reaction force vector (GRFV) passes lateral to the ankle joint and imparts a valgus moment arm on the ankle joint, creating subtalar joint eversion. C, Varus deformity of the distal tibia or ankle moves the GRFV medially. D, Valgus deformity moves the GRFV more laterally, which further increases the load on the lateral aspect of the ankle joint and laterally shifts the talus into the fibula thereby distracting the syndesmosis.

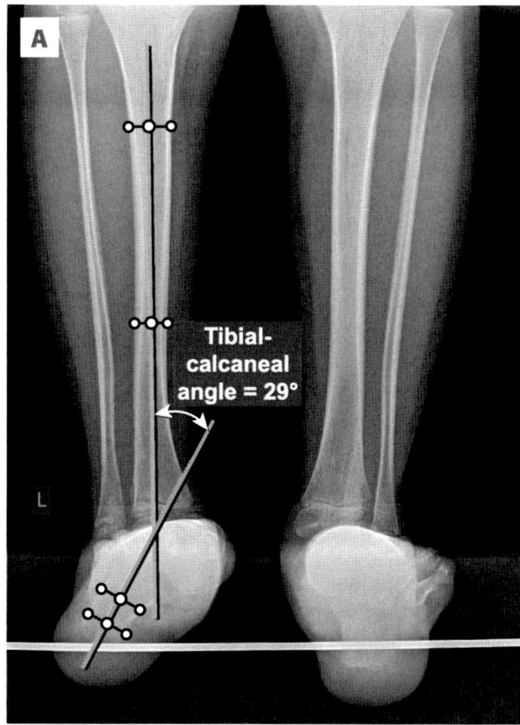


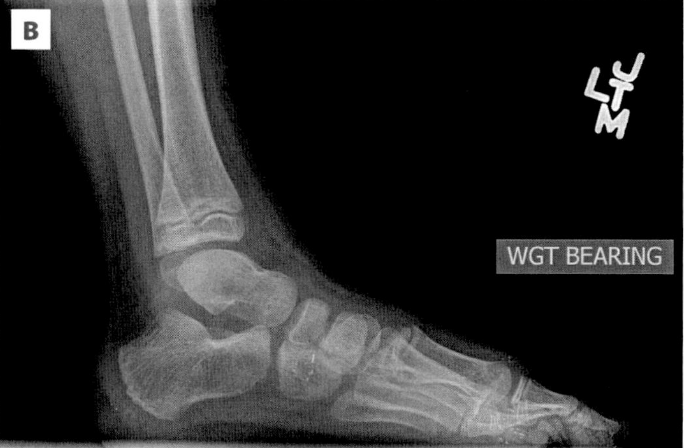


Fig. 6: A, Hindfoot valgus is measured by the tibial-calcaneal angle (29°) on an axial view x-ray. B, Hindfoot valgus can result in compensatory forefoot supinatus (ladder-like metatarsal appearance). Note that the patient is not full weightbearing, thus the calcaneal inclination angle looks normal, not decreased. Also, the forefoot is supinated and does not show the typical superimposition of the metatarsals.

© 2023 Sinai Hospital of Baltimore

### Hindfoot Varus and Valgus Deformity

If hindfoot varus and valgus are seen on the long leg axial calcaneal or hindfoot alignment views, then the forefoot compensates. If hindfoot valgus is present, forefoot supination will occur. If hindfoot varus is present, the forefoot will compensate with pronation. These compensatory mechanisms are designed to allow the foot to be plantigrade with respect to the weightbearing surface of the ground.

- Hindfoot valgus is measured by the tibial-calcaneal angle on an axial view x-ray (Fig. 6).
- Hindfoot valgus can result in a decreased calcaneal inclination angle and compensatory forefoot supinatus (Fig. 6).
- Hindfoot varus will increase the calcaneal inclination angle (Fig. 7) and create compensatory forefoot pronation or plantarflexion of the first metatarsal on a lateral view x-ray.
- Hindfoot valgus creates an increase in Meary's angle on the AP view x-ray (Figs. 8 and 9). A valgus hindfoot also causes talar head uncovering and peritalar lateral/abduction subluxation of the forefoot (Figs. 8 and 9). The opposite is noted in those with a varus hindfoot (Fig. 10).

## Sagittal Plane Axis Planning

Sagittal plane deformity is evaluated on a standing lateral view x-ray (Fig. 11). These deformities are described as procurvatum or recurvatum deformities. The inclination angle of the calcaneus can be useful in determining a calcaneus (>23°) or equinus position (<13°) of the heel.

- Recurvatum deformity is identified by an ADTA less than 78° (Fig. 12A).
- Procurvatum deformity is identified by an ADTA greater than 82° (Figs. 12B and 12C).
- Calcaneal inclination angle greater than 23° signifies a high arch foot type (calcaneus)

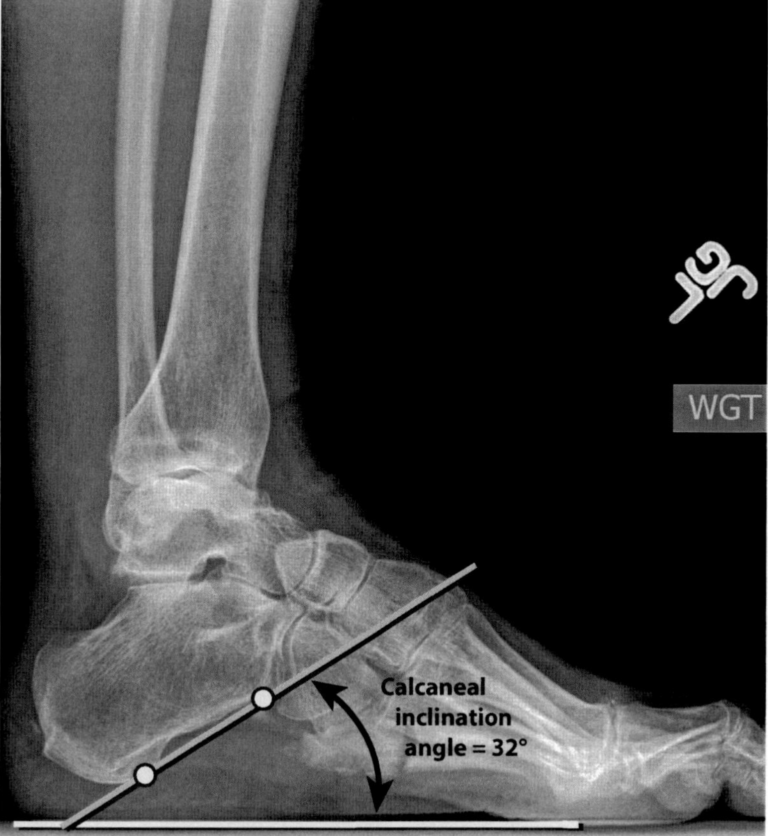


**Fig. 7:** Hindfoot varus will increase the calcaneal inclination angle (32°) and create compensatory forefoot pronation or plantarflexion of the first metatarsal on a lateral view x-ray.

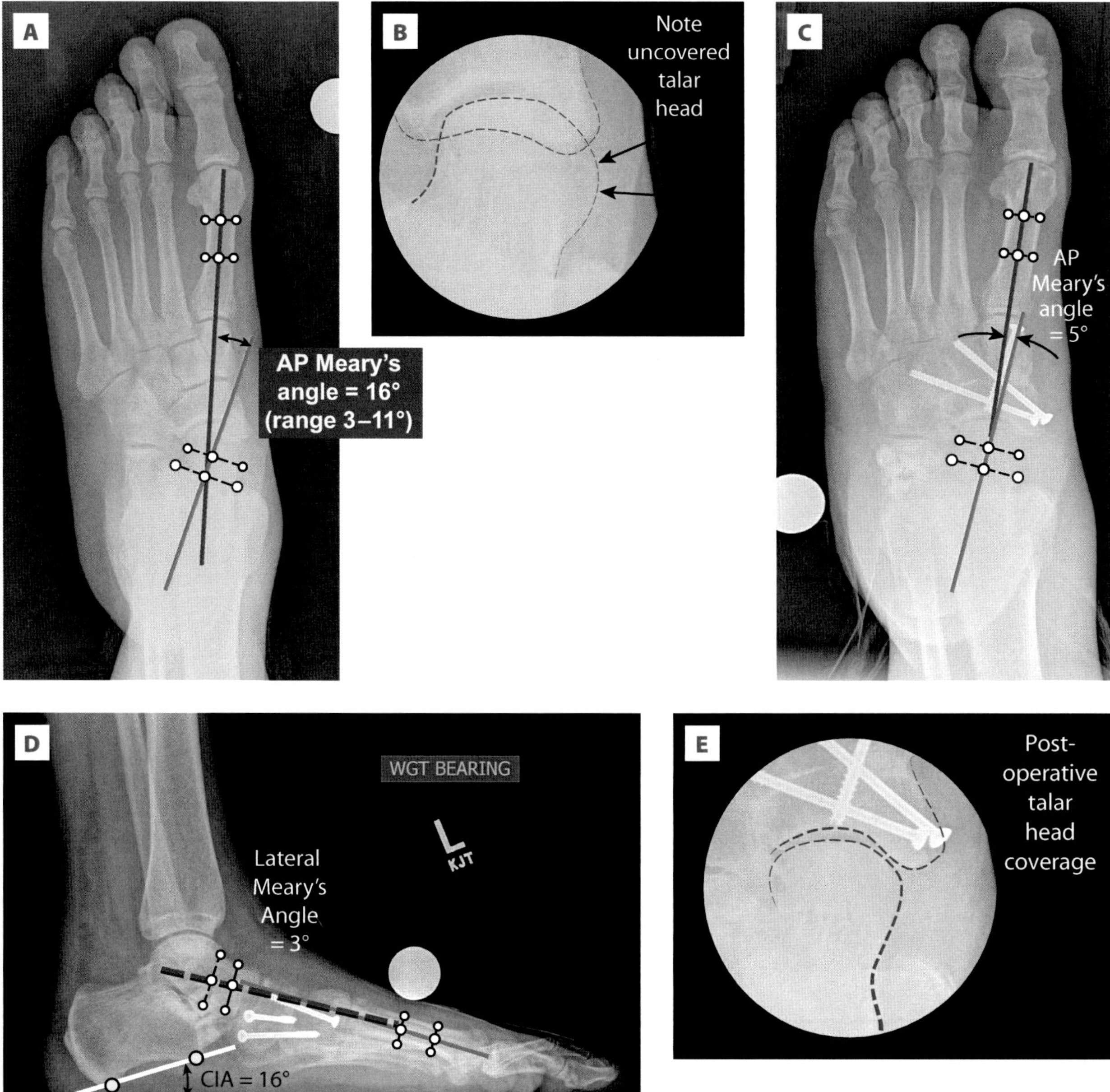


**Fig. 8:** **A** and **B**, Hindfoot valgus creates an increase in Meary's angle (16°) on the AP view x-ray and causes talar head uncovering and peritalar lateral/abduction subluxation of the forefoot. **C**, AP view x-ray after correction was achieved. **D**, Lateral view x-ray after correction was achieved. **E**, After correction was achieved, the talar head was fully covered. CIA, calcaneal inclination angle.

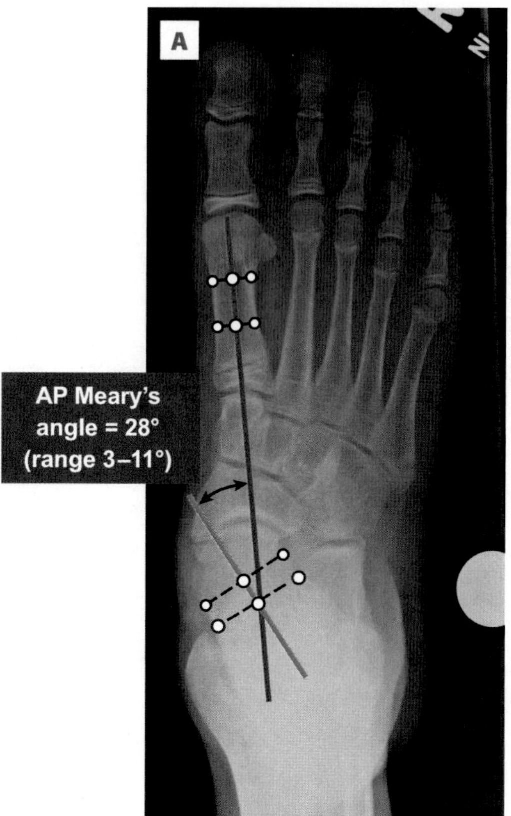


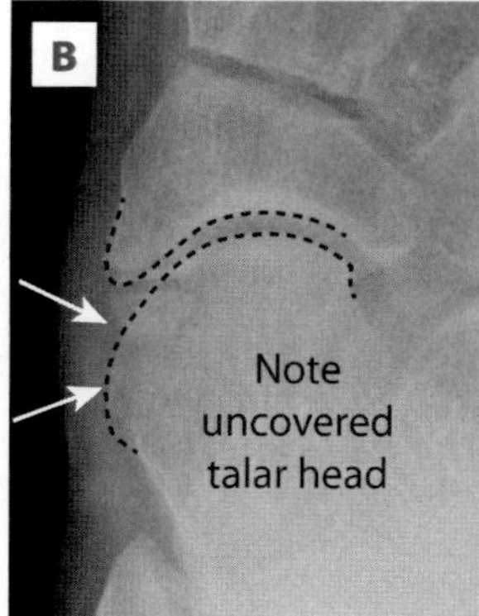


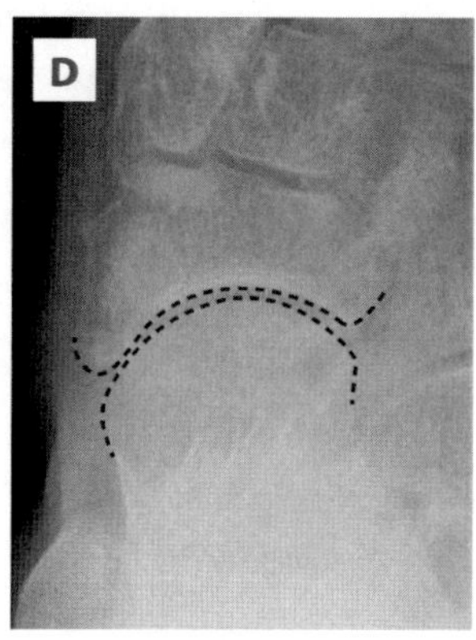


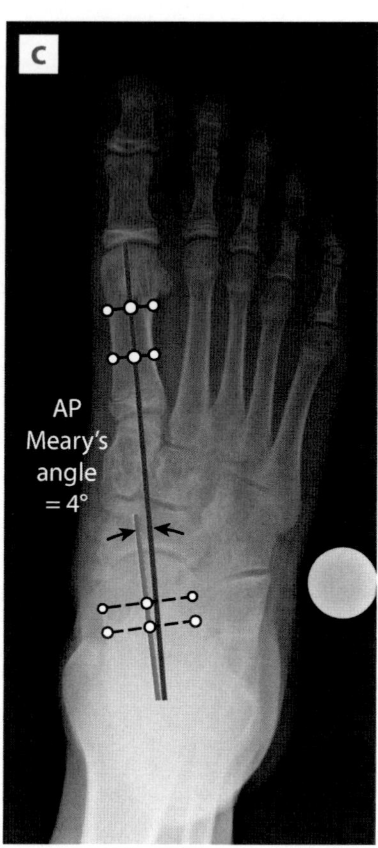


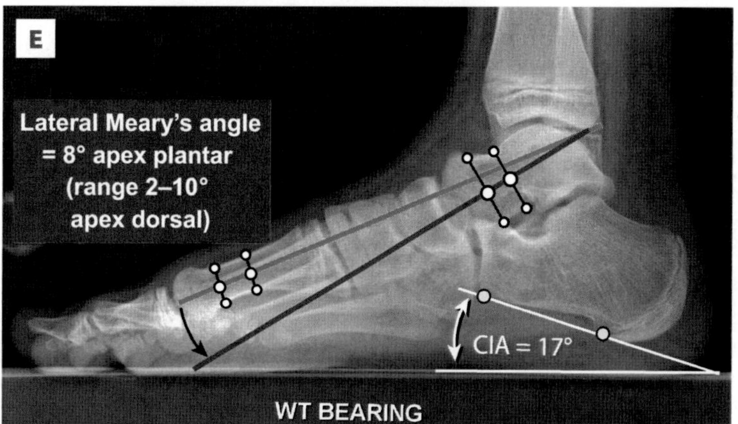


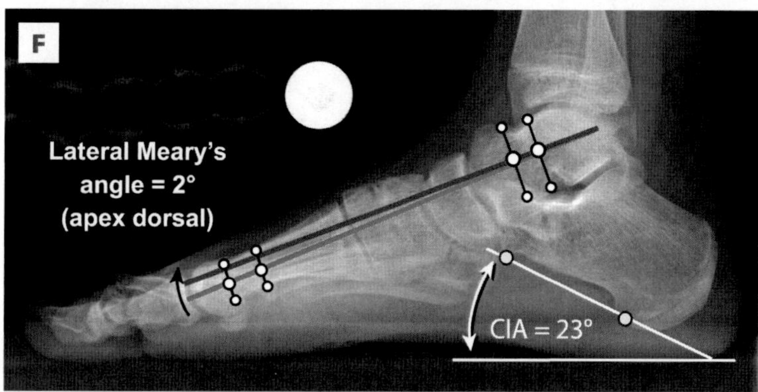


**Fig. 9:** **A** and **B**, Hindfoot valgus creates an increase in Meary's angle (28°) on the AP view x-ray and talar head uncovering. **C**, AP view x-ray after correction was achieved. **D**, After correction was achieved, the talar head was fully covered. **E**, Preoperative lateral view x-ray. **F**, Lateral view x-ray after correction was achieved. CIA, calcaneal inclination angle.

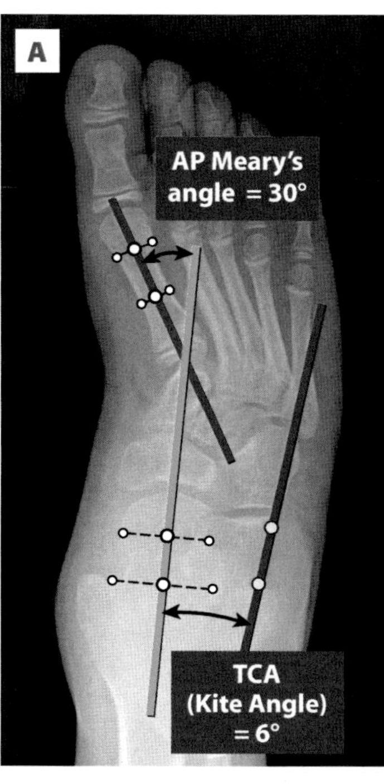


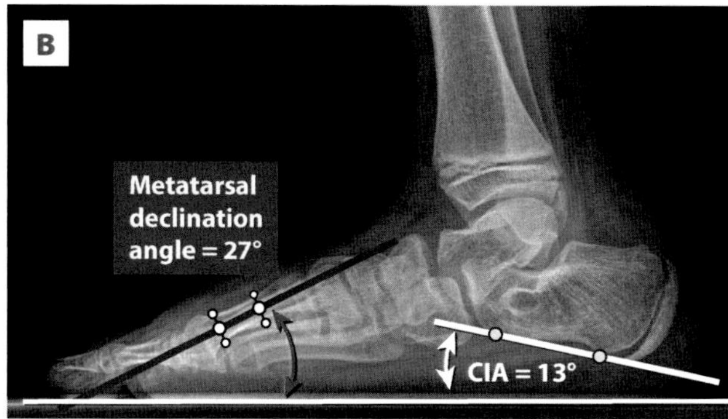


**Fig. 10:** **A**, Hindfoot varus creates a decreased Meary's angle on the AP view x-ray. **B**, Note the increase in the first metatarsal declination angle in the lateral view x-ray. CIA, calcaneal inclination angle.

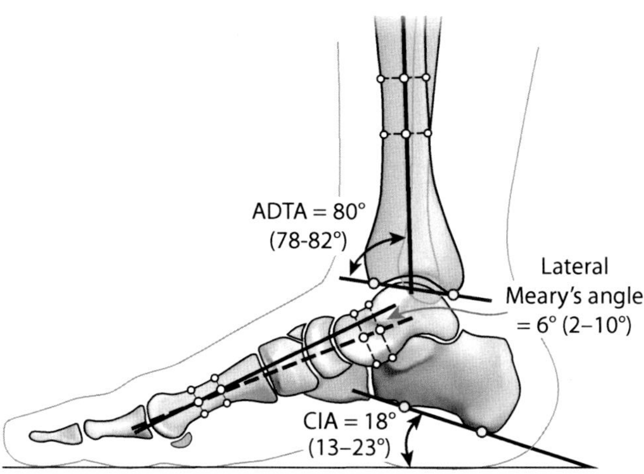


**Fig. 11:** Normal lateral view measurements. CIA, calcaneal inclination angle.

while an inclination less than 13° can be described as a low arch foot type (equinus).

- Lateral Meary's angle is useful to determine the apex of the deformity in pes cavus (high arch), pes planus (flatfoot), or rockerbottom foot types (Fig. 11).
- Patients can clinically present with a pes planus foot type yet have normal angles on the hindfoot alignment view x-ray. In those instances, the deformity can be due to midtarsal or Lisfranc joint pronation and can be noted without a valgus heel position. These feet can be described as high arch flatfoot.

## Compensation for Sagittal Plane Deformity

In the sagittal plane, the foot compensates for procurvatum or recurvatum deformity of the distal tibia by ankle joint dorsiflexion or plantarflexion, respectively. Normal ankle joint range of motion is 50° of plantarflexion and 20° of dorsiflexion. Since greater ankle joint plantarflexion is available, compensation for recurvatum is well tolerated compared with procurvatum.

- Distal tibial recurvatum is more joint destructive because the talar articular surface is uncovered and the talus is displaced anteriorly (Fig. 12A). Typically, this is not painful early on and is recognized only after the condition has significantly progressed.
- Recurvatum of the distal tibia displaces the center of rotation of the ankle joint anteriorly, thus increasing the anterior lever arm of the foot. The triceps surae counter these forces by placing the foot in equinus and decreasing the plantarflexor push off of the foot (Fig. 12A).
- In procurvatum, the articular surface of the ankle joint is well covered in the ankle mortise and is normally spared from deterioration (Fig. 12B).

© 2023 Sinai Hospital of Baltimore

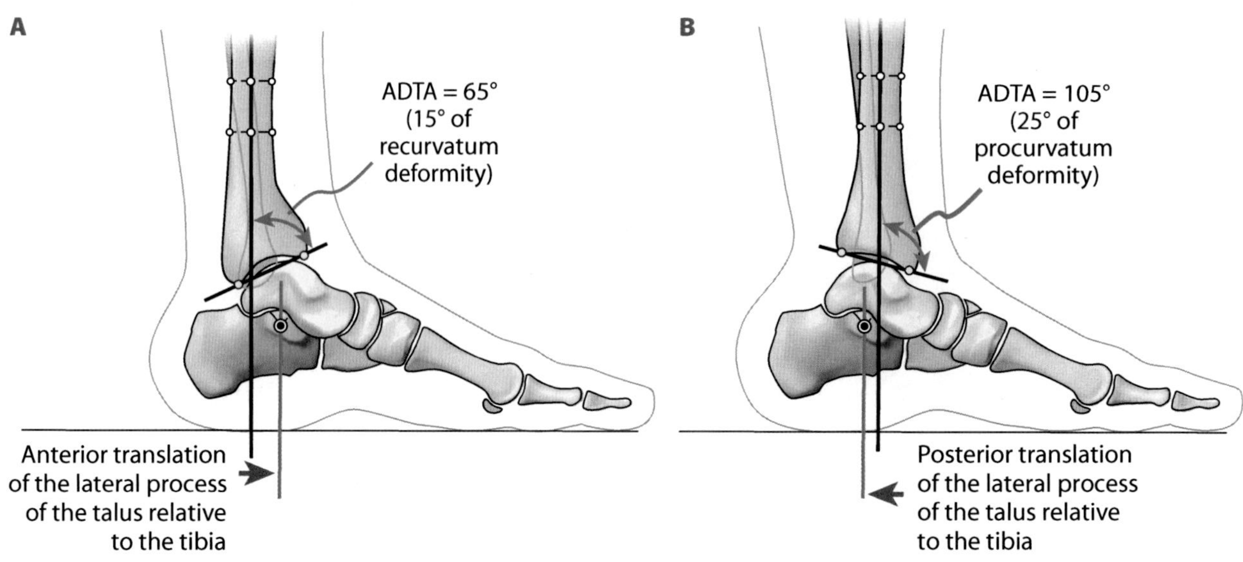


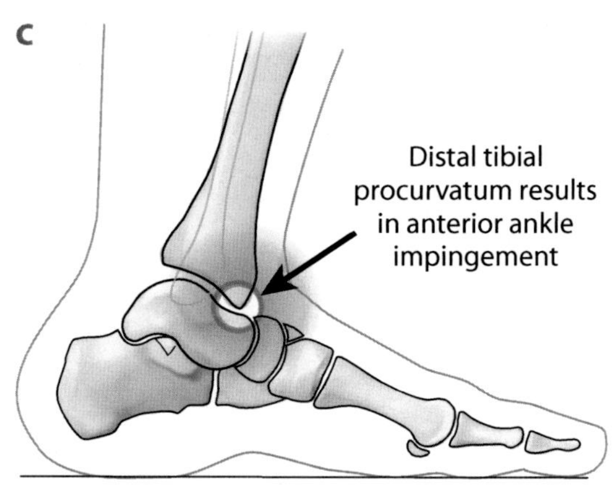


**Fig. 12: A**, Illustration shows distal tibial recurvatum of 15°. The magnitude of the recurvatum deformity is obtained by subtracting the measured value of the ADTA (65°) from the average normal value for ADTA (80°). **B**, Illustration shows distal tibial procurvatum of 25°. The magnitude of the procurvatum deformity is obtained by subtracting the average normal value for ADTA (80°) from the measured value of the ADTA (105°). **C**, Distal tibial procurvatum results in anterior ankle impingement.

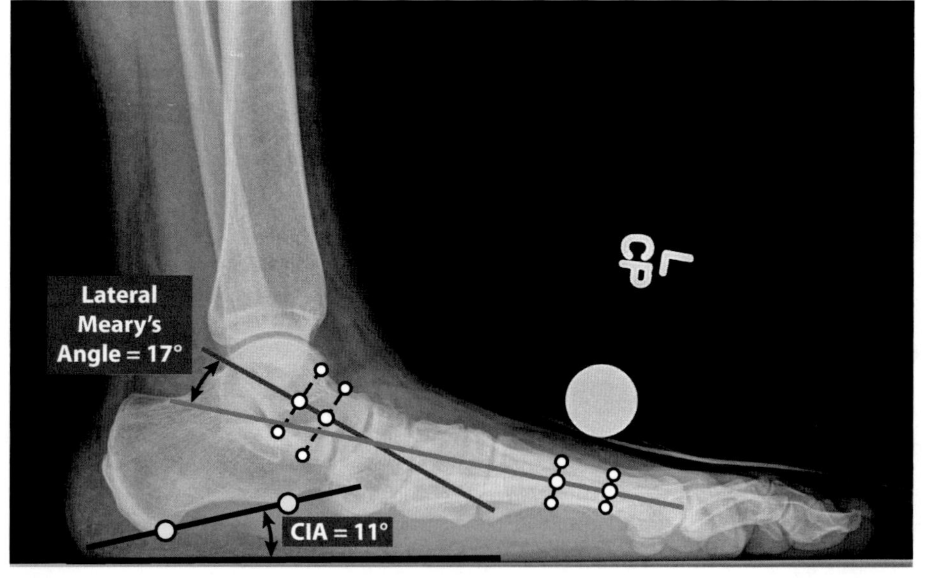


**Fig. 13:** Flatfoot deformity is commonly seen with a combined decreased calcaneal inclination angle and an apex plantar Meary's line. To achieve a plantigrade foot, the forefoot becomes supinated compared with the hindfoot. Note that this is the preoperative x-ray for the same case shown in Figure 8. CIA, calcaneal inclination angle.

- Distal tibial procurvatum is typically more painful because limited dorsiflexion compensation is available through the ankle joint. Distal tibial procurvatum results in anterior ankle joint impingement (Fig. 12C).
- In the sagittal plane, a flatfoot deformity is commonly seen with a combined decreased calcaneal inclination angle and an apex plantar Meary's line. To achieve a plantigrade foot, the forefoot becomes supinated compared with the hindfoot (Fig. 13). On a lateral view x-ray, this will appear as superimposition of the metatarsals.
- A cavus deformity can be a combination of forefoot and hindfoot positioning (Fig. 10). An increased calcaneal inclination angle (>23°) is compensated by plantarflexion of the first ray or forefoot valgus. The apex of Meary's line is more proximal and dorsally located. However, plantarflexion of the first ray can cause compensatory supination of the heel and an increase in the calcaneal inclination angle, thus appearing as hindfoot cavus.

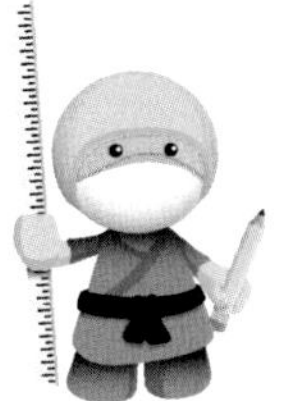

*Sensei says,*

*"A Coleman block test helps distinguish among hindfoot cavus, forefoot cavus, and combined cavus."*

### Rockerbottom Foot Deformity

Rockerbottom foot deformity or a collapsed arch is noted in cases of fracture/dislocation of the midfoot/Lisfranc region. A Charcot or traumatic midfoot/Lisfranc deformity creates a negative lateral Meary's angle. To diagnose and find the apex of a rockerbottom foot deformity:

**Step 1:** Draw the talar bisector line (red line) and the first metatarsal mid-diaphyseal line (blue line) (Fig. 14).

**Step 2:** Measure the calcaneal inclination angle (0°).

**Step 3:** The intersection of the proximal (red) and distal (blue) axis lines defines the apex of deformity. In this case, the magnitude of the deformity is the same angle represented by the lateral Meary's angle (27°).

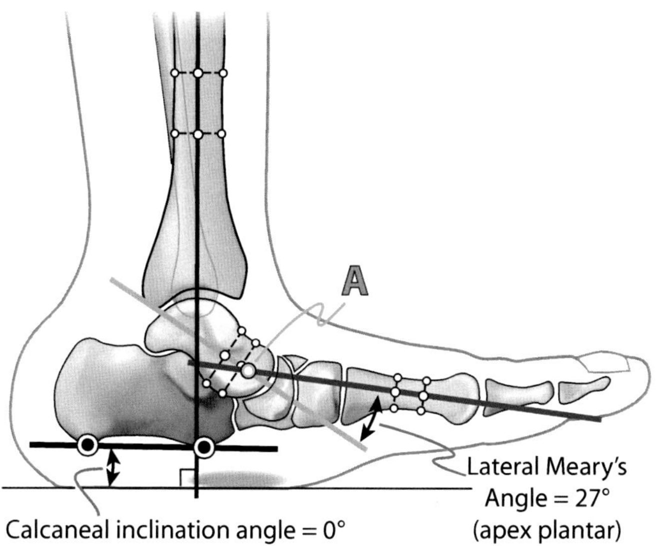


**Fig. 14:** Illustration shows how to find the apex (A) of a rockerbottom deformity.

## Transverse Plane Axis Planning

The foot may also exhibit transverse plane deformity, which is seen in flat feet, metatarsus adductus, and bunion deformities (Fig. 15). In cases of flatfoot, transverse plane deformity is commonly measured by an increase in Kite's or Meary's angle. Those with metatarsus adductus foot types will have an increase in the metatarsus adductus angle (MAA). When the MAA is abnormal, you may need to determine the true intermetatarsal angle. To determine the true intermetatarsal angle, add the number of degrees above the normal MAA to the value of the first intermetatarsal angle.

- In some flatfoot conditions, the talar head will be uncovered and the forefoot will be abducted with respect to the hindfoot. Correction with a calcaneal neck lengthening osteotomy will allow for correction about the midtarsal and subtalar joints, thus realigning the transverse plane deformity (Fig. 15C and 15D).

© 2023 Sinai Hospital of Baltimore

- Note: This correction can also un-mask a compensatory forefoot supination deformity, which would be evident on a lateral view x-ray and present as an elevated first ray/forefoot.
- Note: This correction can also un-mask a metatarsus adductus deformity.

- Metatarsus adductus deformity will generally present with a decrease in the intermetatarsal angles radiographically. The forefoot will appear medially deviated with respect to the tarsus and will have a decreased Kite's angle (Fig. 10).
- Hallux valgus deformity has an increased hallux valgus angle and an increased first IMA.

### Planning for Hallux Valgus Deformities

**Step 1:** Draw the first metatarsal mid-diaphyseal line (red line) (Fig. 15A).

**Step 2:** Draw the second metatarsal mid-diaphyseal line (yellow line) (Fig. 15A).

**Step 3:** The angle formed by these two lines is the first IMA (15°) (Fig. 15A).

**Step 4:** Draw a third line (blue line) that starts at the intersection of the two axes and creates a normal first IMA (8°) (Fig. 15B).

**Step 5:** The apex is located at the intersection of the normal first IMA (8°) (blue line) and the second metatarsal mid-diaphyseal line (yellow line) (Fig. 15B). The magnitude of deformity is 7° (Fig. 15C).

**Step 6:** Measure the translation of the capital fragment required for correction by the perpendicular distance from the red line to the blue line (8 mm shift) at the level of the first metatarsal neck (osteotomy site). Perform the correction (Fig. 15D).

### Compensation for Transverse Plane Deformity

In the transverse plane, abduction of the forefoot is compensated for by toe and/or metatarsal phalangeal joint adduction. Another more common example of transverse plane compensation is the adduction of the first metatarsal (increased intermetatarsal angle ≥ 10°). This adduction of the first metatarsal results in abduction of the hallux or an increase in the hallux abduction angle (bunion).

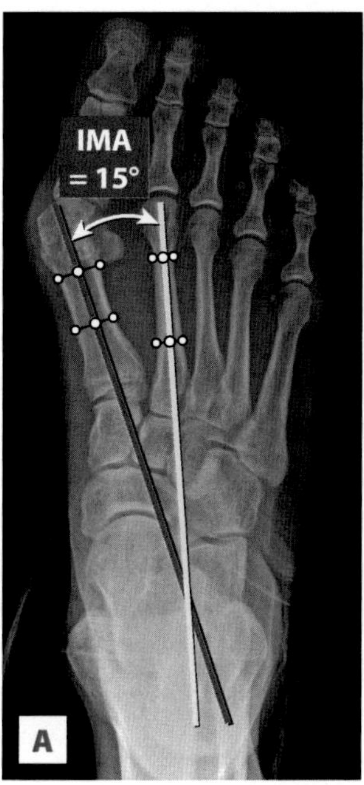


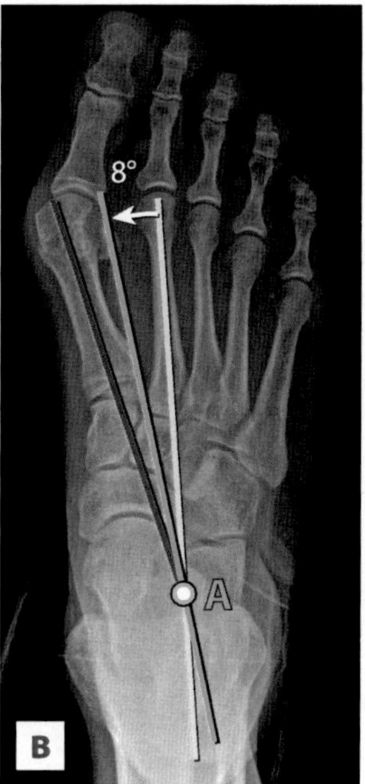


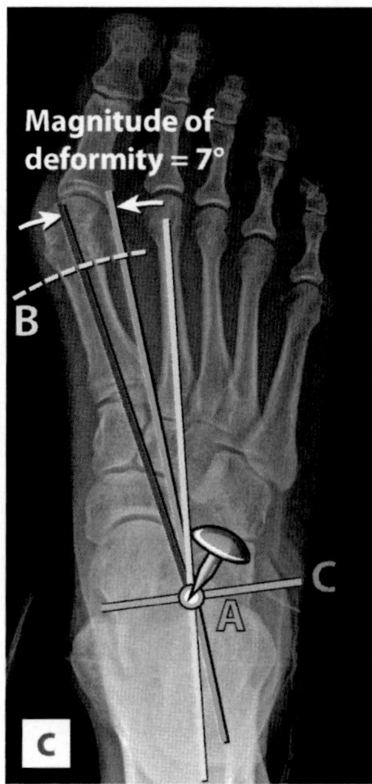


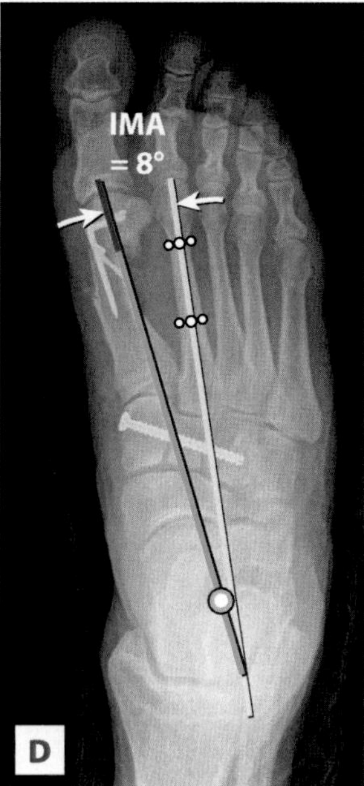


**Fig. 15:** Planning and correction of a hallux valgus deformity. A, apex; B, bone cut; C, C-level.

## Fixed Compensation

The compensatory positions of the ankle, subtalar, and midfoot joints may become fixed if the osseous deformity remains for an extended period of time. For example, chronic valgus deformity of the distal tibia compensated by subtalar inversion may become fixed. In such cases, if the distal tibial deformity is corrected with a supramalleolar osteotomy, then the subtalar inversion contracture is uncovered, producing a varus foot. Similarly, recurvatum deformity of the distal tibia compensated by ankle plantarflexion ends up in equinus after osteotomy correction if the ankle has lost dorsiflexion because of chronic plantarflexion positioning. Therefore, it is essential to identify fixed compensatory motion before performing corrective osteotomy. Usually, this can be accomplished by physical examination. If the foot can be placed in the maximum deformity position, no fixed compensation (contracture) is present. If the foot cannot reach the maximum deformity position, fixed compensatory contracture is present. In the case of recurvatum osseous deformity with fixed compensatory equinus contracture, the equinus needs to be corrected before or simultaneous to the flexion supramalleolar osteotomy.

In summary, clinical examination and radiographic reference lines comprise the foundation for precise surgical planning. An understanding of the standard radiographic lines, points, and angular relationships is critical for appropriate evaluation and identification of the level and extent of deformity. Surgical planning of osseous realignment as well as consideration of concomitant soft-tissue laxity/contracture and adjacent joint compensation are important for successful foot and ankle realignment.

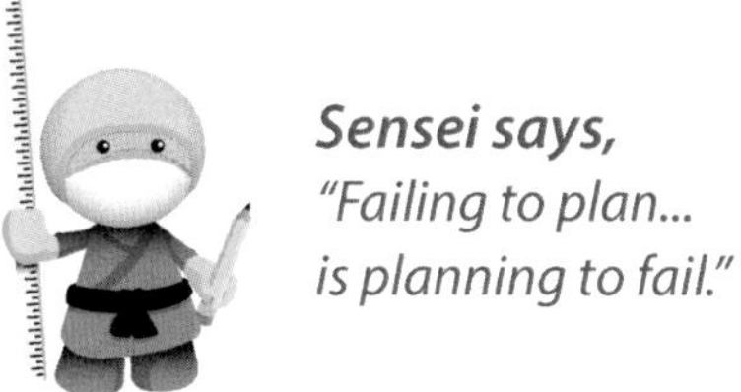

***Sensei says,***
*"Failing to plan...*
*is planning to fail."*

© 2023 Sinai Hospital of Baltimore

# Chapter 15

# Foot and Ankle Deformity Analysis and Surgical Planning

Noman A. Siddiqui, DPM

Kelsey J. Millonig, DPM

Foot and ankle deformity correction can be challenging due to the compensation from the joints within the foot. However, analysis of these deformities can be simplified by applying principles of long bone correction to the foot in addition to understanding the biomechanical considerations. This chapter utilizes the principles of MAP the ABCs for common conditions seen in foot and ankle deformities.

## Pes Planus Foot and Hallux Valgus Deformities

### Preoperative Deformity Analysis and Operative Planning

Frontal plane deformity is best evaluated with hindfoot alignment x-ray.

#### Angle Analysis:

**Step 1:** Draw a mid-diaphyseal line of the distal tibia (*red line*) and calcaneal bisector line (*blue line*) to determine the tibial-calcaneal angle (7° valgus) (Fig. 1).

- Sagittal plane deformity is evaluated on a standing lateral view x-ray of the foot. In the sagittal plane, a flatfoot deformity is commonly seen with a combined decreased calcaneal inclination angle and an apex plantar Meary's line.

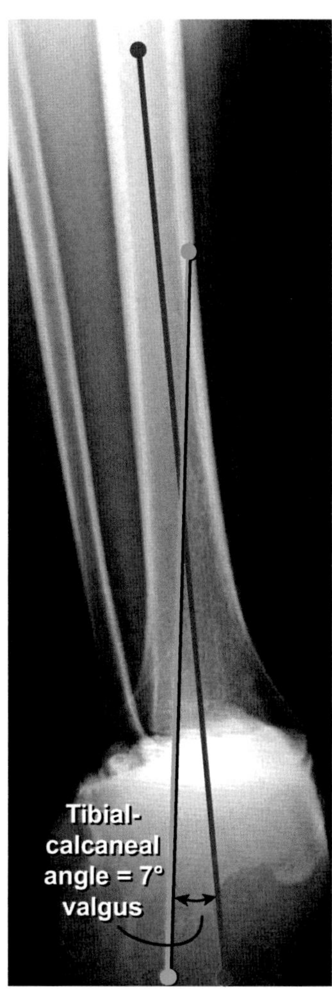


**Fig. 1:** Tibial-calcaneal angle deformity of 7° valgus through subtalar joint motion.

© 2023 Sinai Hospital of Baltimore

**Step 2:** Establish a calcaneal inclination angle (15°) (Fig. 2A).

**Step 3:** Bisect the talar body (*red line*) and bisect the first metatarsal (*blue line*) to establish a lateral Meary's angle (22°) (Fig. 2B).

- Transverse plane deformity is evaluated with a standing AP view x-ray of the foot. An increase in Kite's or Meary's angle as well as hallux valgus deformity are often seen in pes planus deformities.

**Step 4:** Bisect the talar body proximally (*red line*) and bisect the first metatarsal distally (*blue line*) to establish the AP Meary's angle (24°) (Fig. 2C).

## Hindfoot Deformity Correction

**Step 5:** The intersection of the two axes that make up the AP Meary's angle determine the apex (Fig. 3A). The magnitude of deformity is calculated by subtracting the average normal AP Meary's angle (7°) from the value of the AP Meary's angle in this case (24°). The magnitude of the deformity is 17°.

**Step 6:** The osteotomy to correct the deformity cannot be performed at the apex. Therefore, a different location is chosen in the anterior neck of the calcaneus, with the assumption that the correction of the hindfoot will occur through the subtalar and talonavicular joint (Fig. 3B). Since the osteotomy is not performed at the level of the apex, bony translation will occur during the correction.

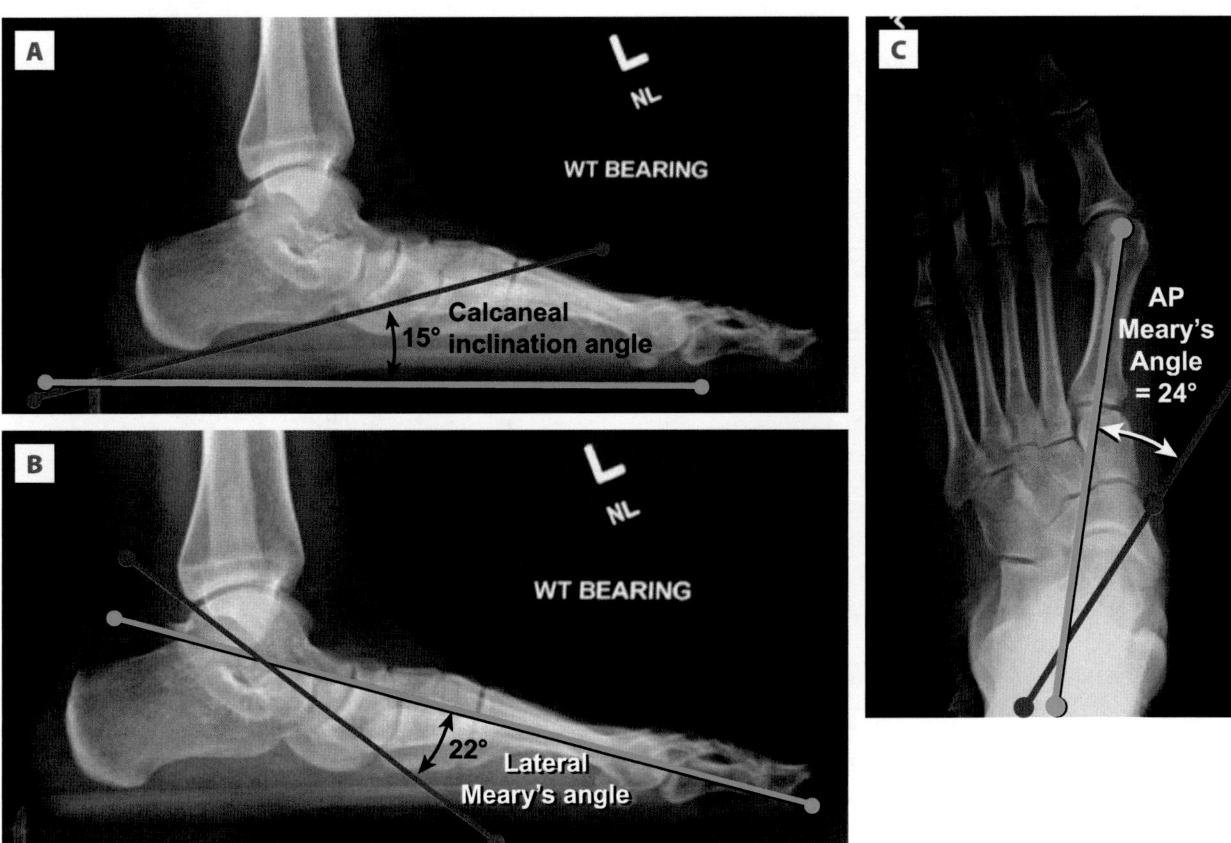


**Fig. 2:** Preoperative deformity planning demonstrating pes planus deformity. **A**, Calcaneal inclination angle (15°). **B**, Lateral Meary's angle (22°). **C**, AP Meary's angle (24°).

**Step 7:** Draw the correction level (C-level) at the apex (Fig. 3C). To draw the C-level, identify the obtuse angle that is created by the intersection of the proximal and distal axes. The C-level bisects this obtuse angle and passes through the apex.

**Step 8:** To achieve correction, the bone segment is angulated about a thumbtack placed on the C-level. Place the thumbtack at the apex along the C-level (Fig. 3D).

**Step 9:** Plan a 23° opening wedge osteotomy (trapezoidal wedge) to restore the angular position (this is commonly known as an Evans procedure) (Fig. 3E). Note that the proximal and distal axes are parallel instead of co-linear after correction due to the function of the joint and the anatomic position of the bone. The new AP Meary's angle is 1°.

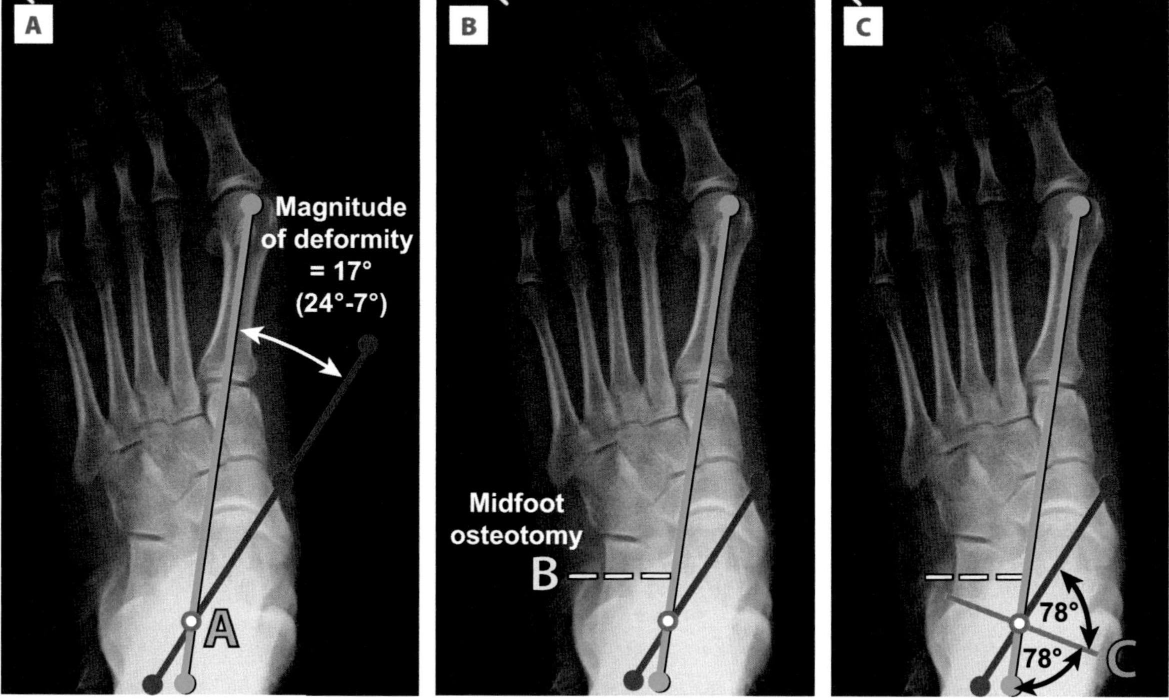


**Fig. 3:** Hindfoot deformity correction. **A**, The apex is located at the intersection of the two axes that make up the AP Meary's angle. The magnitude of deformity is calculated by subtracting the average normal AP Meary's angle (7°) from the value of the AP Meary's angle in this case (24°). The magnitude of the deformity is 17°. **B**, Midfoot osteotomy is placed in the anterior neck of the calcaneus. **C**, The C-level passes through the apex and bisects the obtuse angle that is created by the intersection of the proximal and distal axes. A, apex; B, bone cut; C, C-level.

© 2023 Sinai Hospital of Baltimore

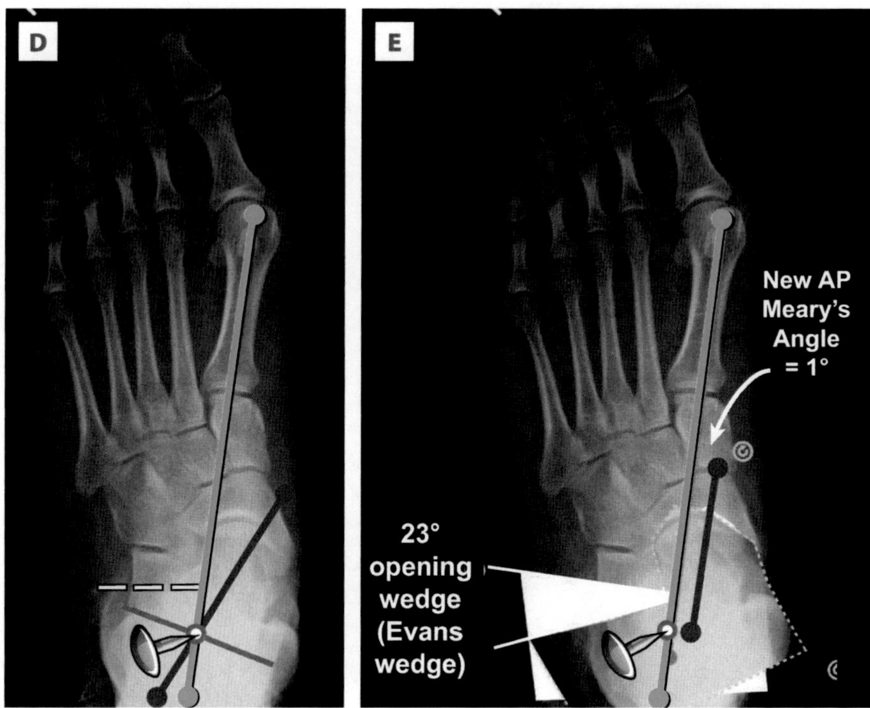


**Fig. 3 (continued): D,** The thumbtack is placed at the apex along the C-level. **E,** A 23° opening wedge osteotomy (trapezoidal wedge) is planned. This is also known as an Evans procedure. The new AP Meary's angle is 1°.

## Hallux Deformity Correction

**Step 10:** Analyze the forefoot hallux valgus deformity. The first mechanical IMA is formed by drawing the mechanical axis of the first metatarsal and second metatarsal (Fig. 4A).

**Step 11:** The intersection of the two axes that make up the first mechanical IMA determine the apex (Fig. 4B). The magnitude of deformity is calculated by subtracting the average normal mIMA (9°) from the value of the mIMA in this case (13°). The magnitude of the deformity is 4°.

**Step 12:** Since the level of the apex in the hindfoot is not acceptable for the osteotomy, an extra-articular osteotomy site is selected in the metatarsal (Figs. 4C). Since the osteotomy is not performed at the level of the apex, bony translation will occur during the correction.

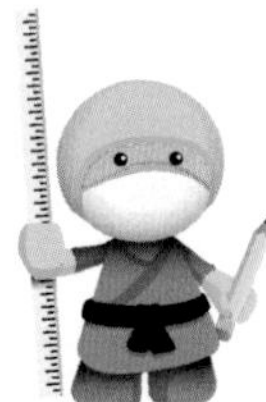

*Sensei says,*

*"In the foot, most osteotomies will not be made at the apex of the deformity; therefore, translation must occur."*

**Step 13:** Draw the C-level at the apex (Fig. 4D). To draw the C-level, identify the obtuse angle that is created by the intersection of the proximal and distal axes. The C-level bisects this obtuse angle and passes through the apex.

**Step 14:** To achieve correction, the bone segment will be angulated about a thumbtack placed on the C-level. Place the thumbtack at the apex along the C-level (Fig. 4E).

**Step 15:** A distal metatarsal osteotomy is performed (Fig. 4F). The metatarsal head is translated to restore the first mIMA to 9°.

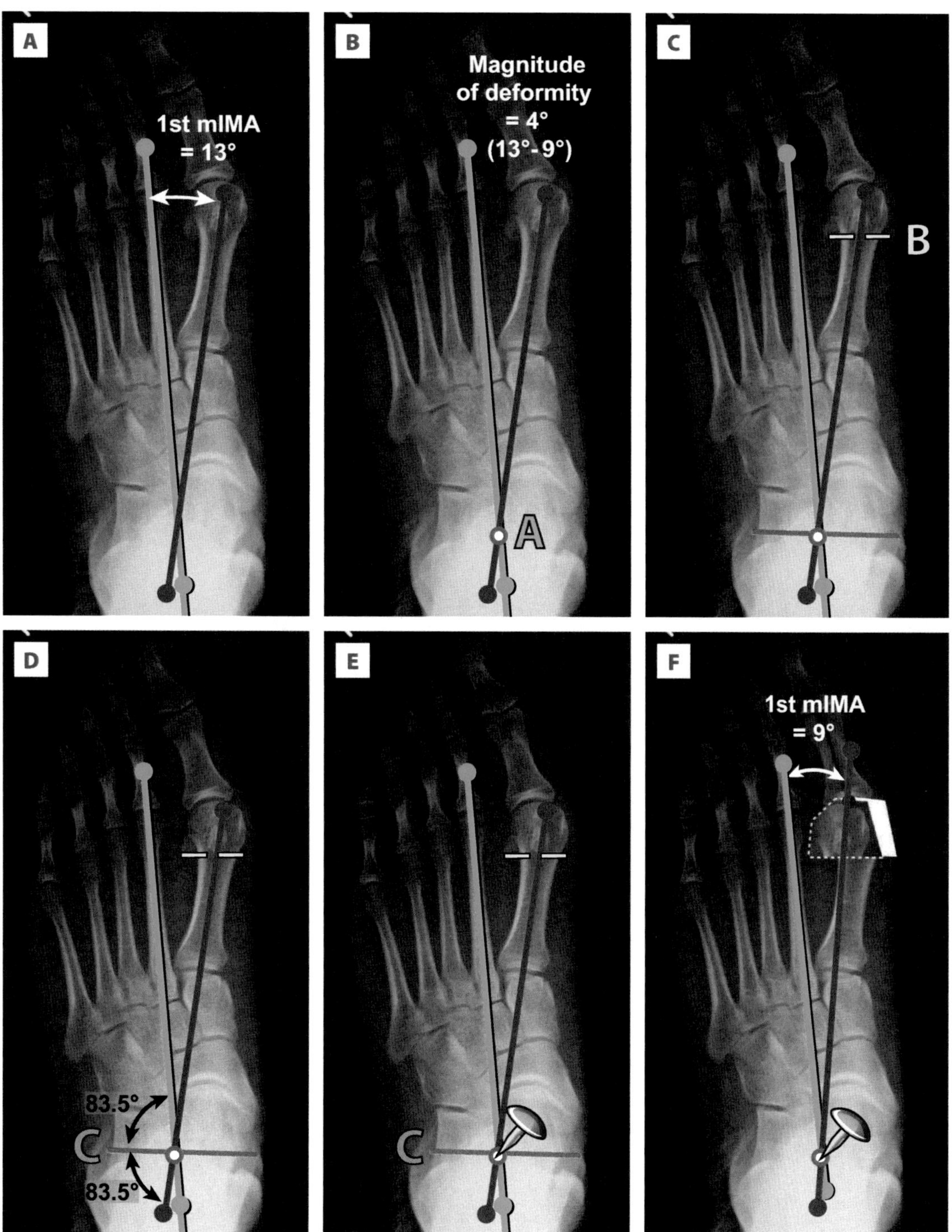


**Fig. 4:** Hallux deformity correction. **A**, To analyze the forefoot hallux valgus deformity, the first mIMA (mechanical intermetatarsal angle) is measured (13°). **B**, The apex is located at the intersection of the two axes that make up the first mIMA. The magnitude of deformity (4°) is calculated by subtracting the average normal mIMA (9°) from the value of the mIMA in this case (13°). **C**, The level of the apex is not acceptable for the osteotomy. An extra-articular osteotomy site is selected in the metatarsal. **D**, The C-level bisects the obtuse angle that is created by the intersection of the proximal and distal axes and it passes through the apex. **E**, The thumbtack is placed at the apex along the C-level. **F**, A distal metatarsal osteotomy is performed. A, apex; B, bone cut; C, C-level.

© 2023 Sinai Hospital of Baltimore

### Proximal Phalanx Correction

**Step 16:** Obtain the hallux abductus angle by drawing the bisection of the phalanx with respect to the metatarsal head mechanical axis (Fig. 5A).

**Step 17:** The intersection of the two axes that make up the hallux abductus angle determine the apex (Fig. 5B). The apex of the deformity is intraarticular. The magnitude of deformity is calculated by subtracting the average normal HAA (8°) from the value of the HAA in this case (25°). The magnitude of the deformity is 17°.

**Step 18:** Since the level of the apex is not acceptable for the osteotomy, a more proximal osteotomy site is selected (Figs. 5C). The osteotomy is not performed at the level of the apex; therefore, bony translation will occur during the correction.

**Step 19:** Draw the C-level at the apex (Fig. 5D). To draw the C-level, identify the obtuse angle that is created by the intersection of the proximal and distal axes. The C-level bisects this obtuse angle and passes through the apex.

**Step 20:** To achieve correction, the bone segment will be angulated about a thumbtack placed on the C-level. Place the thumbtack at the apex along the C-level (Fig. 5E).

**Step 21:** The proximal phalanx osteotomy is performed with a medial closing wedge (Akin osteotomy) (Fig. 5F). The new HAA angle (8°) is within the normal limits.

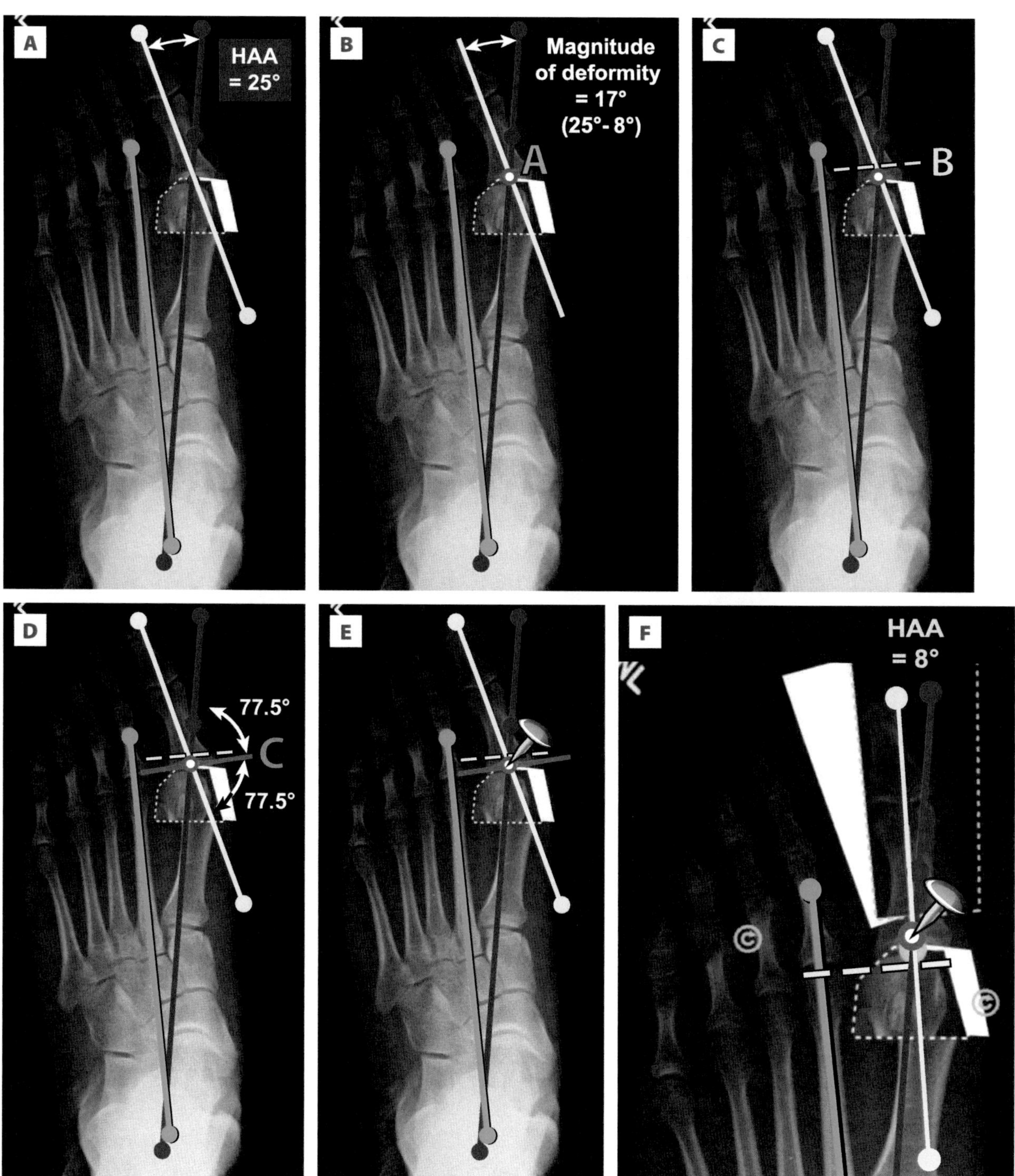


**Fig. 5:** Proximal phalanx correction. **A**, The hallux abductus angle (HAA) is measured (25°). **B**, The apex is located at the intersection of the two axes that make up the HAA. The magnitude of deformity (17°) is calculated by subtracting the average normal HAA (8°) from the value of the HAA in this case (25°). **C**, The level of the apex is not acceptable for the osteotomy. A more proximal osteotomy site is chosen. **D**, The C-level passes through the apex and bisects the obtuse angle that is created by the intersection of the proximal and distal axes. **E**, The thumbtack is placed at the apex along the C-level. **F**, The proximal phalanx osteotomy is performed with a medial closing wedge (Akin osteotomy). A, apex; B, bone cut; C, C-level.

© 2023 Sinai Hospital of Baltimore

**Summary:**

Normal angular relationships have been restored in all planes. Acute realignment of the hindfoot and forefoot is noted on the AP x-ray and fixated with internal fixation (Fig. 6). Postoperative sagittal alignment and frontal plane alignment demonstrate correction with calcaneal inclination (17°), lateral Meary's angle (9°), and tibial-calcaneal angle (0°) (Fig. 7).

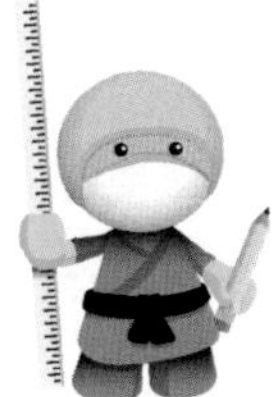

*Sensei says,*

*"Mechanical axis lines can be utilized to determine correction when normal foot anatomy is disrupted."*

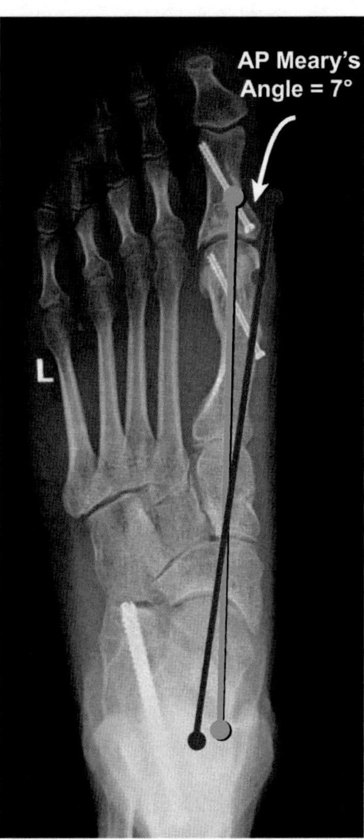


**Fig. 6:** Acute realignment is noted on the AP x-ray with AP Meary's angle (7°).

This example demonstrates how long bone planning principles are applied to the foot. In pedal correction, the ankle, subtalar, and midtarsal joints play an integral role in maintaining alignment. There are some important features in this example.

1. An anterior neck lengthening will restore hindfoot and forefoot alignment by acting on the subtalar joint. Though not obvious to the casual observer, the osteotomy is not at the apex of Meary's angle; therefore, translation must occur. This is seen by the calcaneus obtaining a more rectus position in the frontal and sagittal planes (correction of TCA and CIA). The talus will also restore its position in sagittal plane and transverse planes, which is visualized as coverage of the talar head on the navicular.

2. In bunion correction, the IMA apex is always at a location proximal to the metatarsals while the HAA is always near the first metatarsophalangeal joint or within the first metatarsal head. Both these apexes need to be accounted for during bunion correction. Since an osteotomy is not performed in the hindfoot to restore the IMA, an osteotomy in the metatarsal requires obligatory translation to correct the angular relationship. The further one moves from the apex in the metatarsal, the greater the translation. The HAA can be restored with metatarsophalangeal joint fusion; however, when metatarsophalangeal joint preservation is preferred, an osteotomy in the phalanx assists in restoring the angular relationship, along with the bony and soft-tissue elements of the deformity (e.g., extensor and flexor tendons, sesamoids).

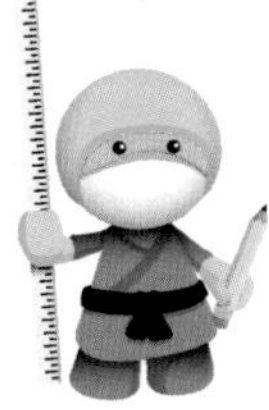

*Sensei says,*

*"Hindfoot valgus creates an increase in Meary's angle on the AP view radiograph with talar head uncovering and peritalar lateral/abduction subluxation of the forefoot."*

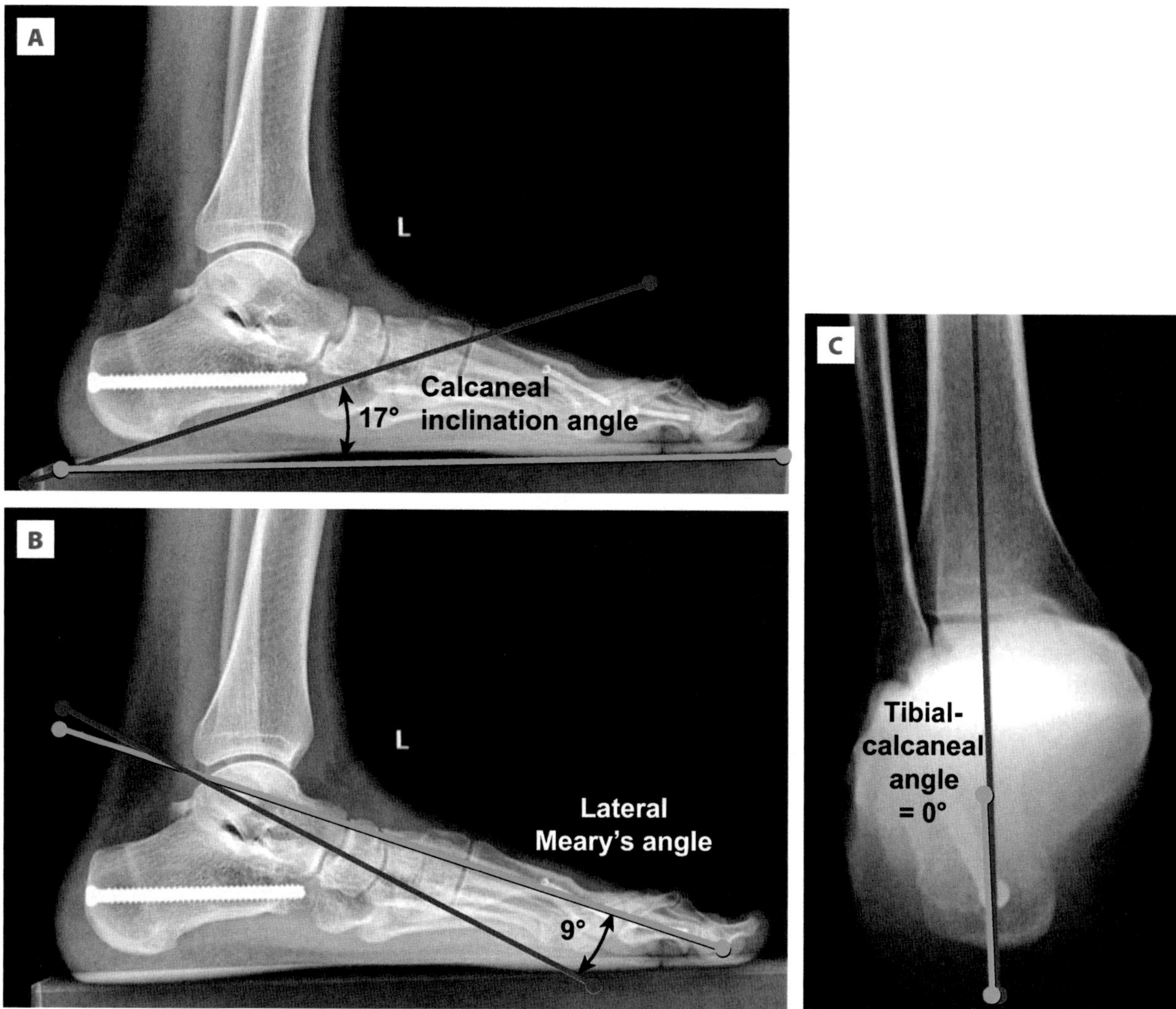


**Fig. 7:** Restoration of normal alignment was achieved in all planes. Postoperative realignment with calcaneal inclination (17°) (**A**), lateral Meary's angle (9°) (**B**), and tibial-calcaneal angle (0°) (**C**).

© 2023 Sinai Hospital of Baltimore

## Cavus Foot Deformity

A cavus deformity can be a combination of forefoot and hindfoot positioning. Trademark identification is an increased calcaneal inclination angle (>23°), which may be compensated by plantarflexion of the first ray or forefoot valgus.

## Preoperative Deformity Analysis and Operative Planning

**Step 1:** Sagittal plane deformity is evaluated on a standing lateral view x-ray of the foot (Fig. 8).

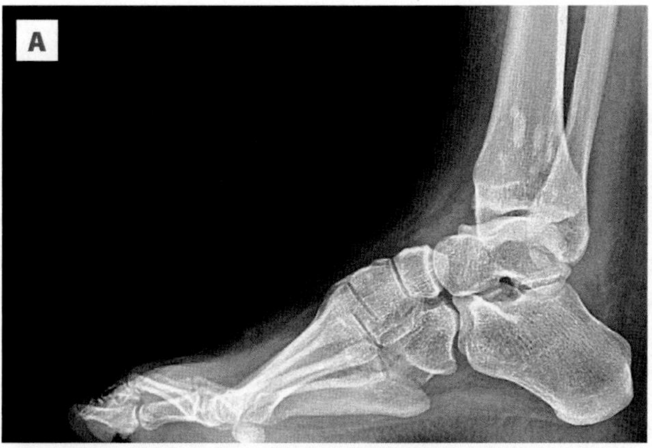


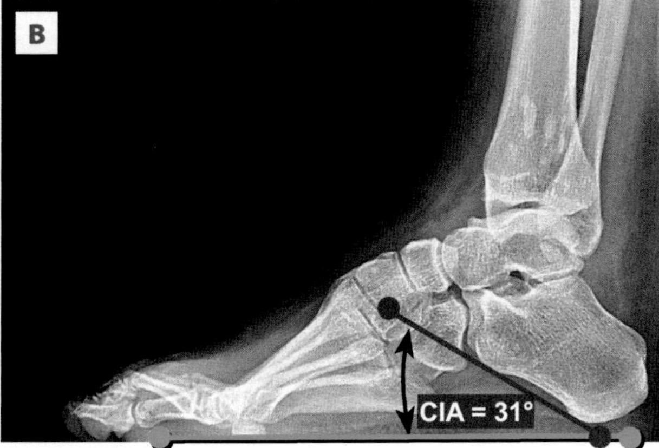


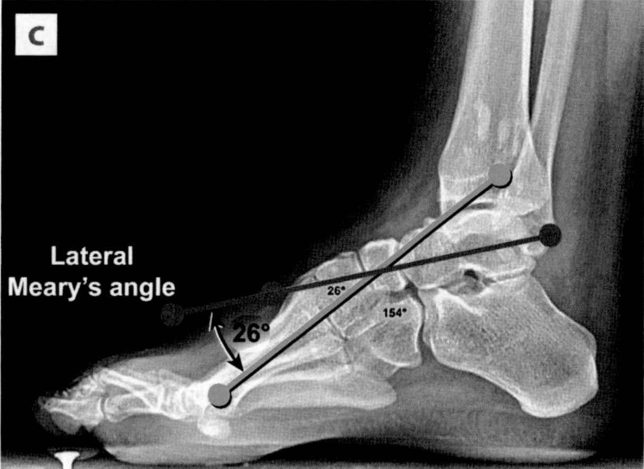


**Fig. 8: A**, Charcot-Marie-Tooth case demonstrates significant calcaneal pitch, external rotation of the ankle, and plantarflexed first ray. **B**, Calcaneal inclination angle (CIA) is 31°. **C**, Lateral Meary's angle is 26°.

**Step 2:** Bisect the talar body (*red line*) and bisect the first metatarsal (*blue line*) to establish the lateral Meary's angle (26°) (Fig. 9A). The intersection of the two axes that make up the lateral Meary's angle determine the apex. The magnitude of deformity is calculated by subtracting the average normal lateral Meary's angle (6°) from the value of the lateral Meary's angle in this case (26°). The magnitude of the deformity is 20° (Fig. 9B).

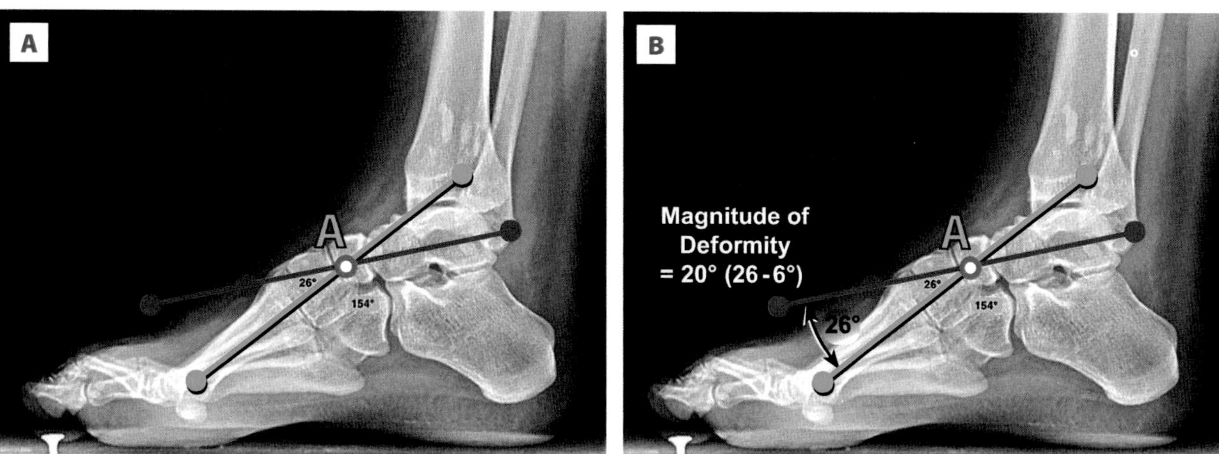


**Fig. 9: A**, The apex of the deformity is at the navicular cuneiform joints at the intersection of the two axes that make up the lateral Meary's angle. **B**, The magnitude of deformity (20°) is calculated by subtracting the average normal lateral Meary's angle (6°) from the value of the lateral Meary's angle in this case (26°). A, apex.

© 2023 Sinai Hospital of Baltimore

**Step 3:** Plan an osteotomy with a closing wedge resection at the level of the apex (Fig. 10A). Since the osteotomy is performed at the level of the apex, bony translation will not occur during the correction.

**Step 4:** Draw the C-level at the apex (Fig. 10B). To draw the C-level, identify the obtuse angle that is created by the intersection of the proximal and distal axes. The C-level bisects this obtuse angle and passes through the apex.

**Step 5:** The thumbtack is placed on the C-level to obtain a closing wedge osteotomy (Fig. 10C).

**Step 6:** Remove the dorsal-based bone wedge with a plantar apex (Fig. 11A).

**Step 7:** Acutely realign the proximal and distal axes (Fig. 11B).

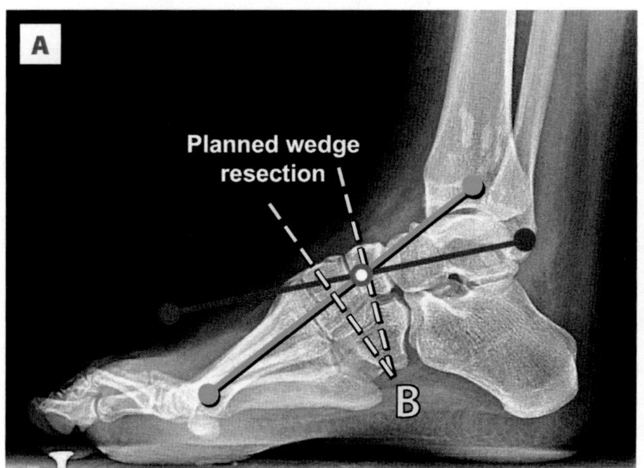


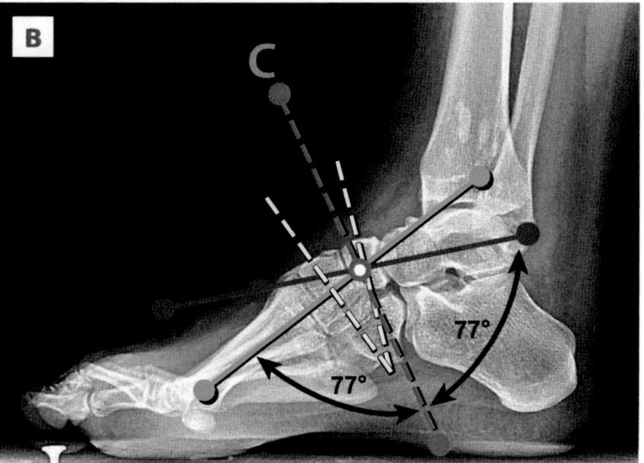


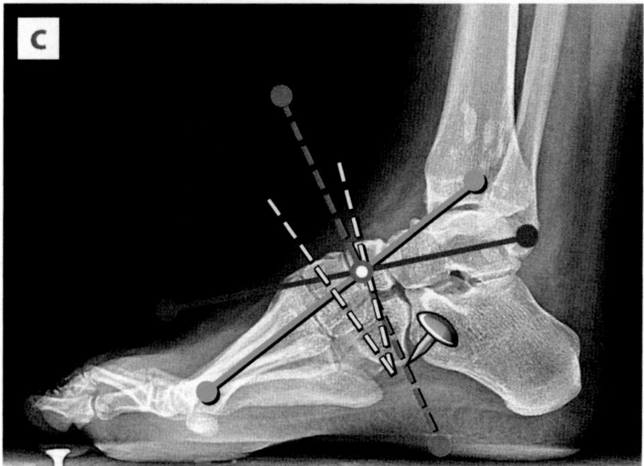


**Fig. 10: A**, A closing wedge resection is planned at the level of the apex through the cuboid and navicular cuneiform bones. **B**, The C-level passes through the apex and bisects the obtuse angle that is created by the intersection of the proximal and distal axes. **C**, The thumbtack is placed on the plantar aspect of the C-level to obtain a closing wedge osteotomy. B, bone cut; C, C-level.

**Step 8:** Fixate with internal fixation (Fig. 12A). A formal arthrodesis was performed of the subtalar joint and tarsal joints along with soft-tissue reconstruction, which included posterior tibial tendon transfer, peroneus longus to brevis transfer, and Steindler stripping. The new calcaneal inclination angle (21°) is within the normal limits (Fig. 12B).

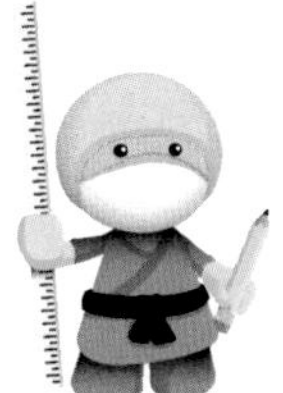

*Sensei says,*

*"When hindfoot varus is present, there will be an increased calcaneal inclination angle and the forefoot will compensate with pronation."*

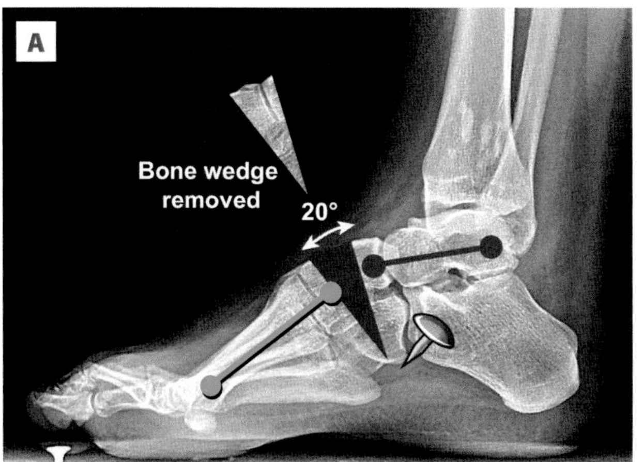


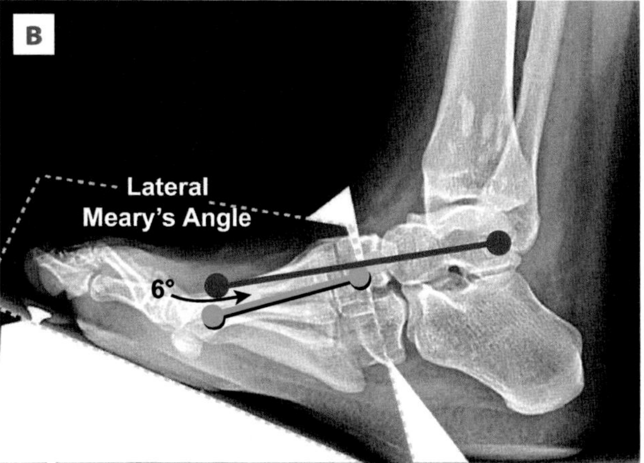


**Fig. 11: A**, The dorsal-based bone wedge is removed. **B**, The proximal and distal axes are acutely realigned. The wedge resection allows for acute correction and realignment of the lateral Meary's angle.

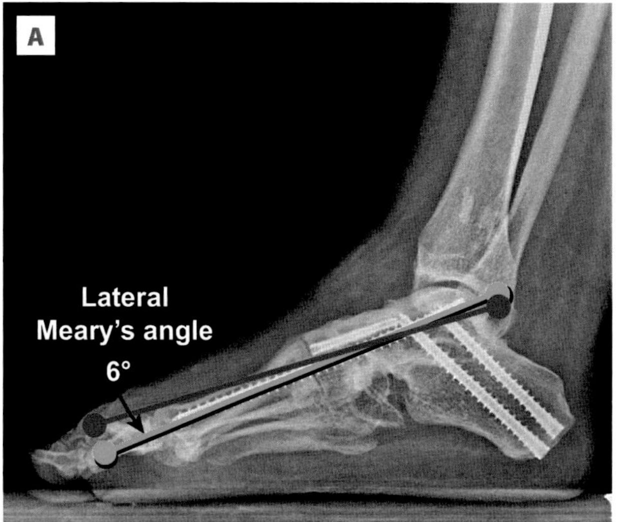


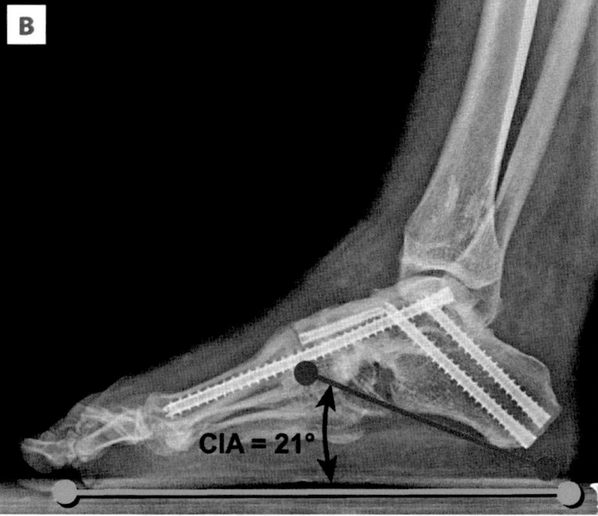


**Fig. 12: A**, The lateral Meary's angle is restored. **B**, The calcaneal inclination angle (CIA) is within the normal limits.

© 2023 Sinai Hospital of Baltimore

## Rockerbottom Midfoot Deformity

Rockerbottom foot deformity is most often noted in cases of fracture/dislocation of the midfoot yielding a negative lateral Meary's angle. This is frequently seen in a Charcot or traumatic midfoot/ Lisfranc deformity. It is essential to determine if the compensation is fixed or not. No fixed compensation (contracture) is present if the foot can be placed in the maximum deformity position.

## Preoperative Deformity Analysis and Operative Planning

**Step 1:** Sagittal plane deformity is evaluated on a standing lateral view x-ray of the foot (Fig. 13A). Determine the calcaneal inclination angle (6°) (Fig. 13B).

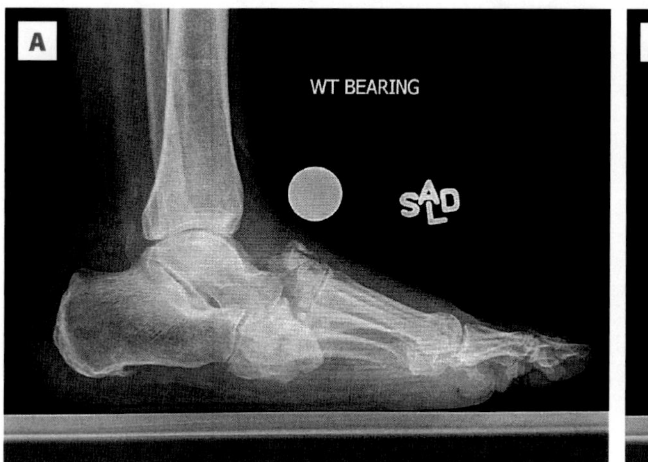


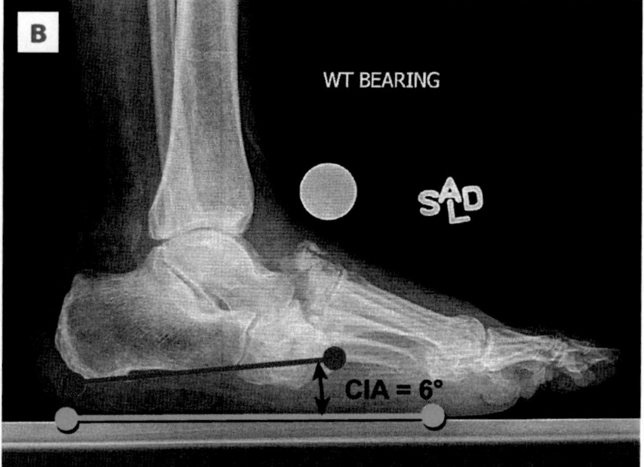


**Fig. 13:** **A**, Preoperative x-ray of a neuropathic fracture dislocation of the midfoot with bayonetting of forefoot onto the midfoot. **B**, Calcaneal inclination angle (CIA) is 6°.

**Step 2:** Bisect the talar body (*red line*) and bisect the first metatarsal (*blue line*) to establish the lateral Meary's angle (17°) (Fig. 14A). The intersection of the two axes that make up the lateral Meary's angle determine the apex (Fig. 14B). The magnitude of deformity is calculated by subtracting the average normal lateral Meary's angle (6°) from the value of the lateral Meary's angle in this case (17°). The magnitude of the deformity is 11° (Fig. 14C).

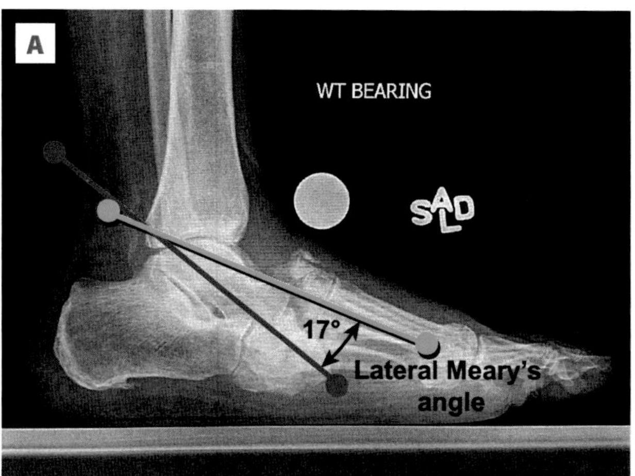


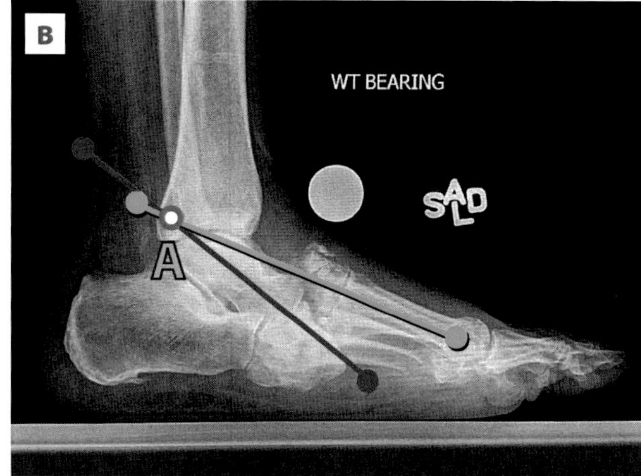


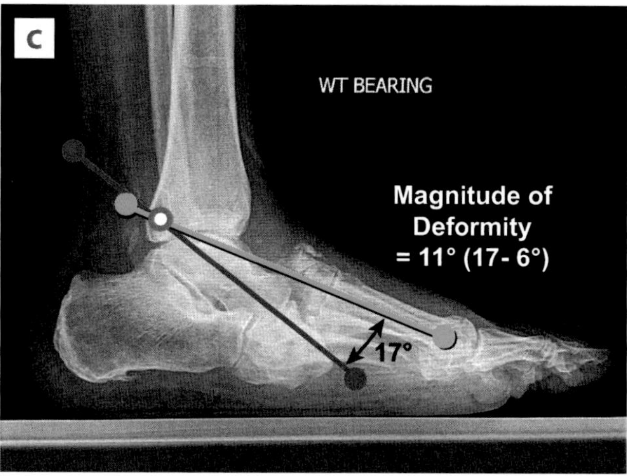


**Fig. 14:** **A**, Lateral Meary's angle is 17°. **B**, The apex of the deformity is at the intersection of the two axes that make up the lateral Meary's angle. In general, the apexes in rockerbottom deformities are in the hindfoot and ankle. **C**, The magnitude of deformity (11°) is calculated by subtracting the average normal lateral Meary's angle (6°) from the value of the lateral Meary's angle in this case (17°). A, apex.

© 2023 Sinai Hospital of Baltimore

**Step 3:** Plan the osteotomy at the level of the midfoot collapse (Fig. 15A). Since the osteotomy is not performed at the level of the apex, bony translation will occur during the correction.

**Step 4:** Draw the C-level (Fig. 15B). Identify the obtuse angle that is created by the intersection of the proximal and distal axes. The C-level bisects this obtuse angle and passes through the apex.

**Step 5:** To achieve correction, the bone segments are angulated about a thumbtack placed on the C-level. This example shows the thumbtack at the apex (Fig. 15C).

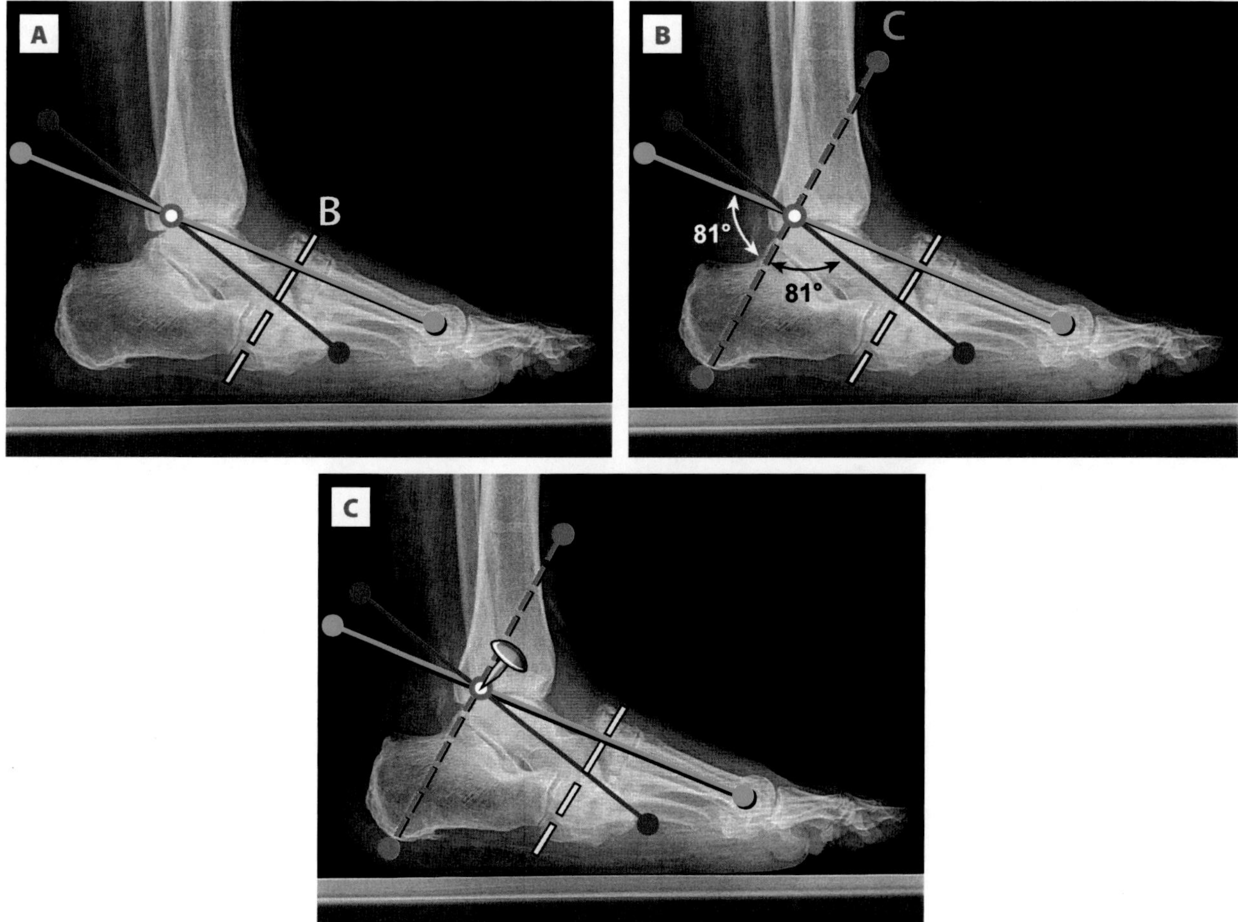


**Fig. 15:** **A**, Due to anatomic constraints, the osteotomy is planned in the midfoot away from the apex. **B**, The C-level passes through the apex and bisects the obtuse angle that is created by the intersection of the proximal and distal axes. **C**, The thumbtack is placed on the apex. B, bone cut; C, C-level.

**Step 6:** Perform acute correction of the midfoot with the distal segment being translated plantarly because the osteotomy was made away from the apex (Fig. 16A).

**Step 7:** Restoration of the hindfoot positioning with soft-tissue correction of equinus deformity (Fig. 16B).

**Step 8:** The hindfoot and midfoot positions have been realigned with normal angular relationships (Fig. 17).

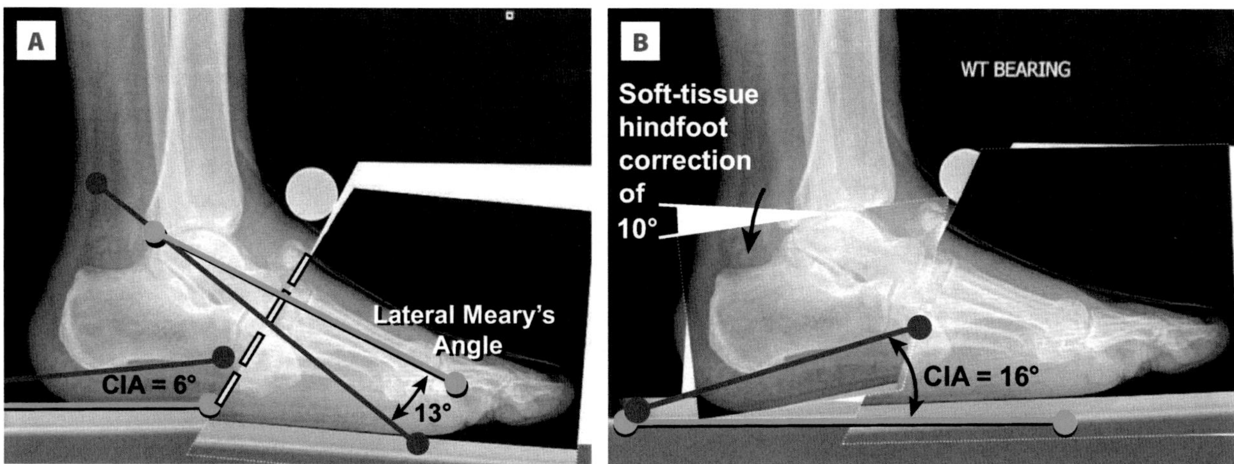


**Fig. 16:** **A**, Acute correction of midfoot. **B**, Hindfoot position is restored and equinus deformity corrected. To improve the calcaneal pitch, a soft-tissue correction was performed that included an Achilles lengthening and posterior tibial lengthening. CIA, calcaneal inclination angle.

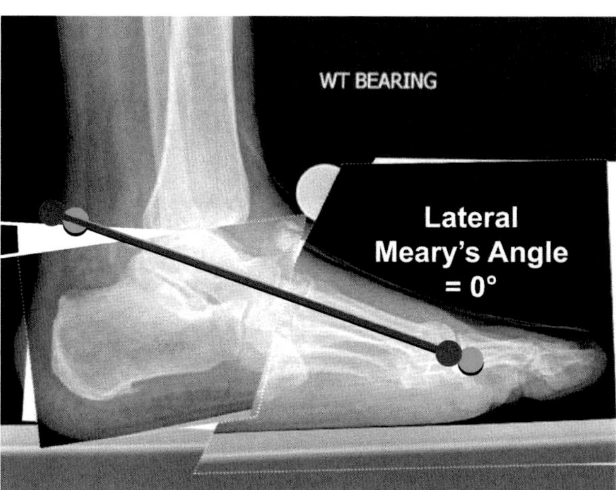


**Fig. 17:** Hindfoot and midfoot are realigned.

© 2023 Sinai Hospital of Baltimore

**Step 9: Correction Option 1 – Acute Correction:** Following definitive fixation of the proximal and distal segments, normal angular relationships were achieved on postoperative x-rays (Fig. 18). Long-term maintenance of the corrected neuropathic fracture dislocation was achieved by arthrodesis.

**Correction Option 2 – Gradual Correction:** Alternatively, the correction of the hindfoot and midfoot can be performed gradually using external fixation (Fig. 19).

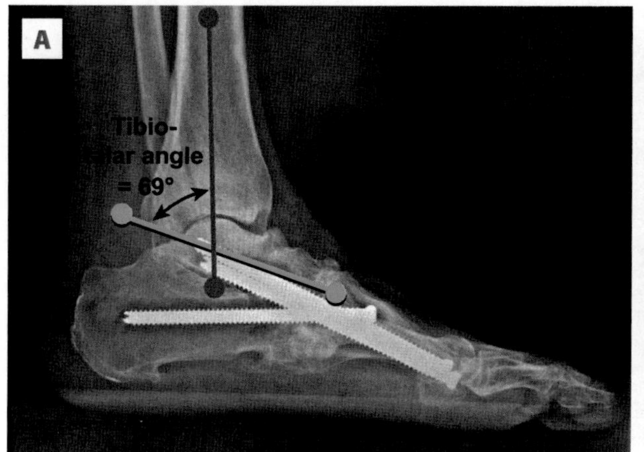


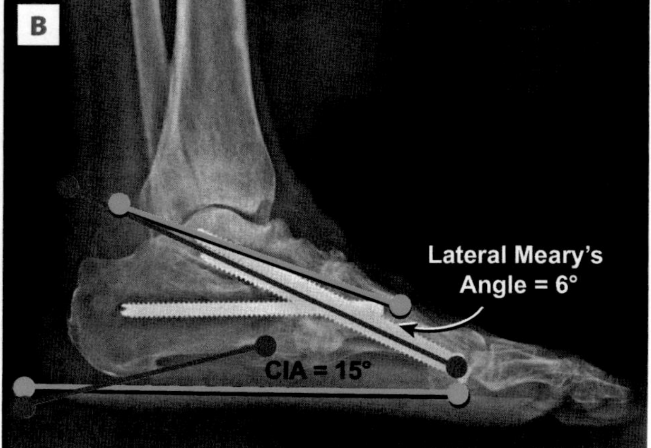


**Fig. 18:** Acute correction and definitive fixation of the proximal and distal segments resulted in a normal tibio-talar angle (**A**), lateral Meary's angle (**B**), and calcaneal inclination angle (**B**). CIA, calcaneal inclination angle.

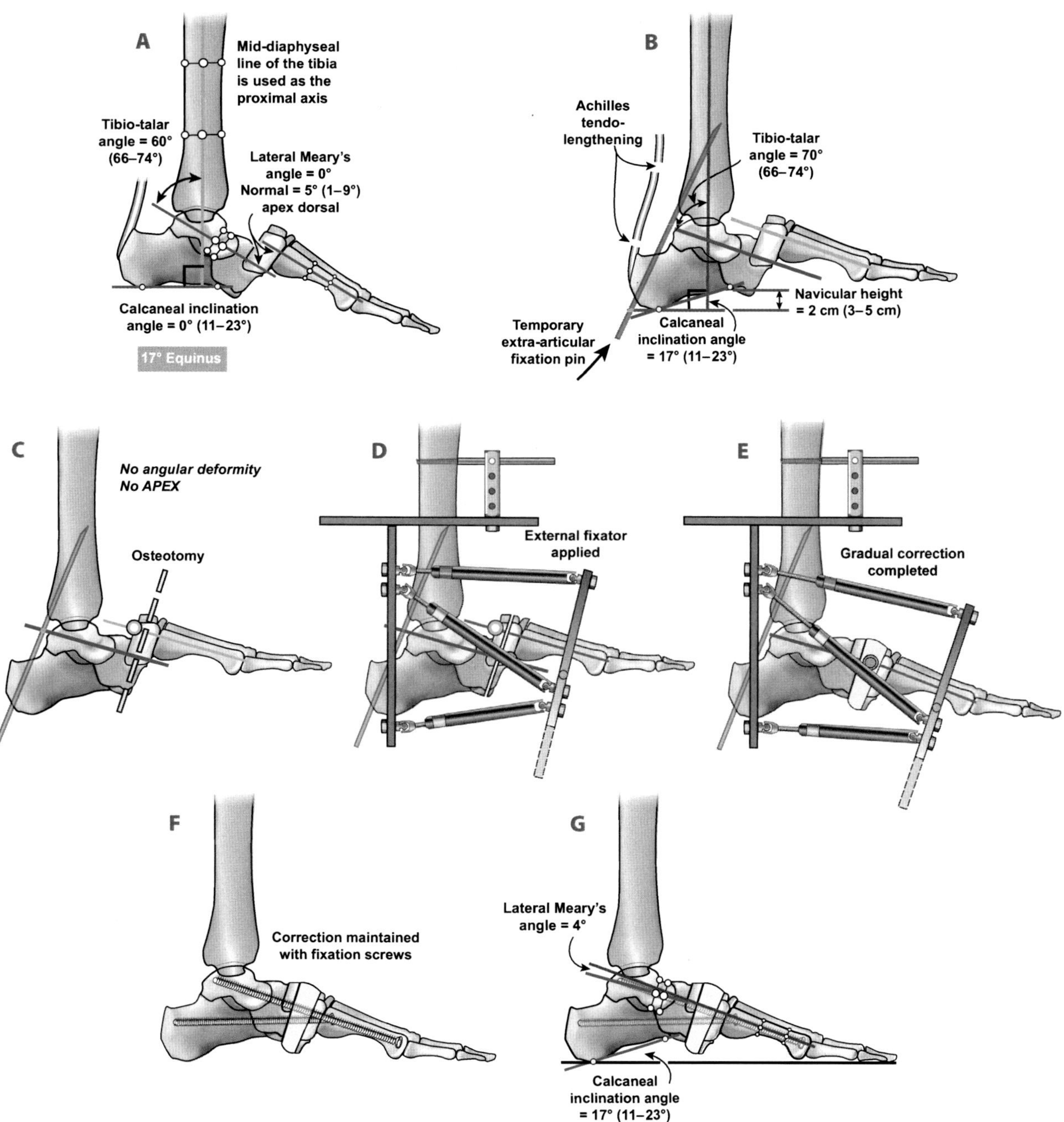


**Fig. 19:** The hindfoot and midfoot can also be corrected gradually using external fixation. Gradual correction will involve distraction and realignment of the midfoot with respect to the hindfoot. **A**, Rockerbottom deformity and bony consolidation are noted. **B**, Achilles tendo-lengthening is performed as well as an extraarticular temporary arthrodesis of the ankle with a large Steinmann pin to restore calcaneal pitch. **C**, No angular deformity is noted in the midfoot. Shortening and dorsal translation is planned. Midfoot osteotomy is performed at consolidated level of collapse. **D**, Hexapod fixator applied with distal reference ring. If done gradually, the soft-tissue correction is performed at the time of frame application. **E**, Gradual distraction and lengthening with plantar translation. **F**, Consolidation and correction achieved (intramedullary fixation recommended to maintain correction).

© 2023 Sinai Hospital of Baltimore

## Ankle Varus Malunion with LLD Deformity

### Preoperative Deformity Analysis and Operative Planning

**Step 1:** Frontal plane deformity is best evaluated with a standing AP view ankle x-ray. (Fig. 20A). Draw the anatomic axis of the tibia (*red line*) and the calcaneal bisector (*blue line*) to determine the tibial-calcaneal angle (10° varus) (Fig. 20B). The intersection of the two axes that make up the tibial-calcaneal angle is the apex (Fig. 20C). The magnitude of the deformity is 10° varus.

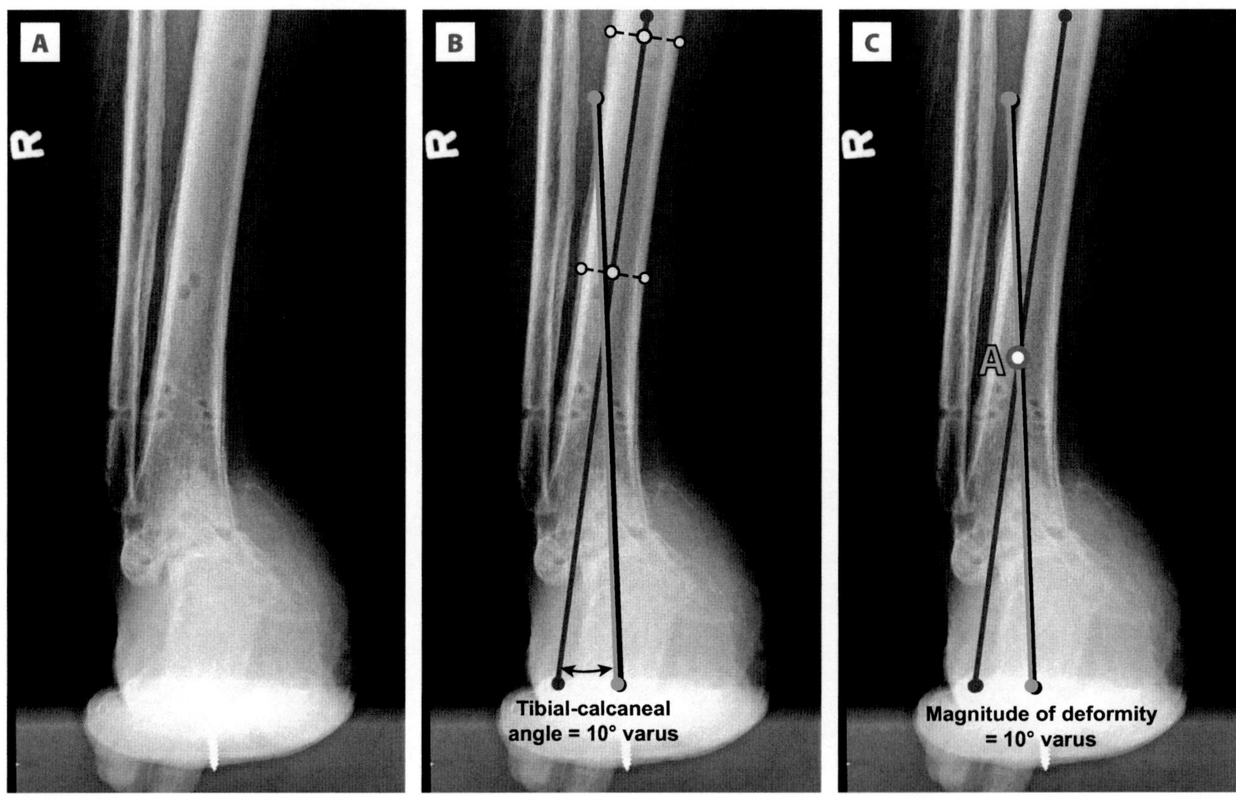


**Fig. 20:** **A**, Ankle varus malunion is noted on the AP view x-ray. **B**, The deformity is 10° varus. **C**, The apex of the deformity is in the distal third of the tibia at the intersection of the two axes that make up the tibial-calcaneal angle. The magnitude of the deformity is 10° varus. A, apex.

**Step 2:** Plan the osteotomy as close to the apex as possible. In this case, the osteotomy is planned distal to the apex at the malunited position of the calcaneus to the distal tibia (Fig. 21A).

**Step 3:** Draw the C-level at the apex (Fig. 21B). Identify the obtuse angle that is created by the intersection of the proximal and distal axes. The C-level bisects this obtuse angle and passes through the apex.

**Step 4:** To achieve correction, the bone segments are angulated about a thumbtack placed on the C-level. This example shows the thumbtack at the apex (Fig. 21C).

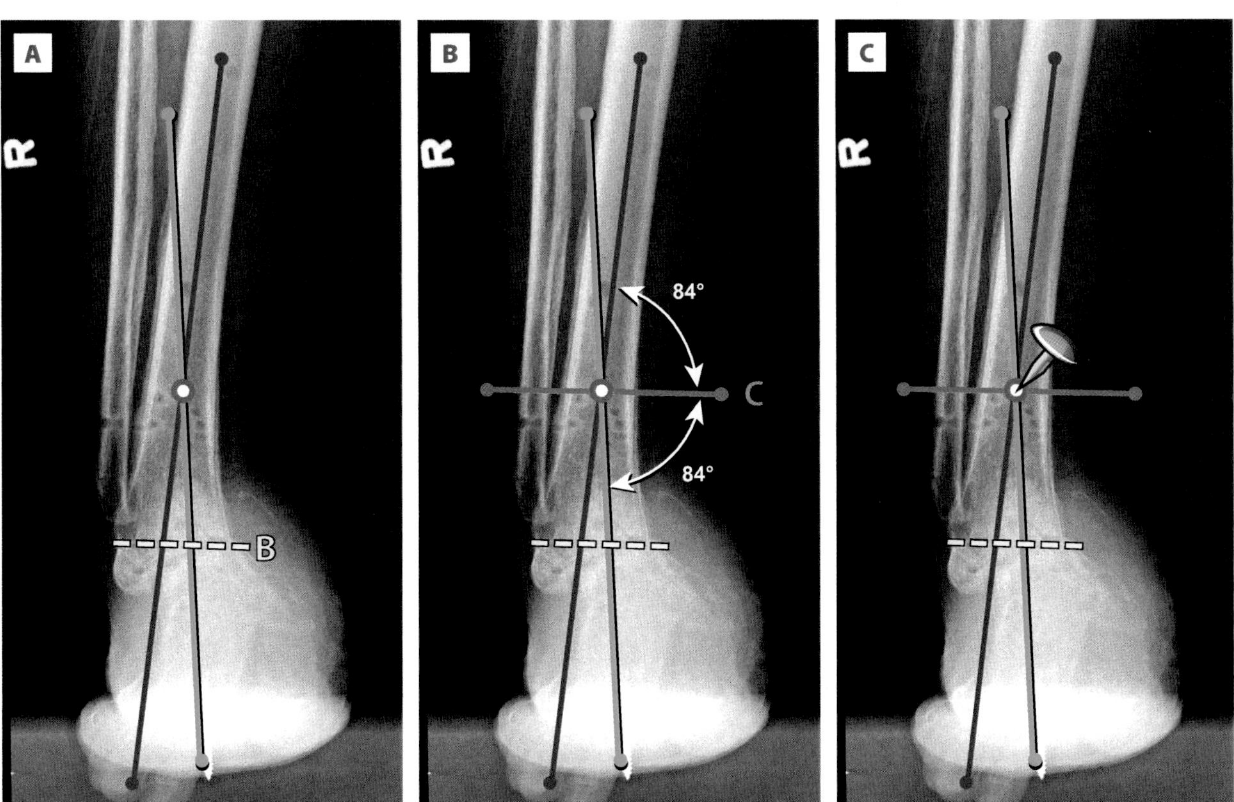


**Fig. 21:** **A**, The osteotomy is planned distal to the apex at the malunited position of the calcaneus to the distal tibia. This osteotomy will be a lateral closing wedge through the arthrodesis site. **B**, The C-level is drawn. **C**, The thumbtack is placed at the apex. B, bone cut; C, C-level.

© 2023 Sinai Hospital of Baltimore

**Step 5:** Tibiotalocalcaneal arthrodesis is planned with correction of the deformity through the fusion sites (Fig. 22A). Additionally, distal tibial lengthening is completed along the normal mechanical axis line to assist with distal arthrodesis and improve the tibial length secondary to bone loss (Fig. 22B and 22C).

**Summary:**

Postoperative x-rays demonstrate that the mechanical axis has been maintained in the sagittal and frontal planes through the fusion site and that the limb length discrepancy has been corrected (Fig. 23). Realignment is noted on the AP view x-ray following the acute realignment of the malunited distal segment (Fig. 23B and C).

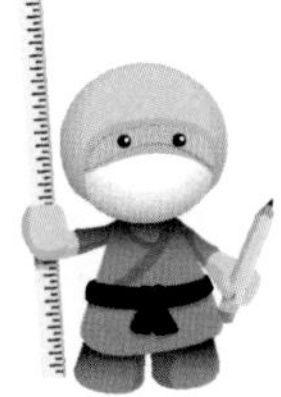

*Sensei says,*
*"The subtalar joint compensates for a varus ankle deformity by eversion. Distal tibial varus deformities that exceed the amount of compensation that is available at the subtalar joint result in compensatory forefoot pronation."*

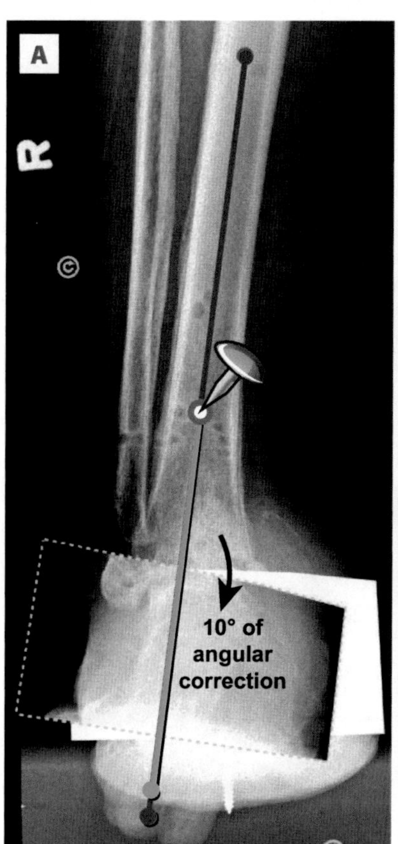


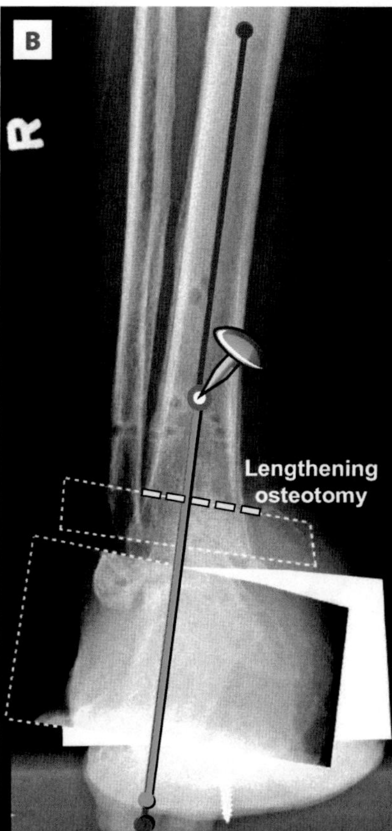


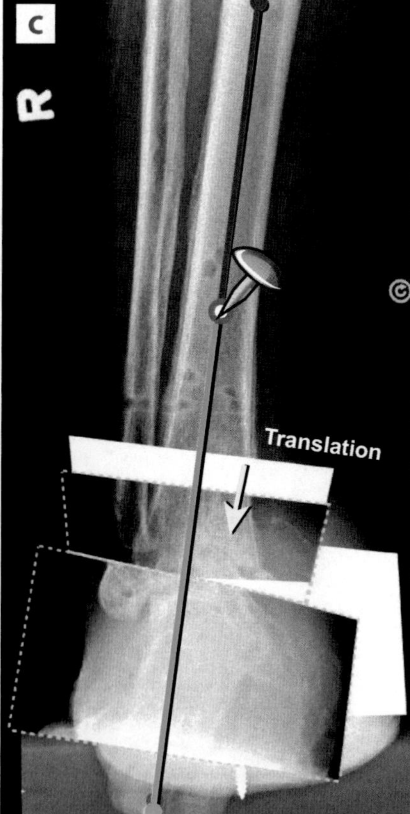


**Fig. 22: A**, Tibiotalocalcaneal arthrodesis is planned. Correction of the deformity is achieved through the fusion sites. **B** and **C**, Distal tibial lengthening and lateral translation of the distal segment are completed.

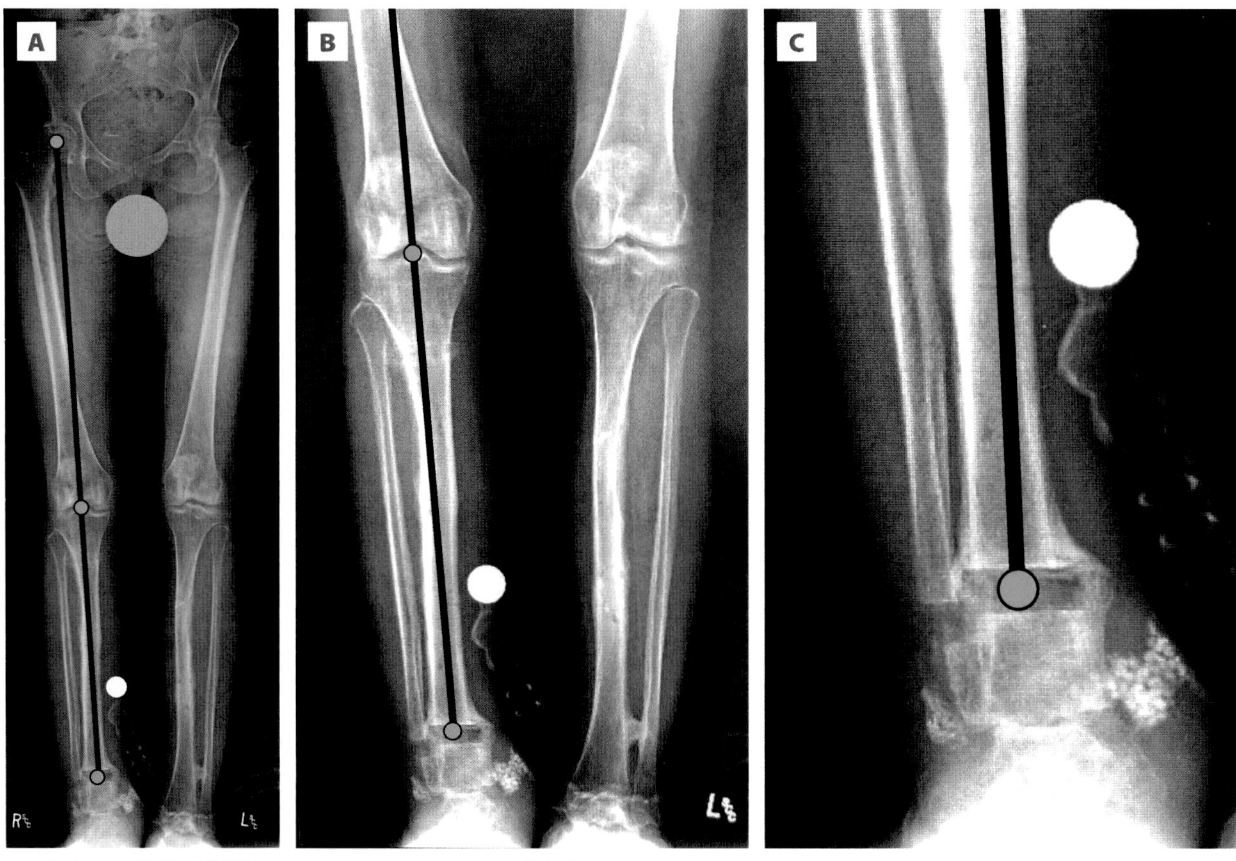

**Fig. 23:** **A**, Limb length discrepancy was corrected and the mechanical axis maintained. **B** and **C**, After acute correction of the malunited distal segment, realignment was achieved. **D**, A normal plantigrade angle was achieved.

© 2023 Sinai Hospital of Baltimore

# Chapter 16

# Intramedullary Lengthening: Planning and Considerations

Michael J. Assayag, MD

Shawn C. Standard, MD

Fundamentally, careful planning is about optimizing the likelihood of a positive outcome. This can be best achieved when following established rules created by those who came before you. Performing distraction osteogenesis with the use of external fixation is going to require different planning than lengthening over a nail or lengthening and then nailing. The principles and rules of limb lengthening are dependent upon the lengthening technique. This chapter is devoted to planning and considerations of mechanical intramedullary lengthening nails (MILNs), a process that may be referred to as "internal lengthening" or "intramedullary lengthening."

Internal lengthening has the distinct advantage of eliminating the external fixation device and concurrent pin and/or wire sites. Avoiding pin sites excludes both the soft tissue tethering that decreases overall patient comfort and any concern for pin site infections. Patients typically find MILNs to be much more comfortable than external fixation. Physical therapy and range of motion, which are essential to limb lengthening, are significantly improved with internal lengthening.

However, there are certain inclusion criteria and disadvantages of internal lengthening. A bone segment must have the adequate length and diameter in order to qualify. Tibial lengthening requires a closed physis. Candidates must be able to comply with postoperative limited weight-bearing and, should magnetic remote controls be used, not have medical conditions that preclude their use (i.e., pacemakers). The disadvantages of internal lengthening are limited weightbearing, an inability to perform gradual deformity correction with lengthening, and the loss of the surgeon's ability to adjust the lengthening axis. Internal lengthening has a limited capacity to correct more complex or multiapical deformities accurately with a single implant. Still, internal lengthening is a viable method to consider for children, adolescents, and skeletally mature patients who simply need length or have a simple deformity that is suitable for correction with a fixator-assisted nailing technique.

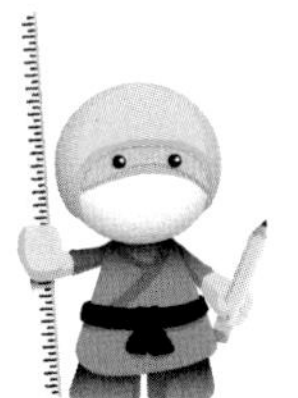

***Sensei says,***
*"One who plans carefully will not be left short!"*

© 2023 Sinai Hospital of Baltimore

## Mechanical Intramedullary Lengthening Nails

### Anatomy of a Nail

Regardless of the nail's mechanism or generation, all MILNs share common traits in their anatomy. It is important for the surgeon to be aware of each portion's name and purpose when doing surgical planning.

The housing or "socket" section is a hollow tube and acts like a sleeve for the mechanism that allows lengthening to occur. The housing is the largest and strongest portion of the MILN. Its end contains variable patterns of locking screw holes that allow for fixation to the bone. The screw hole configuration depends upon both the manufacturer and the bone for which the nail is intended.

The telescopic rod or "plug" segment is a solid piece of metal that is gradually pushed out of the housing by the lengthening mechanism. The telescopic rod is the thinnest part of the nail and is consequently more delicate than the housing. Like the housing at the nail's opposite end, rods will also have varying formations of locking screw holes to affix the rod to bone.

The telescopic junction is the area where the telescopic rod exits out of the housing sleeve. The sudden transition between the two components and subsequent change in bending stiffness/ rotational moment of inertia makes this the most vulnerable part of the entire MILN assembly. The significance of this junction cannot be overstated in surgical planning. As a result of inherent weakness, it is essential that the junction and the regenerate/ lengthening cap never overlap.

Unlike curved intramedullary fixation devices designed for use in trauma surgery, MILNs are straight throughout the diaphyseal segment. All trochanteric, tibial, and humeral nails, as well as certain designs of retrograde femoral nails feature a slight bend (approximately 10°) occurring approximately five cm from the tip of the housing. This bend, called a Herzog bend when occurring in tibial nails, is meant to ease implantation.

Nail types include straight antegrade femoral nails (piriformis start), proximal femoral bent nail (10°, trochanteric start), straight and bent retrograde femoral nails, and bent tibial nails. The exact nail type depends on the clinical situation. For instance, a patient who is skeletally immature will require a proximal femur bent nail for an antegrade femoral lengthening to avoid violating the blood supply to the femoral head.

Each implant has a varied locking screw pattern, including between one and three proximal and distal locking screws. Unlike trauma nails, lengthening implants use locking pegs which are stronger than screws due to their larger core diameter.

### Variety of Nail Mechanisms

For nearly half a century, various types of MILNs have been used to achieve distraction osteogenesis without external fixation. In 1983, Alexander Bliskunov reported on his intramedullary ratcheting nail that was connected to the iliac crest and extended by rotating the hip back and forth. Additional models of nails with ratcheting mechanisms followed over the years. They require the use of a rotational force through the regenerate to allow lengthening. This is typically a painful process and the ratcheting cannot be reversed to shorten the nail.

In 1991, Rainer Baumgart and Augustin Betz developed the first intramedullary nail with an electric motor. These electrical nails use a transcutaneous current via an electrode implanted in a subcutaneous pocket. This style of nail allows for a less painful lengthening when compared with ratcheting MILNs. The inclusion of the electric motor makes shortening possible by reversing the polarity of the electrical current. Another advantage to these nails is that they are viable in the patient with a thick soft tissue envelope. However, the subcutaneous implant can become uncomfortable and may have to be removed early.

As of this writing, the most recent MILN advances have come in the form of magnetic lengthening nails. These rely on a cylindrical magnet inside the nail that is activated by an external magnetic remote control placed over the limb. The distance of communication between the lengthening nail and the remote control is determined by both the implant's magnet size and the remote control's generation. Like electrical nails, shortening is an option, and the lengthening process is reported by patients to be less painful than with ratcheting MILNs. One drawback to these magnetic implants is that some patients have a soft tissue envelope that is too thick to allow for communication between the remote control and the implant.

## General Principles of Intramedullary Lengthening Planning

Several choices must be made when planning an intramedullary bone lengthening. Which segment is being lengthened; the femur, tibia, or both? What direction is best for the nail insertion; antegrade or retrograde? Where is the level of the osteotomy? What nail length is needed? What nail diameter will fit? Although these choices will depend on the circumstances that surround each case, there are a few rules that are universal to the planning of intramedullary lengthening surgeries.

### Osteotomy Placement

When using external fixation for distraction osteogenesis, the optimal location to choose for the osteotomy site is the metaphyseal bone as it creates the best bone regenerate. A diaphyseal osteotomy is preferred for internal lengthening to increase the stability of the construct and prevent malalignment during the lengthening process.

There are two methods to identify the location of the osteotomy. The principles of the first method are available in detail within the chapter entitled "Deformity Analysis and Osteotomy Strategies: Frontal Plane." The second method involves placing the osteotomy according to the length of the implant (Fig. 1) and the presence of a concurrent deformity in the bone segment. This involves an osteotomy site far enough from the MILN's telescopic junction that it does not overlap with the flexible regenerate at the end of lengthening. The desired lengthening must be added to the amount of the telescopic rod protruding from the housing and combined with a safety margin or "buffer."

### Nail Length and Diameter

Because the length of the nail determines the zone of the acceptable osteotomy level, it is crucial to determine the correct length. The choice of length depends on two strategies. The first, the "nail long" strategy, is the insertion of the longest possible nail from the insertion site to the opposite metaphysis. This strategy provides the largest zone of acceptable osteotomy levels and protects the entire bone segment after lengthening. The second method, the "nail short" strategy, is used when a nail does not span the bone segment from metaphysis to metaphysis; instead, the end of the nail stops in the diaphyseal region. The nail short strategy can be used to avoid an underlying bony deformity in the bone segment that does not need to be corrected (i.e., a pronounced distal femoral anterior bow). A disadvantage of the nail short strategy is the area of stress concentration at the end of the nail until its removal.

Nail length is calculated by adding three parameters: the distance from the insertion point to osteotomy, the desired lengthening, and a constant of 8 cm. This constant number is obtained by combining the initial length of the telescopic rod (3 cm) that protrudes from the distal end of the housing prior to distraction and a buffer zone (5 cm). The buffer zone represents the nail housing that will remain on the opposite lengthening segment at the end of distraction. This calculation determines the shortest nail that will accomplish the deformity correction and lengthening. A longer nail can be used if the nail fits the bone segment.

Determining the proper nail length is vital to help prevent hardware failure and non-union. The correct length will also aid in maintaining stability after lengthening concludes. We must ensure that the telescopic junction is not superimposed on the regenerate at any point during the distraction process. Because it is the weakest point of the MILN, an overlap would introduce increased motion at the regenerate and can lead to nonunion or hardware failure.

As mentioned previously, the telescopic junction is the weakest part of the MILN construct. On the other hand, the regenerate is the area where the

© 2023 Sinai Hospital of Baltimore

most stress is transmitted to the implant. If the junction is overlapped with the regenerate at any time during the lengthening, maximal strain will be applied to the implant and the risk of implant failure will be high (Fig. 2).

Nail diameter is dictated by the inner diameter size of the intramedullary canal and the outer diameter of cortical bone. We recommend over-reaming the diameter of the nail by 1–2 mm. A thickness of 3.0–3.5 mm of cortical bone should be maintained on all sides of the nail (Fig. 3). The diameter measurement is performed at the narrowest portion of the bone segment where the nail will be placed. Diameter measurements need to be conducted on both the anteroposterior and lateral radiographic views.

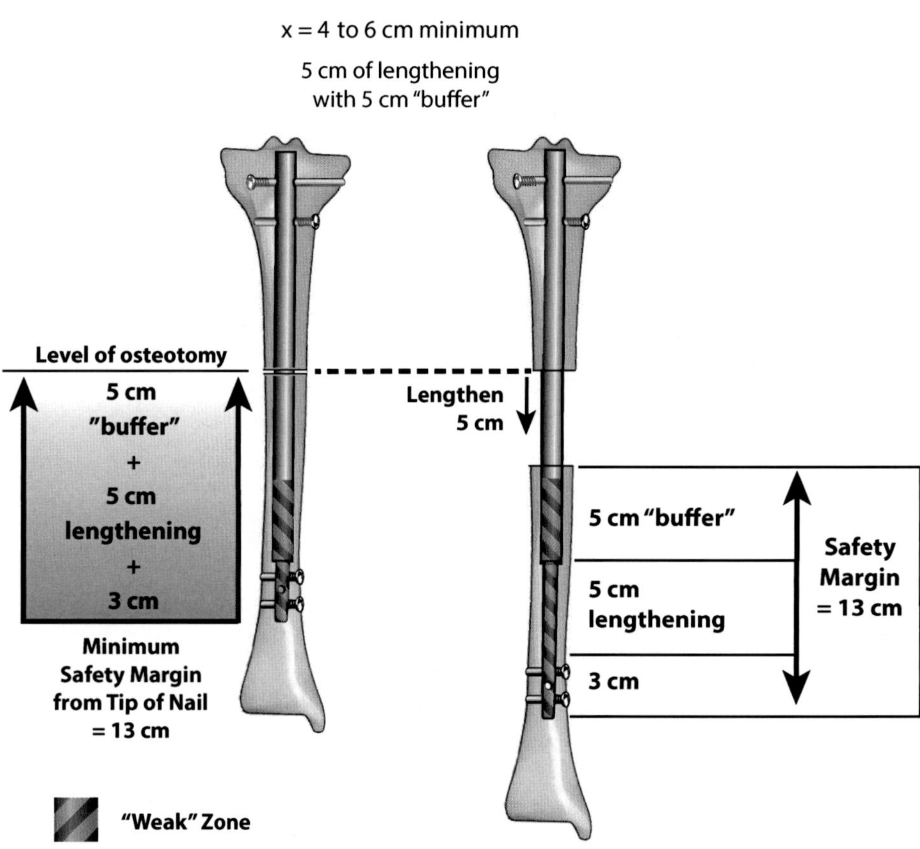


**Fig. 1:** Adding together three numbers will provide the minimum distance away from the tip of the nail for osteotomy placement. These three numbers are derived from the nail's exposed telescopic tip, the anticipated lengthening, and a buffer zone which represents the portion of the nail's housing that remains on the opposite segment. Any osteotomy performed distal to this level will result in a minimal amount of nail housing diameter distal to the regenerate bone. This places the telescopic junction and the rod's thinner diameter in a high-stress zone.

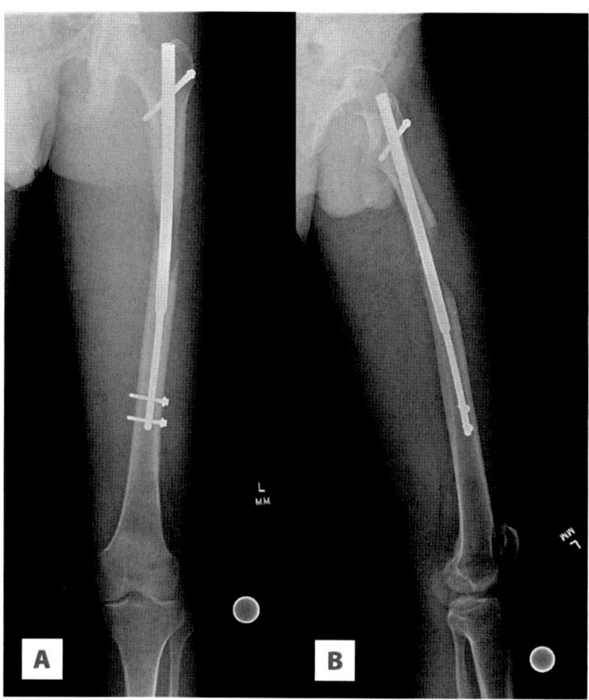


Fig. 2: A, anteroposterior (AP) and B, sagittal radiographs of an osteotomy with an insufficient buffer zone of only 3 cm. Signs of delayed healing and bending are apparent.

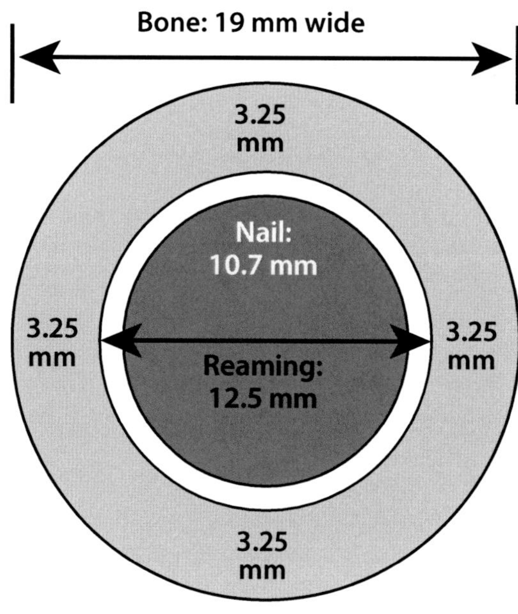


Fig. 3: Intramedullary canal should be over-reamed by approximately 2 mm. This scenario would permit a 10.7 mm nail.

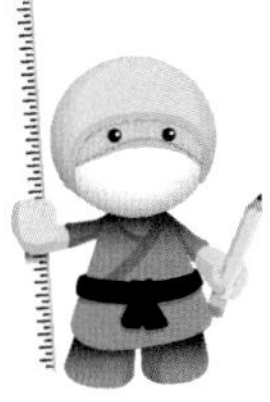

*Sensei says,*
*"Distance to osteotomy + desired lengthening + 8 cm = shortest possible nail length."*

## Femoral Lengthening

### Antegrade Femoral Lengthening

Antegrade femoral lengthening can be done using either a piriformis fossa or trochanteric entry nail. The former is easy to use due to its insertion point directly in-line with the femoral canal. The latter should be used in patients who are skeletally immature to avoid injury to the femoral head blood supply. The correct starting position on the greater trochanter must be chosen depending on the nail's proximal bend. Most trochanteric entry nails have a 10° proximal bend. If the point is placed too lateral, then a proximal femur osteotomy will be shifted into varus with nail insertion. A starting point too medial will create a valgus shift in a proximal femoral osteotomy.

If a straight lengthening is performed in a femur with normal anatomy, the osteotomy should be placed at either the apex of the anterior bow or proximal enough to allow the end of the nail to stop before the anterior bow. The appropriate nail length for either strategy can be calculated as previously described.

A theoretical disadvantage to antegrade lengthening with an internal device is the lengthening axis. Internal lengthening occurs along the anatomic, rather than mechanical, axis. Lengthening along the anatomic axis can result in an alteration of the overall mechanical axis, depending upon the original anatomic-mechanical angle (AMA). If the AMA is convergent, the internal lengthening will shift the mechanical axis laterally (valgus) 1 mm for every 1 cm of length gained. Conversely, if the AMA is divergent, then lengthening along the anatomic axis will instead shift the mechanical axis medially (varus) 1 mm for every 1 cm of

© 2023 Sinai Hospital of Baltimore

length gained. An AMA that is parallel will have no effect on the mechanical axis during internal lengthening. This disadvantage can be avoided by performing retrograde lengthening using the reverse planning method.

### Retrograde Femoral Lengthening

Retrograde femoral lengthening has several advantages over antegrade lengthening. The first is the ability to correct deformities of the distal femur acutely with subsequent lengthening. Second, proximal femoral deformities or retained proximal implants can be avoided. Third, the use of retrograde lengthening and reverse planning can mitigate the change in alignment with antegrade lengthening, as previously mentioned. Retrograde femoral lengthening is strictly for patients who are skeletally mature or have no distal femoral physis.

Retrograde femoral lengthening planning is outlined here with digital planning software. The planning walkthrough for a 25-year-old male case with left genu valgum and 2.5 cm limb length discrepancy (LLD) is provided in Figures 4–8. Post-lengthening radiographs and a comparison of preoperative and post-lengthening photos are also available in Figures 9 and 10.

Please see the chapter entitled "Reverse Planning for Femoral Deformity" for an alternate detailed description of this planning process.

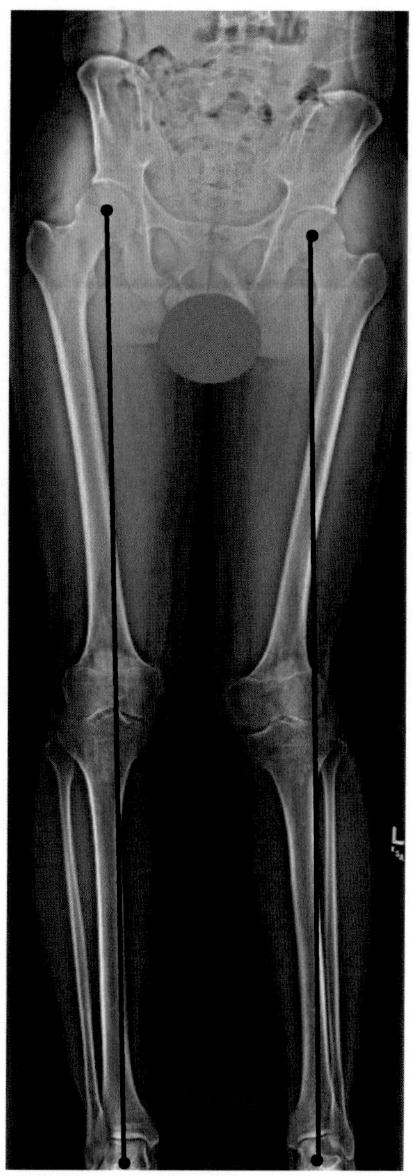

**Fig. 4:** Left leg lateral mechanical axis deviation (MAD) confirms genu valgum alignment.

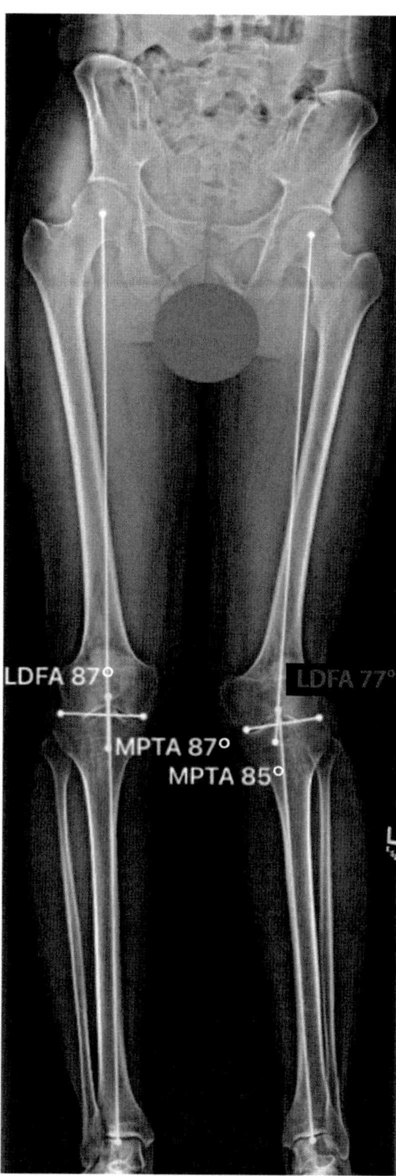


Fig. 5: Joint angles are shown. Red text indicates the abnormal angle. LFDA, lateral distal femoral angle; MPTA, medial proximal tibial angle.

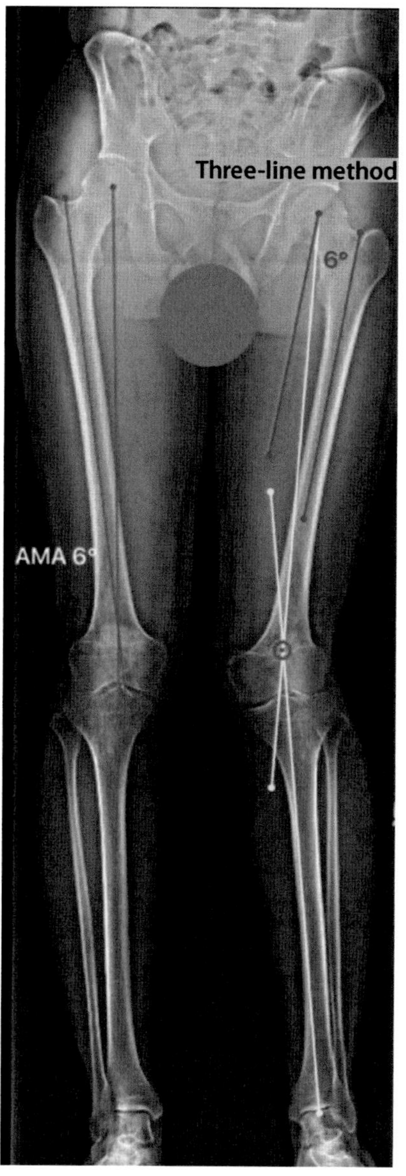


Fig. 6: The apex of deformity is found by using the three-line method to determine the proximal axis and the mechanical axis of the tibia to determine the distal axis. The point at which they intersect is the apex of the deformity. For more information, see the chapter entitled "Femoral Axis Planning: Frontal and Sagittal Planes." The osteotomy is done 8 cm above the joint in order to be extracapsular.

© 2023 Sinai Hospital of Baltimore

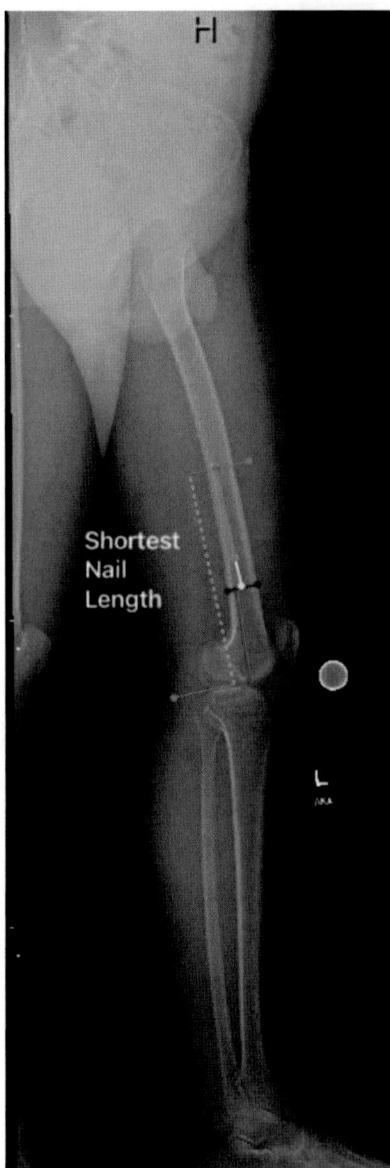


Fig. 7: The red line indicates the distance between the entry point and osteotomy (8 cm). The yellow line indicates the desired lengthening (2.5 cm). The blue line indicates the 8 cm constant. These lines add up to 18.5 cm which indicates the shortest possible nail length.

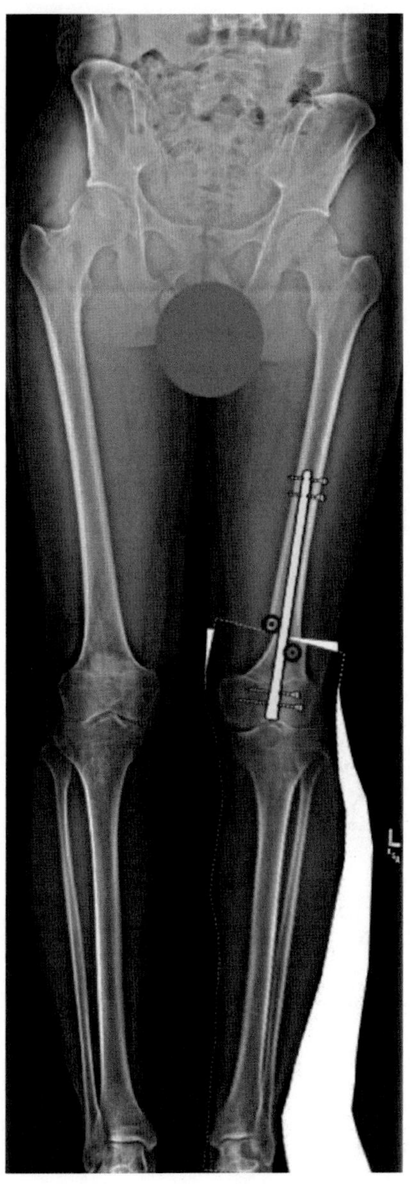


Fig. 8: The anticipated position at the end of lengthening is shown after the osteotomy and nail placement. Black circles on either side of the nail predict placement of blocking screws. This operative plan should be evaluated for feasibility (e.g., osteotomy level, requirement for cortical reaming, need for blocking screws).

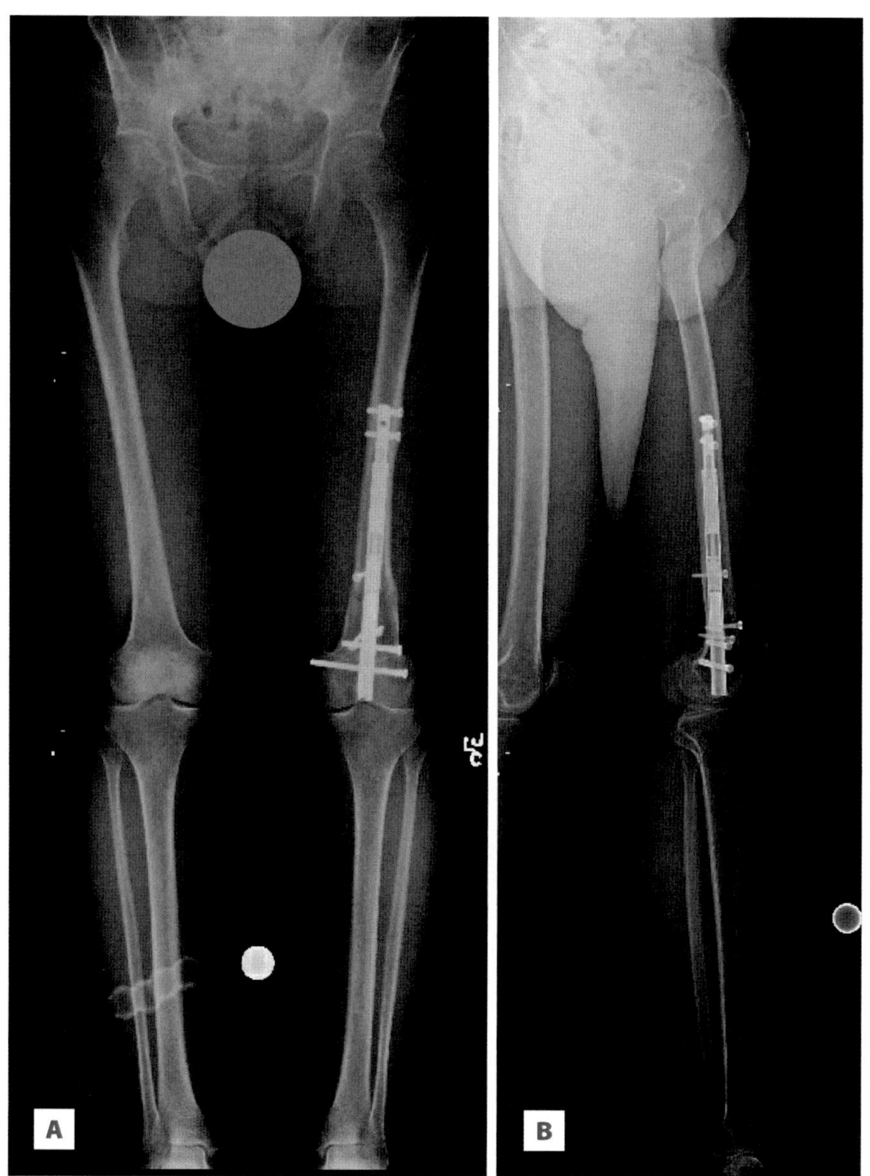


**Fig. 9: A**, AP and **B**, sagittal radiographs captured at 6 months post-lengthening.

© 2023 Sinai Hospital of Baltimore

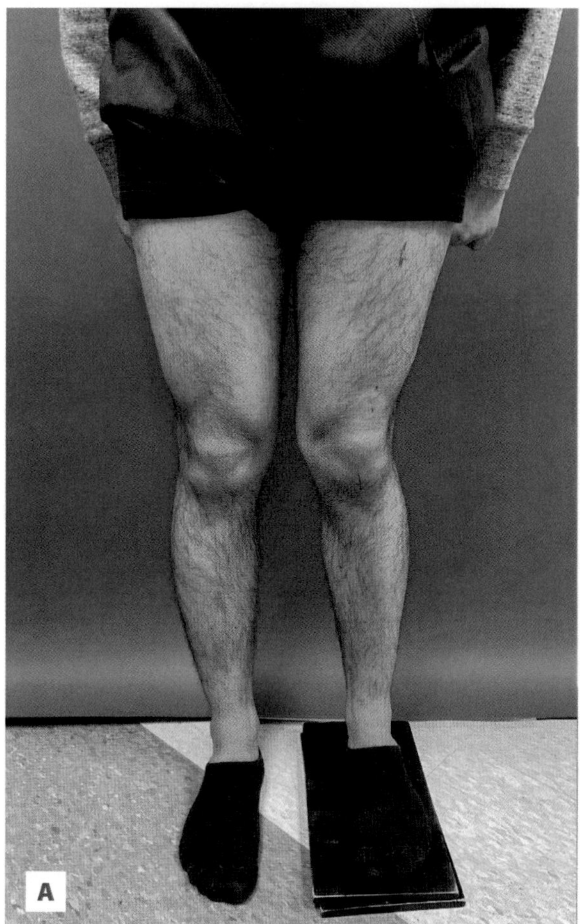

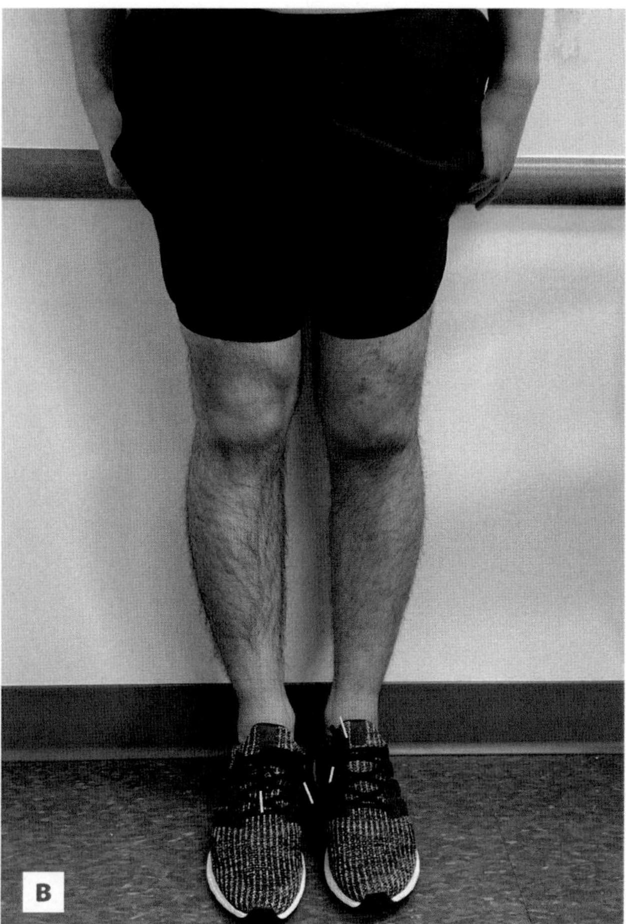

**Fig. 10:** Clinical photos obtained **A**, preoperatively and **B**, at 6 months post-lengthening.

## Tibial Lengthening

Internal lengthening of the tibia is relegated to patients who are skeletally mature or otherwise do not have a proximal tibial physis. The fibula, if present, must be lengthened as well by stabilizing the proximal and distal tibia and fibula joints with screw fixation and performing a midshaft fibular osteotomy.

Tibial lengthening with an MILN can be done with the knee in a deep flexion position or a semi-extended position. In order to maintain a minimally invasive technique from the semi-extended position, the suprapatellar approach requires special instrumentation including long reamers and tubes to protect the patellofemoral joint.

The natural tendency of the proximal tibia osteoplasty lengthening is to drift into valgus and procurvatum deformity. For that reason, the optimal osteotomy location should be 8–10 cm distal to the insertion point at the metaphyseal-diaphyseal junction. At that level, the tibial canal is narrower than at the metaphysis, thus decreasing the risk of inducing a deformity. Therefore, the maximum length nail, or nail long strategy, should always be employed. Concurrent proximal tibial deformity with sequential lengthening is very difficult with the currently available nail designs. If a proximal metaphyseal osteotomy is necessary, then blocking screws must be used to maintain alignment during the insertion and lengthening process.

Blocking screws are a key to success in tibial lengthening using MILNs (Fig. 11). If there is no direct cortical contact with the nail at the level of the osteotomy, a lateral blocking screw should be placed in the proximal fragment to prevent valgus deformity. Similarly, a posterior blocking screw should be placed to prevent apex anterior deformity.

Planning for a tibial lengthening case is outlined in Figures 12–17 and a post-lengthening radiograph is available in Figure 18.

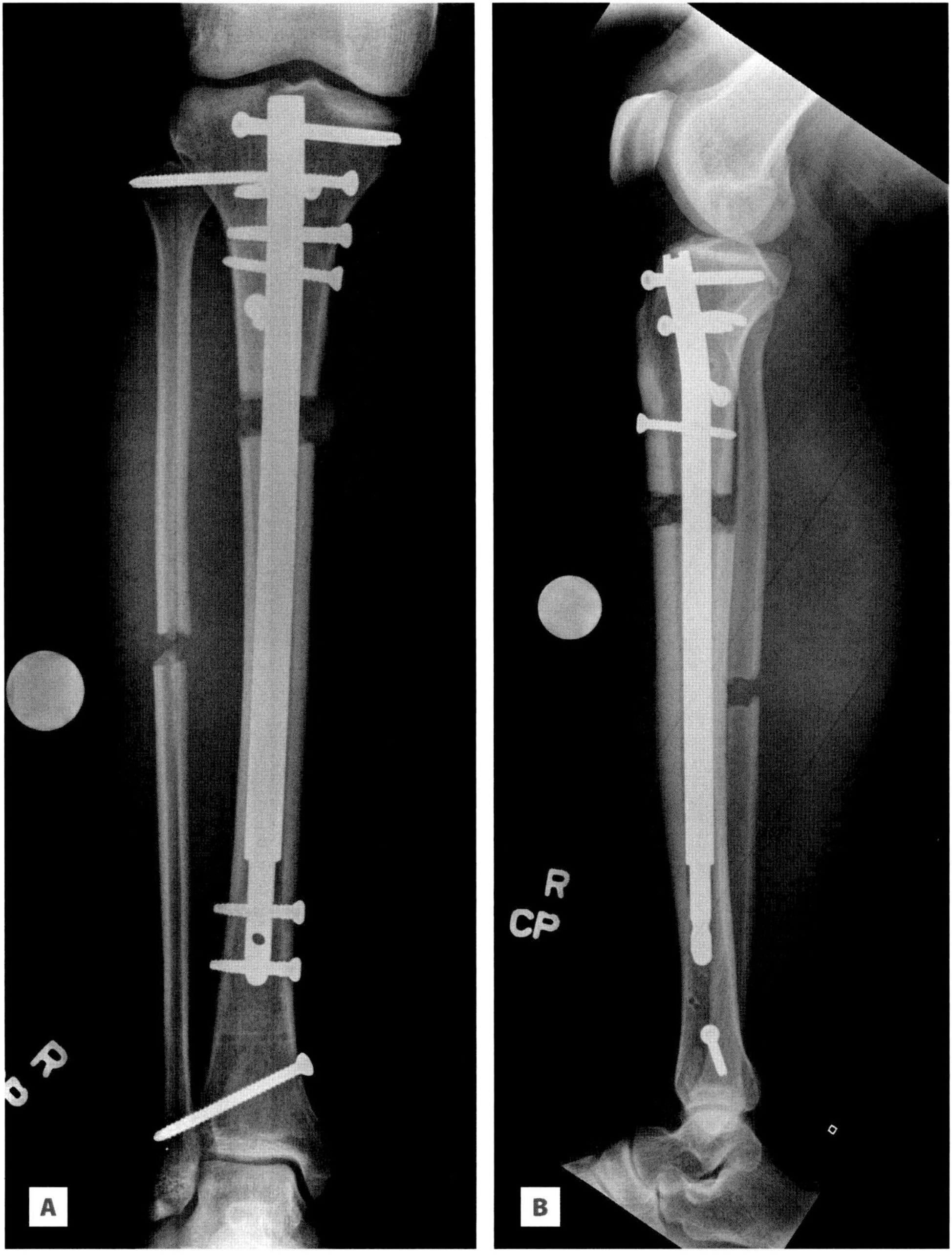


**Fig. 11: A**, AP, and **B**, sagittal radiographs of a right tibia demonstrating posterior and lateral blocking screw placement for syndesmotic fixation.

© 2023 Sinai Hospital of Baltimore

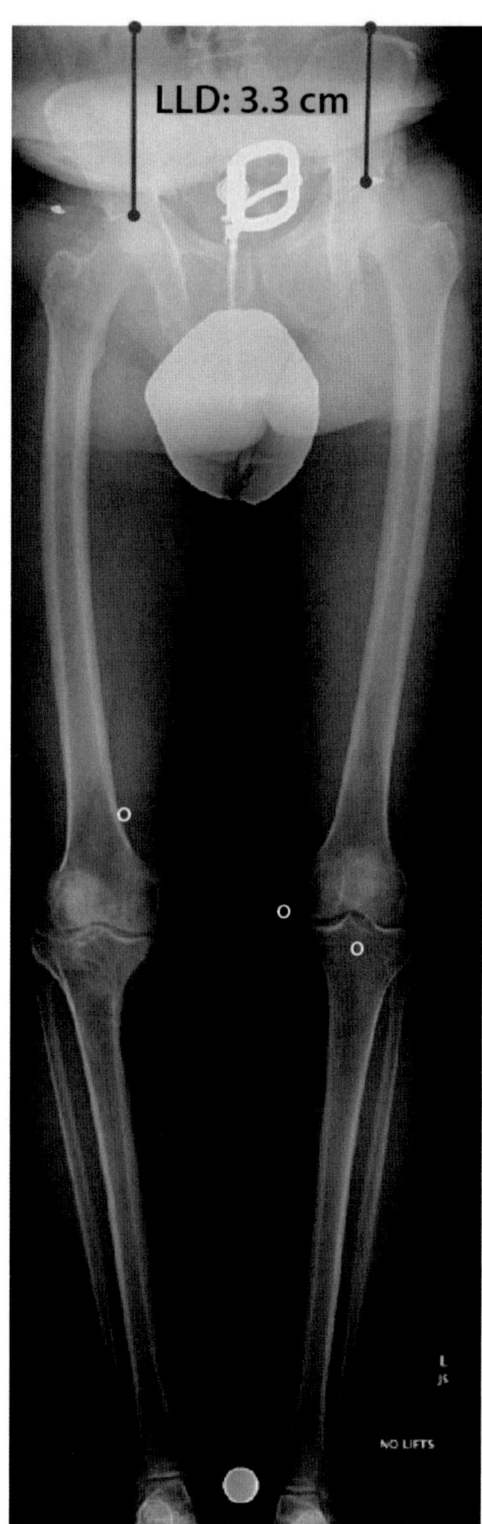


**Fig. 12:** An LLD of 3.3 cm is apparent with the right side shorter than the left. This occurred from a previous injury and right tibial plateau malunion.

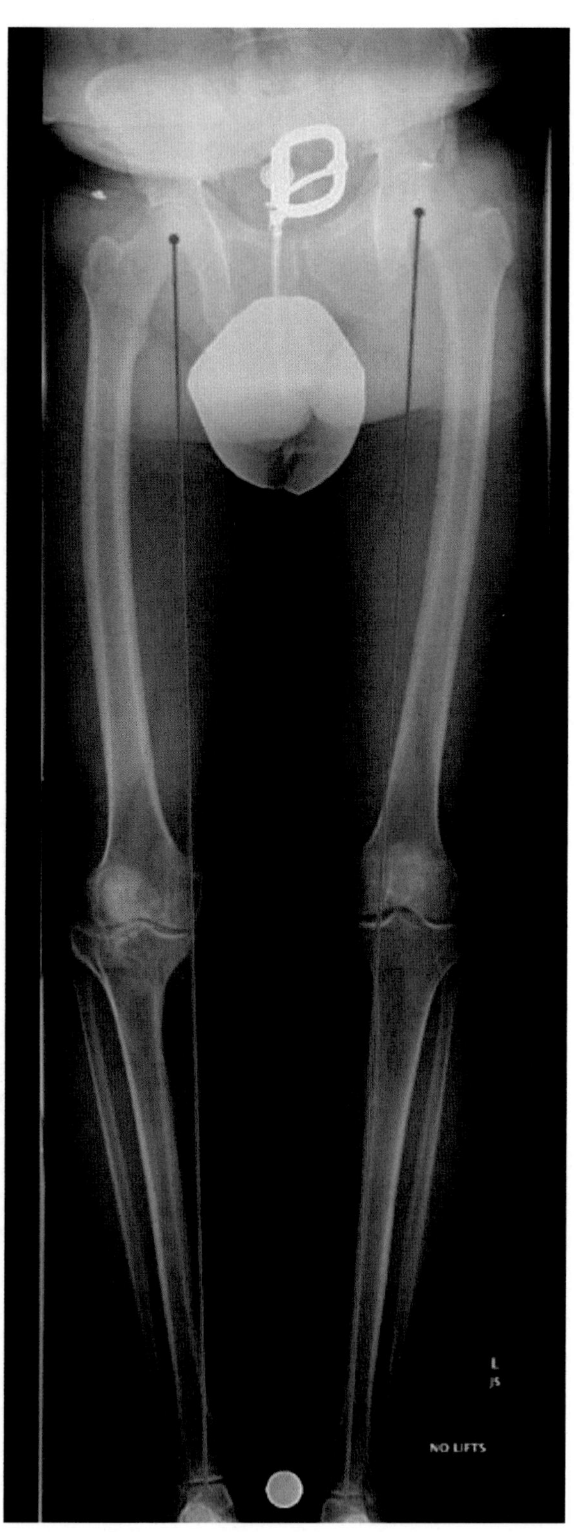


**Fig. 13:** Left leg MAD confirms mild native genu varum. Right leg MAD depicts moderate-to-severe genu varum.

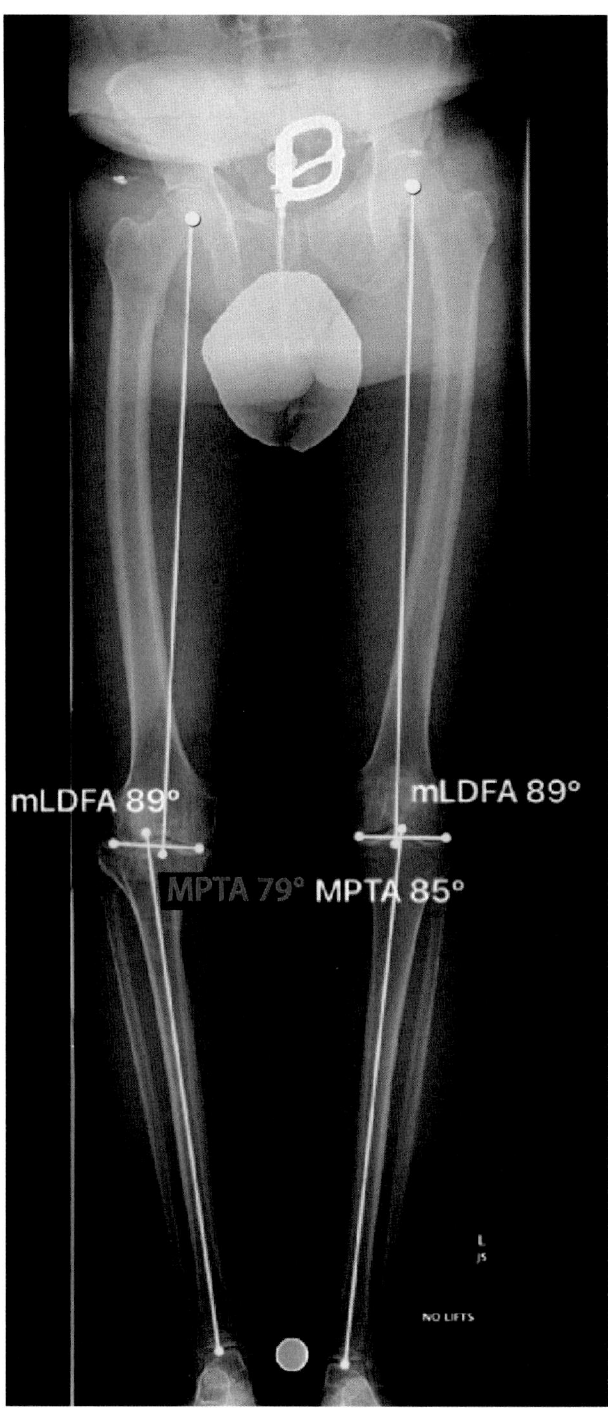


**Fig. 14:** Joint angles are shown. Red text indicates the abnormal angle. mLFDA, mechanical lateral distal femoral angle; MPTA, medial proximal tibial angle.

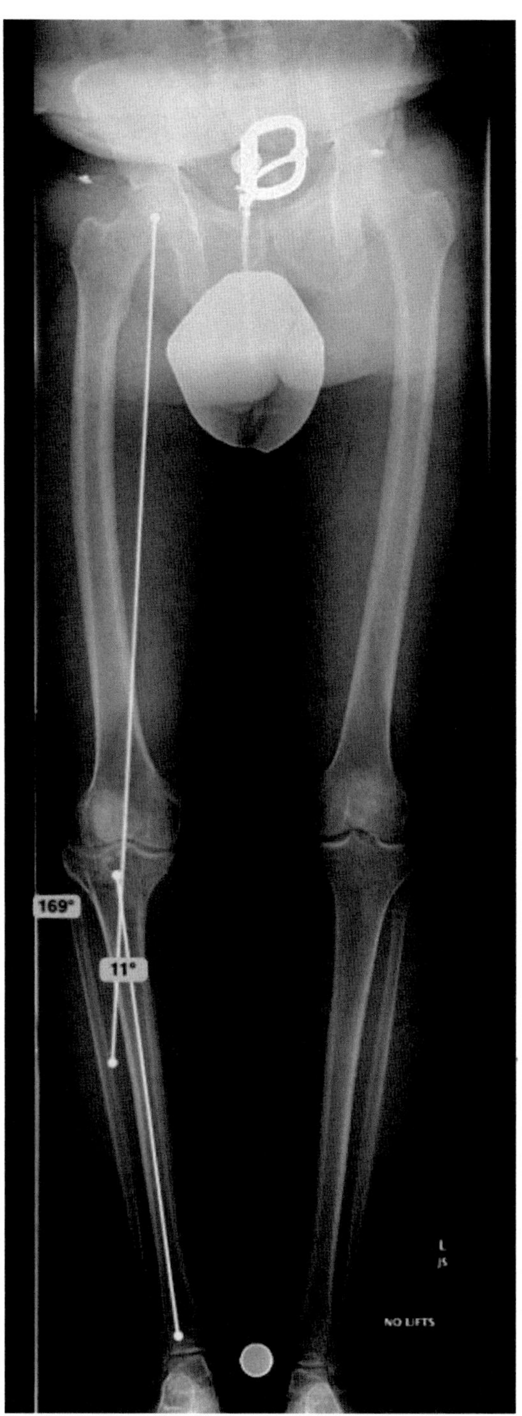


**Fig. 15:** The apex of the deformity is found by using a normal mechanical axis proximally and a long bisector of the tibia distally. There is an 11° varus deformity with an apex where the lines intersect at the right proximal tibia metaphysis.

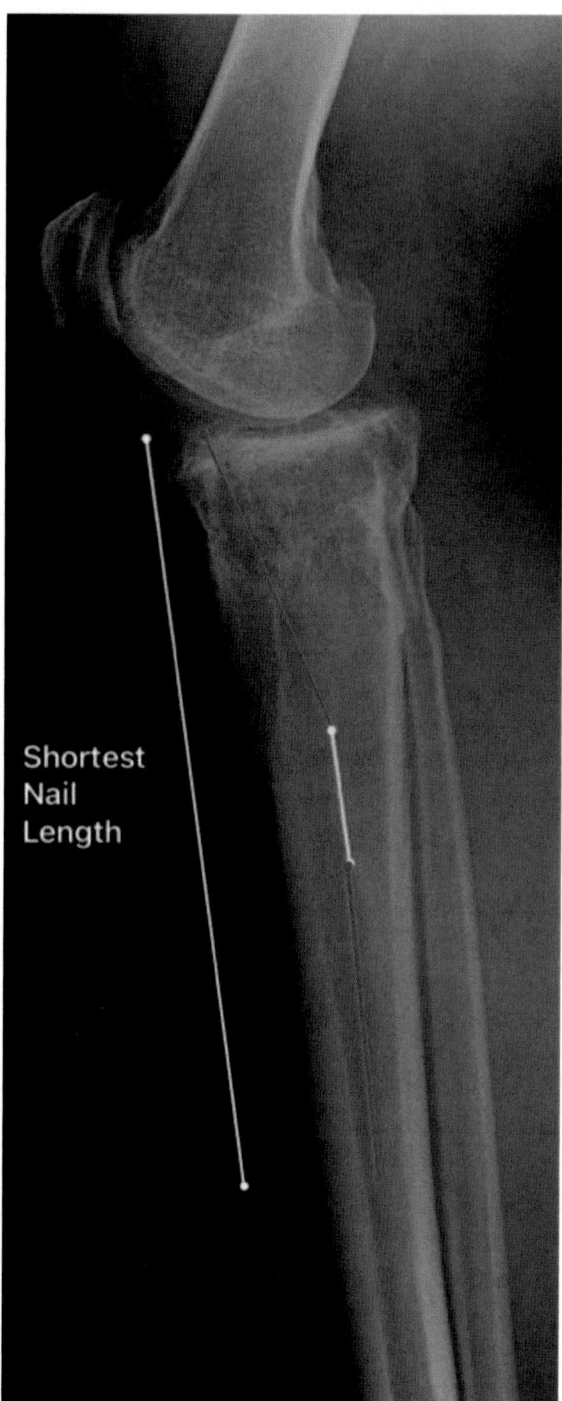


**Fig. 16:** The red line indicates the distance between the entry point and osteotomy (8 cm). The yellow line indicates the desired lengthening (3.3 cm). The blue line indicates the 8 cm constant. These lines add up to 19.3 cm which indicates the shortest possible nail length.

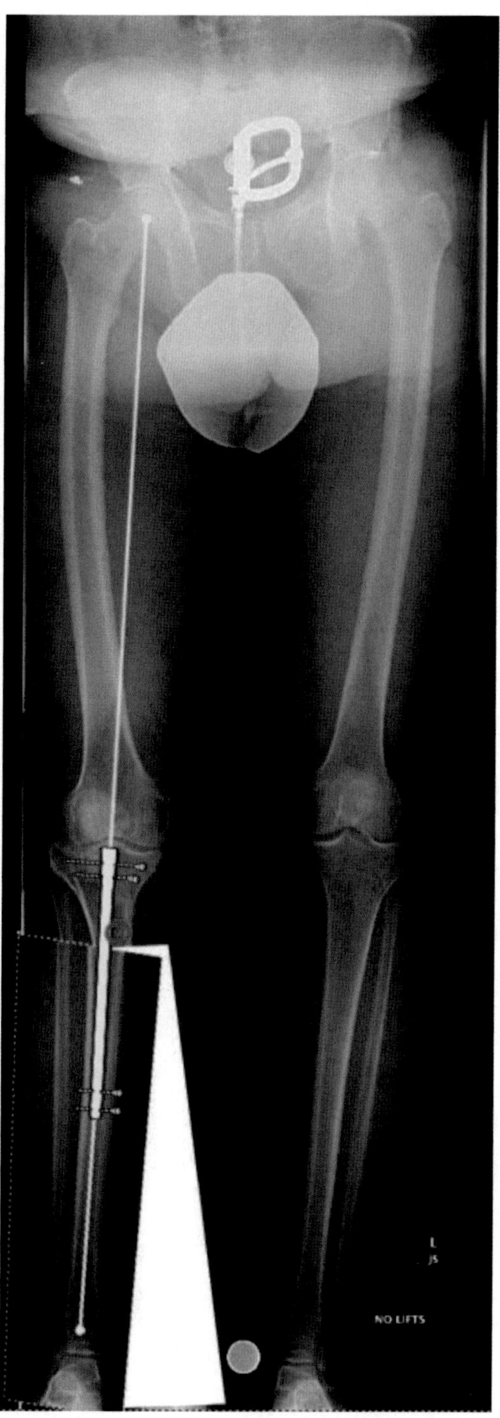


**Fig. 17:** The anticipated position at the end of lengthening is shown after the osteotomy and nail placement. The red circle predicts placement of a blocking screw. This operative plan should be evaluated for feasibility (e.g., osteotomy level, requirement for cortical reaming, need for blocking screws).

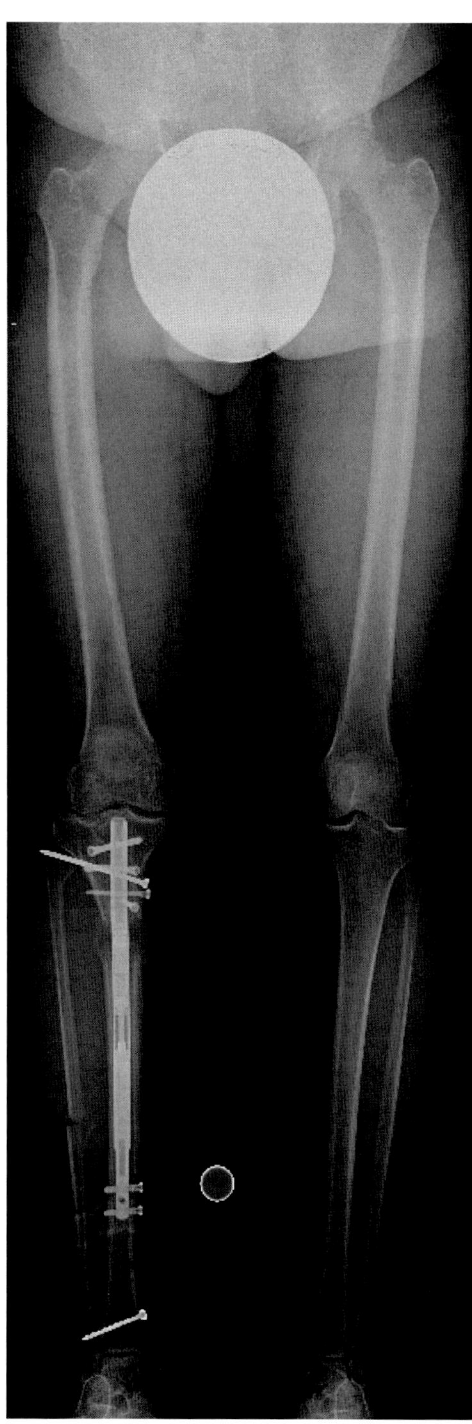

**Fig. 18:** AP radiograph captured at the end of the lengthening phase, six weeks after surgery.

## Osteotomy Technique, Latency, Rate of Distraction, and Rhythm

There are certain factors that are crucial for successful limb lengthening: the type of device used to lengthen the bone, the level of the osteotomy, the osteotomy technique, the latency period before lengthening begins, and the rate of distraction.

The osteotomy technique for internal lengthening is the multiple drill hole osteotomy. This method consists of multiple drill holes created at the level of the osteotomy through a small stab incision. This marks the level of the osteotomy and concurrently vents the intramedullary canal. As the reaming of the canal is performed, the reaming contents egress out of the vent holes, preventing vascular overload of the intramedullary contents while simultaneously providing bone graft at the lengthening site. As the MILN is being inserted, the osteotomy is completed with an osteotome. After completion of the osteotomy, the MILN is driven across the osteotomy site and secured with proximal and/or distal locking screws.

The latency is defined as the amount of time between the osteotomy and the initiation of the distraction. The typical latency period is between 5–10 days. Factors that could affect the latency period include the patient's age, comorbidities that may affect bone healing, the bone segment being lengthened and its health, the osteotomy technique and site (metaphyseal or diaphyseal), the soft-tissue disruption and bony displacement at the time of the osteotomy, and any acute distraction. For example, a 50-year-old male with concurrent diabetes and obesity undergoing a tibial lengthening with an open osteotomy would have a latency period of 10 days. However, a healthy 16-year-old male undergoing a femoral lengthening via a multiple drill hole osteotomy would have a latency period of 5–7 days.

The distraction rate is the amount of daily distraction performed at the osteotomy site after the latency period. It is typically noted as 1 mm per day, however, the rate is variable. This depends upon the bone segment receiving lengthening, the patient's healing potential, the osteotomy location

© 2023 Sinai Hospital of Baltimore

(metaphyseal or diaphyseal), the appearance of the regenerate during interval follow-ups, joint range of motion, pain, and neurologic symptoms. The distraction of a femoral lengthening in a healthy adult is 1 mm per day whereas a metatarsal lengthening in the same patient would be 0.5 mm per day. The rate of distraction should be adjusted as needed during the lengthening period.

Rhythm is defined as the number of lengthening sessions performed daily to accomplish the daily distraction goal. A patient lengthening 1 mm per day may distract 0.25 mm per session and perform 4 lengthening sessions per day. Electrical and magnetic MILNs can provide any combination of distraction and rhythm. The author typically programs 3–5 sessions of 0.2 mm per day.

## Conclusion

The hardware and process of intramedullary lengthening may seem more intuitive and simple than circular fixation. Regardless, any limb lengthening method is complex and presents the potential for numerous complications. Internal lengthening is still lengthening, with all of the possible problems and complications.

## Pediatric Considerations for Intramedullary Lengthening

The advent of internal limb lengthening has drastically changed the surgical approach to limb lengthening in children and adolescents. The use of the external fixation device on children is now relegated to the tibia or femurs that are too short for intramedullary nails. The external fixation lengthening strategy for the femur is now primarily reserved for toddlers and young children.

The limiting factors to internal lengthening in children are the presence of a physis, the length of the bone, and the patient's ability to comply with modified weightbearing. Previously, the diameter of the bone was also a limiting factor. However, the extramedullary internal lengthening technique has afforded this technology to younger children with narrow long bones.

The presence of the physis in the skeletally immature patient does not allow for intramedullary lengthening devices used in retrograde femoral lengthening or antegrade tibial lengthening. The exception to this rule is the presence of a growth arrest where the physis is no longer present (Fig. 19). Retrograde intramedullary tibial lengthening also can be considered in the presence of an ankle and subtalar fusion.

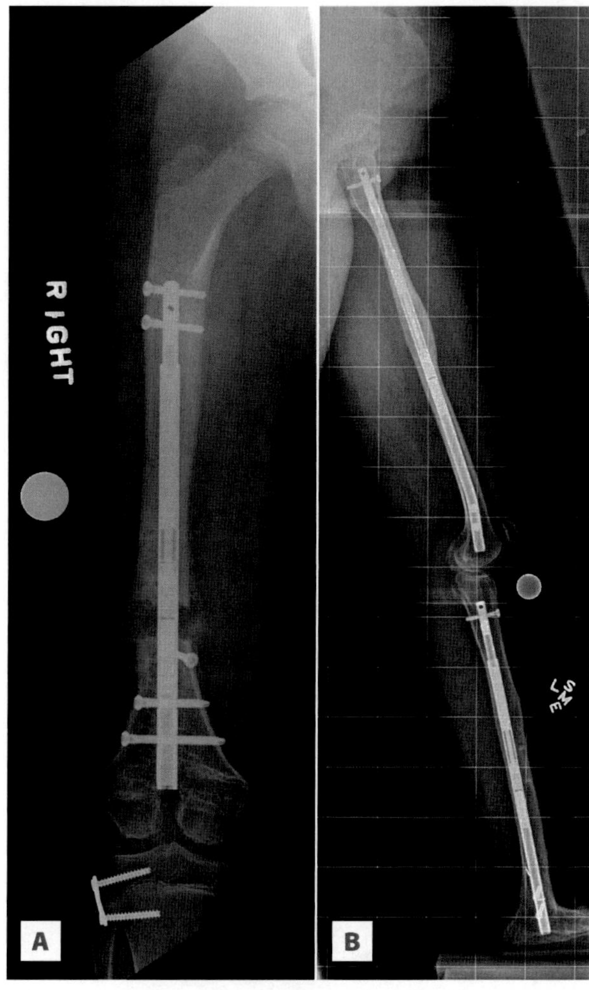


**Fig. 19: A**, AP radiograph of a patient who underwent retrograde femoral lengthening with complete distal femoral physeal arrest. **B**, Long lateral radiograph of a patient with a retrograde tibial lengthening with pantalar arthrodesis.

The length of the bone is also a limiting factor. The shortest internal lengthening device is 160 mm. The shorter nails also are limited to a 50 mm lengthening capacity and have fewer fixation points or locking screw options. The length of the bone will affect both the intramedullary and extramedullary surgical strategies (Fig. 20).

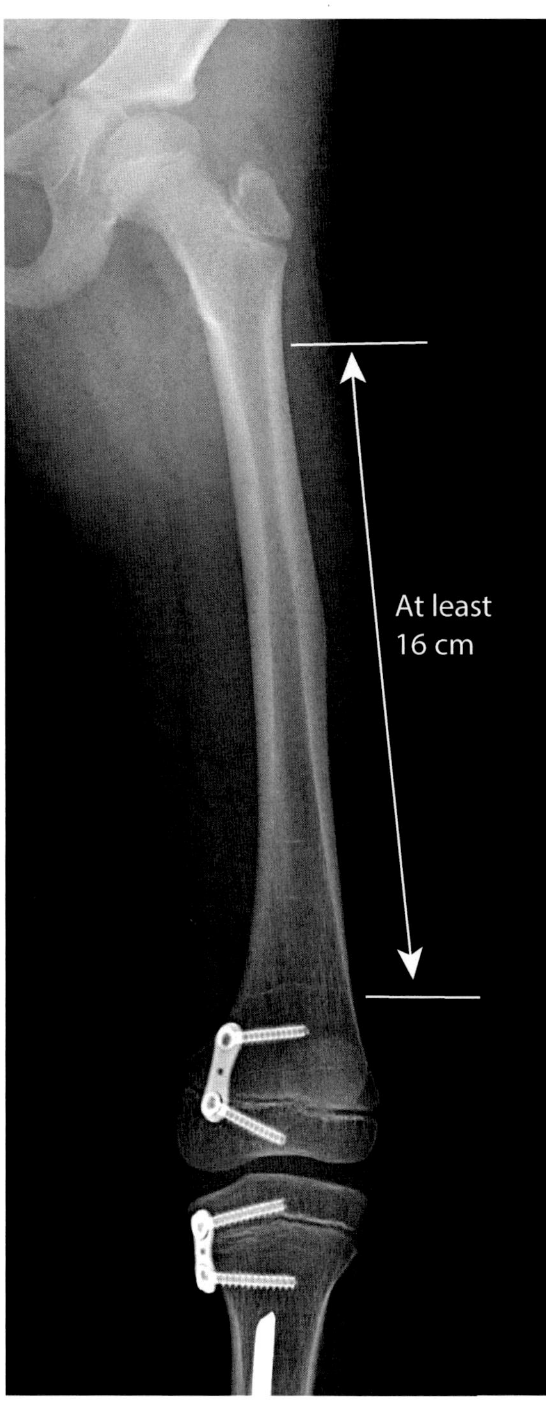


**Fig. 20:** The distance between the base of the greater trochanter and distal femoral metaphyseal flare must be at least 160 mm to accommodate the shortest available mechanical intramedullary lengthening nail.

Although the overall size of a younger child is much less than the typical adult patient, the ability to comply with weightbearing modifications is essential. Typically, the patient is restricted to 50% weightbearing during the lengthening process. For a 5 cm lengthening, this would require 50% weightbearing for approximately 12–16 weeks. Noncompliance with the weightbearing restrictions can result in implant failure and breakage. Also, the inability to comply with postoperative weightbearing restrictions would call into question the patient's compliance with physical therapy and postoperative bracing. The capability of a family and patient to successfully navigate and complete the lengthening reconstruction is multifactorial. The true art of limb lengthening in children is determining when both the family and the child are ready to undertake this complex process. Typically, children at the age of 7-8 years of age can demonstrate the maturity and psychological development to undergo internal lengthening.

Benefits of internal lengthening are eliminating the external fixation device and pin sites. Internal lengthening is more comfortable for the patient during regular activities and especially during physical therapy. Bathing, dressing, and going through day-to-day life feel more normal. Physical therapy yields a better range of motion in the joints above and below the lengthening site without the soft tissue restrictions caused by transfixing external fixation pins. The elimination of pin sites also removes the ever-present possibility of superficial pin site infection. These advantages of internal lengthening make the overall process much easier when compared with lengthening via external fixation. However, the family needs to be reminded that internal lengthening is still a complicated process, and it requires routine physical therapy and close follow-up to avoid complications.

Typical intramedullary lengthening in children follows the same principles as previously described in this chapter. Two considerations specific to planning for children are the femoral entry point and rate of distraction. In the femoral lengthening of the skeletally immature patient, the trochanteric entry point in the proximal femur is always utilized. The piriformis start should never be used in the presence of an open proximal femoral physis. The second item to consider is the rate of distraction during the lengthening process in children. The rate of 1 mm per day is the common reference rate

© 2023 Sinai Hospital of Baltimore

for femoral distraction; it is 0.75 mm per day for the tibia. However, the rate of 0.75 mm per day of bone distraction in children is a better rate for bone formation and avoidance of soft tissue contractures.

The remainder of this chapter describes the more recent development of extramedullary internal lengthening. This technique is used for children and adolescents with significantly narrow intramedullary canals. This approach affords internal lengthening to a younger patient population while simultaneously avoiding over-reaming of the bone or using implants that are too small.

The premise of internal extramedullary lengthening is the utilization of the MILN as an internal "external fixator." The MILN is placed adjacent to the bone being lengthened and secured via locking screws. A smaller simple intramedullary rod (Rush rod) is also used and inserted as a guide rod for the lengthening. This technique works the same way as external fixation lengthening over a trauma intramedullary nail. The only difference is that the entire device is internal and covered by soft tissue.

## Extramedullary Lengthening

### Nail Selection

The distance from the base of the greater trochanter apophysis to the distal femoral flare is measured to ensure it is at least 160 mm, as this length represents the shortest universal femoral magnetic MILN (stroke of 50 mm). For those patients with a distance of at least 215 mm, the corresponding retrograde femoral magnetic MILN (stroke of 50 mm) is used. For those patients with a minimum distance of 245 mm, a longer retrograde femoral magnetic MILN should be selected, which has the benefit of a larger stroke at 80 mm. When allowed by soft tissues, a 10.7 mm diameter nail is preferred, which offers increased strength and resistance to bending forces when compared with its 8.5 mm counterpart. Additionally, the 10.7 mm nail affords larger locking screws.

### Intraoperative Technique (Fig. 21)

Once preoperative planning and implant selection are confirmed, the patient is placed supine on a radiolucent table. Using fluoroscopic guidance, the distance from the base of the greater trochanter apophysis to the distal femoral flare is again confirmed to ensure appropriate implants are available. The osteotomy level is then selected, typically in the subtrochanteric region, and percutaneous multiple drill holes are created in the typical fashion. At this point, a simple Rush rod or slim nail is inserted (typically 4.0–4.8 mm in diameter) antegrade through a greater trochanteric start point to the level of the osteotomy. If any deformity correction or derotation is planned, rotational markers are inserted proximally and distally to guide final alignment. An osteotome is then utilized to partially complete the osteotomy, taking care to leave the medial cortex intact. Next, the simple rod is advanced distally, spanning the length of the entire femur.

A tourniquet is then applied to the thigh and a 5 cm lateral incision starting at the level of the superior pole of the patella is made in a proximal direction. The iliotibial band and lateral intermuscular septum are then visualized and released. Care is taken to avoid injury to the peroneal nerve as it may be found in an unusual location (in cases of congenital femoral deficiency) or be encased in a scar secondary to prior procedures. Through the same incision, the vastus lateralis is lifted off the septum and periosteum using a Cobb elevator, and a tunnel is created in a submuscular fashion retrograde from distal to proximal. The tourniquet is then released, and hemostasis is achieved using electrocautery. Next, a second 5 cm incision is made laterally distal to the greater trochanter. The tensor fascia lata is then divided and a submuscular tunnel is created from proximal to distal under the vastus lateralis muscle, connecting with the retrograde tunnel made previously. A Cobb elevator is introduced from proximal and distal to ensure proper connectivity of the tunnels, with care taken not to dissect posteriorly, risking injury to the perforating arteries to the vastus lateralis muscle.

In the next phase, the MILN which was selected ahead of time is passed from proximal to distal through the tunnel. The MILN is aligned on the bone with the aid of anteroposterior and lateral fluoroscopic images. Two to four 1.8 mm wires are then inserted through the locking holes and directed around the simple Rush rod or slim nail. The MILN is ideally positioned with the proximal screws passing through the lesser trochanter and the distal screws in the metadiaphyseal region of the distal femur. The wires are then over-drilled and appropriately sized fully-threaded locking screws are inserted sequentially. These screws are modified before insertion by a metal burr to remove the proximal larger diameter screw threads and make this region flush with the remaining screw shaft. This ensures the screw can be inserted down to the nail, preventing screw head prominence in the lateral soft tissues.

The medial cortex of the osteotomy is then completed using an osteotomy through a separate anterior stab incision at the appropriate level. Of note, if deformity correction is being performed and rotational markers were used as discussed earlier, the osteotomy may be completed before passing the simple Rush rod or slim nail. The magnet level is then marked on the skin and the nail is tested intraoperatively with fluoroscopic confirmation.

What is the technique?

1. ITB release
2. Create a submuscular tunnel
3. Determine osteotomy level (vent)
4. Insert an intramedullary rod
5. Partial osteotomy
6. Insert extramedullary rod in submuscular tunnel
7. Lock the extramedullary device proximal and distal avoiding intramedullary rod
8. Complete osteotomy
9. Acute distraction of 1–2 mm

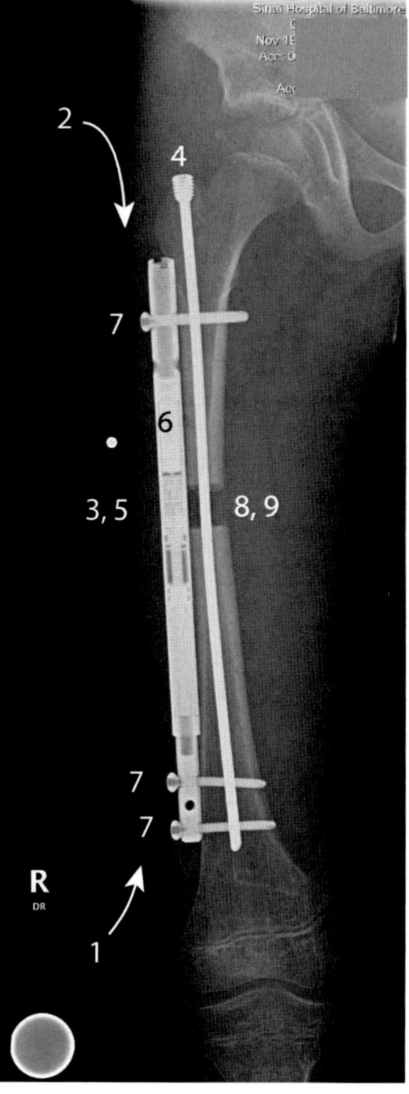


**Fig. 21:** Summary of extramedullary internal lengthening using a mechanical intramedullary lengthening nail. ITB, iliotibial band.

© 2023 Sinai Hospital of Baltimore

### Postoperative Protocol and Complications

The postoperative protocol for extramedullary lengthening is similar to the one prescribed to patients who underwent intramedullary lengthening. The patient is allowed 50% weightbearing, but this can be further limited and is dependent upon the patient's size and weight. The bone segment is allowed to rest after the osteotomy for a typical latency of 7 days. This period may be increased if clinical circumstances dictate possible bone healing issues such as previously lengthened bone, reduced overall surface area at the osteotomy site, traumatic osteotomy, or residual distraction at the osteotomy site. Physical therapy is prescribed 3–5 days per week during the distraction phase of the treatment. Range of motion parameters for femoral lengthening are as follows: the hip must maintain neutral extension and at least 15-20° of hip abduction. The knee must maintain full extension and at least 45° flexion. After the distraction is completed, physical therapy is reduced to 1–2 sessions per week to maintain the range of motion until full healing occurs. Following complete consolidation, the patient is allowed to return to full weightbearing. At this time, physical therapy proceeds with gait training, strengthening, and a return to previous activities. The extramedullary device is removed in 3–6 months with consolidation.

Potential complications and rates of occurrence are comparable to other lengthening techniques. These include infection, loss of length, implant failure, delayed union, joint contracture, joint subluxation, implant bending, and prominent hardware. These complications are uncommon, but lengthening procedures always are accompanied by issues that must be anticipated and managed to have a successful result.

## Conclusion

Internal limb lengthening can be performed in both the pediatric and adolescent populations. The skeletally immature patient requires special consideration for open physes, smaller bone lengths, narrower bone canals, available family support, and physiological development/maturity of the patient.

# Appendix

# Standard Measurements, Landmarks, and Reference Points

© 2023 Sinai Hospital of Baltimore

## Standard Measurements of the Lower Limbs: Frontal Plane

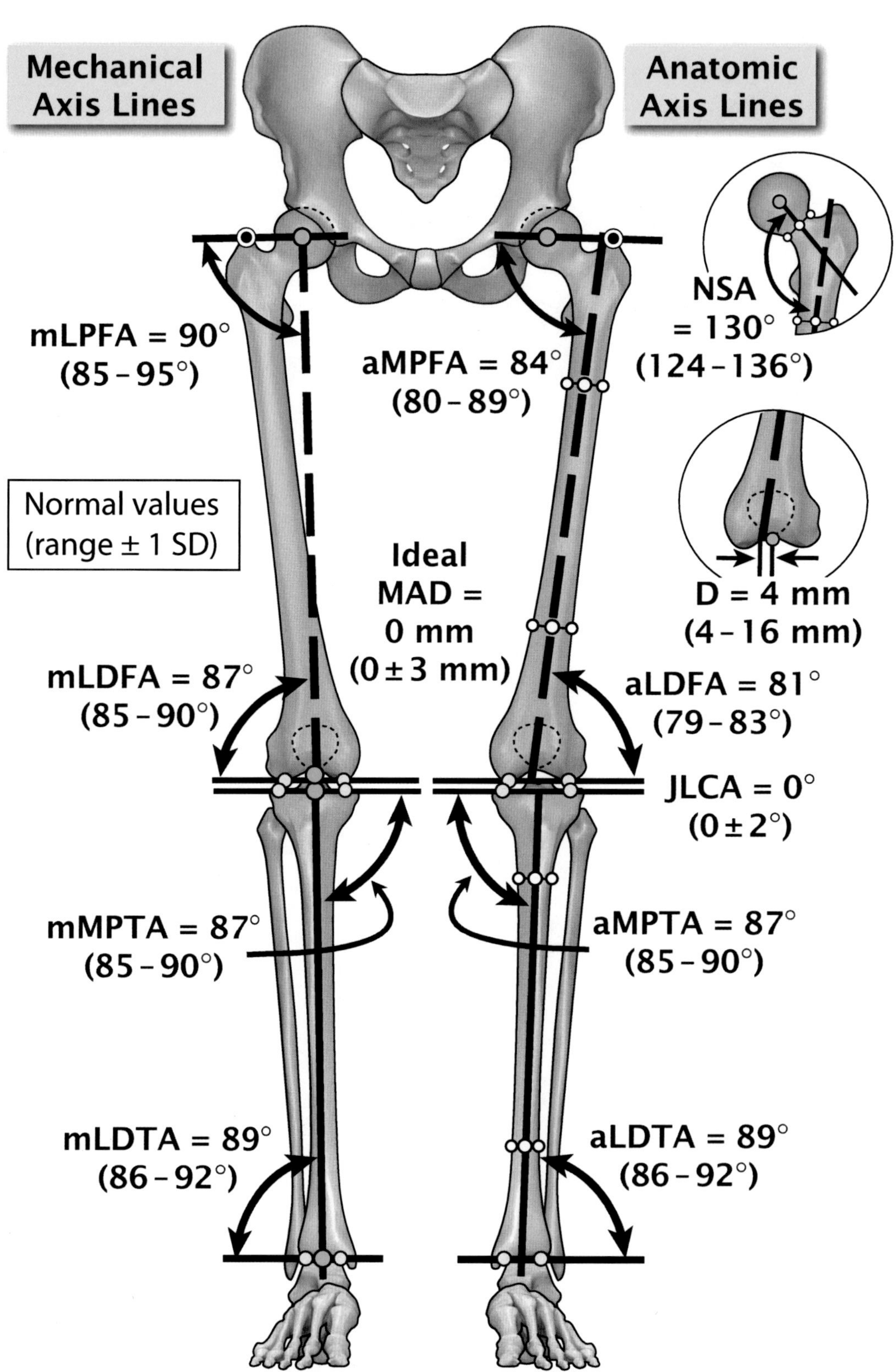

**Frontal Plane Joint Angles Created by the Mechanical Axis Lines**

| Acronym of Joint Angle | Complete Name of Joint Angle | Average Normal Value and Range |
|---|---|---|
| mLPFA | mechanical lateral proximal femoral angle | 90° (85–95°) |
| mLDFA | mechanical lateral distal femoral angle | 87° (85–90°) |
| mMPTA | mechanical medial proximal tibial angle | 87° (85–90°) |
| mLDTA | mechanical lateral distal tibial angle | 89° (86–92°) |

**Frontal Plane Joint Angles Created by the Anatomic Axis Lines**

| Acronym of Joint Angle | Complete Name of Joint Angle | Average Normal Value and Range |
|---|---|---|
| aMPFA | anatomic medial proximal femoral angle | 84° (80–89°) |
| aLDFA | anatomic lateral distal femoral angle | 81° (79–83°) |
| aMPTA | anatomic medial proximal tibial angle | 87° (85–90°) |
| aLDTA | anatomic lateral distal tibial angle | 89° (86–92°) |

*© 2023 Sinai Hospital of Baltimore*

# Standard Measurements of the Lower Limbs: Frontal Plane

**Additional Frontal Plane Joint Angles**

| Acronym of Joint Angle | Complete Name of Joint Angle | Average Normal Value and Range |
|---|---|---|
| JLCA | joint line convergence angle | 0 ± 2° |
| AMA of the femur | anatomic-mechanical angle of the femur | 7° (5–9°) |
| NSA | neck shaft angle | 130° (124–136°) |

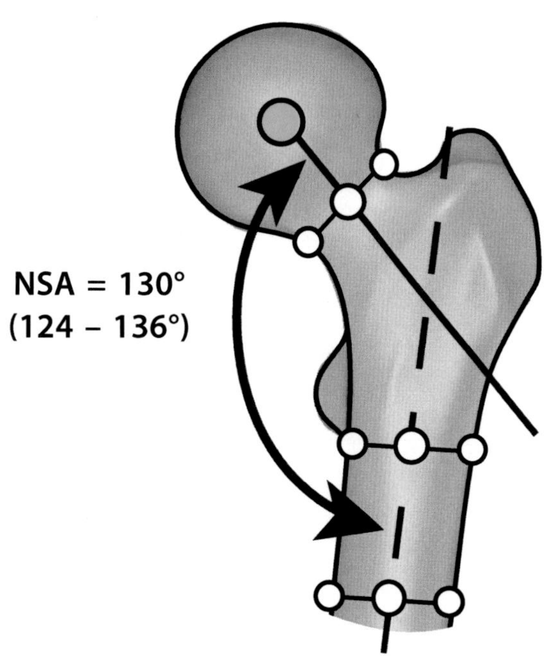


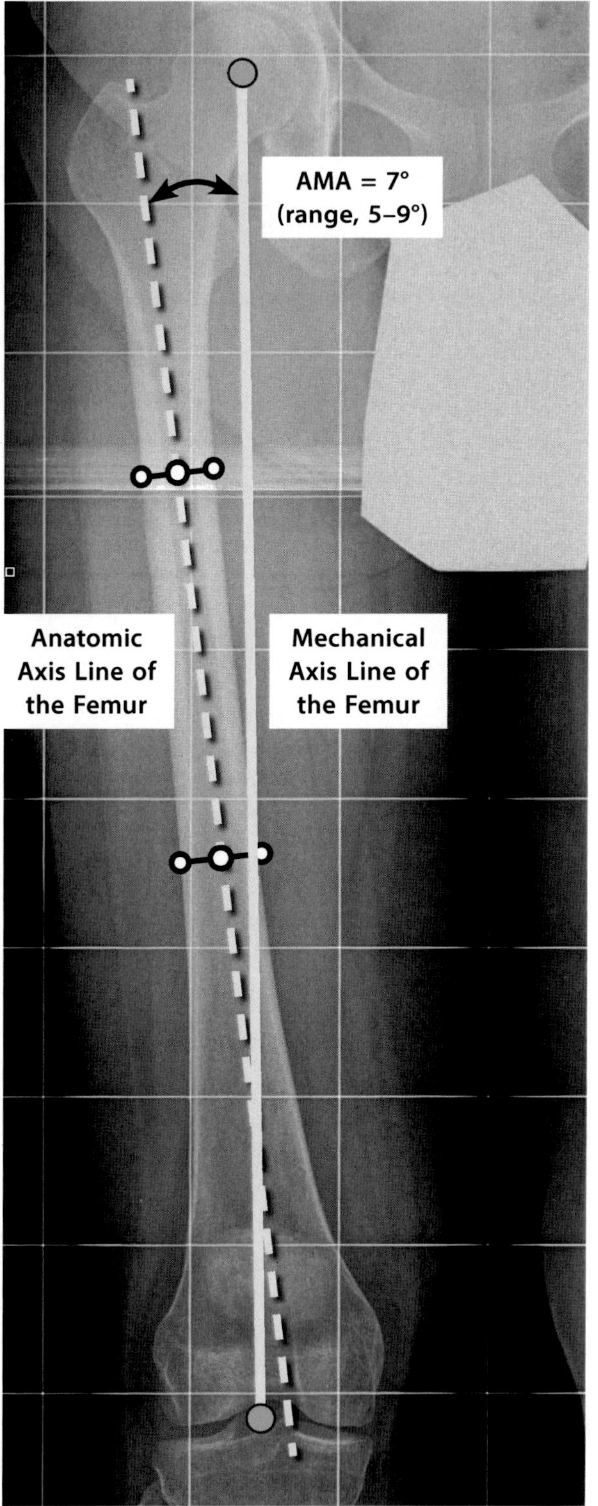

# Standard Measurements of the Lower Limbs: Sagittal Plane

**Sagittal Plane Joint Angles**

| Acronym of Joint Angle | Complete Name of Joint Angle | Average Normal Value and Range |
|---|---|---|
| PDFA | posterior distal femoral angle | 83° (79–87°) |
| PPTA | posterior proximal tibial angle | 81° (77–84°) |
| ADTA | anterior distal tibial angle | 80° (78–82°) |
| SJLA | sagittal joint line angle | 16° ± 3° |
| SMAA | sagittal mechanical axes angle | 0° ± 2° |

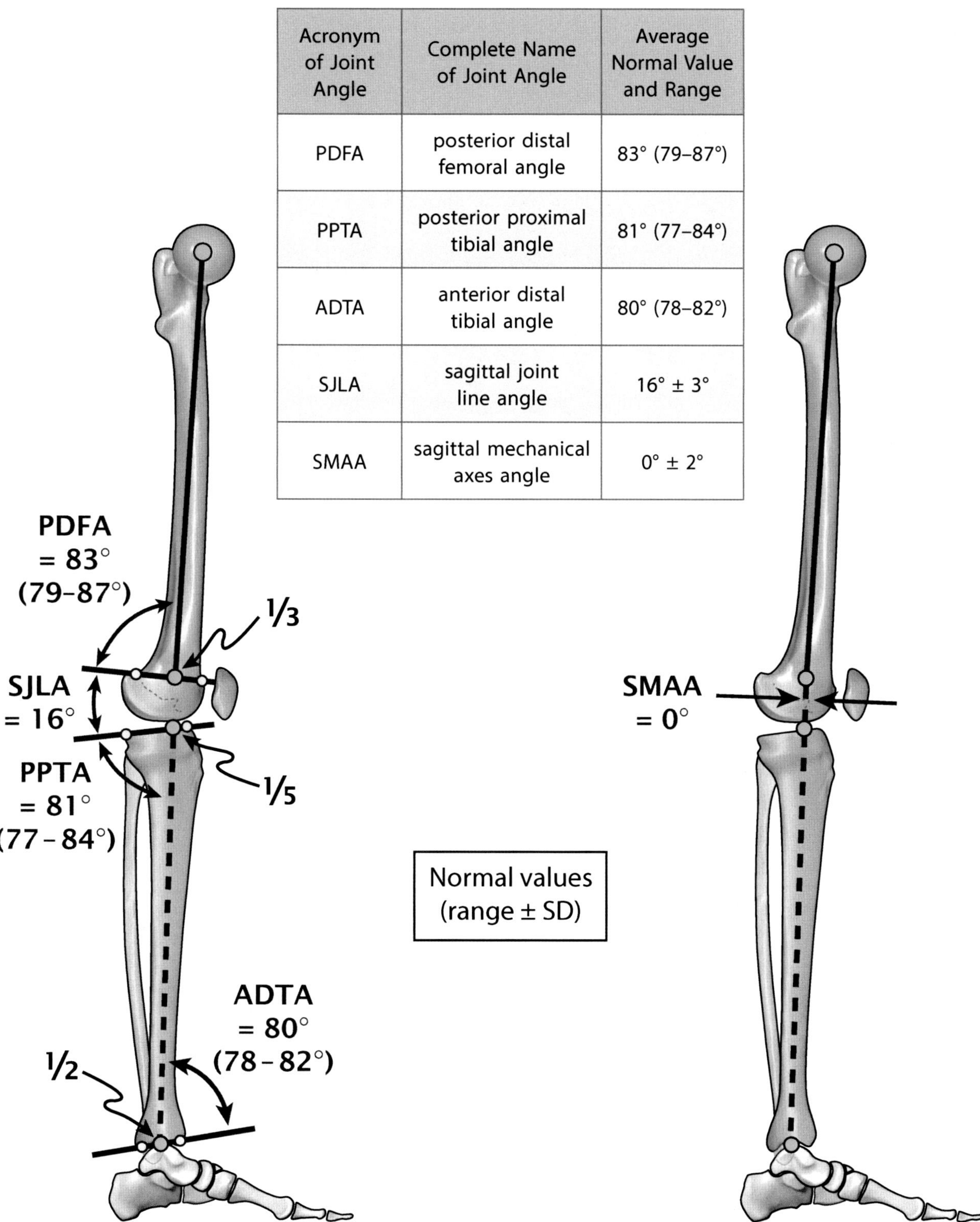


© 2023 Sinai Hospital of Baltimore

## Standard Measurements of the Foot and Ankle: Lateral View

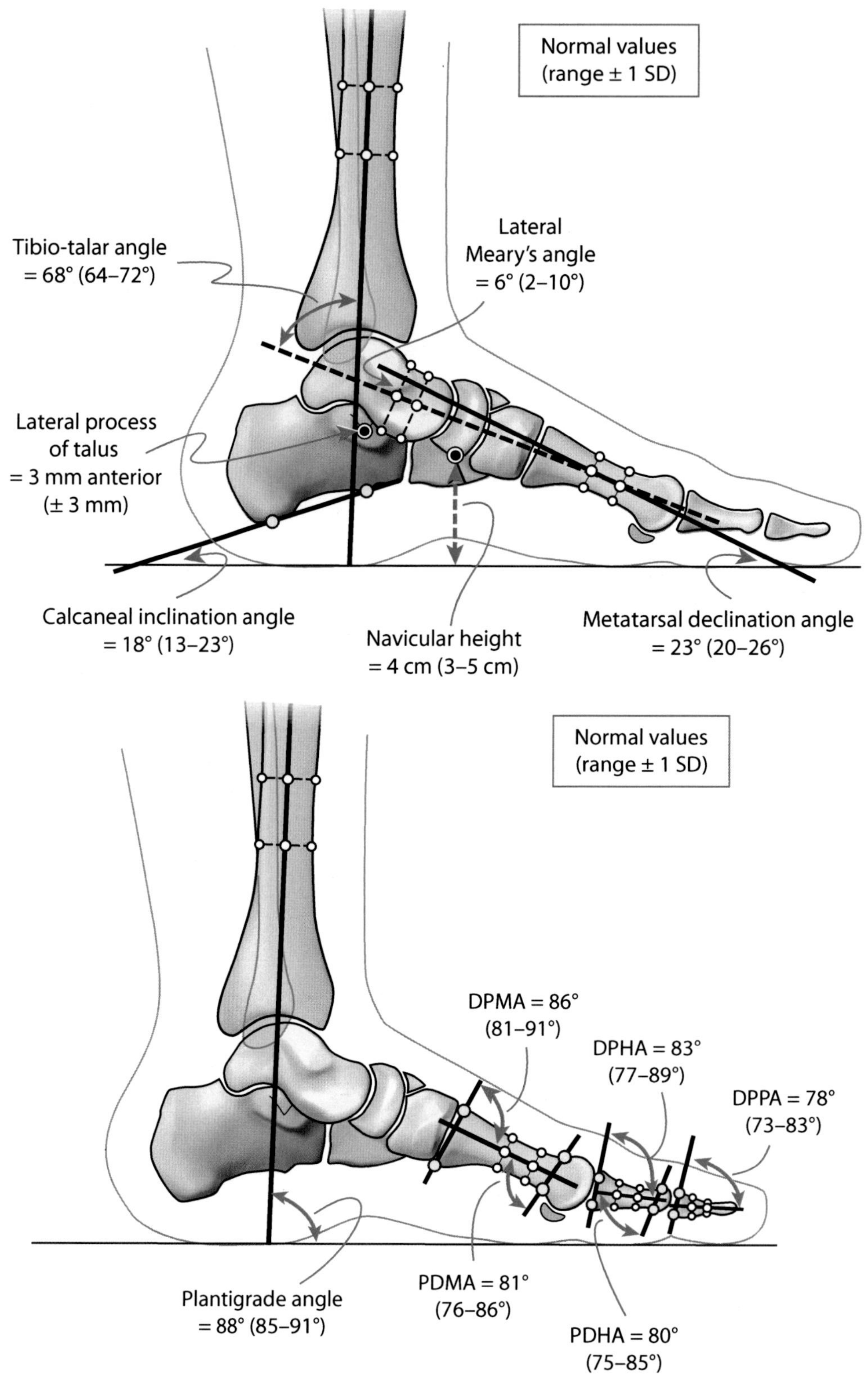

**Lateral View Measurements and Landmarks of the Foot**

| Acronym of Joint Angle | Complete Name of Joint Angle | Average Normal Value (Range ± 1 SD) |
|---|---|---|
| CIA | calcaneal inclination angle | 18° (13–23°) |
| DPHA | dorsal proximal hallux angle | 83° (77–89°) |
| DPMA | dorsal proximal metatarsal angle | 86° (81–91°) |
| DPPA | dorsal proximal phalangeal angle | 78° (73–83°) |
| - | lateral Meary's angle | 6° (2–10°) |
| - | lateral process of talus | 3 mm anterior (± 3 mm) |
| - | metatarsal declination angle | 23° (20–26°) |
| - | navicular height | 4 cm (3–5 cm) |
| PDHA | plantar distal hallux angle | 80° (75–85°) |
| PDMA | plantar distal metatarsal angle | 81° (76–86°) |
| - | plantigrade angle | 88° (85–91°) |
| - | tibio-talar angle | 68° (64–72°) |

© 2023 Sinai Hospital of Baltimore

## Standard Measurements of the Foot: AP View

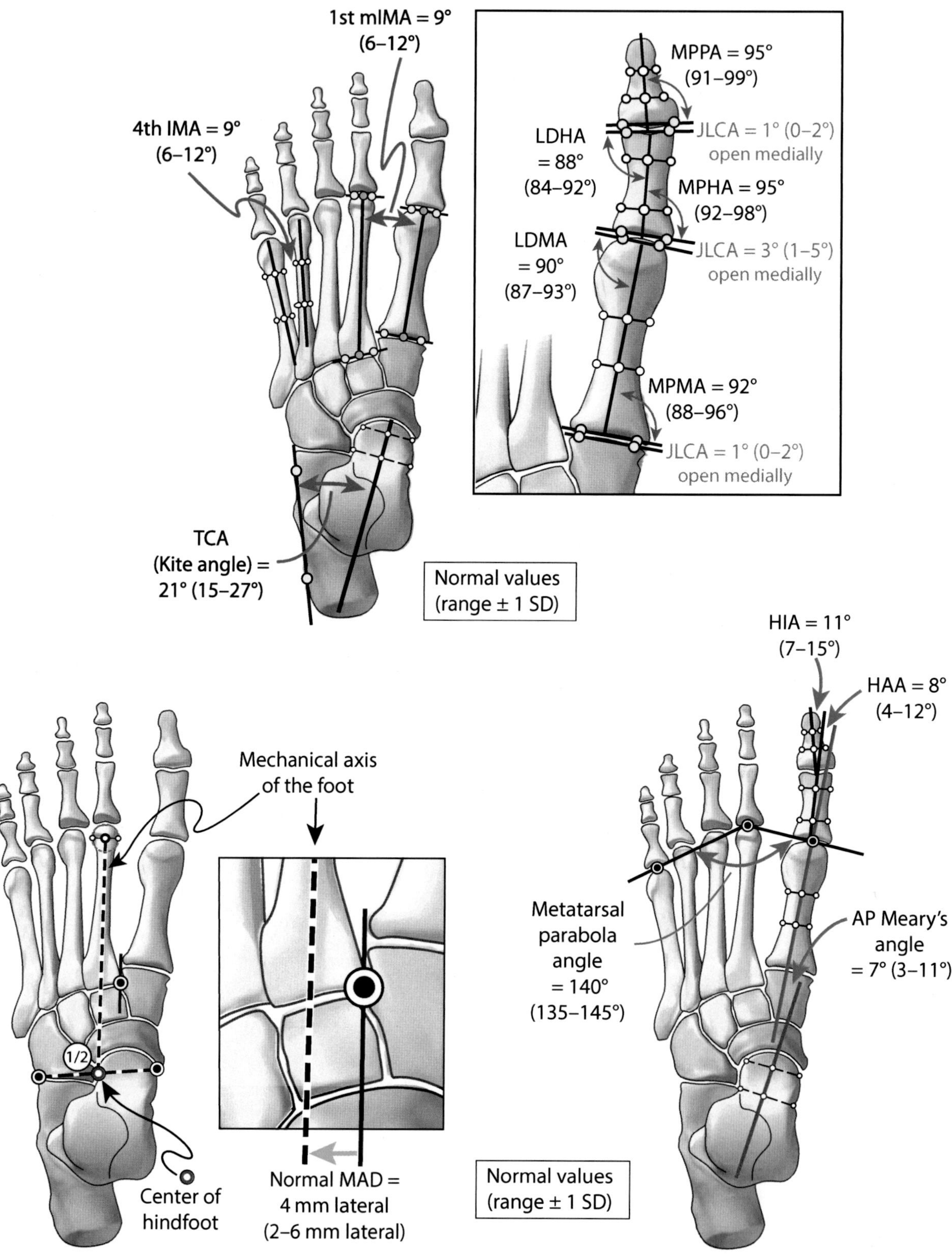

**AP View Joint Line Convergence Angle Measurements of the First Metatarsal**

| Acronym of Joint Angle | Complete Name of Joint Angle | Average Normal Value (Range ± 1 SD) |
|---|---|---|
| JLCA 1st metatarsal cuneiform joint | joint line convergence angle 1st metatarsal cuneiform joint | 1° (0–2°) open medially |
| JLCA 1st metatarsal phalangeal joint | joint line convergence angle 1st metatarsal phalangeal joint | 3° (1–5°) open medially |
| JLCA hallux interphalangeal joint | joint line convergence angle hallux interphalangeal joint | 1° (0–2°) open medially |

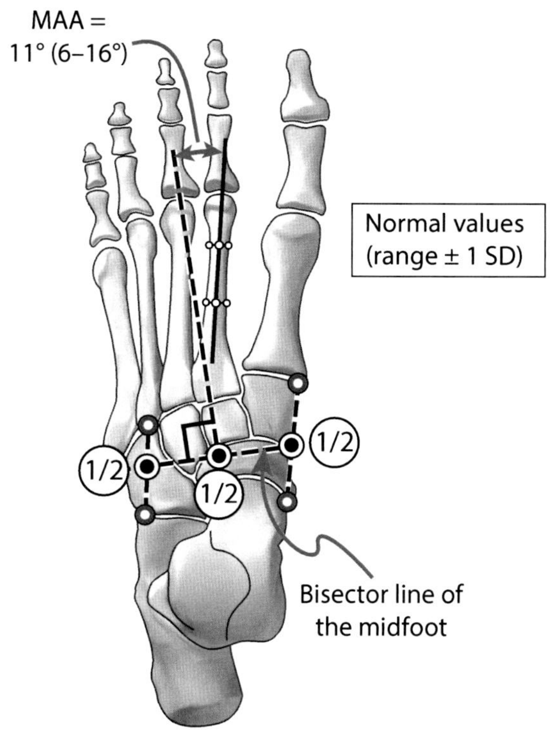


**AP View Measurements and Landmarks of the Foot**

| Acronym of Joint Angle | Complete Name of Joint Angle | Average Normal Value (Range ± 1 SD) |
|---|---|---|
| 1st mIMA | 1st mechanical intermetatarsal angle | 9° (6–12°) |
| 4th IMA | 4th intermetatarsal angle | 9° (6–12°) |
| - | AP Meary's angle | 7° (3–11°) |
| HAA | hallux abductus angle | 8° (4–12°) |
| HIA | hallux interphalangeal angle | 11° (7–15°) |
| LDHA | lateral distal hallux angle | 88° (84–92°) |
| LDMA | lateral distal metatarsal angle | 90° (87–93°) |
| MAD | mechanical axis deviation | 4 mm lateral (2–6 mm lateral) |
| MPHA | medial proximal hallux angle | 95° (92–98°) |
| MPMA | medial proximal metatarsal angle | 92° (88–96°) |
| MPPA | medial proximal phalangeal angle | 95° (91–99°) |
| - | metatarsal parabola angle | 140° (135–145°) |
| MAA | metatarsus adductus angle | 11° (6–16°) |
| TCA | talo-calcaneal angle | 21° (15–27°) |

© 2023 Sinai Hospital of Baltimore

## Standard Measurements of the Foot and Ankle: Axial View

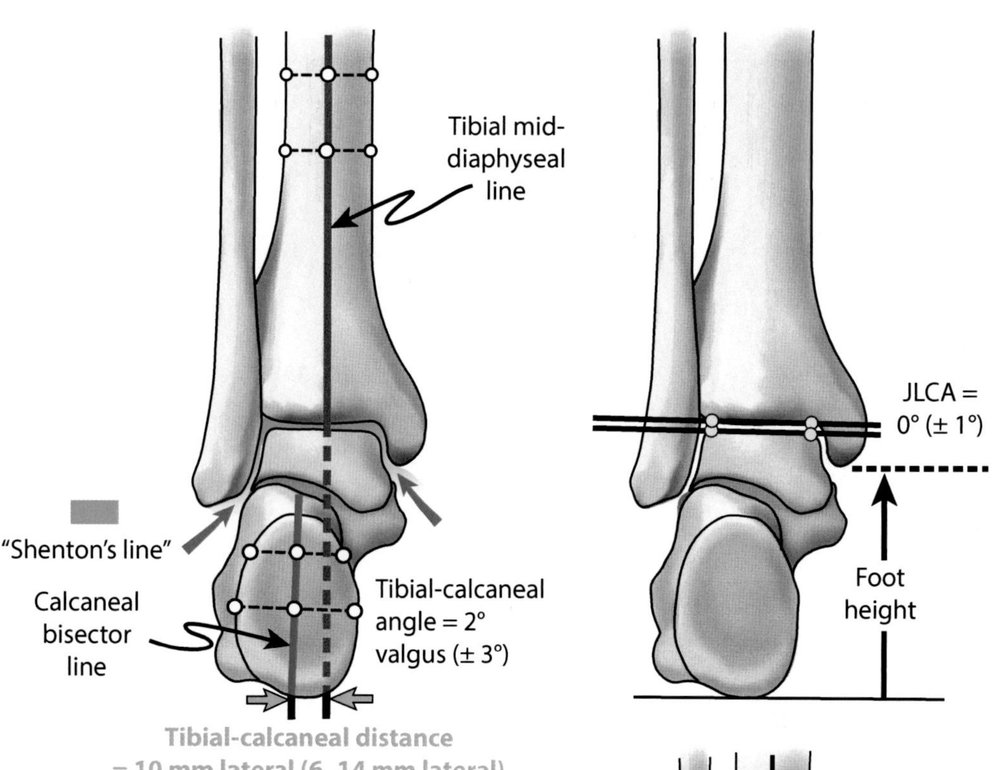


**Axial View Measurements and Landmarks of the Foot**

| Acronym of Joint Angle | Complete Name of Joint Angle | Average Normal Value (Range ± 1 SD) |
|---|---|---|
| JLCA of tibia and talus | joint line convergence angle of tibia and talus | 0° ± 1° |
| PMA | plafond malleolar angle | 15° (13–17°) |
| - | tibial-calcaneal angle | 2° valgus (± 3°) |
| - | tibial-calcaneal distance | 10 mm lateral (6–14 mm lateral) |

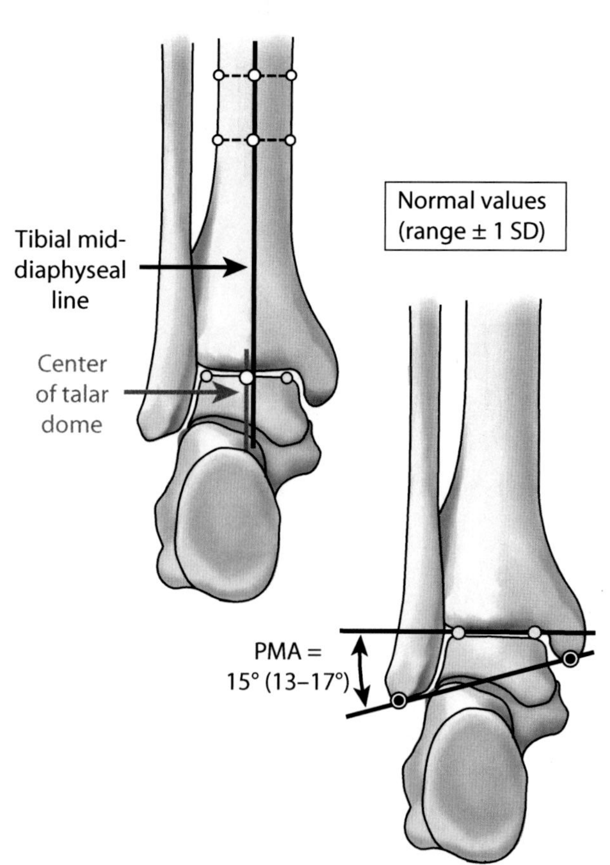

## Using Basic Trigonometry to Calculate Anticipated Contribution of a Bony Sagittal Deformity to the Apparent Knee Deformity

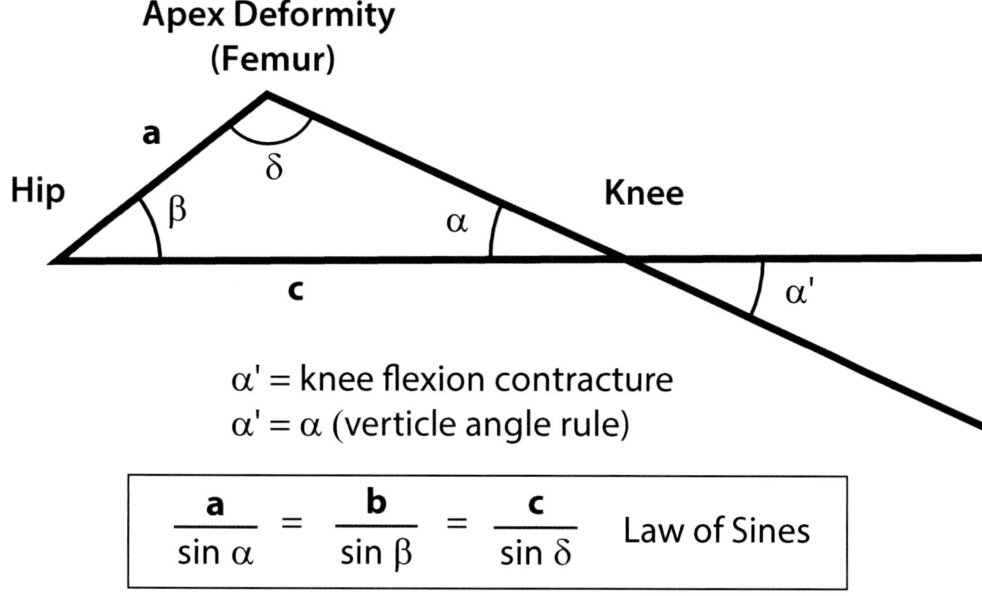


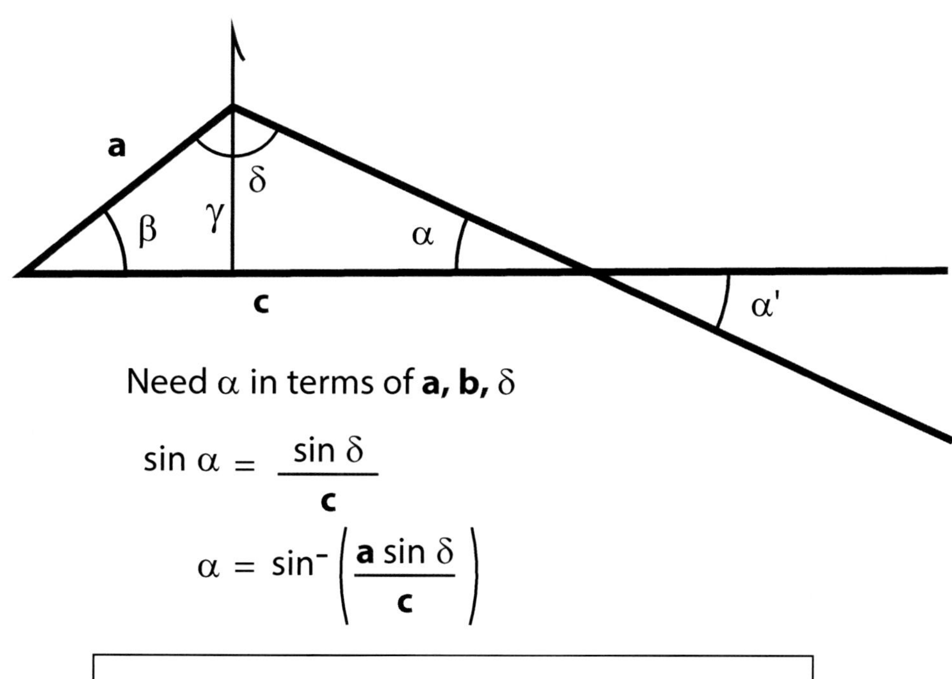


$c^2 = a^2 + b^2 - 2ab\cos(\delta)$ Law of Cosines

$$\alpha = \sin^{-}\left(\frac{\mathbf{a}\sin\delta}{\sqrt{\mathbf{a}^2 + \mathbf{b}^2 - 2ab\cos(\delta)}}\right)$$

© 2023 Sinai Hospital of Baltimore

# Index

© 2023 Sinai Hospital of Baltimore

# Index

## A

## B



## C



© 2023 Sinai Hospital of Baltimore

## D

## E



© 2023 Sinai Hospital of Baltimore

## F

## G



## H



© 2023 Sinai Hospital of Baltimore

## I

## J



## K



## L



© 2023 Sinai Hospital of Baltimore

# Index



## M

## N



© 2023 Sinai Hospital of Baltimore

## O

## P



© 2023 Sinai Hospital of Baltimore

## Q



## R



## S

## T



*© 2023 Sinai Hospital of Baltimore* 

## U



## V

## W



## X



## Y



## Z



© 2023 Sinai Hospital of Baltimore